AF774611

# Advances in Molecular Cytogenetics

# Advances in Molecular Cytogenetics

Editor: Clayton Fisher

FOSTER
ACADEMICS
www.fosteracademics.com

www.fosteracademics.com

FOSTER ACADEMICS

**Cataloging-in-Publication Data**

Advances in molecular cytogenetics / edited by Clayton Fisher.
p. cm.
Includes bibliographical references and index.
ISBN 978-1-63242-697-0
1. Cytogenetics. 2. Molecular genetics. 3. Chromosomes. 4. Medical genetics.
I. Fisher, Clayton.
RB155 .A38 2019
616.042--dc23



Foster Academics,
118-35 Queens Blvd., Suite 400,
Forest Hills, NY 11375, USA

ISBN 978-1-63242-697-0 (Hardback)



Printed and bound in China.

# Contents

# Preface

The field of molecular cytogenetics is concerned with the combination of the fields of cytogenetics and molecular biology, to distinguish normal cells from cancer-causing cells. It is a useful tool for the diagnosis and treatment of malignancies of the brain, blood, etc. Novel techniques known as fluorescence in situ hybridization (FISH) are used for molecular cytogenetic studies. These have DNA labeled with uniquely colored fluorescent tags to image specific regions of the genome. Molecular cytogenetic techniques are crucial for the understanding of the structural and functional organization of the nucleus and the chromosome, genome variation, gene expression and evolution. These also give insight into the contribution of genomic variations and chromosomal abnormalities to tumor genetics and medical genetics. This book is a compilation of chapters that discuss the most vital concepts and emerging trends in the field of molecular cytogenetics. It is an upcoming field of science that has undergone rapid development over the past few decades. Students, researchers, experts and all associated with this field will benefit alike from this book.

The researches compiled throughout the book are authentic and of high quality, combining several disciplines and from very diverse regions from around the world. Drawing on the contributions of many researchers from diverse countries, the book's objective is to provide the readers with the latest achievements in the area of research. This book will surely be a source of knowledge to all interested and researching the field.

In the end, I would like to express my deep sense of gratitude to all the authors for meeting the set deadlines in completing and submitting their research chapters. I would also like to thank the publisher for the support offered to us throughout the course of the book. Finally, I extend my sincere thanks to my family for being a constant source of inspiration and encouragement.

**Editor**

# 1

# Chromosomes of Asian cyprinid fishes: cytogenetic analysis of two representatives of small paleotetraploid tribe Probarbini

Pasakorn Saenjundaeng[1], Marcelo de Bello Cioffi[2*], Ezequiel Aguiar de Oliveira[2,3], Alongklod Tanomtong[1], Weerayuth Supiwong[4], Sumalee Phimphan[1], Maria João Collares-Pereira[5], Alexandr Sember[6], Luiz Antonio Carlos Bertollo[2], Thomas Liehr[7], Cassia Fernanda Yano[2], Terumi Hatanaka[2] and Petr Ráb[6]

**Abstract**

**Background:** Polyploidy, although still poorly explored, represents an important evolutionary event in several cyprinid clades. Herein, *Catlocarpio siamensis* and *Probarbus jullieni* - representatives of the paleotetraploid tribe Probarbini, were characterized both by conventional and molecular cytogenetic methods.

**Results:** Alike most other paleotetraploid cyprinids (with 2n = 100), both species studied here shared 2n = 98 but differed in karyotypes: *C. siamensis* displayed 18m + 34sm + 46st/a; NF = 150, while *P. jullieni* exhibited 26m + 14sm + 58st/a; NF = 138. Fluorescence in situ hybridization (FISH) with rDNA probes revealed two (5S) and eight (18S) signals in *C. siamensis*, respectively, and six signals for both probes in *P. jullieni*. FISH with microsatellite motifs evidenced substantial genomic divergence between both species. The almost doubled size of the chromosome pairs #1 in *C. siamensis* and #14 in *P. jullieni* compared to the rest of corresponding karyotypes indicated chromosomal fusions.

**Conclusion:** Based on our findings, together with likely the same reduced 2n = 98 karyotypes in the remainder Probarbini species, we hypothesize that the karyotype 2n = 98 might represent a derived character, shared by all members of the Probarbini clade. Besides, we also witnessed considerable changes in the amount and distribution of certain repetitive DNA classes, suggesting complex post-polyploidization processes in this small paleotetraploid tribe.

**Keywords:** Fish cytogenetics, Cyprinidae, Chromosomal markers, rDNAs, Microsatellites

## Background

One of the most important evolutionary characteristics of Teleostei is a lineage-specific polyploidization (i.e. teleost-specific whole-genome duplication = TS-WGD) that occurred approximately 226–316 Mya [1], subsequently to its divergence from the remaining actinopterygians (i.e. bichirs, sturgeons, paddlefishes, gars and bowfin) [2, 3]. Furthermore, additional whole-genome duplications (WGDs) took place independently in several other teleostean lineages, such as, e.g., Catostomidae [4], Cobitidae [5], Callichthyidae [6, 7], Salmoniformes [8] and especially Cyprinidae [9–11].

Independent evolutionary tetraploidy and even recurrent hexaploid events of allopolyploid origin have already been evidenced for several cyprinid clades taxonomically recognized as tribes [9]; these are Probarbini, Torini, Smiliogastrini, Cyprinini, Spinibarbini, Schizothoracini, Schizopygopsini and Barbini and overall account for more than 400 polyploid species. Probarbini represents the most early-diverging group [9], with only two genera: (i) the monotypic *Catlocarpio* (*C. siamensis* Boulenger, 1898) being the largest known cyprinid species attaining a length of up to three meters [12, 13], and (ii) the genus *Probarbus*, with three valid species [14] (*P. jullieni* Sauvage, 1880, *P. labeamajor* Roberts, 1992 and *P. labeaminor* Roberts, 1992). These four potamodromous species from large river systems in Southeast Asia have been and are heavily declining in the sizes of populations due to fishery pressures, but also due to

* Correspondence: mbcioffi@ufscar.br
[2]Departamento de Genética e Evolução, Universidade Federal de São Carlos, São Carlos, SP, Brazil
Full list of author information is available at the end of the article

habitat loss and degradation. Thus, since extirpated from most of their native range, these species were considered as "threatened" following IUCN criteria (IUCN Red List of Threatened Species 2012) [15–18].

Irrespective of the evolutionary importance of paleopolyploidy present in various clades of cyprinid fishes [9], its cytogenetic investigation remains practically restricted to reports about diploid chromosome numbers (2n) and karyotype descriptions, rarely complemented with particular chromosome banding protocols [19]. Even less studies applied molecular cytogenetic approaches, such as e.g. the physical mapping of ribosomal genes in Indian species of the genus *Tor*, tribe Torini [20, 21]. The 2n and the karyotypes of the species studied herein were previously reported based exclusively on conventionally Giemsa-stained chromosomes [22, 23]. Based on those reports, two individuals of *P. jullieni* and *C. siamensis*, obtained from aquarium fish dealer, possessed 2n = 98 chromosomes, differing in the proportion of chromosome categories: (18m + 54sm/st + 26a) in *P. jullieni* and (18m + 28sm/st + 52a) in *C. siamensis*. The present study includes in depth cytogenetic analyses of these two species, comprising conventional Giemsa-staining, C-banding and fluorescence in situ hybridization (FISH) approaches with chromosomal mapping of several repetitive DNA classes.

## Results

### Karyotypes

*C. siamensis* possesses 2n = 98 with the karyotype composed of 18m + 34sm + 46st/a elements, with number of chromosomal arms (NF, Nombre Fondamental) being equal to 150. *P. jullieni* shares with the former species 2n = 98, but differs in karyotype composition having 26m + 14sm + 58st/a and NF = 138. The chromosome pairs #1 in *C. siamensis* and #14 in *P. jullieni* were almost doubled in size when compared to the rest of corresponding karyotypes. No differences between male and female karyotypes occur in both species (Fig. 1).

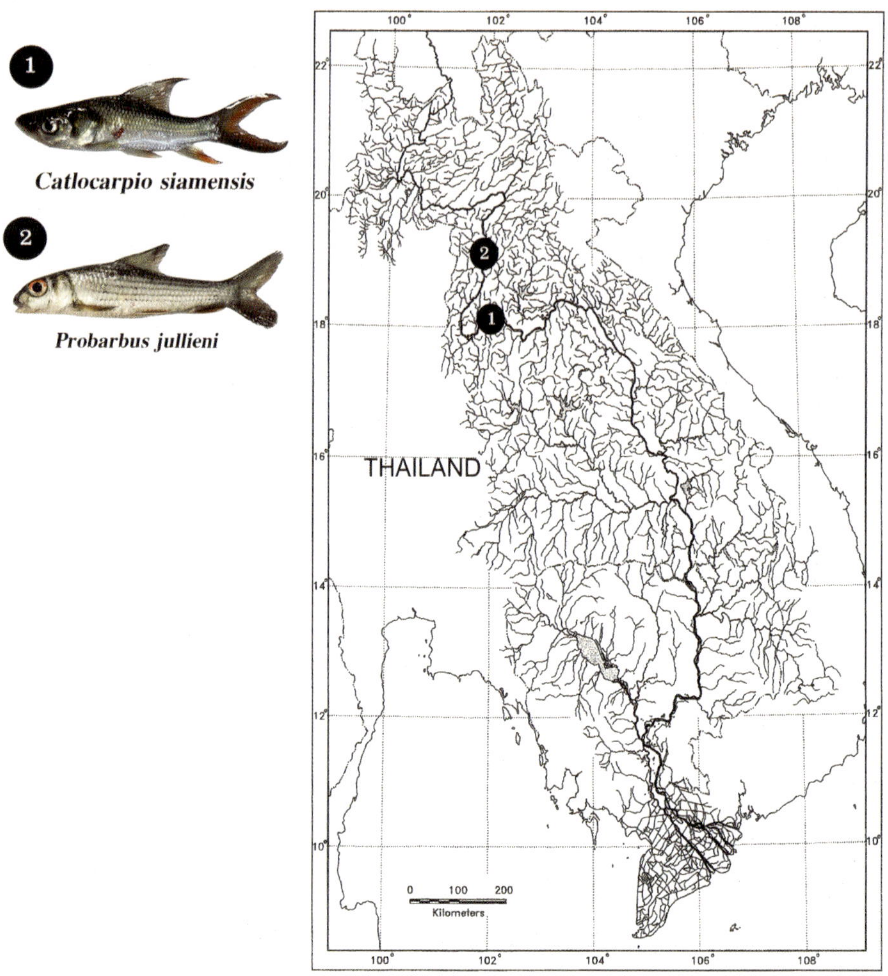


**Fig. 1** Collection sites of *Catlocarpio siamensis* and *Probarbus jullieni* in Thailand examined in the present study (Map of the Mekong River basin modified from Rainboth [13])

### Chromosome mapping of 5S and 18S ribosomal DNA (rDNA) sequences

In the genome of *C. siamensis*, the minor 5S rDNA class is located on a single chromosomal pair (#27), while the major 18S rDNA occurs in four chromosome pairs (#22, #23, #40, #41). By contrast, in *P. jullieni* the 5S rDNA genes are located on three chromosomal pairs (#23, #24, #25), while the 18S rDNA are in another three ones (#19, #35, #36). Consequently, no co-localization of rDNA classes in the genome of either species was detected (Fig. 1).

### Chromosomal mapping of microsatellite sequences

The mapping of the three short repetitive sequences, $(A)_{30}$, $(CA)_{15}$ and $(GA)_{15}$, showed the same hybridization patterns in both species. While $(A)_{30}$ presented a scattered distribution among all chromosomes, the other two motifs $(CA)_{15}$ and $(GA)_{15}$ are both accumulated in the telomeric regions of several chromosome pairs (Fig. 2).

## Discussion

Despite the sporadic occurrence in higher vertebrates, polyploidy was repeatedly documented across several fish lineages and at different taxonomic levels, implying its independent and recurrent origin [24–27]. Out of the four species placed in the tribe Probarbini, just two – *P. jullieni* and *C. siamensis* – have previously been cytogenetically analyzed. Suzuki and Taki [22] reported for the former species 2n = 98 (18m + 54sm/st + 26a) and the follow-up study from the same authors [23] showed 2n = 98 (18m + 28sm/st + 52a) for the latter species. Our results confirmed 2n for both species but with small differences in the karyotype composition. This incongruence reflects probably the small size of the cyprinid chromosomes, especially those of polyploids. Furthermore, cyprinid chromosomes also exhibit a gradual decrease in size, with the centromere positions ranging step-wisely from median to nearly terminal. Indeed, these features make it difficult to assess the chromosomal categories with accuracy [28–30].

Another important aspect of the comparative cytotaxonomy associated with Probarbini species analyzed herein is their slightly reduced 2n = 98 from the usual 2n = 100 that occurs in the overwhelming majority of the polyploid cyprinids [19]. Representatives of the Schizothoracini and Schizopygopsini tribes, the most ones phylogenetically distant from the Probarbini [9], also display a reduced chromosome number ranging from 90 to 98 [31–38]. In this sense, such 2n reductions seem to be a result of independent evolutionary events. As most of other paleotetraploid cyprinine taxa have 2n = 100, 98 chromosomes found in both species examined here likely represent a derived feature. We suppose that the reduced 2n = 98 might be a shared derived character for species of the whole Probarbini clade. Yet, 2n counts for the two remaining members of this group, i.e. *P. labeamajor* and *P. labeaminor*, remain yet to be determined. An obvious but still unclear question is what evolutionary background stands beyond this 2n reduction? Probarbini are highly potamodromous fishes, while the representatives of the other two lineages are confined to high altitudes in Qinghai–Tibetan plateau, forming small, highly fragmented populations [39]. These lineages also contain hexaploid forms [33] or even triploid derivative of this hexaploid level [40] suggesting complex evolutionary processes.

Rapid changes for content in polyploid genomes represent an integral part of very complex processes leading to both immediate and long-term post-polyploidization

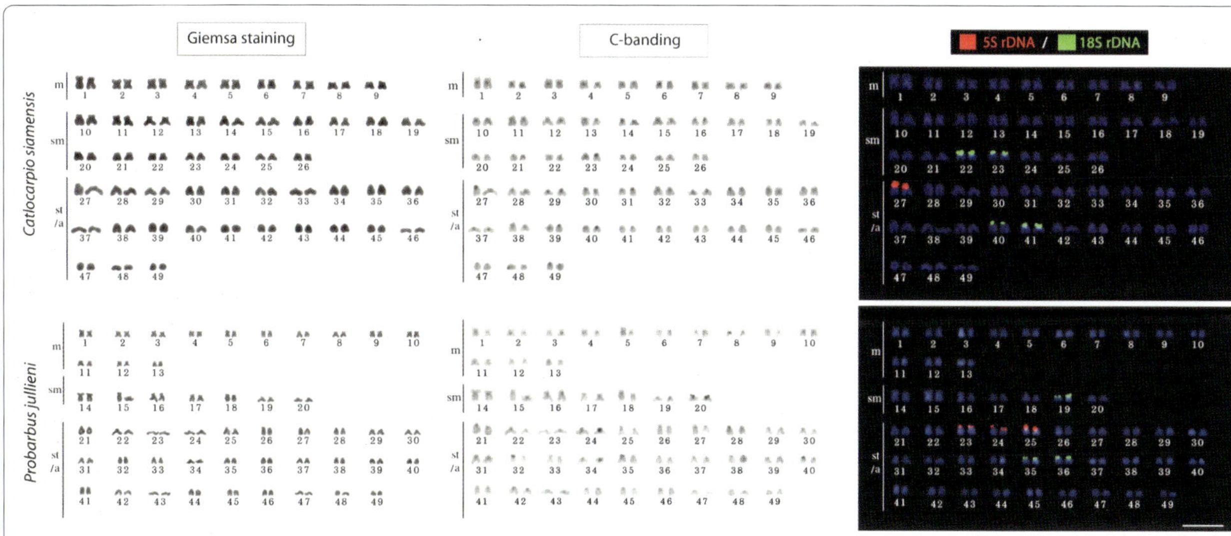


**Fig. 2** Karyotypes of *Catlocarpio siamensis* and *Probarbus jullieni* arranged from Giemsa-stained, C-banded chromosomes and after dual-colour FISH with 5S (red) and 18S (green) rDNA probes. Scale bar = 5 μm

alterations, involving restructuring of genome architecture, epigenetic landscape and gene expression patterns. These processes lead to gradual re-diploidization, i.e. re-establishment of genome balance and diploid-like inheritance [41–49]. Repetitive DNA sequences may be either lost during the process of the so-called genome downsizing, or they can be amplified and/or accumulated in gene-poor regions. Such changes may be driven by illegitimate (non-homologous) recombination and deregulated control of (retro) transposition activity [43, 44, 47, 50–52].

Therefore, the mapping of repetitive DNA classes might provide a useful tool for elucidating the dynamics of (especially young) post-polyploid genomes. Alike the comprehensive cytogenetic maps produced for plant neopolyploids e.g. [53–55], similar research in fishes is mainly restricted to mapping of tandemly-repeated clusters of major (nucleolus-forming, 45S) and minor (5S) rDNA classes as they are the most utilized markers in fish cytotaxonomy in general [28, 56–59]. However, studies performing cytogenetic mapping of e.g. several markers such as *Hox* genes or satellite DNAs, in conjunction with recent advances in genome sequencing and bioinformatics, are also starting to be implemented typically in non-teleost acipenserids [60, 61]. Regarding rDNA profiles, they proved useful especially in deciphering the origin of rather recent homoploid or polyploid hybrids, because the intermediate pattern might help to identify the parental species [62–66]. Moreover, if the numbers of rDNA sites remain additive in polyploids of uncertain origin, the mechanism of either auto- or allopolyploidy might be inferred [67–69]. However, both rDNA classes are subjected to dynamic and complementary evolutionary forces leading either to intragenomic sequence homogenization (concerted evolution), or to the emergence of new repeat variants (birth-and-death evolution) [70–76]. In polyploids, these processes are further modified by the nature of polyploidy, with nucleolar dominance [71, 77, 78] and chimeric sequence variants (described also in cyprinids [72–75]) being a typical example found in allopolyploids. Finally, deregulated control of (retro) transposition activity, especially in hybrid genomes, may further greatly contribute to rDNA site number instability/ hypervariability [76], as both rDNA classes are known to be frequent targets for insertion of various mobile elements [79–83]. All these processes are adding complexity to rDNA dynamics and may disable smooth usage of these markers for examination of karyotype differentiation processes. To name a few examples, high polymorphism and/or rapid amplification of rDNA sites were found in homoploid or polyploid cyprinid fishes [29, 62, 84–86] as well as in other paleo- or neopolyploid fish taxa across the teleost phylogeny [58, 87]. However, also some diploid cyprinids might pose a challenge in terms of rDNA site number analysis due to varied degree of intra- or interindividual polymorphism [88, 89] and interspecific variability [90, 91].

In this study, the number and distribution of ribosomal genes were not conserved among both analyzed species. Thus, whereas two and eight 5S and 18S rDNA signals, respectively, were mapped on the chromosomes of *C. siamensis*, a total of six signals for both rDNA classes was observed in the *P. jullieni* karyotype (Fig. 1). Considering only the strictly polyploid taxa, the distribution patterns of the rDNA sites among the cyprinid lineages remain poorly covered [29, 30], except for some representatives of the Torini and Cyprinini tribes. The available data for five Indian species of the genus *Tor* (Torini) [21, 84, 85] demonstrate very similar pattern as found in our present study, i.e., either single or multiple chromosome pairs carrying both ribosomal clusters. However, the genomes of several members of the clade Cyprinini were examined more thoroughly for these markers [19]; also they exhibit variable site numbers for both rDNA classes. As an example, the common carp *Cyprinus carpio*, with a (paleo) tetraploid karyotype 2n = 100, exhibits a re-diploidized pattern for 45S rDNA, with only a single chromosome pair carrying such sites [92, 93]. Also four to eight 5S rDNA loci [94] can be observed there, while in the (paleo-) tetraploid crucian carp *Carassius carassius* the major rDNA sites occupy two different chromosomal pairs, and the minor rDNA encompasses a variable number of 8–18 loci [29, 30]. Besides, a comparable variability of rDNA distribution was also present in several polyploid forms of *C. auratus* complex [63, 67, 95]. While some reports have evidenced co-localized sites of 5S and 45S rDNA clusters in several either diploid or polyploid cyprinids [62, 86, 94, 96], this is not the case for the species studied herein. Finally, the multiple 45S rDNA sites in both Probarbini species display only slight site-number changes, while 5S rDNA shows a re-diploidized condition in *C. siamensis* - accompanied, however, by apparently larger sizes of both homologous loci. Complementary analyses in the remaining Probarbini species, *P. labeamajor* and *P. labeaminor*, will complete the picture of the post-polyploid rDNA dynamics in this clade. However, from the current data, probable mechanisms such as unequal crossing overs, illegitimate recombination and also transpositions might account for the observed patterns, possibly facilitated by the allopolyploid/hybrid origin of the species.

Microsatellites or simple sequence repeats (SSRs) are oligonucleotides of 1–6 base pairs in length, forming excessive tandem repeats of usually four-to-40 units [97–99]. They show abundant distribution throughout eukaryotic genomes, being dispersed or clustered both in euchromatin or heterochromatin. They are highly polymorphic regarding copy number variations [98]. In the fish genomes, microsatellites are usually abundant in the centromeric and telomeric regions, and they can also localize preferentially to sex chromosomes [56, 100, 101]. In our study, both species exhibited the same general hybridization pattern for all applied probes, with the motif $(A)_{30}$ showing moderate abundance and dispersed hybridization pattern throughout the genomes. Otherwise, the dinucleotides $(CA)_{15}$ and $(GA)_{15}$ accumulated exclusively in telomeric and subtelomeric chromosomal regions, corroborating findings from other fish groups studied to date [101–107]. While the bearing of the observed patterns to the dynamics of polyploidy remains unclear, some authors [104, 107] suggested that the preferential targeting of $(CA)_{15}$ and $(GA)_{15}$ and other microsatellite motifs to telomeric and subtelomeric regions might be functionally linked with the structural formation of telomeres. As microsatellites can be found to be embedded within rDNA clusters [108] and all rDNA sites turned out to be terminal in both species under study, we suppose that $(CA)_{15}$ and $(GA)_{15}$ dinucleotides might have contributed to the dynamic behavior of rDNA sites in these Probarbini representatives.

## Methods

### Animals

Individuals of *Catlocarpio siamensis* (12♂ and 6♀) and *Probarbus jullieni* (8♂ and 8♀) from different tributaries of the Mekong River basin (Thailand) were analyzed (Fig. 3). The specimens were caught using a hand-net, placed in sealed plastic bags containing oxygen and clean water, and transported to the laboratory. Experiments were performed in accordance with ethical protocols, and anesthesia using clove oil was administered prior to sacrificing the animals, as approved by the Ethics Committee of Khon Kaen University and by the RGJ committee under no. PHD/K0081/2556 (Thailand). The specimens were deposited in the fish collection of the Cytogenetic Laboratory, Department of Biology Faculty of Science, Khon Kaen University (Thailand).

### Chromosome preparation and C-banding

Mitotic chromosomes were obtained from the anterior kidney, cell suspensions dropped onto microscopic slides and air-dried [109]. Conventional staining was done by 5% Giemsa solution in phosphate buffer (pH 6.8) for 10 min. The distribution of constitutive heterochromatin on chromosomes was demonstrated by C-banding method [110].

### The probe preparation and FISH experiments

Two tandemly arrayed rDNA sequences, namely 5S and 18S, were obtained via PCR from the nuclear DNA of *C. siamensis*. The 5S repeat copy encompassing 120 base pairs (bp) of the 5S rRNA coding region and 200 bp of the non-transcribed spacer (NTS) was produced according to Pendas et al. [111]. The 18S rDNA fragment, with 1,400-bp in length including the 18S rRNA gene coding sequence, was prepared according to Cioffi et al. [112]. Both rDNA fragments were cloned into plasmid vectors and propagated in DH5α *Escherichia coli* competent cells (Invitrogen, San Diego, CA, USA). The final 5S and 18S rDNA probes were directly labeled with SpectrumOrange-dUTP and SpectrumGreen-dUTP, respectively, by Nick translation kit (Roche, Mannheim, Germany) according to the manufacturer's recommendations. FISH was performed under high stringency conditions following the protocol of Yano et al. [113].

FISH with the set of probes corresponding to three microsatellite motifs $(A)_{30}$, $(CA)_{15}$ and $(GA)_{15}$ was performed as described in [114], with slight modifications.

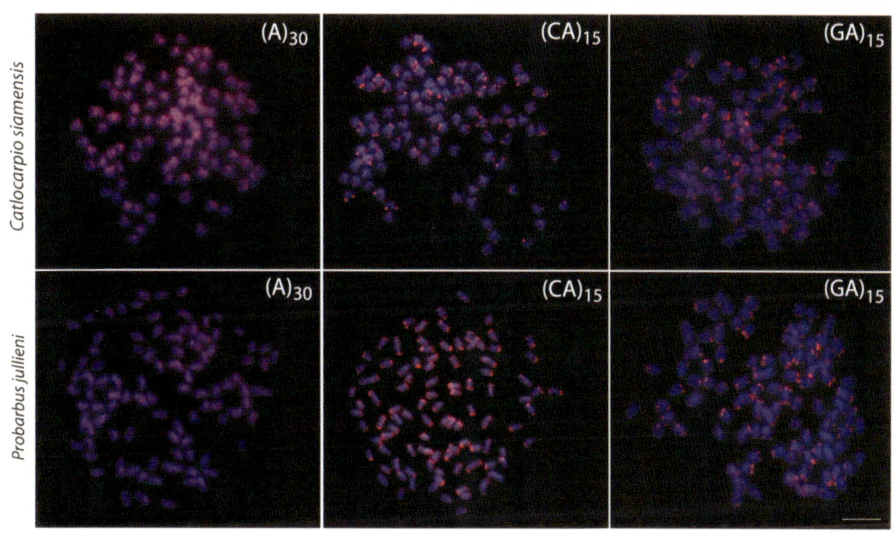


**Fig. 3** Metaphase plates of *Catlocarpio siamensis* and *Probarbus jullieni* after FISH with different microsatellite motifs. Scale bar = 5 μm

These sequences were directly labeled by Cy3 at the 5′ terminus during synthesis (Sigma, St. Louis, MO, USA).

Chromosomes were counterstained with DAPI (1.2 μg/ml) and mounted in antifading solution (Vector, Burlingame, CA, USA,) in both experiments.

### Image processing

At least 30 metaphase spreads per individual were analyzed to confirm the diploid number, karyotype structure and FISH data. Images were captured using an Olympus BX50 microscope (Olympus Corporation, Ishikawa, Japan) with CoolSNAP and processed using Image Pro Plus 4.1 software (Media Cybernetics, Silver Spring, MD, USA). Chromosomes were classified according to centromere position as metacentric (m), submetacentric (sm) and subtelocentric (st)/acrocentric (a) ones [115], with the st and a chromosome pairs being scored together in one st-a category. For the chromosomal arm number (NF; Nombre Fondamental) to be calculated, m + sm were scored as bi-armed while st + as mono-armed.

## Conclusions

Here we hypothesized that the karyotype characterized by 2n = 98 in both analyzed species might represent a derived character, probably also shared by all members of the Probarbini clade. Besides, we also witnessed considerable changes in the amount and distribution of certain repetitive DNA classes, hence suggesting complex post-polyploidization processes in this small paleotetraploid tribe.

#### Abbreviations

2n: Diploid number; a: acrocentric chromosome; DAPI: 4′,6-diamidino-2-phenylindole; dUTP: 2′-Deoxyuridine-5′-Triphosphate; FISH: Fluorescence in situ hybridization; m: metacentric chromosome; NF: Nombre Fondamental; NTS: Non-transcribed spacer; PCR: Polymerase chain reaction; rDNA: ribosomal DNA; rRNA: ribosomal RNA; sm: submetacentric chromosome; st: subtelocentric chromosome

#### Funding

This work was financially supported by: The Thailand Research Fund (TRF) through the Royal Golden Jubilee Ph.D. Program Grant No. PHD/0140/2557 and Toxic Substances in Livestock and Aquatic Animals Research Group, Khon Kaen University; scholarship under the Post-Doctoral Trainning Program from Research Affairs and Graduate School (Grant No. 59255). The funders had no role in study design, data collection; Project EXCELLENCE CZ.02.1.01/0.0/0.0/15_003/0000460 OP RDE (PR) and with the institutional support RVO: 67985904 (PR, AS) by the Czech Academy of Sciences; Conselho Nacional de Desenvolvimento Científico e Tecnológico - CNPq (Proc. nos 401962/2016–4 and 304992/2015–1), Fundação de Amparo à Pesquisa do Estado de São Paulo-FAPESP (Proc. No 2016/22196–2) and CAPES/Alexander von Humboldt (Proc. No. 88881.136128/2017– 01).

#### Authors' contributions

PS, EAO, CFY and TH carried out the cytogenetic analysis and drafted the manuscript, MBC, AT, WS and SP helped in the cytogenetic analysis, drafted and revised the manuscript. MJCP, AS, LACB, TL and PR drafted and revised the manuscript. MBC, AT and PR coordinated the study, drafted and revised the manuscript. All authors read and approved the final version of the manuscript.

#### Competing interests

The authors declare that they have no competing interests.

#### Author details

[1]Toxic Substances in Livestock and Aquatic Animals Research Group, Department of Biology, Faculty of Science, Khon Kaen University, Muang District, Khon Kaen, Thailand. [2]Departamento de Genética e Evolução, Universidade Federal de São Carlos, São Carlos, SP, Brazil. [3]Secretaria de Estado de Educação de Mato Grosso – SEDUC-MT, Cuiabá, MT, Brazil. [4]Faculty of Applied Science and Engineering, Khon Kaen University, Nong Kai Campus, Muang, Nong Kai, Thailand. [5]Faculdade de Ciencias, Centre for Ecology, Evolution and Environmental Changes, Universidade de Lisboa, Campo Grande, PT–1749-016 Lisbon, Portugal. [6]Laboratory of Fish Genetics, Institute of Animal Physiology and Genetics, Czech Academy of Sciences, Rumburská 89, 277 21 Liběchov, Czech Republic. [7]Institute of Human Genetics, Jena University Hospital, Am Klinikum 1, D-07747 Jena, Germany.

#### References

1. Hurley IA, Mueller RL, Dunn KA, Schmidt EJ, Friedman M, Ho RK, et al. A new time-scale for ray-finned fish evolution. Proc R Soc London B Biol Sci. 2007;274:489–98.
2. Braasch I, Postlethwait JH. Polyploidy in fish and the teleost genome duplication. In: Soltis PS, Soltis DE, editors. Polyploidy and genome evolution. Berlin: Springer; 2012. p. 341–83.
3. Sallan LC. Major issues in the origins of ray-finned fish (Actinopterygii) biodiversity. Biol Rev. 2014;89:950–71.
4. Uyeno T, Smith GR. Tetraploid origin of the karyotype of catostomid fishes. Science. 1972;175:644–6.
5. Saitoh K, Chen W-J, Mayden RL. Extensive hybridization and tetrapolyploidy in spined loach fish. Mol Phylogenet Evol. 2010;56:1001–10.
6. Alexandrou MA, Oliveira C, Maillard M, McGill RAR, Newton J, Creer S, et al. Competition and phylogeny determine community structure in Müllerian co-mimics. Nature. 2011;469:84.
7. Marburger S, Alexandrou MA, Taggart JB, Creer S, Carvalho G, Oliveira C, et al. Whole genome duplication and transposable element proliferation drive genome expansion in Corydoradinae catfishes. Proc R Soc B. 2018;285:20172732.
8. Macqueen DJ, Johnston IA. A well-constrained estimate for the timing of the salmonid whole genome duplication reveals major decoupling from species diversification. Proc R Soc B Biol Sci. 2014;281:20132881.
9. Yang L, Sado T, Vincent Hirt M, Pasco-Viel E, Arunachalam M, Li J, et al. Phylogeny and polyploidy: resolving the classification of cyprinine fishes (Teleostei: Cypriniformes). Mol Phylogenet Evol. 2015;85:97–116.
10. Schmidt RC, Bart HL Jr. Nomenclatural changes should not be based on equivocally supported phylogenies: reply to Yang et al. 2015. Mol Phylogenet Evol. 2015;90:193–4.
11. Wang X, Gan X, Li J, Chen Y, He S. Cyprininae phylogeny revealed independent origins of the Tibetan plateau endemic polyploid cyprinids and their diversifications related to the Neogene uplift of the plateau. Sci China Life Sci. 2016;59:1149–65.
12. Smith HM. The freshwater fishes of Siam, or Thailand. Bull - United States Natl Museum. 1945;188:1–633.

13. Rainboth WJ. Fishes of the cambodian mekong. Rome: Food & Agriculture Org.; 1996.
14. Robert TR. Revision of the southeast Asian cyprinid fish genus *Probarbus*, with two new species threatened by proposed construction of dams on the Mekong River. Ichthyol Explor Freshwaters. 1992;3:37–48.
15. Hogan Z, Baird I. *Probarbus jullieni*. The IUCN Red List of Threatened Species. 2011. https://doi.org/10.2305/IUCN.UK.2011-1.RLTS.T18182A7742599.en. Accessed 6 Sep 2017.
16. Baird I. Probarbus labeamajor. The IUCN Red List of Threatened Species. 2011. https://doi.org/10.2305/IUCN.UK.2011-1.RLTS.T18183A7744836.en. Accessed 6 Sep 2017.
17. Baird I. Probarbus labeaminor. The IUCN Red List of Threatened Species 2012. https://doi.org/10.2305/IUCN.UK.2012-1.RLTS.T18184A1728617.en. Accessed 6 Sep 2017.
18. Hogan Z. Catlocarpio siamensis. The IUCN Red List of Threatened Species. 2011. https://doi.org/10.2305/IUCN.UK.2011-1.RLTS.T180662A7649359.en. Accessed 6 Sep 2017.
19. Arai R. Fish karyotypes: a check list. Tokio: Springer Science & Business Media; 2011.
20. Singh M, Kumar R, Nagpure NS, Kushwaha B, Gond I, Lakra WS. Chromosomal localization of 18s and 5s rDNA using FISH in the genus *Tor* (Pisces, Cyprinidae). Genetica. 2009;137:245–52.
21. Mani I, Kumar R, Singh M, Nagpure NS, Kushwaha B, Srivastava PK, et al. Nucleotide variation and physical mapping of ribosomal genes using FISH in genus *Tor* (Pisces, Cyprinidae). Mol Biol Rep. 2011;38:2637–47.
22. Suzuki A, Taki Y. Chromosomes and DNA values of two cyprinid fishes of the subfamily Barbinae. Japanese J Ichthyol. 1986;32:459–62.
23. Suzuki A, Taki Y. Karyotype and DNA content in the cyprinid *Catlocarpio siamensis*. Japanese J Ichthyol. 1988;35:389–91.
24. Otto SP, Whitton J. Polyploid incidence and evolution. Annu Rev Genet. 2000;34:401–37.
25. Le Comber SC, Smith C. Polyploidy in fishes: patterns and processes. Biol J Linn Soc. 2004;82:431–42.
26. Mable BK, Alexandrou MA, Taylor MI. Genome duplication in amphibians and fish: an extended synthesis. J Zool. 2011;284:151–82.
27. Glasauer SMK, Neuhauss SCF. Whole-genome duplication in teleost fishes and its evolutionary consequences. Mol Gen Genomics. 2014;289:1045–60.
28. Ráb P, Collares-Pereira MJ. Chromosomes of European cyprinid fishes (Cyprinidae, Cypriniformes). A review. Folia Zool. 1995;44:193–214.
29. Spoz A, Boron A, Porycka K, Karolewska M, Ito D, Abe S, et al. Molecular cytogenetic analysis of the crucian carp, *Carassius carassius* (Linnaeus, 1758)(Teleostei, Cyprinidae), using chromosome staining and fluorescence in situ hybridisation with rDNA probes. Comp Cytogenet. 2014;8:233–48.
30. Knytl M, Kalous L, Rylková K, Choleva L, Merilä J, Ráb P. Morphologically indistinguishable hybrid *Carassius* female with 156 chromosomes: a threat for the threatened crucian carp, *C. carassius*, L. PLoS One. 2018;13:e0190924.
31. Rishi KK, Singh J, Kaul MM. Chromosome analysis of *Schizothoracichthys progastus* (McCll) (Cypriniformes). Chromosom Inform Serv. 1983;34:12–3.
32. Rishi KK, Rishi S. Karyotype study on six Indian hill-stream fishes. Chromosom Sci. 1998;2:9–13.
33. Zan RG, Liu WG, Song Z. Tetraploid-hexaploid relationship in Schizothoracinae. Acta Genet Sin. 1985;12:137–42.
34. Mazik EJ, Toktosunovic A, Ráb P. Karyotype study of four species of the genus *Diptychus* (Pisces, Cyprinidae), with remarks on polyploidy of schizothoracine fishes. Folia Zool. 1989;38:325–32.
35. Ahmad F, Yousuf AR, Tripathi NK, Zargar UR. On the chromosomes of two cyprinid fishes of the subfamily Schizothoracinae from Kashmir. Nat Sci. 2011;9:53–61.
36. Yu X, Zhou T, Li K, Li Y, Zhou M. On the karyosystematics of cyprinid fishes and a summary of fish chromosome studies in China. Genetica. 1987;72:225–35.
37. Yu XJ, Zhou T, Li YC, Li K, Zhou M. Chromosomes of Chinese freshwater fishes. Beijing: Science Press; 1989.
38. Yu XY, Li YC, Zhou T. Karyotype studies of cyprinid fishes in China-comparative study of the karyotypes of 8 species of schizothoracine fishes. Wuhan Univ J Nat Sci. 1990;2:97–104.
39. He D, Chen Y, Chen Y, Chen Z. Molecular phylogeny of the specialized schizothoracine fishes (Teleostei: Cyprinidae), with their implications for the uplift of the Qinghai-Tibetan Plateau. Chin Sci Bull. 2004;49:39–48.
40. Yu XY, Yu XJ. A schizothoracine fish species, *Diptychus dipogon*, with a very high number of chromosomes. Chromosom Inf Serv. 1990;48:17–8.
41. Wolfe KH. Yesterday's polyploids and the mystery of diploidization. Nat Rev Genet. 2001;2:333–41.
42. Comai L. The advantages and disadvantages of being polyploid. Nat Rev Genet. 2005;6:836–46. https://doi.org/10.1038/nrg1711.
43. Ma X-F, Gustafson JP. Genome evolution of allopolyploids: a process of cytological and genetic diploidization. Cytogenet Genome Res. 2005; 109:236–49.
44. Leitch IJ, Hanson L, Lim KY, Kovarik A, Chase MW, Clarkson JJ, et al. The ups and downs of genome size evolution in polyploid species of *Nicotiana* (Solanaceae). Ann Bot. 2008;101:805–14.
45. Parisod C, Holderegger R, Brochmann C. Evolutionary consequences of autopolyploidy. New Phytol. 2010;186:5–17.
46. Madlung A. Polyploidy and its effect on evolutionary success: old questions revisited with new tools. Heredity. 2013;110:99–104.
47. Tayalé A, Parisod C. Natural pathways to polyploidy in plants and consequences for genome reorganization. Cytogenet Genome Res. 2013;140:79–96.
48. Wertheim B, Beukeboom LW, Van de Zande L. Polyploidy in animals: effects of gene expression on sex determination, evolution and ecology. Cytogenet Genome Res. 2013;140:256–69.
49. Soltis DE, Visger CJ, Marchant DB, Soltis PS. Polyploidy: pitfalls and paths to a paradigm. Am J Bot. 2016;103:1146–66.
50. Schwarzacher T, Leitch AR, Bennett MD, Heslop-Harrison JS. *In situ* localization of parental genomes in a wide hybrid. Ann Bot. 1989;64:315–24.
51. Leitch IJ, Bennett MD. Genome downsizing in polyploid plants. Biol J Linn Soc. 2004;82:651–63.
52. Parisod C, Alix K, Just J, Petit M, Sarilar V, Mhiri C, et al. Impact of transposable elements on the organization and function of allopolyploid genomes. New Phytol. 2010;186:37–45.
53. Chester M, Leitch AR, Soltis PS, Soltis DE. Review of the application of modern cytogenetic methods (FISH/GISH) to the study of reticulation (polyploidy/hybridisation). Genes (Basel). 2010;1:166–92.
54. Xiong Z, Pires JC. Karyotype and identification of all homoeologous chromosomes of allopolyploid *Brassica napus* and its diploid progenitors. Genetics. 2011;187:37–49.
55. Cuadrado Á, de Bustos A, Jouve N. On the allopolyploid origin and genome structure of the closely related species *Hordeum secalinum* and *Hordeum capense* inferred by molecular karyotyping. Ann Bot. 2017;120:245–55.
56. Cioffi MB, Bertollo LAC. Chromosomal distribution and evolution of repetitive DNAs in fish. In: Garrido-Ramos MA, editor. Genome dynamics. Basel: Karger; 2012. p. 197–221.
57. Gornung E. Twenty years of physical mapping of major ribosomal RNA genes across the teleosts: a review of research. Cytogenet Genome Res. 2013;141:90–102.
58. Maneechot N, Yano CF, Bertollo LAC, Getlekha N, Molina WF, Ditcharoen S, et al. Genomic organization of repetitive DNAs highlights chromosomal evolution in the genus *Clarias* (Clariidae, Siluriformes). Mol Cytogenet. 2016;9:4.
59. Sochorová J, Garcia S, Gálvez F, Symonová R, Kovařík A. Evolutionary trends in animal ribosomal DNA loci: introduction to a new online database. Chromosoma. 2018;127:141–50.
60. Biltueva LS, Prokopov DY, Makunin AI, Komissarov AS, Kudryavtseva AV, Lemskaya NA, et al. Genomic organization and physical mapping of tandemly arranged repetitive DNAs in sterlet (*Acipenser ruthenus*). Cytogenet Genome Res. 2017;152:148–57.
61. Symonová R, Havelka M, Amemiya CT, Howell WM, Kořínková T, Flajšhans M, et al. Molecular cytogenetic differentiation of paralogs of Hox paralogs in duplicated and re-diploidized genome of the north American paddlefish (*Polyodon spathula*). BMC Genet. 2017;18:19.
62. Gromicho M, Coutanceau J-P, Ozouf-Costaz C, Collares-Pereira MJ. Contrast between extensive variation of 28S rDNA and stability of 5S rDNA and telomeric repeats in the diploid-polyploid *Squalius alburnoides* complex and in its maternal ancestor *Squalius pyrenaicus* (Teleostei, Cyprinidae). Chromosom Res. 2006;14:297–306.
63. Zhu H-P, Gui J-F. Identification of genome organization in the unusual allotetraploid form of *Carassius auratus gibelio*. Aquaculture. 2007;265:109–17.
64. Da Silva M, Matoso DA, Ludwig LAM, Gomes E, Almeida MC, Vicari MR, et al. Natural triploidy in *Rhamdia quelen* identified by cytogenetic monitoring in Iguaçu basin, southern Brazil. Environ Biol Fish. 2011;91:361–6.
65. Zhang C, Ye L, Chen Y, Xiao J, Wu Y, Tao M, et al. The chromosomal constitution of fish hybrid lineage revealed by 5S rDNA FISH. BMC Genet. 2015;16:140.

66. Ribeiro LB, Moraes Neto A, Artoni RF, Matoso DA, Feldberg E. Chromosomal mapping of repetitive sequences (Rex3, Rex6, and rDNA Genes) in hybrids between *Colossoma macropomum* (Cuvier, 1818) and *Piaractus mesopotamicus* (Holmberg, 1887). Zebrafish. 2017;14:155–60.
67. Zhu HP, Ma DM, Gui JF. Triploid origin of the gibel carp as revealed by 5S rDNA localization and chromosome painting. Chromosom Res. 2006;14:767–76.
68. Li Y-J, Tian Y, Zhang M-Z, Tian P-P, Yu Z, Abe S, et al. Chromosome banding and FISH with rDNA probe in the diploid and tetraploid loach *Misgurnus anguillicaudatus*. Ichthyol Res. 2010;57:358–66.
69. Qin Q, Wang J, Hu M, Huang S, Liu S. Autotriploid origin of *Carassius auratus* as revealed by chromosomal locus analysis. Sci China Life Sci. 2016;59:622–6.
70. Eickbush TH, Eickbush DG. Finely orchestrated movements: evolution of the ribosomal RNA genes. Genetics. 2007;175:477–85.
71. Feliner GN, Rosselló JA. Concerted evolution of multigene families and homoeologous recombination. In: Wendel JF, editor. Plant genome diversity volume 1. Vienna: Springer-Verlag; 2012. p. 171–93.
72. Qin Q, He W, Liu S, Wang J, Xiao J, Liu Y. Analysis of 5S rDNA organization and variation in polyploid hybrids from crosses of different fish subfamilies. J Exp Zool Part B Mol Dev Evol. 2010;314:403–11.
73. He W, Qin Q, Liu S, Li T, Wang J, Xiao J, et al. Organization and variation analysis of 5S rDNA in different ploidy-level hybrids of red crucian carp × topmouth culter. PLoS One. 2012;7:e38976.
74. Huang P, Xiao A, Tong X, Lin S, Zhang B. Targeted mutagenesis in zebrafish by TALENs. In: Clifton NJ, editor. Methods in molecular biology. New Jersey: Human Press; 2016. p. 191–206.
75. Ye L, Zhang C, Tang X, Chen Y, Liu S. Variations in 5S rDNAs in diploid and tetraploid offspring of red crucian carp × common carp. BMC Genet. 2017;18:75.
76. Fontdevila A. Hybrid genome evolution by transposition. Cytogenet Genome Res. 2005;110:49–55.
77. Volkov RA, Komarova NY, Hemleben V. Ribosomal DNA in plant hybrids: inheritance, rearrangement, expression. Syst Biodivers. 2007;5:261–76.
78. Kovarik A, Dadejova M, Lim YK, Chase MW, Clarkson JJ, Knapp S, et al. Evolution of rDNA in *Nicotiana allopolyploids*: a potential link between rDNA homogenization and epigenetics. Ann Bot. 2008;101:815–23.
79. Rebordinos L, Cross I, Merlo A. High evolutionary dynamism in 5S rDNA of fish: state of the art. Cytogenet Genome Res. 2013;141:103–13.
80. Zhang X, Eickbush MT, Eickbush TH. Role of recombination in the long-term retention of transposable elements in rRNA gene loci. Genetics. 2008;180:1617–26.
81. Cioffi MB, Martins C, Bertollo LAC. Chromosome spreading of associated transposable elements and ribossomal DNA in the fish *Erythrinus erythrinus*. Implications for genome change and karyoevolution in fish. BMC Evol Biol. 2010;10:271.
82. Symonová R, Majtánová Z, Sember A, Staaks GBO, Bohlen J, Freyhof J. Genome differentiation in a species pair of coregonine fishes: an extremely rapid speciation driven by stress - activated retrotransposons mediating extensive ribosomal DNA multiplications. BMC Evol Biol. 2013;13:42.
83. Sember A, Bohlen J, Šlechtová V, Altmanová M, Symonová R, Ráb P. Karyotype differentiation in 19 species of river loach fishes (Nemacheilidae, Teleostei): extensive variability associated with rDNA and heterochromatin distribution and its phylogenetic and ecological interpretation. BMC Evol Biol. 2015;15:251.
84. Singh M, Kumar R, Nagpure NS, Kushwaha B, Mani I, Chauhan UK, et al. Population distribution of 45S and 5S rDNA in golden mahseer, *Tor putitora*: population-specific FISH marker. J Genet. 2009;88:315–20.
85. Singh M, Kumar R, Nagpure NS, Kushwaha B, Mani I, Lakra WS. Extensive NOR site polymorphism in geographically isolated populations of golden mahseer, *Tor putitora*. Genome. 2009;52:783–9.
86. Pereira CSA, Aboim MA, Ráb P, Collares-Pereira MJ. Introgressive hybridization as a promoter of genome reshuffling in natural homoploid fish hybrids (Cyprinidae, Leuciscinae). Heredity. 2014;112:343–50.
87. Śliwińska-Jewsiewicka A, Kuciński M, Kirtiklis L, Dobosz S, Ocalewicz K, Jankun M. Chromosomal characteristics and distribution of rDNA sequences in the brook trout *Salvelinus fontinalis* (Mitchill, 1814). Genetica. 2015;143:425–32.
88. Collares-Pereira MJ, Ráb P. NOR polymorphism in the Iberian species *Chondrostoma lusitanicum* (Pisces: Cyprinidae)–re-examination by FISH. Genetica. 1999;105:301–3.
89. Libertini A, Sola L, Rampin M, Rossi AR, Iijima K, Ueda T. Classical and molecular cytogenetic characterization of allochthonous European bitterling *Rhodeus amarus* (Cyprinidae, Acheilognathinae) from northern Italy. Genes Genet Syst. 2008;83:417–22.
90. Pereira CSA, Ráb P, Collares-Pereira MJ. Chromosomes of European cyprinid fishes: comparative cytogenetics and chromosomal characteristics of ribosomal DNAs in nine Iberian chondrostomine species (Leuciscinae). Genetica. 2012;140:485–95.
91. Rossi AR, Milana V, Hett AK, Tancioni L. Molecular cytogenetic analysis of the Appenine endemic cyprinid fish *Squalius lucumonis* and three other Italian leuciscines using chromosome banding and FISH with rDNA probes. Genetica. 2012;140:469–76.
92. Li Y-J, Gao Y-C, Zhou H, Liu B, Gao M, Wang Y-S, et al. Molecular cytogenetic study of genome ploidy in the German mirror carp *Cyprinus carpio*. Fish Sci. 2014;80:963–8.
93. Kumar R, Baisvar VS, Kushwaha B, Waikhom G, Nagpure NS. Cytogenetic investigation of *Cyprinus carpio* (Linnaeus, 1758) using giemsa, silver nitrate, CMA 3 staining and fluorescence in situ hybridization. Nucl. 2017;60:1–8.
94. Inafuku J, Nabeyama M, Kikuma Y, Saitoh J, Kubota S, Kohno S. Chromosomal location and nucleotide sequences of 5S ribosomal DNA of two cyprinid species (Osteichthyes, Pisces). Chromosom Res. 2000;8:193–9.
95. Murakami M, Fujitani H. Characterization of repetitive DNA sequences carrying 5S rDNA of the triploid ginbuna (Japanese silver crucian carp, *Carassius auratus langsdorfi*). Genes Genet Syst. 1998;73:9–20.
96. Phillips RB, Reed KM. Localization of repetitive DNAs to zebrafish (*Danio rerio*) chromosomes by fluorescence in situ hybridization (FISH). Chromosom Res. 2000;8:27–35.
97. Tautz D, Renz M. Simple sequences are ubiquitous repetitive components of eukaryotic genomes. Nucleic acids Res Acids Res. 1984;12:4127–38.
98. Ellegren H. Microsatellites: simple sequences with complex evolution. Nat Rev Genet. 2004;5:435–45.
99. Chistiakov DA, Hellemans B, Volckaert FAM. Microsatellites and their genomic distribution, evolution, function and applications: a review with special reference to fish genetics. Aquaculture. 2006;255:1–29.
100. Yano CF, Bertollo LAC, Liehr T, Troy WP, Cioffi MDB. W chromosome dynamics in *Triportheus* species (Characiformes, Triportheidae): an ongoing process narrated by repetitive sequences. J Hered. 2016;107:342–8.
101. Oliveira EA, Sember A, Bertollo LAC, Yano CF, Ezaz T, Moreira-Filho O, et al. Tracking the evolutionary pathway of sex chromosomes among fishes: characterizing the unique XX/XY1Y2 system in *Hoplias malabaricus* (Teleostei, Characiformes). Chromosoma. 2018;127:115–28.
102. Cioffi MB, Kejnovsky E, Bertollo LAC. The chromosomal distribution of microsatellite repeats in the genome of the wolf fish *Hoplias malabaricus*, focusing on the sex chromosomes. Cytogenet Genome Res. 2011;132:289–96.
103. Xu D, Lou B, Bertollo LAC, Cioffi MDB. Chromosomal mapping of microsatellite repeats in the rock bream fish *Oplegnathus fasciatus*, with emphasis of their distribution in the neo-Y chromosome. Mol Cytogenet. 2013;6:12.
104. Terencio ML, Schneider CH, Gross MC, Vicari MR, Farias IP, Passos KB, et al. Evolutionary dynamics of repetitive DNA in *Semaprochilodus* (Characiformes, Prochilodontidae): a fish model for sex chromosome differentiation. Sex Dev. 2013;7:325–33.
105. Yano CF, Poltronieri J, Bertollo LAC, Artoni RF, Liehr T, Cioffi MDB. Chromosomal mapping of repetitive DNAs in *Triportheus trifurcatus* (Characidae, Characiformes): insights into the differentiation of the Z and W chromosomes. PLoS One. 2014;9:e90946.
106. Oliveira EA, Bertollo LAC, Yano CF, Liehr T, Cioffi MDB. Comparative cytogenetics in the genus *Hoplias* (Characiformes, Erythrinidae) highlights contrasting karyotype evolution among congeneric species. Mol Cytogenet. 2015;8:56.
107. Pucci MB, Barbosa P, Nogaroto V, Almeida MC, Artoni RF, Scacchetti PC, et al. Chromosomal spreading of microsatellites and (TTAGGG)n sequences in the *Characidium zebra* and *C. gomesi* genomes (Characiformes: Crenuchidae). Cytogenet Genome Res. 2016;149:182–90. https://doi.org/10.1159/000447959.
108. Piscor D, Parise-Maltempi PP. Microsatellite organization in the B chromosome and a chromosome complement in *Astyanax* (Characiformes, Characidae) species. Cytogenet Genome Res. 2016;148:44–51.
109. Bertollo LAC, Cioffi MB, Moreira-Filho O. Direct chromosome preparation from freshwater teleost fishes. In: Ozouf-Costaz C, Pisano E, Foresti F, Almeida Toledo LF, editors. Fish cytogenetic techniques. Enfield USA: CRC Press; 2015. p. 21–6. https://doi.org/10.1201/b18534-4.
110. Sumner AT. A simple technique for demonstrating centromeric heterochromatin. Exp Cell Res. 1972;75:304–6.
111. Pendás AM, Móran P, Freije JP, Garcia-Vásquez E. Chromosomal location and nucleotide sequence of two tandem repeats of the Atlantic salmon 5S

rDNA. Cytogenet Cell Genet. 1994;67:31–6. https://doi.org/10.1159/000133792.
112. Cioffi MB, Martins C, Centofante L, Jacobina U, Bertollo LAC. Chromosomal variability among allopatric populations of erythrinidae fish *Hoplias malabaricus*: mapping of three classes of repetitive DNAs. Cytogenet Genome Res. 2009;125:132–41.
113. Yano CF, Bertollo LAC, Cioffi MB. FISH-FISH: molecular cytogenetics in fish species. In: Liehr T, editor. Fluorescence in situ hybridization (FISH) - application guide. 2nd ed. Berlin: Springer; 2017. p. 429–43.
114. Kubat Z, Hobza R, Vyskot B, Kejnovsky E. Microsatellite accumulation on the Y chromosome in *Silene latifolia*. Genome. 2008;51:350–6.
115. Levan A, Fredga K, Sandberg AA. Nomenclature for centromeric position on chromosomes. Hereditas. 1964;52:201–20.

2

# Pallister-Killian syndrome: clinical, cytogenetic and molecular findings in 15 cases

Birsen Karaman[1*], Hülya Kayserili[1,2], Asadollah Ghanbari[1], Zehra Oya Uyguner[1], Güven Toksoy[1], Umut Altunoglu[1] and Seher Basaran[1]

**Abstract**

**Background:** Pallister Killian syndrome (PKS, OMIM 601803) is a rare genetic disorder with a distinct phenotype caused by tissue- limited mosaicism tetrasomy of the short arm of chromosome 12, which usually cytogenetically presents as an extra isochromosome 12p.

Wide phenotypic variability in PKS has been reported, ranging from pre-to perinatal death due to multiple congenital anomalies, especially diaphragmatic hernia, and classic phenotypes including seizures, severe developmental delay, macrosomia at birth, deafness, and distinct dysmorphic features, such as coarse face, temporal alopecia, a small nose with anteverted nostrils, long philtrum, and hypo–/hyper- pigmented streaks on the skin.

**Results:** Karyotypes obtained from cultured peripheral lymphocytes of 13 cases, who were diagnosed as PKS, were normal, while karyotypes obtained from cultured skin samples and buccal mucosa revealed the supernumerary mosaic i(12p). Mosaic karyotype was found in both fibroblast and buccal mucosa in 14 of 15 patients in our series, whereas in one stillbirth, following the clinical diagnosis of PKS, skin and buccal smear samples were taken, and all karyotypes from cultured fibroblasts revealed a supernumerary i(12p), while I-FISH study showed 60% mosaicism in mucosal cells.

**Conclusions:** We here share the clinical, cytogenetic and molecular cytogenetic findings of 15 cases with PKS phenotype and the parental origin of seven i(12p) identified by molecular analyses. To our knowledge, this is the largest series of PKS patients with parental origin study from a single center. We believe that our study makes a significant contribution to the literature because we specifically found no differences in the phenotypes of cases with either a maternal or paternal origin of the extra element and differential imprinting appeared not to be a factor.

**Keywords:** OMIM 601803, Pallister-Killian syndrome, Somatic mosaicism, Mosaic tetrasomy 12p, Isochromosome 12p, Parental origin, Small supernumerary marker chromosome

## Background

Pallister-Killian syndrome (PKS) was first described an adult phenotype by Pallister in 1977 and independently a childhood phenotype by Killian and Teschler-Nicola in 1981 [1, 2]. In both instances, cytogenetic examinations of blood cells did not reveal any abnormality. Later observations by Schinzel in 1991 confirmed a distinct phenotype. In 1987, PKS was shown to be caused by somatic mosaicism of an extra chromosome, which was not primarily not detected since mosaicism was limited to fibroblasts and not present in lymphocytes [3, 4]. Using banded karyotypes, and after several mis-interpretations, the extra element was identified as an isochromosome 12p.

The clinical phenotype of PKS is quite homogeneous for the dysmorphic pattern, but highly variable for developmental delay, congenital malformations, and survival. There is a wide range of congenital malformations that occur rarely including anal atresia/stenosis and atlanto-occipital fusion. Areas of hyper- or hypo-pigmentation are often found and reflect the mosaic pattern of the skin, with different proportions of hyperdiploid cells [5].

* Correspondence: bkaraman@istanbul.edu.tr
[1]Department of Medical Genetics, Istanbul Medical Faculty, Istanbul University, Millet cad.34039 Capa, İstanbul, Turkey
Full list of author information is available at the end of the article

The developmental delay in patients with PKS is quite variable, and although most reported patients with PKS have severe to profound mental retardation, milder phenotypes have also been reported [6–13]. A large number of patients with i(12p) were reported in the literature, and also their clinical and cytogenetic information routinely posted in a database (http://ssmc-tl.com/sSMC.html http://ssmc-tl.com/chromosome-12.html http://ssmc-tl.com/chromosome-12.html#iso) [14].

Here, we report the cytogenetic, and molecular cytogenetic findings in 15 cases with PKS phenotype and parental origin analysis results of 7 cases with i(12p) chromosome. To our knowledge, this series is the first series from Turkey and the largest series of PKS patients with parental origin study from a single center.

## Methods

All cases were evaluated at Medical Genetics Department outpatients' clinics, Istanbul Medical Faculty, Istanbul University. Cytogenetic and molecular cytogenetic analyses were performed in the laboratory of the department. Before the implementation of the FISH technique, in presence of the clinical features of PKS, cytogenetic studies were performed from cultured fibroblasts from skin biopsies in parallel to the peripheral lymphocyte cultures. Following the introduction of the interphase FISH (I-FISH) study using chromosome 12 centromeric probe (D12Z3, Aquarius®, Cytocell Cambridge, UK), I-FISH test on mucosal cells from buccal smear were applied- in parallel to the lymphocyte cultures (Fig. 1).

De novo supernumerary i(12p) was further confirmed by FISH using chromosome 12 specific wcp, centromeric and subtelomeric probes.

To determine the parental origin and formation mechanism, 7 cases with i(12p) were investigated with gel-electrophoresis technique using 15 microsatellite markers on 12p (D12S352, D12S99, D12S77, D12S269, D12S320, D12S364, D12S1303, D12S373, D12S301, D12S1669, D12S1650, D12S799, D12S823, D12S1053, D12S345,) and 2 markers on 12q (D12S72, D12S43).

## Results

### Clinical findings

Fifteen cases were cytogenetically evaluated due to their phenotypic features (Fig. 2).

The mean age at the time of diagnosis was about 2.5 years of age (ranging between one day-7 years 10/12).

Karyotypes of fibroblast cultures in 15 cases revealed the supernumerary mosaic i(12p), while cultured peripheral blood lymphocytes of those cases were normal. The 12 p tetrasomic metaphases were observed 10% to 100% of cells analyzed in fibroblasts. Although the level of +i(12p) in cultured fibroblasts was low (11%), I-FISH indicated higher level of i(12p) (40%) in the mucosal cells in one case. In one stillborn, following the clinical diagnosis of PKS, skin and buccal smear samples were taken, and a supernumerary i(12p) was present in all metaphases of cultured fibroblasts, while I-FISH study showed mosaicism of 60% in mucosal cells (Table 1).

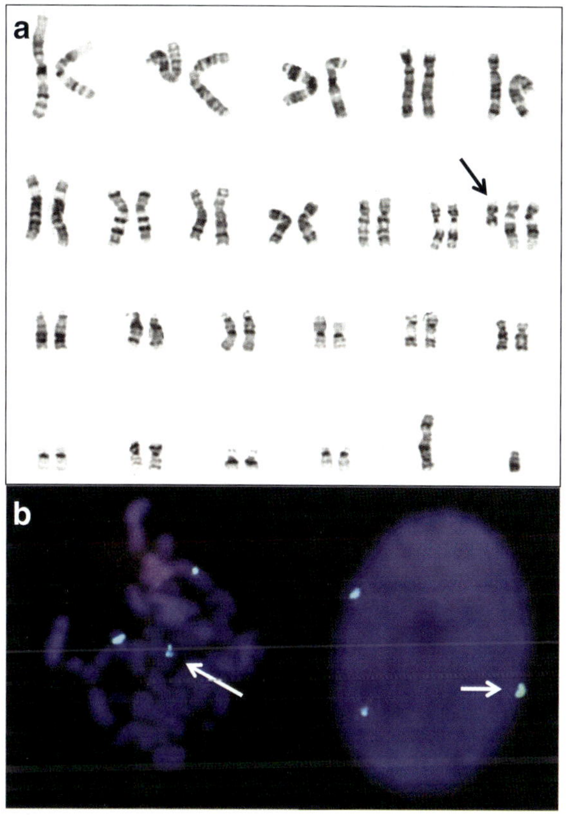


**Fig. 1 a** G-banding karyotype of the fibroblasts. The arrow shows the isochromosome 12p. **b** FISH analysis using 12 centromere specific D12Z3 probe (Aquarius®, Cytocell Cambridge, UK) in the fibroblasts. The white arrow shows a supernumerary chromosome in the metaphase and interphase

The clinical findings of the cases with tetrasomy 12p are summarized in Table 2. Almost all cases with tetrasomy 12p had coarse facial features, bitemporal alopecia, anteverted nostrils and everted lower lip, hypertelorism, epicanthus, long philtrum and hypo/hyperpigmented skin changes. Intellectual disability was observed in all patients over 8 months of age except one case with near normal intelligence at adult age (case 7), and three newborns.

Parental origin was determined by STR analysis as maternal in 6 cases (85.7%), paternal in one case (14.22%).

## Discussion

Classical PKS is a rare condition caused by mosaic tetrasomy 12p presenting with an additional isochromosome of 12p, which is usually not present in blood lymphocyte cultures, but can be shown in skin

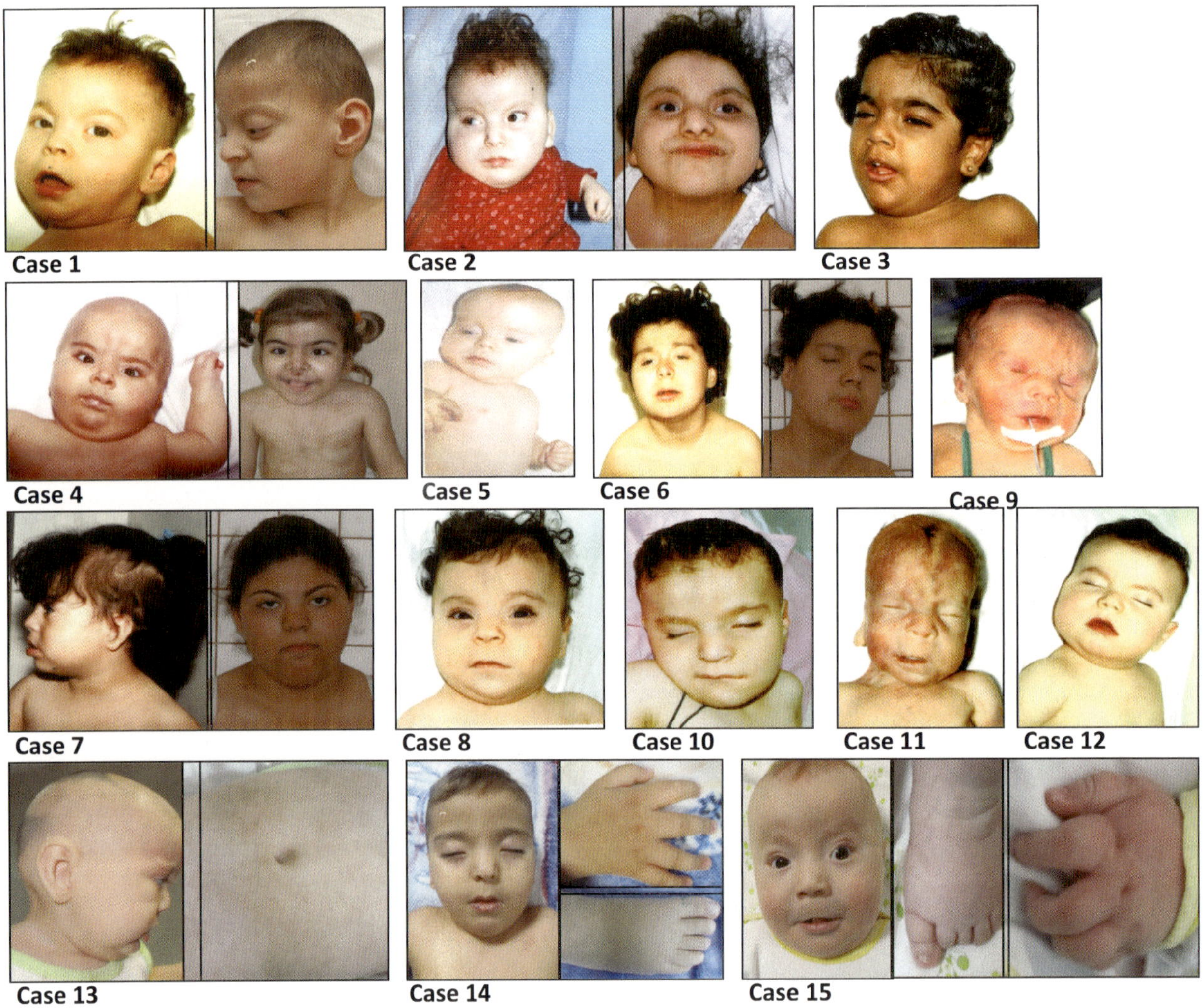


**Fig. 2** Facial appearance of the patients. Alopecia/Sparse temporal hair, hypo- or hyper pigmented areas and other stigmata such as epicanthic folds and slightly low-set ears, prominent forehead, hypertelorism, up- slanting palpebral fissures, anteverted nostrils, long philtrum, everted lower lip, short neck and short hands and toes

fibroblasts [3, 4] and other tissues such as buccal smears, chorionic villi and amniocytes. The clinical phenotype is characterized by a pattern of dysmorphic features, hypo- or hyperpigmentation areas of the skin, progressive coarsening of the face with advancing age and moderate to severe- profound intellectual disability accompanied with different types of seizures. Congenital malformations have been found in a minority of live births.

The dysmorphic pattern is age-dependent and includes brachycephaly, temporal balding during the first years of life, a short nose with flat bridge and anteverted nostrils giving the false impression of hypertelorism, microstomia, progressive macroglossia, prominent everted lower lip, small mandible and short neck. Supernumerary nipples are frequent as are hypoplastic male external genitalia. Hands and fingers, feet and toes are proportionately small. Pigmentation anomalies of the skin are due to mosaicism with different expression of pigmentation genes with predominance of one or the other cell line. This is well known for mosaicism in general [14–23].

Although there are limited number of reports on the mosaicism of the isochromosome in peripheral blood cells in PKS patients by I-FISH, microarray studies, and karyotype analysis [24–27]. Studies have shown that phytohaemagglutinin used in lymphocyte cultures promotes the growth of the normal cells, which leads to under- representation or disappearing of the abnormal cells [28–31]. Furthermore tissues with a shorter turnover period seem to lose the cells with additional chromosomes, either due to longer duration of cell division, the instability of (submicroscopically) dicentric chromosomes or the abnormal cell line going through apoptosis or necrosis at a higher rate than the normal cells [32].

**Table 1** Karyotypes and FISH findings in different tissues

| Case no | Karyotypes on cultured lymphocytes | Karyotype on fibroblast | % | I-FISH results on buccal swap sample | % | Parental origin |
|---|---|---|---|---|---|---|
| 1 | 46,XY | mos 46,XY/47,XY,+i(12)(p10)[33/17] | 34 | – | | P |
| 2 | 46,XX | mos 46,XX/47,XX,+i(12)(p10)[18/2] | 10 | – | | M |
| 3 | 46,XX | mos 46,XX/47,XX,+i(12)(p10)[100/11] | 9.9 | .ish (D12Z2x2/D12Z2x3)[50/13] | 20.6 | |
| 4 | 46,XX | mos 46,XX/47,XX,+i(12)(p10)[28/12] | 30 | – | | |
| 5 | 46,XY | mos 46,XY/47,XY,+i(12)(p10)[65/35] | 35 | – | | M |
| 6 | 46,XX | mos 46,XX/47,XX,+i(12)(p10)[24/9] | 27.3 | – | | M |
| 7 | 46,XX | mos 46,XX/47,XX,+i(12)(p10)[15/5] | 25 | – | | M |
| 8 | 46,XX | mos 46,XX/47,XX,+i(12)(p10)[31/4] | 11.4 | .ish (D12Z2x2/D12Z2x3)[64/41] | 39 | |
| 9 | 46,XY | mos 46,XY/47,XY,+i(12)(p10)[21/9] | 30 | .ish (D12Z2x2/D12Z2x3)[5/13] | 72 | |
| 10 | 46,XY | mos 46,XY/47,XY,+i(12)(p10)[20/20] | 50 | .ish (D12Z2x2/D12Z2x3)[25/30] | 54.5 | |
| 11 | – | 47,XY,+i(12)(p10) | 100 | .ish (D12Z2x2/D12Z2x3)[40/60] | 60 | M |
| 12 | 46,XY | mos 46,XY/47,XY,+i(12)(p10)[25/5] | 16.6 | .ish (D12Z2x2/D12Z2x3)[7/25] | 78.1 | M |
| 13 | 47,XY,+mar.ish(14/22)(q10;q10)mat | 48,XY,+mar.ish(14/22)(q10;q10) mat, +i(12(p10) | 100 | – | | |
| 14 | – | mos 46,XY/47,XY,+i(12)(p10)[45/40] | 47 | .ish (D12Z2x2/D12Z2x3)[71/68] (F)<br>.ish (D12Z2x2/D12Z2x3)[50/53] (BS) | 49<br>51.4 | |
| 15 | 46,XY | – | | mos.ish (D12Z2x2/D12Z2x3)[180/20] | 10 | |

*F* Fibroblast, *BS* Buccal swap, *M* Maternal, *P* Paternal

At present I-FISH using chromosome 12 centromeric probes on buccal mucosa cells is a very useful, non-invasive, reliable, rapid and cost-effective test for the definite diagnosis [33, 34]. It is suggested that all live born tetrasomy 12 cases are mosaic, even it could not be shown in one tissue. Therefore, it is helpful to investigate different tissues by different techniques to enlighten the mosaicism like in our case 11 (Table 2). However, in all similar cases from the literature only one or at most two different tissues had been analysed and thus mosaicism in non-examined tissues or even in a second skin biopsy from another area of the body was not excluded. In a few cases with clinical diagnosis of PKS normal karyotype both in blood and fibroblast cultures derived from one or two skin biopsies mosaicism could not be excluded.

#### Early cytogenetic misinterpretations

Prior to and during the early banding era of cytogenetics, several patients were published as tetrasomy 21 (an aberration which seems incompatible with life) [35–39] and the extra chromosome was also classified as chromosome 12 with deletion of about ¾ of the long arm [40].

#### Mechanism (s) of formation of the additional i(12p)

Molecular marker analysis favored the following steps: Initial maternal meiosis II nondisjunction (evidenced by centromere-near homozygosity of the maternal markers) leading to trisomy 12. Trisomy 12 zygotes will spontaneously abort; the few exceptions are those conceptuses in which a secondary structural aberration, isochromosome formation, results in loss of the acentric long arms and subsequent formation of an +i(12p) [41–45]. Ravel et al. published a mosaic case with trisomy 12 and + i(12p) diagnosed prenatally and proposed a formation mechanism for +i12p [46]. Pauli et al. discussed the mechanisms of formation based on the data of their monozygotic twins and suggested that prezygotic or postzygotic error (both before the twinning event) in the inner cell mass may have happened. [47].

The increased mean maternal age at conception suggests this mechanism [43]. In a few cases paternal origin of the i(12p) could be demonstrated [25, 42, 48], obviously caused by a different cascade of events. To the best of our knowledge, there seems to be no difference in phenotype between the cases of maternal versus paternal origin of the extra element and thus no effect of differential imprinting [6, 10].

#### Karyotype-phenotype correlation

It has been suggested that no correlation could be established between the proportion of tetrasomic cells and the severity of clinical presentation [5]. Our observation supports this suggestion, because of the technical limitations, the severity of the phenotype was independent from the degree of mosaicism in karyotyping. However, fibroblast cultures were analyzed from only one biopsy in all cases. As mentioned above, the incidence of hyperdiploid cells may grossly vary among

**Table 2** Clinical finding of Pallister Killian patients

| Case No | 1 | 2 | 3 | 4 | 5 | 6 | 7 | 8 | 9 | 10 | 11 | 12 | 13 | 14 | 15 |
|---|---|---|---|---|---|---|---|---|---|---|---|---|---|---|---|
| Sex | m | f | f | f | m | f | f | f | m | m | m | m | m | m | m |
| Age at diagnosis (days/months (m)/year) | $7^{7/12}$ | $10^{8/12}$ | $6^{8/12}$ | $12^{10/12}$ | 9 m | $7^{1/12}$ | $2^{11/12}$ | 8 m | 1 day | $5^{10/12}$ | 22 days | 11 m | 1 day | 1 | $1^{1/12}$ |
| Gestation age at birth | 'term' | 38 | 37 | 40 | 39 | 'term' | 'term' | 36 | 33 | 41 | 37 | 'term' | 40 | 32 | 38 |
| Maternal/paternal age at conception | 18/25 | 32/33 | 22/22 | 23/28 | 28/29 | 38/38 | 19/25 | 35/42 | 31/31 | 21/23 | 33/31 | 28/29 | 39/33 | 32/32 | 33/41 |
| Weight/length at birth | 2100/? | 3500/47 | 3500/50 | 2600/45 | 3450/54 | 4250/? | 3250/? | 2250/45 | 2500/44 | 4750/? | 2950/49 | 3800/ | 3200/53 | 2800/? | 3830/53 |
| Intellectual disability | + | + | + | + | + | + | -(near norma) | + | ? | + | ? | + | ? | + | + |
| Seizures | – | – | + | + | – | – | – | – | – | – | – | – | – | + | + |
| Hypotonia | + | + | + | – | + | + | – | + | – | – | – | – | + | + | + |
| Prominent forehead | + | + | – | + | + | + | + | + | – | – | – | + | + | + | + |
| Bitemporal alopecia/sparse temporal hair | + | + | + | + | + | + | + | + | + | + | + | + | + | + | + |
| Coarse facial features | + | + | + | + | + | + | + | + | + | + | + | + | + | + | + |
| Flat occiput | + | – | – | – | – | – | – | – | – | – | – | – | – | + | – |
| Hypertelorism | + | + | borderline | + | + | + | – | + | – | – | + | – | + | + | + |
| Epicanthus | – | – | – | – | – | – | – | – | – | – | – | – | + | + | – |
| Dysmorphic ears | + | + | – | – | + | + | – | + | + | + | + | + | + | + | + |
| Short nose | – | – | + | – | + | – | + | + | + | + | + | + | + | + | + |
| Anteverted nostrils | + | – | + | + | + | + | + | + | + | + | + | + | + | + | + |
| Long philtrum | + | – | – | + | + | – | + | + | + | + | + | + | + | + | + |
| Macroglossia | – | – | – | – | – | – | – | + | – | – | – | – | – | + | |
| Micrognathia | – | – | – | – | + | – | – | + | – | – | – | + | + | + | – |
| Everted lower lip | + | + | + | + | + | + | + | + | + | + | + | + | + | + | + |
| Short neck | – | + | + | + | + | – | + | – | + | + | – | – | + | + | + |
| Accessory nipples | – | – | – | + | – | – | – | + | – | – | – | – | – | – | – |
| Hypo/hyperpigmented areas of skin | +/+ | +/+ | +/+ | +/+ | +/+ | +/+ | +/+ | +/+ | –/– | +/+ | –/– | +/+ | +/+ | +/+ | –/– |
| Short hands and feet | + | + | – | + | + | – | + | + | – | + | – | + | – | + | + |
| CHD | – | – | – | PDA,PFO,VSD | – | – | – | – | PDA | – | PFO, PDA | – | | ASD | – |

*Abbr*: *CHD* congenital heart defect, *PDA* patent ductus arteriosus, *PF O* patent foramen ovale, *VSD* ventricular septal defect, *ASD* atrial septal defect

fibroblast cultures, derived from different areas of pigmentation state even in the same individual [6, 10, 49]. Moreover, tissues whose mosaic constitution is the most important for the degree of developmental delay, i.e. CNS cells, cannot be investigated.

To date a few cases have been reported with only mild psychomotor delay and minor facial anomalies [49]. In our series, only one patient (case 7) presented with minor facial manifestations and near normal intelligence and after 20 years of follow up she has married and after an uneventful pregnancy had a normal baby.

The mechanism of the formation of isochromosomes is still not fully clear. Various mechanisms during prezygotic mitosis or meiosis or even postzygotic mitosis have been proposed. Hunter et al. proposed five different mechanisms for the formation of i(12p) and the issue was summarized by Struthers et al. [45, 50].

Our study was in agreement with the literature data on predominance of maternal inheritance in + i(12p) cases [42, 45, 46, 48, 51, 52].

It has been reported that the risk for +i(12p) increases with advanced maternal age [53–55]. The mean maternal age was 28.6 years (range: 18–39) in our cohort, however maternal age was over 33 for all the cases with maternal origin. Our findings are in agreement with the hypothesis that the increase in risk of having +i(12p) conceptus correlates with advanced maternal age.

## Conclusion

Phenotypic and cytogenetic variability of PKS may be challenging for the differential diagnosis. Karyotyping on lymphocytes usually do not reveal the supernumerary i(12p). Therefore, we suggest that in cases with suspicion of clinical diagnosis of PKS, when pigmentation anomalies of the skin and temporal balding is noted as accompanying features, I-FISH on buccal mucosa cells and karyotyping from peripheral lymphocytes should be performed as a first tier test.

#### Abbreviations

CNS: Central Nervous System; FISH: Florescence In Situ Hybridization; I-FISH: Interphase FISH; PKS: Pallister-Killian syndrome; STR: Short Tandem Repeats

#### Acknowledgments

The authors cordially thank to emeritus Prof. Albert Schinzel for his critical review of the manuscript. We share our gratitude to the families for their cooperation which made this work possible.

#### Authors' contributions

BK, HK, AG, ZOU, GT, UA, and SB wrote the manuscript. All authors read and approved the final manuscript.

#### Competing interests

The authors declare that they have no competing interests.

#### Author details

[1]Department of Medical Genetics, Istanbul Medical Faculty, Istanbul University, Millet cad.34039 Capa, İstanbul, Turkey. [2]Medical Genetics Department & Genetic Diagnosis Center, Koç University School of Medicine, 34010 İstanbul, Turkey.

#### References

1. Pallister PD, et al. The pallister mosaic syndrome. Birth Defects Orig Artic Ser. 1977;13(3B):103–10.
2. Teschler-Nicola M, Killian W. Case report 72: mental retardation, unusual facial appearance, abnormal hair. Synd Ident. 1981;7(1):6–7.
3. Peltomäki P, et al. Pallister-Killian syndrome: cytogenetic and molecular studies. Clin Genet. 1987;31(6):399–405.
4. Warburton D, Anyane-Yeboa K, Francke U. Mosaic tetrasomy 12p: four new cases, and confirmation of the chromosomal origin of the supernumerary chromosome in one of the original Pallister-mosaic syndrome cases. Am J Med Genet. 1987;27(2):275–83.
5. Schinzel A. Tetrasomy 12p (Pallister-Killian syndrome). J Med Genet. 1991; 28(2):122–5.
6. Bielanska MM, Khalifa MM, Duncan AM. Pallister-Killian syndrome: a mild case diagnosed by fluorescence in situ hybridization. Review of the literature and expansion of the phenotype. Am J Med Genet. 1996; 65(2):104–8.
7. Blyth M, et al. Pallister Killian syndrome: a study of 22 British patients. J Med Genet. 2015;52(7):454–64.
8. Filloux FM, et al. Occurrence and clinical features of epileptic and non-epileptic paroxysmal events in five children with Pallister-Killian syndrome. Eur J Med Genet. 2012;55(5):367–73.
9. Kostanecka A, et al. Developmental and behavioral characteristics of individuals with Pallister-Killian syndrome. Am J Med Genet A. 2012; 158A(12):3018–25.
10. Schaefer GB, et al. Clinical variability of tetrasomy 12p. Clin Genet. 1997; 51(2):102–8.
11. Vogel I, et al. Pallister-Killian syndrome in a girl with mild developmental delay and mosaicism for hexasomy 12p. Am J Med Genet A. 2009; 149A(3):510–4.
12. Izumi K, Krantz ID. Pallister-Killian syndrome. Am J Med Genet C Semin Med Genet. 2014;166C(4):406–13.
13. Wilkens A, et al. Novel clinical manifestations in Pallister-Killian syndrome: comprehensive evaluation of 59 affected individuals and review of previously reported cases. Am J Med Genet A. 2012;158A(12):3002–17.
14. Liehr, T., Small supernumerary marker chromosomes. 2018. http://ssmc-tl.com/sSMC.html, http://ssmc-tl.com/chromosome-12.html, http://ssmc-tl.com/chromosome-12.html#iso [accessed 08/07/2018]. 2018.
15. Chitayat D, Friedman JM, Johnston MM. Hypomelanosis of Ito--a nonspecific marker of somatic mosaicism: report of case with trisomy 18 mosaicism. Am J Med Genet. 1990;35(3):422–4.
16. Donnai D, Read AP. Hypomelanosis of Ito. Lancet. 1992;339(8796):819–20.
17. Donnai D, et al. Hypomelanosis of Ito: a manifestation of mosaicism or chimerism. J Med Genet. 1988;25(12):809–18.
18. Happle R. Genetic interpretation of linear skin abnormalities. Hautarzt. 1978; 29(7):357–63.
19. Harrod MJ, Howard-Peebles PN, Friedman JM. Tetrasomy 12p: differential degree of mosaicism in fibroblasts from normal and abnormally pigmented skin. Proc Greenwood Genet Center. 1986;6:107.
20. Liehr T, et al. Clinical impact of somatic mosaicism in cases with small supernumerary marker chromosomes. Cytogenet Genome Res. 2013; 139(3):158–63.
21. Read AP, Donnai D. Association of pigmentary anomalies with chromosomal and genetic mosaicism and chimerism. Am J Hum Genet. 1990;47(1):166–8.
22. Thomas IT, et al. Association of pigmentary anomalies with chromosomal and genetic mosaicism and chimerism. Am J Hum Genet. 1989;45(2): 193–205.
23. Ward BE, Hayden MW, Robinson A. Isochromosome 12p mosaicism (Pallister-Killian syndrome): newborn diagnosis by direct bone marrow analysis. Am J Med Genet. 1988;31(4):835–9.

24. Cobben JM, Engelen M, Polstra A. Array CGH on unstimulated blood does not detect all cases of Pallister-Killian syndrome: buccal smear analysis should remain the diagnostic procedure of first choice. Am J Med Genet A. 2013;161A(6):1517–9.
25. Conlin LK, et al. Utility of SNP arrays in detecting, quantifying, and determining meiotic origin of tetrasomy 12p in blood from individuals with Pallister-Killian syndrome. Am J Med Genet A. 2012;158A(12):3046–53.
26. Harrison V, et al. Diagnosis of Pallister-Killian syndrome by array comparative genome hybridization from a spleen sample. Clin Dysmorphol. 2011;20(1):58–60.
27. Lloveras E, et al. Supernumerary ring chromosome: an etiology for Pallister-Killian syndrome? Fetal Diagn Ther. 2013;34(3):172–5.
28. Kayser M, et al. Blaschkolinear skin pigmentary variation due to trisomy 7 mosaicism. Am J Med Genet. 2000;95(3):281–4.
29. Kulharya AS, Lovell CM, Flannery DB. Unusual mosaic karyotype resulting from adjacent 1 segregation of t(11;22): importance of performing skin fibroblast karyotype in patients with unexplained multiple congenital anomalies. Am J Med Genet. 2002;113(4):367–70.
30. Lessick ML, Szego K, Wong PW. Trisomy 22 mosaicism with normal blood chromosomes. Case report with literature review. Clin Pediatr (Phila). 1988; 27(9):451–4.
31. Pagon RA, et al. Abnormal skin fibroblast cytogenetics in four dysmorphic patients with normal lymphocyte chromosomes. Am J Hum Genet. 1979; 31(1):54–61.
32. Tang W, Wenger SL. Cell death as a possible mechanism for tissue limited mosaicism in Pallister-Killian syndrome. J Assoc Genet Technol. 2005;31(4):168–9.
33. Manasse BF, et al. The Pallister-Killian syndrome is reliably diagnosed by FISH on buccal mucosa. Clin Dysmorphol. 2000;9(3):163–5.
34. Ohashi H, Ishikiriyama S, Fukushima Y. New diagnostic method for Pallister-Killian syndrome: detection of i(12p) in interphase nuclei of buccal mucosa by fluorescence in situ hybridization. Am J Med Genet. 1993;45(1):123–8.
35. Chiesa J, et al. Pallister-Killian syndrome [i(12p)]: first pre-natal diagnosis using cordocentesis in the second trimester confirmed by in situ hybridization. Clin Genet. 1998;54(4):294–302.
36. Fryns JP, et al. Mosaic tetrasomy 21 in severe mental handicap. Eur J Pediatr. 1982;139(1):87–9.
37. Gilgenkrantz S, et al. Mosaic tetrasomy 12p. Clin Genet. 1985;28(6):495–502.
38. Kunz J, et al. Tetrasomy 12p (Pallister-Killian syndrome): difficulties in prenatal diagnosis. Arch Gynecol Obstet. 2009;280(6):1049–53.
39. Park IY, et al. Prenatal diagnosis of Pallister-Killian syndrome associated with pulmonary stenosis and right ventricular dilatation. Korean J Lab Med. 2009; 29(4):366–70.
40. Karki CB, Walters RM. Trisomy 12p mosaicism syndrome. J Ment Defic Res. 1990;34(Pt 1):75–80.
41. Bugge M, et al. Tetrasomy 18p de novo: parental origin and different mechanisms of formation. Eur J Hum Genet. 1996;4(3):160–7.
42. Cormier-Daire V, et al. Prezygotic origin of the isochromosome 12p in Pallister-Killian syndrome. Am J Med Genet. 1997;69(2):166–8.
43. Kotzot D, et al. Isochromosome 18p results from maternal meiosis II nondisjunction. Eur J Hum Genet. 1996;4(3):168–74.
44. Shen JD, et al. Pallister-Killian syndrome: meiosis II non-disjunction may be the first step in the formation of isochromosome 12p. Chin Med J. 2010; 123(23):3482–5.
45. Struthers JL, Cuthbert CD, Khalifa MM. Parental origin of the isochromosome 12p in Pallister-Killian syndrome: molecular analysis of one patient and review of the reported cases. Am J Med Genet. 1999;84(2):111–5.
46. de Ravel TJ, et al. Post-zygotic origin of isochromosome 12p. Prenat Diagn. 2004;24(12):984–8.
47. Pauli S, et al. Discordant phenotype in monozygotic twins with mosaic trisomy 12p in lymphocytes. Eur J Med Genet. 2012;55(8–9):480–4.
48. Turleau C, et al. Parental origin and mechanisms of formation of three cases of 12p tetrasomy. Clin Genet. 1996;50(1):41–6.
49. Genevieve D, et al. Mild phenotype in a 15-year-old boy with Pallister-Killian syndrome. Am J Med Genet A. 2003;116A(1):90–3.
50. Hunter AG, Clifford B, Cox DM. The characteristic physiognomy and tissue specific karyotype distribution in the Pallister-Killian syndrome. Clin Genet. 1985;28(1):47–53.
51. Los FJ, et al. Prenatal diagnosis of mosaic tetrasomy 12p/trisomy 12p by fluorescent in situ hybridization in amniotic fluid cells: a case report of Pallister-Killian syndrome. Prenat Diagn. 1995;15(12):1155–9.
52. Schubert R, et al. Report of two new cases of Pallister-Killian syndrome confirmed by FISH: tissue-specific mosaicism and loss of i(12p) by in vitro selection. Am J Med Genet. 1997;72(1):106–10.
53. Rivera H, Rivas F, Cantu JM. On the origin of extra isochromosomes. Clin Genet. 1986;29(6):540–1.
54. Van Dyke DL, Babu VR, Weiss L. Parental age, and how extra isochromosomes (secondary trisomy) arise. Clin Genet. 1987;32(1):75–9.
55. Wenger SL, Boone LY, Steele MW. Mosaicism in Pallister i(12p) syndrome. Am J Med Genet. 1990;35(4):523–5.

3

# An improved method for inducing prometaphase chromosomes in plants

Agus Budi Setiawan[1], Chee How Teo[2], Shinji Kikuchi[1], Hidenori Sassa[1] and Takato Koba[1*]

**Abstract**

**Background:** Detailed karyotyping using metaphase chromosomes in melon (*Cucumis melo* L.) remains a challenge because of their small chromosome sizes and poor stainability. Prometaphase chromosomes, which are two times longer and loosely condensed, provide a significantly better resolution for fluorescence in situ hybridization (FISH) than metaphase chromosomes. However, suitable method for acquiring prometaphase chromosomes in melon have been poorly investigated.

**Results:** In this study, a modified Carnoy's solution II (MC II) [6:3:1 (*v/v*) ethanol: acetic acid: chloroform] was used as a pretreatment solution to obtain prometaphase chromosomes. We demonstrated that the prometaphase chromosomes obtained using the MC II method are excellent for karyotyping and FISH analysis. We also observed that a combination of MC II and the modified air dry (ADI) method provides a satisfactory meiotic pachytene chromosome preparation with reduced cytoplasmic background and clear chromatin spreads. Moreover, we demonstrated that pachytene and prometaphase chromosomes of melon and *Abelia* × *grandiflora* generate significantly better FISH images when prepared using the method described. We confirmed, for the first time, that *Abelia* × *grandiflora* has pairs of both strong and weak 45S ribosomal DNA signals on the short arms of their metaphase chromosomes.

**Conclusion:** The MC II and ADI method are simple and effective for acquiring prometaphase and pachytene chromosomes with reduced cytoplasm background in plants. Our methods provide high-resolution FISH images that can help accelerate molecular cytogenetic research in plants.

**Keywords:** Prometaphase, Pachytene, Chloroform, FISH, *Cucumis melo*, *Abelia* × *grandiflora*

## Background

Chromosome preparation is crucial for cytogenetic studies. Fluorescence in situ hybridization (FISH), a molecular cytogenetic technique, requires properly dispersed metaphase or prometaphase chromosomes for its application. Melon (*Cucumis melo* L.) belongs to the *Cucurbitaceae* family and is a diploid species having $2n = 2x = 24$ chromosomes [1]. Detailed karyotype analysis in the *Cucumis* genus, particularly in melon, has been difficult to achieve because of their small chromosome sizes and poor stainability [2, 3]. In addition, the identification of secondary constrictions and the procurement of more detailed chromatin images are also difficult, even when using properly dispersed metaphase chromosomes, because of their highly condensed status. For these reasons, we propose the use of prometaphase chromosomes for FISH analyses in melon. Prometaphase chromosomes are effective and preferable for cytogenetic analyses and identification of individual chromosomes because the chromosomes are easily distinguishable due to the uneven condensation of chromatin fibers along chromosomes [4]. FISH using prometaphase chromosomes has been successfully applied in studies involving *Brassica* [5], rice [6–8], *Catharanthus roseus* [9], and *Lablab purpureus* [10]. However, suitable methods to induce prometaphase chromosomes in other plants have been poorly investigated.

Prometaphase chromosomes in *Brassica* [5] and rice [7] have been successfully induced using ethanol and acetic acid (3:1) without pretreatment. Other methods to accumulate metaphase and prometaphase chromosomes, such as with ice water (ice) treatment for 24 h [11] or 0. 002 M 8-hydroxyquinoline (8-Hq) [12, 13] have also

* Correspondence: koba@faculty.chiba-u.jp
[1]Laboratory of Genetics and Plant Breeding, Graduate School of Horticulture, Chiba University, Matsudo, Chiba 271-8510, Japan
Full list of author information is available at the end of the article

been reported. Although FISH studies have also been reported in melon [12–15], most of them used metaphase chromosomes, which are shorter and more compact than prometaphase chromosomes.

Modified Carnoy's solution II (MC II) made up of ethanol: acetic acid: chloroform (6:3:1) has been previously used to produce super-stretched pachytene chromosomes in maize [16]. However, its efficiency in inducing prometaphase chromosomes in mitotic cells in other plant species has not yet been reported. Here, using melon, we compared the effectiveness of MC II with other methods including Carnoy's solution (ethanol: acetic acid (3:1)), 24-h ice water treatment and 0.002 M 8-Hq for the induction of properly dispersed prometaphase and metaphase chromosomes. We demonstrated that MC II can be used for FISH analysis with enhanced chromosome distribution in melon. Furthermore, we provide a protocol for obtaining pachytene chromosomes from melon and *Abelia* × *grandiflora* flower buds without the need to squash the slides. This is achieved by a combination of MC II and the modified air dry (ADI) methods.

## Methods

### Plant materials

*Cucumis melo* L. subsp. *melo* var. cantalupo Ser. cultivar 'Baladewa' (local name, Blewah), a commercial melon in Indonesia, was used in this study for FISH analyses. *Abelia* × *grandiflora*, a hybrid plant between *Abelia chinensis* and *Abelia uniflora*, was also used to test the effectiveness of MC II and ADI methods in obtaining pachytene chromosomes. The plant was grown and maintained at the Graduate School of Horticulture, Chiba University, Matsudo, Japan.

### Experimental design

The present experiment was performed using a completely randomized design (CRD) with four treatments as follows: (1) Melon root tips from germinated seeds were treated with the MC II method [16]. In this method, the root tips were pretreated with freshly prepared 6:3:1 (v/v) ethanol: acetic acid: chloroform for 3–4 h at room temperature (RT), and then fixed in 3:1 (v/v) ethanol: acetic acid solution (C3:1) for 5 days at 4 ° C. (2) Root tips were pre-treated with 0.002 M 8-Hq for 4 h at RT and then fixed in C3:1 (v/v) for 5 days at 4 °C. (3) Root tips were pretreated with Ice for 24 h and then fixed in C3:1 for 5 days at 4 °C. (4) Root tips were directly fixed in C3:1 for 5 days at 4 °C. Each treatment was replicated three times using 10 root tips per replication. Three slides of each replication from each treatment were chosen for chromosome data analysis.

### Mitotic chromosome preparations

The seeds were germinated on moistened filter paper kept in petri dishes in a growth chamber at 25 °C. The main root tips (0.5–1 cm) were cut, and the germinated seeds were transplanted into potting trays maintained in a greenhouse. Additional root tips could be harvested from the transplanted melon plants. The root tips of each treatment were washed in 1 ml of enzyme buffer (40 ml of 100 mM citric acid + 60 ml of 100 mM sodium citrate, pH 4.8) for 10 min [11]. The meristematic root tips were cut and macerated in 15 μl of enzyme mixture containing 4% Cellulose Onozuka RS (Yakult), 2% Pectinase (Sigma), and 1% Pectolyase Y-23 (Kyowa Chemical, Osaka, Japan) at 37 °C for 1 h. The enzyme mixture was cleaned off from the meristematic root tips using Kimwipe tissues. Then, 10 μl of 60% acetic acid was added onto the root tips and left until the root tips became transparent or pale, and an 18 × 18 mm cover slip was placed over the slide. The slides were tapped using probe needles to spread the cells, squashed, and flame-dried over an alcohol flame for a few seconds. Finally, the slides were kept at − 81 °C for 1–2 days, and the cover slips were removed before FISH.

### Meiotic chromosome preparations

We selected MC II for pachytene chromosome preparation as we found it to be preferable for inducing prometaphase and metaphase in melon cells when combined together with the ADI method [17]. The melon and *Abelia* × *grandiflora* flower buds were pretreated with 6:3:1 (v/v) ethanol: acetic acid: chloroform for 3–4 h at RT and fixed in C3:1 for 5 days at 4 °C. The flower buds were washed in 1 ml of enzyme buffer (40 ml of 100 mM citric acid + 60 ml of 100 mM sodium citrate, pH 4.8) for 10 min. The anthers were dissected using the forceps under a stereomicroscope and macerated in 15 μl of the enzyme mixture described above at 37 °C for 1 h. The enzyme mixture surrounding the meristematic anthers was cleaned using Kimwipe tissues. The ADI method consisted of three main solutions, namely, fixative I [60% of 1:1 (*v*/v) acetic acid:ethanol in distilled water; 3 ml of glacial acetic acid + 3 ml ethanol (> 99.5%) + 4 ml distilled water], fixative II [4 ml absolute 1: 1 (v/v) acetic acid: ethanol; 2 ml glacial acetic acid + 2 ml ethanol (> 99.5%)], and fixative III (2 ml glacial acetic acid). Fixatives I and II were freshly prepared before use; Fixative I should not be stored overnight because it degrades rapidly into ethyl acetate, which is detrimental to cells [17]. Fixative I was applied (5 μl) to the anthers, and the anthers were rapidly macerated using forceps to spread the pollen mother cells (PMCs). Fixative I was applied once again (5 μl), and most of it spread out to the edge of the slide. After 1–2 min, fixative I had evaporated. To avoid drying of the slide, 5 μl of fixative II was quickly applied and left to spread to the edge of the slide. Finally, 5 μl of fixative III was applied, and the slide was air dried. The excess fixative on the edge of the slide was removed using filter paper. The slides can be stored in a slide box at RT up to 6 months without noticeable degradation.

#### Probe preparations

Wheat 45S ribosomal DNA (rDNA; pTa71) and melon centromere satellite DNA (Cmcent) were used as the probes [18, 19]. The Cmcent probe was labeled with the dig-nick translation mix (Roche) or biotin-nick translation mix (Roche), while the 45S rDNA probe was labeled with the dig-nick translation mix (Roche).

#### FISH analysis

Slides containing melon chromosomes were pretreated with 200 μl RNase A solution per slide [2 μl of 10 mg/ml RNase A + 20 μl of 20× saline sodium citrate (SSC) + 178 μl of sterile distilled water (SDW)], incubated at 37 °C for 1 h, washed in 2× SSC for 2 min and air dried. The slides were further pretreated with 150 μl of pepsin solution per slide (1.5 μl of 500 μg/ml pepsin + 0.25 μl of 6 N hydrochloride acid + 148.25 μl of SDW), incubated at 37 °C for 30 min, washed in 2× SSC for 2 min and air dried. The slides were re-fixed with 100 μl of 1% paraformaldehyde per slide for 10 min at RT, washed in 2× SSC for 2 min and air dried. The slides were hybridized with 10 μl of hybridization cocktail (5 μl of formamide + 2 μl of 50% dextran sulfate + 1 μl of 20× SSC + 1–2 μl probe) per slide and covered with a cover slip (22 × 22 mm). The edges of the cover slips were sealed with rubber cement and denatured on a hot plate at 80 °C for 2–3 min. Finally, the slides were placed in a humidity chamber and incubated at 37 °C overnight. Following hybridization, the slides were washed in 2× SSC for 2 min to remove the cover slips, washed in milliQ water for 1 min, and air dried. Following this, 126 μl detection solution [125 μl of 1% BSA in 4× SSC + 0.5 μl of 0.4 μg/ml anti-digoxigenin rhodamine (Roche) + 0.5 μl of 0.5 μg/ml biotinylated streptavidin-FITC (vector laboratories)] was applied for detection and the slides were incubated at 37 °C for 30 min. The slides were then washed in 2× SSC for 2 min, in milliQ water for 1 min, and air dried. Finally, the slides were counter-stained using 5 μg/ml 4,6-diamidino-2-phenylindole (DAPI) in a VectaShield antifade solution (Vector Laboratories). The slides were observed under a fluorescence microscope (Olympus BX53) equipped with a cooled CCD camera (Photometrics CoolSNAP MYO), processed by Metamorph, Metavue imaging series version 7.8 and edited with Adobe Photoshop CS 6.

#### Data analysis

Total chromosome length and percentage of cells showing properly dispersed chromosomes per slide were measured for each treatment. Total chromosome length was measured in 20 properly dispersed cells. The total number of cells having properly dispersed chromosomes per slide was determined by tracing the entire slide using 40× magnification. The data were analyzed using analysis of variance according to CRD and Duncan's multiple range test. The statistical analyses were performed using SAS 9.3 software package (SAS Institute, USA).

## Results

#### Modified Carnoy's solution II increases the prometaphase index

Four methods, namely, MC II, 0.002 M 8-Hq for 4 h, ice treatment for 24 h, and C3:1 were compared for their effectiveness in obtaining properly dispersed prometaphase and metaphase chromosomes in melon. The root tips were harvested between 7 am and 9 am and treated as mentioned above. The total chromosome lengths obtained using MC II (3.17 μm) were significantly longer than those obtained using the other three methods (1.1–1.7 μm, Fig. 1a). This result suggests that melon chromosomes obtained using MC II are twice as longer as those with the other methods. In addition, the total number of cells having properly dispersed chromosomes per slide using MC II was significantly higher than those obtained using the 8-Hq, ice, and C3:1 methods (Fig. 1b). Thus, these results suggest that the MC II method is effective for increasing the prometaphase index in pretreated root tips. Cells with numerous chromosomes that are properly dispersed are essential for FISH in order to properly visualize the chromosomes.

#### Prometaphase chromosomes offer details on melon chromosome morphology

Prometaphase chromosomes were successfully arrested in melon by the MC II method (Fig. 2a). These chromosomes were larger and less condensed than the metaphase chromosomes obtained using the 8-Hq, ice, and C3:1 methods (Fig. 2b, c, and d). Using MC II-treated prometaphase chromosomes, we were able to clearly detect the heterochromatic and euchromatic regions. Most of the metaphase chromosomes obtained using the 8-Hq, ice, and C3:1 methods had almost the same sizes for each individual chromosome, and no difference was observed in the total chromosome lengths (Fig. 2b, c, and d). In contrast, prometaphase chromosomes treated by the MC II method showed different chromosome lengths for each individual chromosome (Fig. 2a). The ease of identifying individual chromosomes by size, as a result of uneven condensation

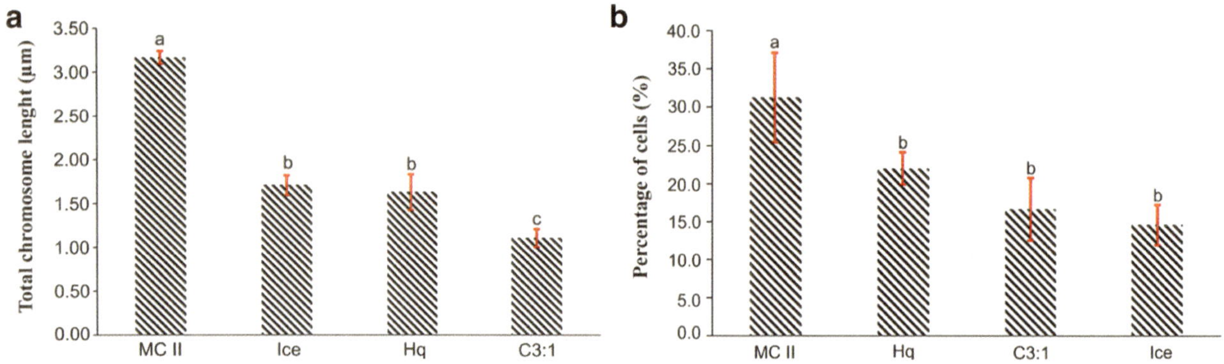


**Fig. 1** The total chromosome length (**a**) and percentage of cells showing properly dispersed chromosomes per slide (**b**) that were obtained by four methods, i.e., MC II, 8-Hq, ice, and C3:1. Note: bars with the same letters are not significantly different at $P \leq 0.05$. Red lines depict standard deviations

of each individual prometaphase chromosome, is an advantage of using prometaphase chromosomes for karyotyping [4]. Prometaphase chromosomes with different degrees of condensation can be used for initial karyotyping of a plant in cases where DNA probes are not available to distinguish individual chromosomes, particularly for newly karyotyped plant species with small chromosome sizes.

### Preparation of pachytene chromosomes using a combination of MC II and ADI methods

The high degree of cytoplasm present in PMCs caused a reduction in FISH resolution and was the primary obstacle for chromosome preparation when using the squash method. The ADI method for karyotyping ant chromosomes was developed by Dr. Hirotami T. Imai [17]. In this

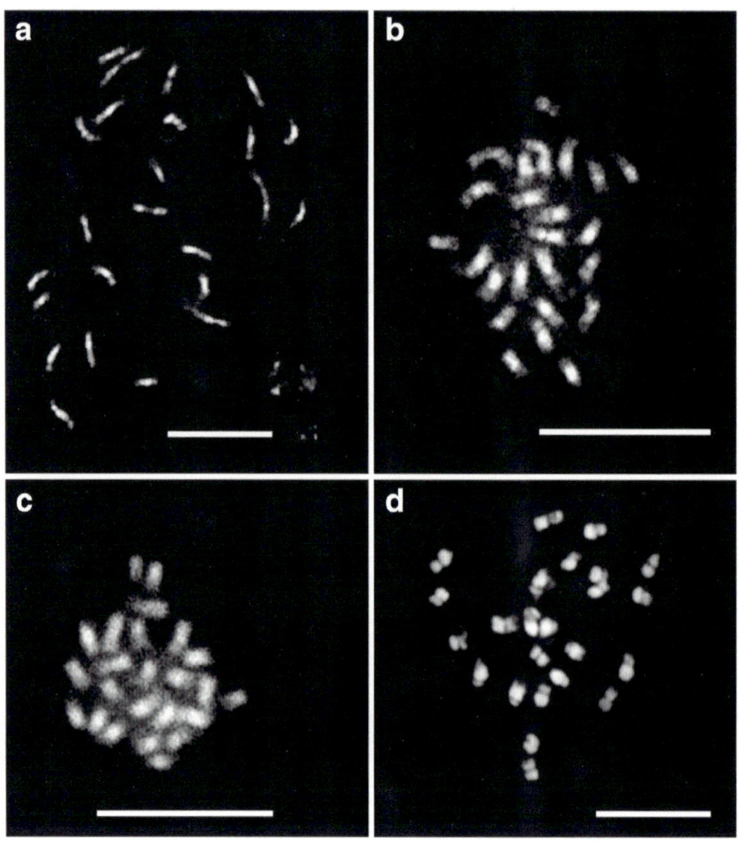


**Fig. 2** Melon chromosomes obtained by the four treatments: prometaphase chromosomes using the MC II method (**a**), metaphase chromosomes using the ice treatment (**b**), metaphase chromosomes using the C3:1 treatment (**c**), and metaphase chromosomes using the 8-Hq treatment (**d**). Scale bars = 10 μm

experiment we used a combination of the MC II and ADI methods to prepare pachytene chromosome slides from melon and *Abelia* × *grandiflora* flower buds (Figs. 3, 4b1 and c1). These pachytene cells showed reduced cytoplasm and clear chromosomes. We also obtained properly dispersed metaphase II and interphase cells with no cytoplasmic background in *Abelia* × *grandiflora*, and confirmed that it had 32 chromosomes (Fig. 4a1). In this method, freezing the slides at an ultralow temperature is unnecessary, and the slides can be directly used for FISH after being inspected using phase-contrast microscopy.

### FISH analyses of melon and *Abelia* × *grandiflora* chromosomes

Chromosome spreads obtained from root tips and PMCs prepared by the MC II method alone as well as a combination of the MC II and ADI methods, were evaluated for their applicability for FISH analysis of somatic metaphase and meiotic pachytene chromosomes of *Abelia* × *grandiflora* and melon. FISH performed on somatic metaphase and pachytene chromosomes of *Abelia* × *grandiflora* using a 45S rDNA probe revealed four metaphase and two pachytene hybridization signals (Fig. 4a3 and b3). One pair of metaphase chromosomes had strong signals, whereas the rest had weak signals, with both signals being located on the short arms. FISH performed on interphase nuclei also showed four signals of 45S rDNA in *Abelia* × *grandiflora* (Fig. 4a3). These results suggest the conservation of 45S rDNA on two pairs of chromosomes in *Abelia* × *grandiflora*.

Twelve signals of Cmcent located at heterochromatic blocks were detected in melon pachytene chromosomes

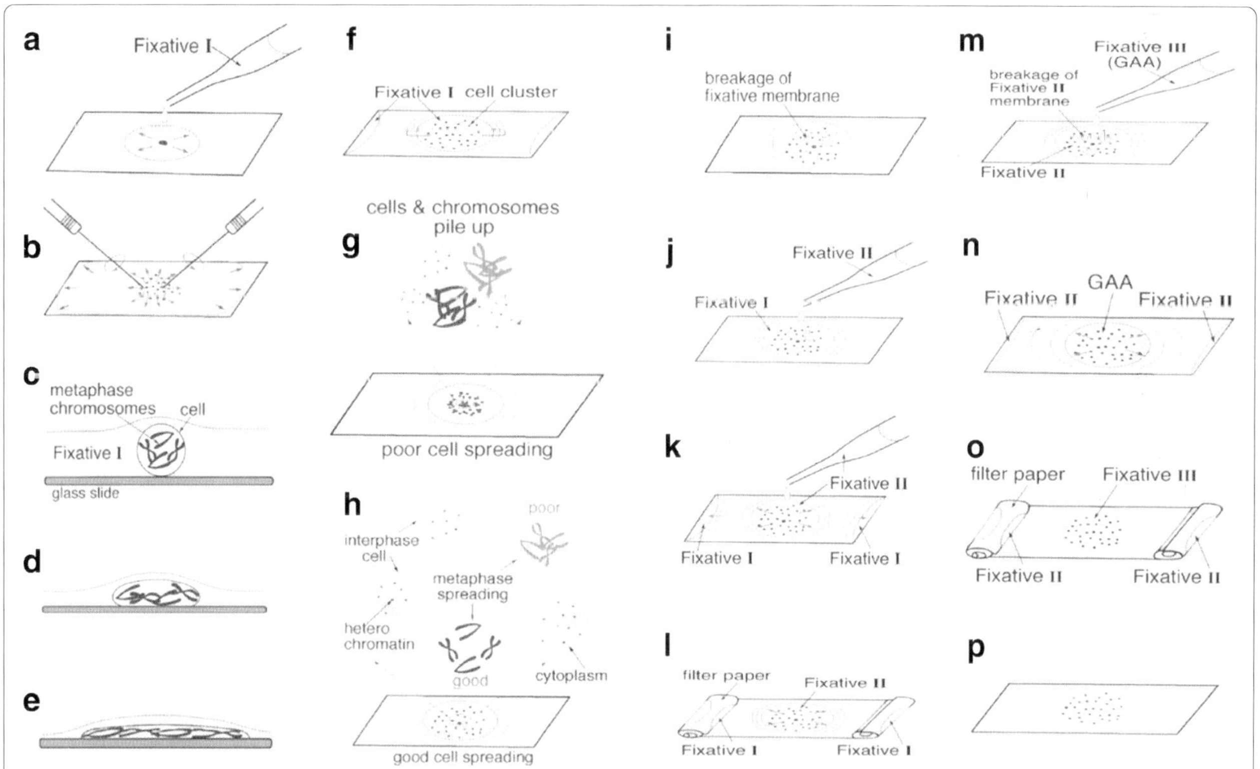


**Fig. 3** Illustration of the ADI method. The figures are modified with permission [17]. The anthers are treated with enzyme mixtures and incubated at 37 °C for 1–2 h. After incubation, the enzyme surrounding the anther is cleaned using a Kimwipe tissue. Fixative I solution (5-10 μl) is applied directly onto the anther (**a**). The anther is macerated as quickly as possible using dissected needles (**b**). Most of fixative I spreads out to the edge of the slide but partially remains around the cells. After a few minutes, the fixative I evaporates, leaving behind a thin layer, and the spherical cells floating in the fixative adhere to the slide by surface tension (**c-f**). If the humidity is less than 50%, most of the fixative evaporates before the cell becomes flat, and the chromosomes aggregate together (**g**). If the temperature is > 25 °C and humidity is > 80%, the fixative retracts again to the center of the slide (**f**). If the temperature is 20 °C with 65%–70% humidity, the evaporation speed of the fixative and flattening of the cell by surface tension are balanced (**h**). When the breakage of the fixative membrane covers approximately half of the area of the spreading cells (**i**), 5–10 μl of freshly prepared fixative II is added (**j**). Fixative I (60%, 1:1) then moves to the edge of the slide immediately (**k**) and is replaced by fixative II (absolute, 1:1). Fixative II should be applied before the breakage of the fixative membrane to allow expansion of the chromosomes. Fixative I accumulation at the edge of the slide can be removed with rolled filter paper (**l**). When the breakage of the fixative II membrane covers approximately half of the area of the spreading cells, 5–10 μl of freshly prepared fixative III is added (**m**), and fixative II moves to the edge of the slide (**n**). Fixative III is effective in removing cytoplasm and cleaning up the background of metaphase spreads. Fixative II accumulation at the edge of the slide can be removed with rolled filter paper (**o**) to dry the slide completely (**p**)

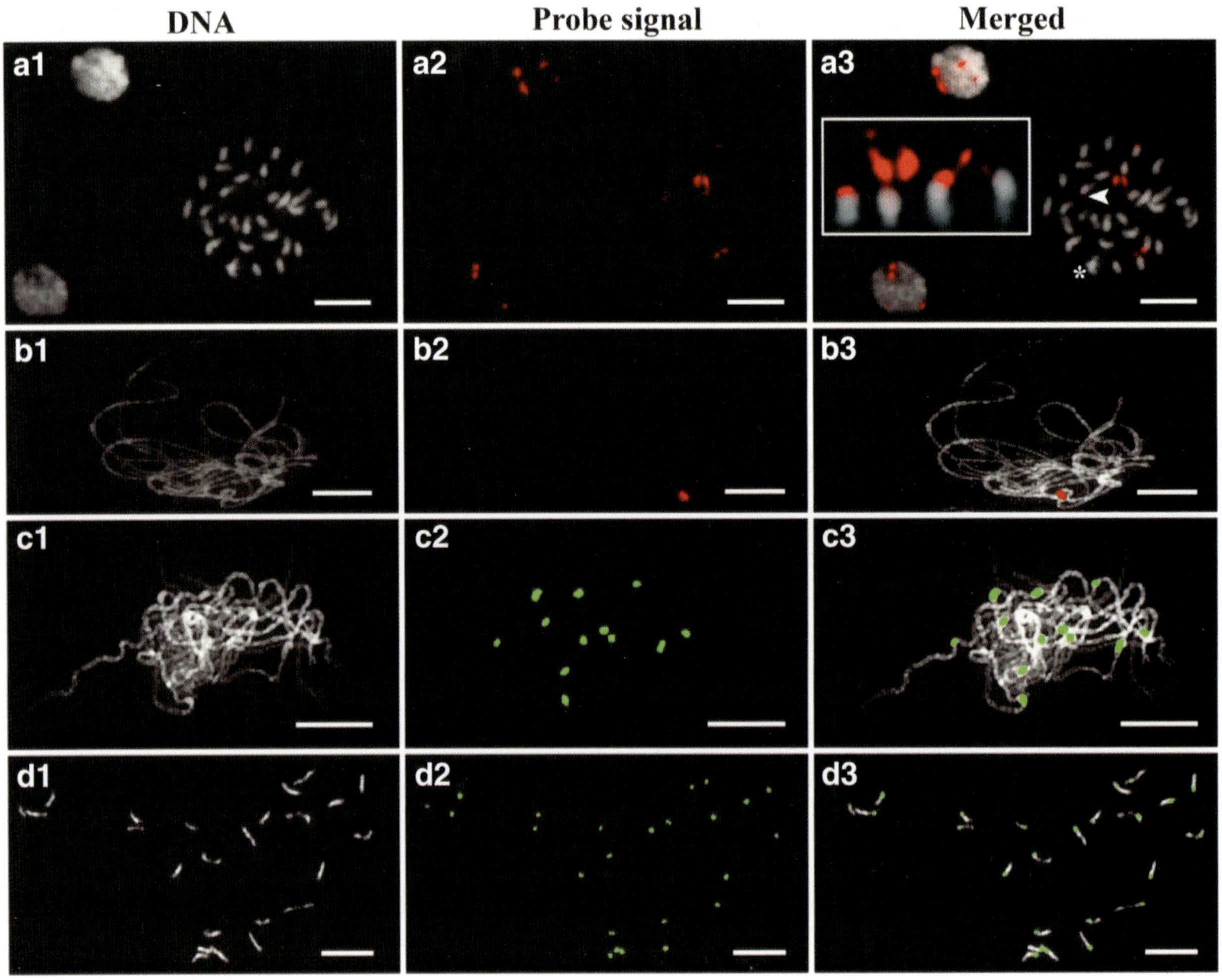


**Fig. 4** Prometaphase and pachytene chromosomes of *Abelia* × *grandiflora* (**a** and **b**) and *Cucumis melo* (**c** and **d**). FISH detection of 45S rDNA in somatic metaphase (**a1**-**a3**) and pachytene (**b1**-**b3**) chromosomes of *Abelia* × *grandiflora*. Arrowhead shows a weak signal of 45S rDNA. Asterisk shows overlapped chromosomes, and inset shows the arrangement of two pairs of chromosomes with 45S rDNA signals (**a3**). FISH detection of melon centromeres in pachytene cells (**c1**-**c3**) and prometaphase cells (**d1**-**d3**). Somatic metaphase and pachytene chromosome of *Abelia* × *grandiflora* (**a1** and **b1**) and melon pachytene chromosomes (**c1**) were acquired using a combination of MC II and ADI methods. Melon prometaphase chromosome spread (**d1**) was obtained using the germinated root with the MC II method. Red signals in **a2** and **b2** are 45S rDNA. Green signals in **c2** depict Cmcent labeled with digoxigenin. Green signals in **d2** are Cmcent labeled with biotin. Scale bars = 10 μm

(Fig. 4c3), similar to previously reported results [14]. Cmcent, a marker associated with the melon centromere, was successfully hybridized to melon prometaphase chromosomes. The signal positions on the chromosomes were consistent with previously described results [18]. In addition, the chromosome morphology prior to the FISH experiment (DAPI images) was preserved even after FISH. Different chromosome morphologies are typically observed during FISH experiments, caused by the effect of heat treatment on chromosomes, inducing changes in chromatin conformation. Another method reported that using the steam-drop method can induce chromatin protrusion and requires a pretreatment before proceeding to FISH [20]. In this study, we demonstrate that prometaphase chromosomes obtained using the MC II method are satisfactory for FISH experiments in plant species.

## Discussion

Chromosome preparation is a key factor in FISH experiments and karyotyping. Every plant species has different chromosome sizes and intracellular components [21] that may affect the choice of chromosome preparation techniques used to obtain a satisfactory chromosome slide. Many researchers use different fixative solutions to arrest metaphase or prometaphase chromosomes, such as 2.5 μM amiprophos-methyl in *Vicia faba* L. [22], 0. 002 M 8-Hq in melon [14], and α-bromonaphthalene in *S. formosissima* [21] and orchids [23]. Metaphase chromosomes have been used for karyotyping and FISH in melon [12–14, 18]. Chromosome sizes in melon are small, and the metaphase chromosomes are too condensed for FISH karyotyping analysis. Therefore, we chose prometaphase chromosomes, which are less condensed and display more detail than metaphase chromosomes. Because of uneven condensation patterns, prometaphase chromosomes have been found to be more convenient for karyotyping in plant species with small chromosome sizes [4].

The MC II method was effective in arresting the prometaphase chromosomes in the present study. In addition, using this method, the prometaphase index was increased, i.e., the number of properly dispersed chromosomes per slide and the total length of chromosomes were both significantly increased. The pretreatment was conducted between 7.00 am and 9. 00 am at which time the root meristem was actively growing. In contrast to the MC II treatment, results obtained using the 8-Hq, ice, and C3:1 treatments were consistent with those of previous studies, where metaphase chromosomes were mostly arrested as reported in *Humulus japonicus* [20], *Hippeastrum puniceum* [24], *Passiflora* [25], melon [26, 27], *Papaver* sp. [28], and *Triticale* [29]. Therefore, timing of the pretreatment along with MC II treatment was found to be significantly important for arresting most of the cells in prometaphase condition. In addition, the morphologies of prometaphase and pachytene chromosomes before performing FISH (DAPI images) were preserved even after the completion of FISH. This may be due to the combination of ethanol, acetic acid, and chloroform, which prevents the considerable shrinking of tissue with hydrogen bonding that stabilizes and preserves the tissue structures [30].

MC II can be used to prepare super-stretched pachytene chromosomes in maize, that are more robust and durable compared with those acquired by other fixative solutions [16], whereas the ADI method was developed primarily for ant chromosomes [17]. We demonstrated that a method combining the MC II and ADI methods can be used for plant species. We obtained satisfactory pachytene chromosomes with reduced cytoplasm in melon and *Abelia* × *grandiflora*. Furthermore, we reduced the time required for FISH by skipping the slide-freezing step used in the chromosome squash method. The ADI method consists of three main fixative solutions; fixative I is important to spread the chromosomes evenly on the slide, fixative II is critical to obtain satisfactory and properly dispersed metaphase and pachytene chromosomes, and fixative III is used to remove the cytoplasmic background of the metaphase and pachytene chromosome cells [17].

## Conclusions

The results reported here demonstrate the effectiveness of the MC II method for inducing prometaphase chromosomes in plant species. The root tips treated by this method demonstrate an increased prometaphase index. In addition, the prometaphase chromosome distribution prepared with this method reveals more distinct patterns of heterochromatic, euchromatic, and centromere regions than metaphase chromosomes. The combination of the MC II and ADI methods also provides high-resolution pachytene chromosomes with reduced cytoplasmic background. Physical mapping of 45S rDNA and Cmcent was used to test the applicability of chromosome distribution prepared by those methods. The signals of those probes were easily detected and different chromatin conformations were not found after completion of FISH experiment.

### Abbreviations

ADI: Air dry Imai; ANOVA: Analysis of variance; C3:1: 3:1 (v/v) ethanol: acetic acid; DAPI: 4,6-diamidino-2-phenylindole; FISH: Fluorescence in situ hybridization; HCl: Hydrochloride acid; Hq: 8 hydroxyquinoline; Ice: Ice water; MC II: Modified Carnoy's solution II; PMC: Pollen mother cell; rDNA: Ribosomal DNA; RT: Room temperature; SDW: Sterile distilled water; SSC: Saline sodium citrate

### Funding

This work was supported in part by Grants-in-Aid for Scientific Research (No. 16K07588) from the Ministry of Education, Culture, Sports, Science and Technology, Japan.

### Authors' contributions

ABS designed the study, performed the research, analyzed data, and wrote the manuscript. CHT performed the research and wrote the manuscript. SK and HS interpreted the data and reviewed the manuscript. TK designed the study, interpreted the data, and wrote and reviewed the manuscript. All authors read and approved the final manuscript.

### Competing interests

The authors declare that they have no competing interests.

### Author details

[1]Laboratory of Genetics and Plant Breeding, Graduate School of Horticulture, Chiba University, Matsudo, Chiba 271-8510, Japan. [2]Center for Research in Biotechnology for Agriculture, University of Malaya, 50603 Kuala Lumpur, Malaysia.

### References

1. Pitrat M. Melon. In: Prohens J, Nuez F, editors. Handbook crop breeding vol I vegetables. New York: Springer; 2008. p. 283–315.

2. Chen J-F, Zhou X-H. Cucumis. In: Kole C, editor. Wild crop relatatives: genomic breeding resources vegetables. Berlin: Springer; 2011. p. 67–90.
3. Koo D, Hur Y, Jin D, Bang J. Karyotype analysis of a korean cucumber cultivar (*Cucumis sativus* L. cv. Winter long) using C-banding and bicolor fluorescence *in situ* hybridization. Mol Cells. 2002;13:413–8.
4. Fukui K, Mukai Y. Condensation pattern as a new image parameter for identification of small chromosomes in plants. Japanese J Genet. 1988; 63:359–66.
5. Fukui K, Nakayama S, Ohmido N, Yoshiaki H, Yamabe M. Quantitative karyotyping of three diploid brassica species by imaging methods and localization of 45s rDNA loci on the identified chromosomes. Theor Appl Genet. 1998;96:325–30.
6. Ohmido N, Fukui K. Visual verification of close disposition between a rice a genome-specific DNA sequence (TrsA) and the telomere sequence. Plant Mol Biol. 1997;35:963–8.
7. Ohmido N, Akiyama Y, Fukui K. Physical mapping of unique nucleotide sequences on identified rice chromosomes. Plant Mol Biol. 1998;38:1043–52.
8. Fukui K, Iijima K. Somatic chromosome map of rice by imaging methods. Theor Appl Genet. 1991;81:589–96.
9. Guimarães G, Cardoso L, Oliveira H, Santos C, Duarte P, Sottomayor M. Cytogenetic characterization and genome size of the medicinal plant *Catharanthus roseus* (L.) G. Don. AoB Plants. 2012;12:1–10.
10. She C-W, Jiang X-H. Karyotype analysis of *Lablab purpureus* (L .) sweet using fluorochrome banding and fluorescence *in situ* hybridisation with rDNA probes. Czech J Genet Plant Breed. 2015;2015:110–6.
11. Schwarzacher T, Heslop-Harrison P. Practical in situ hyridization. New York: Springer; 2000; pp. 203.
12. Liu C, Liu J, Li H, Zhang Z, Han Y, Huang S, et al. Karyotyping in melon (*Cucumis melo* L.) by cross-species fosmid fluorescence *in situ* hybridization. Cytogenet Genome Res. 2010;129:241–9.
13. Zhang Z-T, Yang S, Li Z-A, Zhang Y, Wang Y, Cheng C, et al. Comparative chromosomal localization of 45S and 5S rDNAs and implications for genome evolution in *Cucumis*. Genome. 2016;59:449–57.
14. Han Y, Zhang Z, Liu C, Liu J, Huang S, Jiang J, et al. Centromere repositioning in cucurbit species: implication of the genomic impact from centromere activation and inactivation. Proc Natl Acad Sci U S A. 2009;106: 14937–41.
15. Zhang Y, Cheng C, Li J, Yang S, Wang Y, Li Z, et al. Chromosomal structures and repetitive sequences divergence in *Cucumis* species revealed by comparative cytogenetic mapping. BMC Genomics. 2015;16:730.
16. Koo DH, Jiang J. Super-stretched pachytene chromosomes for fluorescence *in situ* hybridization mapping and immunodetection of DNA methylation. Plant J. 2009;59:509–16.
17. Imai HT. A manual for ant chromosome preparations (an improved air-drying method) and Giemsa staining. Chromosom Sci. 2016;19:57–66.
18. Koo D-H, Nam Y-W, Choi D, Bang J-W, de Jong H, Hur Y. Molecular cytogenetic mapping of *Cucumis sativus* and *C. melo* using highly repetitive DNA sequences. Chromosom Res. 2010;18:325–36.
19. Gerlach WL, Bedbrook JR. Cloning and characterization of ribosomal RNA genes from wheat and barley. Nucleic Acids Res. 1979;7:1869–85.
20. Kirov I, Divashuk M, Van Laere K, Soloviev A, Khrustaleva L. An easy "SteamDrop" method for high quality plant chromosome preparation. Mol Cytogenet. 2014;7:21.
21. Rodríguez-Domínguez J, Ríos-Lara L, Tapia-Campos E, Barba-Gonzalez R. An improved technique for obtaining well-spread metaphases from plants with numerous large chromosomes. Biotech Histochem. 2017;92:159–66.
22. Dolezel J, Cihalíková J, Lucretti S. A high-yield procedure for isolation of metaphase chromosomes from root tips of *Vicia faba* L. Planta. 1992; 188:93–8.
23. Daviña JR, Grabiele M, Cerutti JC, Hojsgaard DH, Almada RD, Insaurralde IS, et al. Chromosome studies in *Orchidaceae* from Argentina. Genet Mol Biol. 2009;32:811–21.
24. Poggio L, Realini MF, Fourastié MF, García AM, González GE. Genome downsizing and karyotype constancy in diploid and polyploid congeners: a model of genome size variation. AoB Plants. 2014;6:1–11.
25. Souza MM, Urdampilleta JD, Forni-Martins ER. Improvements in cytological preparations for fluorescent in situ hybridization in *Passiflora*. Genet Mol Res. 2010;9:2148–55.
26. Zhang W, Hao H, Ma L, Zhao C, Yu X. Tetraploid muskmelon alters morphological characteristics and improves fruit quality. Sci Hortic. 2010; 125:396–400.
27. Ezura H, Amagai H, Yoshioka K, Oosawa K. Highly frequent appearance of tetraploidy in regenerated plants, a universal phenomenon, in tissue cultures of melon (*Cucumis melo* L.). Plant Sci. 1992;85:209–13.
28. Osalou AR, Daneshvar Rouyandezagh S, Alizadeh B, Er C, Sevimay CS. A comparison of ice cold water pretreatment and α-bromonaphthalene cytogenetic method for identification of *Papaver* species. Sci World J. 2013;608650.
29. Merker A. A Giemsa technique for rapid identification of chromosomes in *Triticale*. Hereditas. 1973;75:280–2.
30. Puchtler H, Sweat Waldrop F, Conner HM, Terry MS. Carnoy fixation: practical and theoretical considerations. Histochemie. 1968;16:361–71.

# 4

# Identification of genomic copy number variations associated with specific clinical features of head and neck cancer

Boris Zagradišnik[1*], Danijela Krgović[1], Špela Stangler Herodež[1], Andreja Zagorac[1], Bogdan Ćižmarević[2] and Nadja Kokalj Vokač[1]

**Abstract**

**Background:** Copy number variations (CNSs) of large genomic regions are an important mechanism implicated in the development of head and neck cancer, however, for most changes their exact role is not well understood. The aim of this study was to find possible associations between gains/losses of genomic regions and clinically distinct subgroups of head and neck cancer patients.

**Results:** Array comparative genomic hybridization (aCGH) analysis was performed on DNA samples in 64 patients with cancer in oral cavity, oropharynx or hypopharynx. Overlapping genomic regions created from gains and losses were used for statistical analysis. Following regions were overrepresented: in tumors with stage I or II a gain of 2. 98 Mb on 6p21.2-p11 and a gain of 7.4 Mb on 8q11.1-q11.23; in tumors with grade I histology a gain of 1.1 Mb on 8q24.13, a loss of a large part of p arm of chromosome 3, a loss of a 1.24 Mb on 6q14.3, and a loss of terminal 32 Mb region of 8p23.3; in cases with affected lymph nodes a gain of 0.75 Mb on 3q24, and a gain of 0.9 Mb on 3q26.32-q26. 33; in cases with unaffected lymph nodes a gain of 1.1 Mb on 8q23.3, in patients not treated with surgery a gain of 12. 2 Mb on 7q21.3-q22.3 and a gain of 0.33 Mb on 20q11.22.

**Conclusions:** Our study identified several genomic regions of interest which appear to be associated with various clinically distinct subgroups of head and neck cancer. They represent a potentially important source of biomarkers useful for the clinical management of head and neck cancer. In particular, the *PIK3CA* and *AGTR1* genes could be singled out to predict the lymph node involvement.

**Keywords:** Head and neck cancer, Copy number variations, Array comparative genomic hybridization, Biomarkers

## Background

The head and neck squamous cell carcinomas (HNSCCs) are among the most common cancers, affecting approximately 530,000 new patients and causing 293,000 deaths worldwide every year [1]. The overall survival rate of around 50% is an important indicator that this type of cancer represents a major medical problem [2]. An improvement in disease management can be expected from better understanding of molecular mechanisms underlying this medical condition. Acquired DNA mutations which range from epigenetic DNA methylation alterations, single nucleotide changes to variations in whole chromosomal copy number are a well-established cause of cancer. An important subset represent copy number variations (CNVs) which can include large chromosomal regions or gene-size changes [3–5]. Gains and losses of particular genomic segments usually contain important oncogenes and tumor suppressor genes. These include such regions as a gain of 11q13 (*CCND1* gene, cyclin D1), a gain of 7p11 (*EGFR* gene, epidermal growth factor receptor), a loss of 9p (*CDKN2A* gene, cyclin dependent kinase 2a / p16), among many others [3, 6, 7]. The development of array comparative genomic hybridization provided further evidence for the role of frequent and characteristic gains and losses in HNSCCs. The accumulating data clearly reveal great heterogeneity apparent from a long list of

* Correspondence: boris.zagradisnik@ukc-mb.si
[1]Laboratory of Medical Genetics, University Medical Centre Maribor, Ljubljanska 5, 2000 Maribor, Slovenia
Full list of author information is available at the end of the article

genomic regions harboring gains (1q, 3p, 3q, 5p, 7p, 7q, 8q, 9q, 11q, 14q, 16p, 19q, 20q) and losses (2p, 3p, 3q, 4q, 8p, 10p, 16q, 18q) [8–11]. These are all excellent tumor markers which when present clearly and unequivocally identify a tissue sample as cancerous. However, the adoption of CNV detection for other roles in disease management is not easy because data supporting associations with various clinical parameters are often sparse or even contradictory [12, 13]. Consequently, these genetic biomarkers remain the interest of research with few of them nearing clinical practice of head and neck cancer treatment [14]. Nevertheless, they are of great importance in a quest to refine the current clinical description of tumors based on the TNM classification [15]. High heterogeneity exhibited by HNSCC may not always be sufficiently accounted for by the disease staging and pathomorphologic characterization. Therefore, it is important to continue the search for additional parameters which may help improve the categorization of individual cases of HNSCC. A hypothesis-free whole genome analysis is the modern approach to conduct such an examination [16].

This study identifies possible associations between gains/losses of genomic regions and clinical features characteristic for two distinct subgroups of head and neck cancer patients, those with early disease vs. those with loco-regionally advanced cancer.

## Methods

### Patients

The study included 64 patients (50 males, 78.1%; 14 females, 21.9%) with the diagnosis of head and neck cancer located in oral cavity, oropharynx or hypopharynx, who underwent treatment at the Department of Otorhinolaryngology, Cervical and Maxillofacial Surgery, University Medical Centre Maribor, Slovenia. They were recruited between November 2010 and March 2015. Clinical information about age, gender, age at diagnosis, follow-up and survival time, and disease recurrence was collected from medical records. The stage of the disease was determined from the TNM status of the tumor; however, not all patients received surgical treatment and postoperative evaluation was not available for all tumors. Histologic grade was also obtained. In addition, the treatment regimens in patients were recorded as surgery, chemotherapy, radiotherapy or the combinations thereof.

This study was approved by the Ethics committee of the University Medical Centre Maribor, where the study was conducted. Each patient signed an informed consent prior to the study enrollment.

### Tumor samples

Tumor samples were excised from primary tumor sites and not from metastatic sites or affected lymph nodes. All samples were specimens for pathological confirmation following surgery or diagnostic biopsy of which a small part was obtained for the long term storage at −80 °C.

### DNA extraction

At least 10 mg of tumor tissue was thoroughly disrupted with the TissueLyzer (Qiagen G.m.b.h., Hilden, Germany). The lysate was then used for the extraction of genomic DNA with the Qiaamp DNA Mini Kit on QIACUBE (both Qiagen G.m.b.h., Hilden, Germany). All procedures were performed according to the manufacturer's instructions.

### Human papilloma virus detection

In order to ascertain the presence of human papilloma virus (HPV) DNA in tumor samples a simple duplex polymerase chain reaction protocol was developed. A 10 μL reaction contained 10 μM of primers MY09 (5'-CGTCCMARRGGAWACTGATC-3′) and MY11 (5'-GC MCAGGGWCATAAYAATGG-3′) [17], 1 μM of control locus primers (Forward: 5'-CTATCCCACTGTATTATT CAGGGC-3′; Reverse: 5′-TGAGTCTCCAGGTTGCAG GTGACA-3′), 50 ng of tumor genomic DNA in 1× Multiplex PCR Master Mix Kit (Qiagen G.m.b.h., Hilden, Germany). The temperature protocol was: 15 min of initial denaturation/enzyme activation at 95 °C, followed by 35 cycles of 30 s denaturation at 94 °C, 1 min annealing at 55 °C and 1 min elongation at 72 °C. The amplification products were detected with agarose gel electrophoresis after staining with SYBR Green I.

### Array comparative genomic hybridization analysis

Array CCH analysis was performed using the BlueGnome Cytochip ISCA 8x60K platform (BlueGnome Ltd., Cambridge, United Kingdom). The assay was performed according to the manufacturer's instructions. Data were obtained using the BlueFuse Multi software tool. Automatic assessment provided by the software was used to acquire genetic variations. A minimal size of 20,000 base pairs (20kbp) was adopted as an inclusion criterion. The data were arranged according to chromosomal location to obtain the extent and frequency of overlapping regions, which were then used for further analysis. Gains and losses were analyzed separately. The GRCh37/hg19 was used for genomic data analysis and representation.

### Statistical analysis

The odds ratios (ORs) and chi-squared test (Chi2) with Yates correction were used to evaluate differences in copy number variation frequencies stratified by the patients' characteristics. Patients were grouped according to the disease stage (stage I & II vs. stage III & IV), histological grade (grade 1 vs. grade 2 & 3), tumor size (T1 & T2 vs, T3 & T4), lymph node involvement (cases N0 vs. cases N1 or higher) and surgical treatment (surgery used vs. no surgery used). A 2 × 2 contingency table was generated between each of the five clinical feature groups and each genomic region involved. 95% confidence intervals (CI) were computed where applicable and a $p$ value <0.05 was considered statistically significant. All analyses were done in OpenOffice, org Calc spreadsheet application.

## Results

Our study included 64 patients, mostly men (50, 78.1%, male to female ratio 3.57:1). with similar median age at diagnosis for both gender groups (Table 1). Since the study enrollment 42 patients have died (33 due to cancer, 9 from other causes) and 3 were lost to follow-up. Histologically verified squamous cell carcinoma was present in all patients. Most patients were affected with HNSCC for the first time; however, in 3 patients the cancer has re-occurred after a prolonged disease free interval. The tumors were positioned in oral cavity (34 patients), oropharynx (25 patients), and hypopharynx (5 patients) (Table 1), although for some large tumors their locations could not be precisely determined because they affected multiple adjacent anatomic regions. Most cancers were locally advanced (47 stage IV cases) and lymph node involvement was also frequent (42 cases) (Table 1). Distant metastases were a rare event observed in 3 cases (two in the lung; one in the brain) (Table 1). Various combinations of radical surgery, radiotherapy and chemotherapy were used for cure or palliative care in 62 patients,

**Table 1** Clinical data of patients with HNSCC

| | # (%) | Median age at diagnosis (range) | | Median observation time (range) | |
|---|---|---|---|---|---|
| Women | 14 (21.9%) | 56.5 (48–76) years | | 13 (2–53) months | |
| Men | 50 (78.1%) | 57 (34–78) years | | 22 (2–61) months | |
| Deceased | 42 (65.6%) | | | | |
| Status unknown | 3 (4.7%) | | | | |
| Disease reoccurrence | 3 (4.7%) | | | | |
| Tumor locations | # (%) | | | | |
| Oral cavity | 34 (53.1%) | | | | |
| Oropharynx | 25 (39.1%) | | | | |
| Hypopharynx | 5 (7.8%) | | | | |
| TNM classification | | | | | |
| Tumor | # (%) | Lymph node status | # (%) | Distant metastases | # (%) |
| T1 | 8 (12.5%) | N0 | 22 (34.4%) | M0 | 61 (95.3%) |
| T2 | 16 (25.0%) | N1 or higher | 42 (65.6%) | M1 | 3 (4.7%) |
| T3 | 7 (10.9%) | | | | |
| T4 | 33 (51.6%) | | | | |
| Disease stage | # (%) | | Histologic grading | # (%) | |
| I | 6 (9.4%) | | grade 1 | 12 (18.7%) | |
| II | 8 (12.5%) | | grade 2 | 36 (56.3%) | |
| III | 3 (4.7%) | | grade 3 | 16 (25.0%) | |
| IVA | 37 (57.8%) | | | | |
| IVB | 7 (10.9%) | | | | |
| IVC | 3 (4.7%) | | | | |
| Cancer treatment applied | # (%) | | | | |
| Radical surgery | 13 (20.3%) | | | | |
| Radical surgery & Chemotherapy & Radiotherapy | 13 (20.3%) | | | | |
| Radical surgery & Radiotherapy | 18 (28.1%) | | | | |
| Chemotherapy & Radiotherapy | 10 (15.6%) | | | | |
| Radiotherapy | 8 (12.5%) | | | | |
| No therapy | 2 (3.1%) | | | | |

whereas in 2 patients their very poor general condition precluded the treatment of cancer (Table 1).

The aCGH analysis detected a total of 689 CNVs, 438 (63.6%) were identified as gains (additional copies of genetic material present) and 251 (33.4%) were losses (deficit of genetic material). Most variations were classified by the BlueFuse Multi software as potentially pathogenic, 483 out of 689 (70.1%), whereas 50 variations (7.3%) were declared as benign CNVs and the rest, 156 (22.6%) as unknown. The size of variations ranged between the cut-off value of 20 kb and whole chromosomes. The level of gain/loss, the log2 ratio, also included a wider range of values, which is clearly the consequence of the presence of tumor DNA with substantial amount of somatic mosaicism. Only 2 samples have not yielded any variations. Summarized data are presented in Table 2.

The association analysis between overlapping genomic regions constructed from obtained variations and stratified clinical data revealed several statistically significant results (Table 3). Each genomic region statistical data is complemented with the range of Log2 ratios values as well as sizes of CNVs that overlap at the particular region. In low stage tumors (stage I and II) a 2.98 Mb region from 6p21.2-p11 and a 7.4 Mb region from 8q11.1-q11.23 were overrepresented in comparison to higher stage tumors. Within the latter locus a smaller 1.4 Mb genomic region has a higher association (Table 3).

A 1.1 Mb region on 8q24.13 was overrepresented in well-differentiated tumors (grade 1) compared to poorly differentiated tumors (grades 2 & 3). The loss of a large part of a short arm of chromosome 3 was significantly more common in grade 1 tumors. This approximately 80 Mb long continuous region from 3p was found to be associated with a varying degree of statistical significance as indicated in Table 3 (entry loss 1). The data for this genomic region are displayed only as ranges includeing maximal and minimal values from all smaller overlapping genomic regions that constitute the entire entry loss 1. The loss of further genomic regions associated with well differentiated tumors included a 1.24 Mb region on 6q14.3 and a 32 Mb terminal region of chromosome 8 (8p23.3).

Furthermore, genomic regions that were significantly overrepresented in cases with lymph node involvement were a gain of 0.75 Mb region on 3q24 and a gain of 0.9 Mb region on 3q26.32-q26.33. Genomic regions overrepresented in cases without lymph node involvement included a gain 1.1 Mb region on 8q23.3.

Additional genomic regions were identified when patients were stratified according the use of surgery for treating of their cancer. On 7q21.3-q22.3 a 12.2 Mb large gain was overrepresented in patients without surgical treatment. A short 0.33 Mb overlapping gain region on 20q11.22 was also significantly more frequent in patients with no surgical treatment.

No significant overrepresentations of gains or losses were found when tumors were stratified according to their size in TNM classification.

The HPV genetic material was present in 5 samples out of 64. A more detailed characterization of these samples is presented in Table 4.

## Discussion

The role of gains and losses of large chromosomal regions in cancer has been and still is a major field of research. In our study we analyzed possible associations between CNVs and two clinically distinct groups of head and neck squamous cell carcinomas, early disease and locoregionally advanced cancer. We identified 12 regions from 5 different chromosomes to be significantly overrepresented in 4 different subgroups stratified according to selected clinical parameters (Table 3). We consider overrepresentation of gains of two regions from chromosome 3 in cases with confirmed cancer in local lymph nodes to be important. In the first instance, the region of interest contains a known oncogene, *PIK3CA* (Gain 6, Table 3, Fig. 1), which has a well-established role in cancer development [18]. The product of this gene is a catalytic unit of the PI3K kinase and in most cancer cases harbors activating mutations [19]. The signaling pathway, PI3K/AKT, is also very frequently mutated in HNSCCs [20]. Copy number gain of the *PIK3CA* region has been documented to be important in HNSCC, but the reported finding [21] is somewhat contradictory to our results because it conferred poor survival to metastatic HNSCCs with unaffected lymph nodes, whereas our study showed more *PIK3CA* copy number gains in cancers with affected lymph nodes (Table 3). Earlier studies have identified the *PIK3CA* gains in the HNSCCs [22], as well as in other major cancers; i.e. breast cancer [23], lung cancer [24] or urothelial cancer [25]. However, PIK3CA gains influencing the spreading of metastases to the lymph nodes have not been reported for HNSCCs. The *PIK3CA* alterations appear to be present in squamous cell carcinomas regardless from which organ they originate [26]. Not surprisingly we were able to associate

**Table 2** Summary data on observed copy number variations

| | # | Pathogenic (%) | Benign (%) | Unknown (%) | Log2 range | Size range (bp) |
|---|---|---|---|---|---|---|
| Gains | 438 | 321 (73.3%) | 24 (5.5%) | 93 (21.2%) | 0.22 – 2.82 | 20,486–155,171,772 |
| Losses | 251 | 162 (64.5%) | 26 (10.4%) | 63 (25.1%) | −3.62 – -0.25 | 23,615–127,293,063 |

2/64 samples without CNVs: male, oropharynx, stage IVA, pT4pN2, survival time 45 months; female, tongue, stage II, pT2pN0, alive after 40 months

**Table 3** Genomic regions associated with specific clinical features in HNSCC patients

| | | | | | | | |
|---|---|---|---|---|---|---|---|
| Stage I&II vs III&IV | | | | | | | |
| | Locus | # | OR (95% CI) | p(Chi2)[a] | Log2 ratio range | CNV sizes[c] | # of genes |
| gain 1 | chr6: 38,729,522–41,698,277 | 3/11 vs. 0/50 | – | 0.084 | 0.54–0.62 | 18.6–19.5 Mb | 35 |
| gain 2 | chr8: 46,942,986–54,391,986 | 4/10 vs. 2/48 | 0.104 (0.017–0.649) | 0.0232 | 0.29–0.9 | 1.56–146 Mb | 20 |
| gain 3 | chr8: 49,091,330–50,447,801 | 6/8 vs. 3/47 | 0.085 (0.018–0.411) | 0.0021 | 0.29–0.9 | 1.56–146 Mb | 5 |
| Histological grade 1 vs. grade 2 & 3 | | | | | | | |
| | Locus | # | OR (95% CI) | p(Chi2)[a] | Log2 ratio range | CNV sizes[c] | # of genes |
| gain 4 | chr8: 122,449,344–123,538,355 | 5/7 vs. 6/46 | 5.476 (1.312–22.851) | 0.0385 | 0.28–0.58 | 1.0–145 Mb | 2 |
| loss 1[b] | chr3: 93,979–80,817,252 | 5/7 vs. 2/50; 4/8 vs. 3/49 | 17.86 (2.891–110.3) 8.167 (1.532–43.52) | 0.0011–0.024 | −0.64 – −0.26 | 1.4–93 Mb | 647 |
| loss 2 | chr6: 85,683,523–86,925,006 | 2/10 vs. 0/52 | – | 0.0384 | −0.7 – −0.26 | 1.24–40 Mb | 6 |
| loss 3 | chr8: 221,641–32,847,282 | 3/9 vs. 1/51 | 17 (1.587–182.1) | 0.0205 | −0.64 – −0.26 | 6.8–43 Mb | 309 |
| Node lymph involvement vs. cases without affected lymph nodes | | | | | | | |
| | Locus | # | OR (95% CI) | p(Chi2)[a] | Log2 ratio range | CNV sizes[c] | # of genes |
| gain 5 | chr3: 147,963,947–148,708,961 | 9/33 vs. 0/22 | – | 0.0495 | 0.28–0.96 | 5.6–109 Mb | 3 |
| gain 6 | chr3: 178,764,078–179,689,394 | 14/28 vs. 1/21 | 9.414 (1.141–77.65) | 0.0349 | 0.27–0.96 | 5–109 Mb | 13 |
| gain 7 | chr8: 108,460,956–109,567,888 | 3/39 vs. 7/15 | 0.165 (0.038–0.723) | 0.0264 | 0.28–0.8 | 0.2–146 Mb | 4 |
| Cases treated with surgery vs. cases without surgical treatment | | | | | | | |
| | Locus | # | OR (95% CI) | p(Chi2)[a] | Log2 ratio range | CNV sizes[c] | # of genes |
| gain 8 | chr7: 92,828,329–105,027,875 | 2/42 vs. 5/15 | 0.143 (0.025–0.816) | 0.0457 | 0.35–0.83 | 21–78 Mb | 196 |
| gain 9 | chr20: 33,690,620–34,021,768 | 0/44 vs. 3/17 | – | 0.0462 | 0.35–0.67 | 33-34 Mb | 9 |

[a]degree of freedom = 1
[b]values in categories # and OR correspond to the p(Chi2) values which are the lower and upper boundary of observed statistical significance in this region; values in categories Locus, Log2 ratio range and CNV size are range boundaries that do not correspond to the displayed statistical data for the entry loss1
[c]column CNV sizes displayes the range of sizes of CNVs that include the region of each particular entry

a member of a gene signature specific for squamous cell carcinoma with a clinically distinct subtype. It is important to note that the aggressive behavior of tumors with altered PIK3CA gene function is not the only possible consequence, because the role as good prognostic marker is also known for the activated PI3K/AKT signalling pathway [27].

Secondly, the overrepresentation of a region containing the gene for angiotensin II receptor type 1 (*AGTR1*) (Gain 5, Table 3, Fig. 1) in HNSCC cases with metastases in local lymph nodes was observed. Although this association was weaker in comparison to previously described *PIK3CA* association, it nevertheless identified a very interesting gene, *AGTR1*, as a tumor biomarker for HNSCC. This observation is in line with the increased expression of *AGTR1* in head and neck cancer [28]. Also, the *AGTR1* gene was found to be implicated in other important cancers, i.e. colorectal or breast cancer [29, 30].

**Table 4** Clinical characteristics of patients with HPV positive tumor DNA samples

| Gender | Age at diagnosis | Tumor location | TNM classification | Histology | Treatment | Status |
|---|---|---|---|---|---|---|
| male | 67 | oral cavity | pT4 N0 | grade 3 | surgery, radiotherapy | deceased |
| male | 58 | oropharynx | pT4 pN2 M1 | grade 1 | surgery, radiotherapy | alive |
| male | 51 | oropharynx | T4 N1 | grade 2 | chemotherapy, radiotherapy | alive |
| male | 60 | oral cavity | pT4 pN2 | grade 1 | surgery | deceased |
| male | 55 | oropharynx | pT4 pN2 | grade 3 | surgery, chemotherapy, radiotherapy | deceased |

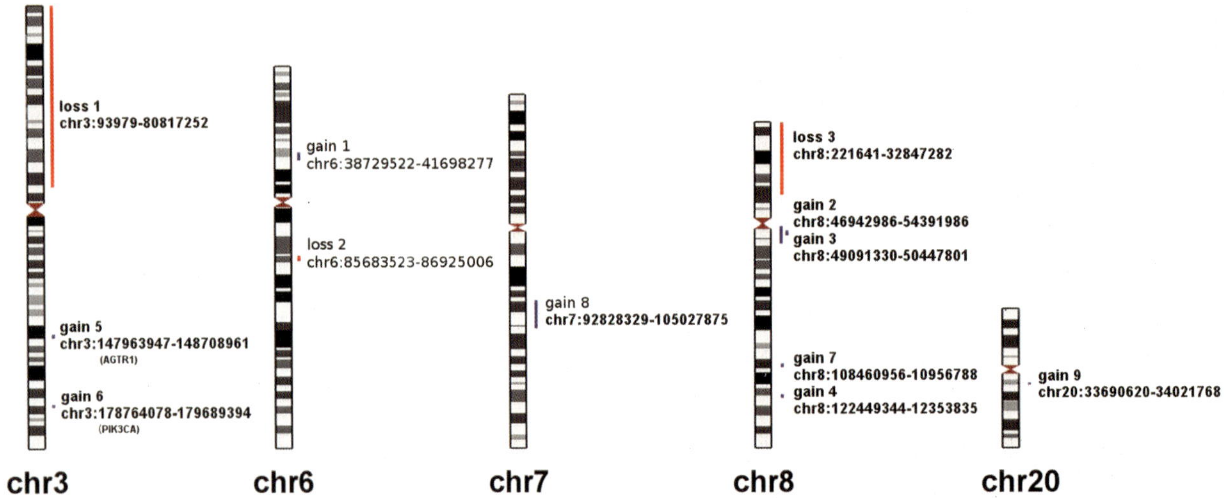


**Fig. 1** Chromosomal locations of genomic regions associated with various subgroups of patients

The association of the *AGTR1* gene with advanced head and neck cancer is important because it identifies an additional target for chemotherapy as there are several different blocking agents already in use for the treatment of hypertension. Such therapeutic approach was proposed for breast cancer cases overexpressing AGTR1 [31] and the effect of the drugs is known from in-vitro cell line experiments [32]. Because comparable data is not available for head and neck cancers, further inquiries into AGTR1 expression changes and underlying genetic alterations may help establish this gene and its signalling pathway as a legitimate therapeutic target.

We found gains of two genomic regions (Gain 8 and 9, Table 3, Fig. 1) to be overrepresented in a subgroup of patients who have not undergone radical surgery. These individuals either had an inoperable tumor, were in very poor general condition with additional other ailments, or they declined the operation because the procedure was deemed too mutilating. Their tumors were all large lesions with local invasion and extensive lymph node involvement. The first region from chromosome 7 (gain 8) overlaps with the 7q21 chromosomal region previously reported to be present in additional copies in head and neck cancer [33]. Although it contains many interesting genes which are continuously studied with respect to their role in cancer development in an ever increasing body of research, a well-established biomarker has not emerged so far. The second region (Gain 9) is from 20q which has also been implicated in HNSCC [34]. The Gain 9 is a much smaller region than Gain 8 region, but it contains several genes which may contribute to aggressive tumor growth when they are overexpressed. Specific reports for HNSCC may not be available for all the genes of interest but published studies clearly document the cancer involvement for *MMP24, EIF6 FAM83C* and *GDF5* [35–38]. These genes together with the large number of genes from the Gain 8 region warrant further analysis because they are potential biomarkers for aggressive tumor growth.

The remaining genomic regions were all overrepresented in subgroups of patients with a less aggressive or less advanced form of HNSCC. The gains (Gain 1, 2, 3, 4, 7) and losses (Loss 1, 2, 3) are presented in Table 3 and showed in Fig. 1. Such significant increase, that is not associated with a higher malignancy but with less malignant cases of HNSCC may indicate a possible role in earlier phases of cancer progression. Among the many genes included in the described variations, several genes were already studied for their role in cancer development. For most of these candidate genes the available information does not derine from studies on HNSCC but from studies focusing on other types of cancer. In less advanced cancers with stage I and II the overrepresented region gain 1 contained at least 2 genes of interest: overexpressed *TREM2* gene known to be implicated in cell proliferation, was observed in early cases of esophageal cancer [39, 40] whereas the *TFEB* gene, a transcription factor for lysosomal biogenesis, is part of a well- documented cancer specific translocation t(6;11) [41, 42]. The genomic region Gain 2 from chromosome 8 also contains additional genes important for cancer development. Thus, the overexpression of *MCM4* gene was detected in laryngeal squamous cell carcinoma and this gene was also implicated in other cancers because it codes for an important component of the DNA replication machinery [43, 44]. Inside the genomic region Gain 2 a continuous segment, named Gain 3, was obverved, which showed an even a higher level of association and contained the *SNAI2* gene. This is a transcription factor with a demonstrated role as an oncogene in HNSCC [45].

Notwithstanding, we did observe overrepresented gains in less malignant cases (stage I & II) while the gene was found to contribute to poor disease survival [46]. This is contradictory but it may be that an overexpressed *SNAI2* is required early in HNSCC development to gain malignant potential.

The largest genomic region exhibiting significant association comprises almost the entire short arm of the chromosome 3 (Loss 1, Table 3, Fig. 1). The loss of this region was overrepresented in well-differentiated grade 1 classified tumors. Thus, our observation identifies a well documented chromosomal aberration as a biomarker for a subgroup of tumors which retained good differentiation. As noted previously, earlier studies identified frequent presence of the 3p deletion in head and neck cancers [47, 48]. Then the 3p deletion was described in early displastic lesions [49]. More recently, when *p53* mutations were detected in combination with 3p deletions worse survival was observed in such cancer cases [50]. Therefore our result identifies a novel facet of this particular genetic alteration, namely its presence in well differentiated HNSCCs, which has not been reported so far.

Furthermore, additional three genomic regions were also overrepresented in well differentiated grade 1 tumors (Table 3, Fig. 1), whereas the Gain 4 region comprises only of 2 possible genes/transcribed regions (*HAS2-AS1, LOC105375734*) - with little available information. The loss of a region from chromosome 6 (Loss 2) overlaps with a 6q14 region previously described to be deleted in HNSCC [51]. This region was studied for its role in many different cancer types but it was only recently demonstrated that the 2 genes coding for small nuclear RNA, *SNORD50A* and *SNORD50B*, directly affect the activity of K-Ras, because both snoRNAs bind to it and when deleted, K-Ras activity is increased [52]. Finally, we observed a deletion of the large part of the short arm of chromosome 8 (Loss 3) to be significantly more frequent in grade 1 tumors than in poorly differentiated tumors. This particular aberration is also well known in HNSCC; however, we detected an overabundance in a well differentiated subgroup of tumors which appears to be a novel observation [47, 48]. The 8p deletions are characteristic for HNSCC but their role is not well understood. Although from other cancers a more malignant behavior was observed when its presence was detected [53].

Our study found several genomic regions (Gain 1, 2, 3, 4, 7, Loss 1, 2, 3; listed in Table 3, presented in Fig. 1) with CNVs to be more frequent in tumor subgroups with less malignant properties. Such findings suggest that certain genetic variations may have a more transitory role in cancer progression. They may be crucial for the tumor to reach a certain stage in its development and are then less important for the further disease course. It is also possible that such variations remain present in the tumor but their existence is masked by the clonal expansion of other cancer cells. Consequently when tumor samples are obtained for a study, relevant sections of tumor may not be included and a single sample from large, advanced tumor may not contain all cancer cell clones. Also the aCGH analysis requires the use of extracted DNA from a highly heterogeneous tumor sample where low percentage CNVs may be masked by normal DNA. The protocol implemented in our study certainly introduced further variability into the analysis of HNSCCs, which are considered highly heterogeneous tumors. As a consequence, it is not particularly surprising that associations were not observed for the most common and typical genomic regions implicated in HNSCC. I.e., the gain of 11q13 region containing the *CCND1* gene, was the most frequent CNV in our sample for which we did not detect any significant association (data not shown). Several other genomic regions with important genes showed frequent CNVs (i.e. 7p12, *EGFR* gene) but associations were not present (data not shown) [54]. Such findings can be attributed to a small sample size available for this study which in combination with highly heterogeneous clinical presentation of HNSCC restricts the ability to detect significant associations between genetic markers and clinical parameters. Consequently, we were not able to observe significant differences in survival and this analysis was omitted from the study. In addition, we detected HPV DNA in 5 out of 64 samples (clinical data presented in Table 4) which is significantly below the rate of approximately 20% reported HNSCC cases in Slovenia [55]. Therefore, it was not possible to detect CNVs that are specifically associated with the HPV infection and HNSCC.

## Conclusions

This analysis compared frequencies of genomic copy number variations in subgroups of HNSCC patients which were stratified according to clinical parameters characteristic for early or advanced cancer. We identified gains of genomic regions from 3q containing *PIK3CA* and *AGTR1* genes with significantly higher frequencies in cases with lymph node involvement. The cancer cases which were not treated with surgery also harbored gains of 7q21 and 20q genomic regions significantly more often. Interestingly, other gaines and losses with significant associations were overrepresented in subgroups defined by parameters characteristic for early HNSCC. Nevertheless, many different genes could be implicated in HNSCC development and they all represent a potentially important source of biomarkers useful for clinical management of this cancer and targets for further research.

#### Abbreviations

aCGH: Array comparative genomic hybridization; CNV: Copy number variation; HNSCC: Head and neck squamous cell carcinoma; HPV: Human papilloma virus

#### Acknowledgments

Not applicable.

#### Funding

The study was supported by the University Medical Centre Maibor internal research project IRP-13-01-04.

#### Authors' contributions

B.Z. performed the statistical analysis and drafted the manuscript. D.K. performed DNA extraction, aCGH analysis and helped to draft the manuscript. Š.S.H. performed DNA extraction, HPV typing and helped to draft the manuscript. A.Z. performed aCGH analysis and helped to draft the manuscript. B.Ć. recruited the patients, provided tumor samples, clinical data for each partcipant and helped to draft the manuscript. N.K.V. designed the study, provided the funding, performed aCGH analysis and helped to draft the manuscript. All authors read and approved the final manuscript.

#### Competing interests

The authors declare that they have no competing interests.

#### Author details

[1]Laboratory of Medical Genetics, University Medical Centre Maribor, Ljubljanska 5, 2000 Maribor, Slovenia. [2]Department of Otorhinolaryngology, University Medical Centre Maribor, Ljubljanska 5, 2000 Maribor, Slovenia.

#### References

1. Ferlay J, Soerjomataram I, Dikshit R, Eser S, Mathers C, Rebelo M, Parkin DM, Forman D, Bray F. Cancer incidence and mortality worldwide: sources, methods and major patterns in GLOBOCAN 2012. Int J Cancer. 2015; 136:E359–86.
2. Psyrri A, Licitra L, Lacombe D, Schuuring E, Budach W, Ozsahin M, Knecht R, Vermorken JB, Langendijk JA. Strategies to promote translational research within the European Organization for Research and Treatment of cancer (EORTC) head and neck cancer group: a report from the translational research subcommittee. Ann Oncol. 2010;21:1952–60.
3. Schuuring E. The involvement of the chromosome 11q13 region in human malignancies: cyclin D1 and EMS1 are two new candidate oncogenes–a review. Gene. 1995;159:83–96.
4. Kim HS, Chung WB, Hong SH, Kim JA, Na SY, Jang HJ, Sohn YK, Kim JW. Inactivation of p16INK4a in primary tumors and cell lines of head and neck squamous cell carcinoma. Mol Cells. 2000;10:557–65.
5. Riethdorf S, Friedrich RE, Ostwald C, Barten M, Gogacz P, Gundlach KK, Schlechte H, Becker J, Bregenzer T, Riethdorf L, Löning T. p53 gene mutations and HPV infection in primary head and neck squamous cell carcinomas do not correlate with overall survival: a long-term follow-up study. J Oral Pathol Med. 1997;26:315–21.
6. Grandis JR, Tweardy DJ. Elevated levels of transforming growth factor alpha and epidermal growth factor receptor messenger RNA are early markers of carcinogenesis in head and neck cancer. Cancer Res. 1993;53:3579–84.
7. González MV, Pello MF, López-Larrea C, Suárez C, Menéndez MJ, Coto E. Deletion and methylation of the tumour suppressor gene p16/CDKN2 in primary head and neck squamous cell carcinoma. J Clin Pathol. 1997;50: 509–12.
8. Freier K, Knoepfle K, Fleichtenmacher C, Pungs S, Devens F, Toedt G, Hofele C, Joos S, Lichter P, Radlwimmer B. Recurrent copy number gain of transcription factor SOX2 and corresponding high expression in oral squamous cell carcinoma. Genes Chromosome Canc. 2010;49:9–16.
9. Uchida K, Oga A, Mano T, Mihara M, Kawauchi S, Furuya T, Ueyama Y, Sasaki K. Loss of 3q26.3 is an independent prognostic factor in patients with oral squamous cell carcinoma. Oncol Rep. 2011;26:463–9.
10. Hao JJ, Shi ZZ, Zhao ZX, Zhang Y, Gong T, Li CX, Zhan T, Cai Y, Dong JT, SB F, Zhan QM, Wang MR. Characterization of genetic rearrangements in esophageal squamous carcinoma cell lines by a combination of M-FISH and array-CGH: further confirmation of some split genomic regions in primary tumours. BMC Cancer. 2012;12:367.
11. Baldwin C, Garnis C, Zhang L, Rosin MP, Lam WL. Multiple microalterations detected at high frequency in oral cancer. Cancer Res. 2005;65:7561–7.
12. Kaminagakura E, Werneck da Cunha I, Soares FA, Nishimoto IN, Kowalski LP. CCND1 amplification and protein overexpression in oral squamous cell carcinoma of young patients. Head Neck. 2011;33:1413–9.
13. Rainsbury JW, Ahmed W, Williams HK, Roberts S, Paleri V, Mehanna H. Prognostic biomarkers of survival in oropharyngeal squamous cell carcinoma: systematic review and meta-analysis. Head Neck. 2013;35:1048–55.
14. Reiter M, Baumeister P, Hartmann M, Schwenk-Zieger S, Harréus U. Chemoprevention by celecoxib and mutagen sensitivity of cyclin d1 in patients with oropharyngeal carcinoma. In Vivo. 2014;28:49–53.
15. Pan Q, Gorin MA, Teknos TN. Pharmacotherapy of head and neck squamous cell carcinoma. Expert Opin Pharmacother. 2009;10:2291–302.
16. Lunde ML, Roman E, Warnakulasuriya S, Mehrotra R, Laranne J, Vasstrand EN, Ibrahim SO. Profiling of chromosomal changes in potentially malignant and malignant oral mucosal lesions from south and South-East Asia using array-comparative genomic hybridization. Cancer Genomics Proteomics. 2014;11: 127–40.
17. Qu W, Jiang G, Cruz Y, Chang CJ, Ho GY, Klein RS, Burk RD. PCR detection of human papillomavirus: comparison between MY09/MY11 and GP5+/GP6+ primer systems. J Clin Microbiol. 1997;35:1304–10.
18. Lai K, Killingsworth MC, Lee CS. Gene of the month: PIK3CA. J Clin Pathol. 2015;68:253–7.
19. Samuels Y, Waldman T. Oncogenic mutations of PIK3CA in human cancers. Curr Top Microbiol Immunol. 2010;347:21–41.
20. Lui VW, Hedberg ML, Li H, Vangara BS, Pendleton K, Zeng Y, Lu Y, Zhang Q, Du Y, Gilbert BR, Freilino M, Sauerwein S, Peyser ND, Xiao D, Diergaarde B, Wang L, Chiosea S, Seethala R, Johnson JT, Kim S, Duvvuri U, Ferris RL, Romkes M, Nukui T, Kwok-Shing Ng P, Garraway LA, Hammerman PS, Mills GB, Grandis JR. Frequent mutation of the PI3K pathway in head and neck cancer defines predictive biomarkers. Cancer Discov. 2013;3:761–9.
21. Suda T, Hama T, Kondo S, Yuza Y, Yoshikawa M, Urashima M, Kato T, Moriyama H. Copy number amplification of the PIK3CA gene is associated with poor prognosis in non-lymph node metastatic head and neck squamous cell carcinoma. BMC Cancer. 2012;12:416.
22. Liu CJ, Lin SC, Chen YJ, Chang KM, Chang KW. Array-comparative genomic hybridization to detect genomewide changes in microdissected primary and metastatic oral squamous cell carcinomas. Mol Carcinog. 2006;45:721–31.
23. Wu G, Xing M, Mambo E, Huang X, Liu J, Guo Z, Chatterjee A, Goldenberg D, Gollin SM, Sukumar S, Trink B, Sidransky D. Somatic mutation and gain of copy number of PIK3CA in human breast cancer. Breast Cancer Res. 2005;7:R609–16.
24. Toschi L, Finocchiaro G, Nguyen TT, Skokan MC, Giordano L, Gianoncelli L, Perrino M, Siracusano L, Di Tommaso L, Infante M, Alloisio M, Roncalli M, Scorsetti M, Jänne PA, Santoro A, Varella-Garcia M. Increased SOX2 gene copy number is associated with FGFR1 and PIK3CA gene gain in non-small cell lung cancer and predicts improved survival in early stage disease. PLoS One. 2014;9:e95303.
25. Bellmunt J, Werner L, Leow JJ, Mullane SA, Fay AP, Riester M, Van Hummelen P, Taplin ME, Choueiri TK, Van Allen E, Rosenberg J. Somatic copy number abnormalities and mutations in PI3K/AKT/mTOR pathway have prognostic significance for overall survival in platinum treated locally advanced or metastatic Urothelial tumors. PLoS One. 2015;10:e0124711.
26. Schwaederle M, Elkin SK, Tomson BN, Carter JL, Kurzrock R. Squamousness: next-generation sequencing reveals shared molecular features across squamous tumor types. Cell Cycle. 2015;14:2355–61.
27. Hashimoto K, Tsuda H, Koizumi F, Shimizu C, Yonemori K, Ando M, Kodaira M, Yunokawa M, Fujiwara Y, Tamura K. Activated PI3K/AKT and MAPK pathways are potential good prognostic markers in node-positive, triple-negative breast cancer. Ann Oncol. 2014;25:1973–9.
28. Mitra S, Mukherjee N, Das S, Das P, Panda CK, Chakrabarti J. Anomalous altered expressions of downstream gene-targets in TP53-miRNA pathways in head and neck cancer. Sci Rep. 2014;4:6280.

29. Zhou L, Luo Y, Sato S, Tanabe E, Kitayoshi M, Fujiwara R, Sasaki T, Fujii K, Ohmori H, Kuniyasu H. Role of two types of angiotensin II receptors in colorectal carcinoma progression. Pathobiology. 2014;81:169–75.
30. Rhodes DR, Ateeq B, Cao Q, Tomlins SA, Mehra R, Laxman B, Kalyana-Sundaram S, Lonigro RJ, Helgeson BE, Bhojani MS, Rehemtulla A, Kleer CG, Hayes DF, Lucas PC, Varambally S, Chinnaiyan AM. AGTR1 overexpression defines a subset of breast cancer and confers sensitivity to losartan, an AGTR1 antagonist. Proc Natl Acad Sci U S A. 2009;106:10284–9.
31. Singh A, Nunes JJ, Ateeq B. Role and therapeutic potential of G-protein coupled receptors in breast cancer progression and metastases. Eur J Pharmacol. 2015;763:178–83.
32. Du N, Feng J, Hu LJ, Sun X, Sun HB, Zhao Y, Yang YP, Ren H. Angiotensin II receptor type 1 blockers suppress the cell proliferation effects of angiotensin II in breast cancer cells by inhibiting AT1R signaling. Oncol Rep. 2012;27:1893–903.
33. Hannen EJ, Macville MV, Wienk SM, Slootweg PJ, Manni JJ, Hanselaar AG, de Wilde PC. Different chromosomal imbalances in metastasized and nonmetastasized tongue carcinomas identified by comparative genomic hybridization. Oral Oncol. 2004;40:364–71.
34. Martin CL, Reshmi SC, Ried T, Gottberg W, Wilson JW, Reddy JK, Khanna P, Johnson JT, Myers EN, Gollin SM. Chromosomal imbalances in oral squamous cell carcinoma: examination of 31 cell lines and review of the literature. Oral Oncol. 2008;44:369–82.
35. de la Peña S, Sampieri CL, Ochoa-Lara M, León-Córdoba K, Remes-Troche JM. Expression of the matrix metalloproteases 2, 14, 24, and 25 and tissue inhibitor 3 as potential molecular markers in advanced human gastric cancer. Dis Markers. 2014;2014:285906.
36. Pinzaglia M, Montaldo C, Polinari D, Simone M, La Teana A, Tripodi M, Mancone C, Londei P, Benelli D. EIF6 over-expression increases the motility and invasiveness of cancer cells by modulating the expression of a critical subset of membrane-bound proteins. BMC Cancer. 2015;15:131.
37. Cipriano R, Miskimen KL, Bryson BL, Foy CR, Bartel CA, Jackson MW. Conserved oncogenic behavior of the FAM83 family regulates MAPK signaling in human. Mol Cancer Res. 2014;12:1156–65.
38. Margheri F, Schiavone N, Papucci L, Magnelli L, Serratì S, Chillà A, Laurenzana A, Bianchini F, Calorini L, Torre E, Dotor J, Feijoo E, Fibbi G, Del Rosso M. GDF5 regulates TGFß-dependent angiogenesis in breast carcinoma MCF-7 cells: in vitro and in vivo control by anti-TGFß peptides. PLoS One. 2012;7:e50342.
39. Wang XQ, Tao BB, Li B, Wang XH, Zhang WC, Wan L, Hua XM, Li ST. Overexpression of TREM2 enhances glioma cell proliferation and invasion: a therapeutic target in human glioma. Oncotarget. 2016;7:2354–66.
40. Warnecke-Eberz U, Metzger R, Hölscher AH, Drebber U, Bollschweiler E. Diagnostic marker signature for esophageal cancer from transcriptome analysis. Tumour Biol. 2016;37:6349–58.
41. Sardiello M, Palmieri M, di Ronza A, Medina DL, Valenza M, Gennarino VA, Di Malta C, Donaudy F, Embrione V, Polishchuk RS, Banfi S, Parenti G, Cattaneo E, Ballabio AA. Gene network regulating lysosomal biogenesis and function. Science. 2009;325:473–7.
42. Tan PH, Cheng L, Rioux-Leclercq N, Merino MJ, Netto G, Reuter VE, Shen SS, Grignon DJ, Montironi R, Egevad L, Srigley JR, Delahunt B, Moch H, Renal Tumor ISUP. Panel. Renal tumors: diagnostic and prognostic biomarkers. Am J Surg Pathol. 2013;37:1518–31.
43. Lian M, Fang J, Han D, Ma H, Feng L, Wang R, Yang F. Microarray gene expression analysis of tumorigenesis and regional lymph node metastasis in laryngeal squamous cell carcinoma. PLoS One. 2013;8:e84854.
44. Bruck I, Perez-Arnaiz P, Colbert MK, Kaplan DL. Insights into the initiation of eukaryotic DNA replication. Nucleus. 2015;6(6):449–54.
45. Katafiasz D, Smith LM, Wahl JK 3rd. Slug (SNAI2) expression in oral SCC cells results in altered cell-cell adhesion and increased motility. Cell Adhes Migr. 2011;5:315–22.
46. Zhang J, Cheng Q, Zhou Y, Wang Y, Chen X. Slug is a key mediator of hypoxia induced cadherin switch in HNSCC: correlations with poor prognosis. Oral Oncol. 2013;49:1043–50.
47. Hermsen MA, Joenje H, Arwert F, Braakhuis BJ, Baak JP, Westerveld A, Slater R. Assessment of chromosomal gains and losses in oral squamous cell carcinoma by comparative genomic hybridisation. Oral Oncol. 1997;33:414–8.
48. Garnis C, Baldwin C, Zhang L, Rosin MP, Lam WL. Use of complete coverage array comparative genomic hybridization to define copy number alterations on chromosome 3p in oral squamous cell carcinomas. Cancer Res. 2003;63: 8582–5.
49. Chakraborty SB, Dasgupta S, Roy A, Sengupta A, Ray B, Roychoudhury S, Panda CK. Differential deletions in 3p are associated with the development of head and neck squamous cell carcinoma in Indian patients. Cancer Genet Cytogenet. 2003;146:130–8.
50. Gross AM, Orosco RK, Shen JP, Egloff AM, Carter H, Hofree M, Choueiri M, Coffey CS, Lippman SM, Hayes DN, Cohen EE, Grandis JR, Nguyen QT, Ideker T. Multi-tiered genomic analysis of head and neck cancer ties TP53 mutation to 3p loss. Nat Genet. 2014;46:939–43.
51. Wreesmann VB, Shi W, Thaler HT, Poluri A, Kraus DH, Pfister D, Shaha AR, Shah JP, Rao PH, Singh B. Identification of novel prognosticators of outcome in squamous cell carcinoma of the head and neck. J Clin Oncol. 2004;22:3965–72.
52. Siprashvili Z, Webster DE, Johnston D, Shenoy RM, Ungewickell AJ, Bhaduri A, Flockhart R, Zarnegar BJ, Che Y, Meschi F, Puglisi JD, Khavari PA. The noncoding RNAs SNORD50A and SNORD50B bind K-Ras and are recurrently deleted in human cancer. Nat Genet. 2016;48:53–8.
53. Lebok P, Mittenzwei A, Kluth M, Özden C, Taskin B, Hussein K, Möller K, Hartmann A, Lebeau A, Witzel I, Mahner S, Wölber L, Jänicke F, Geist S, Paluchowski P, Wilke C, Heilenkötter U, Simon R, Sauter G, Terracciano L, Krech R, von der Assen A, Müller V, Burandt E. 8p deletion is strongly linked to poor prognosis in breast cancer. Cancer Biol Ther. 2015;16:1080–7.
54. The Cancer Genome Atlas Network. Comprehensive genomic characterization of head and neck squamous cell carcinomas. Nature. 2015;517:576–82.
55. Strojan P, Zadnik V, Šifrer R, Lanišnik B, Didanović V, Jereb S, Poljak M, Kocjan BJ, Gale N. Incidence trends in head and neck squamous cell carcinoma in Slovenia, 1983-2009: role of human papillomavirus infection. Eur Arch Otorhinolaryngol. 2015;272:3805–14.

# 5

# Analysis of the accuracy of Z-scores of non-invasive prenatal testing for fetal Trisomies 13, 18, and 21 that employs the ion proton semiconductor sequencing platform

Yuan Tian[1], Linlin Zhang[1], Weifang Tian[1], Jinshuang Gao[1], Liting Jia[1*] and Shihong Cui[2]

**Abstract**

**Background:** Non-invasive prenatal testing (NIPT) is frequently being used to screen for trisomies 13, 18 and 21 for prenatal diagnosis. However, NIPT performs poorly when compared with invasive testing and thus should not be used to diagnose trisomies. The result of NIPT for an individual woman in most genome-wide methods is calculated as a Z-score. The aim of this study was to assess the correlation between Z-scores of NIPT results and the accuracy of non-invasive prenatal testing.

**Results:** We evaluated 108 pregnant women with positive NIPT results, which were validated through karyotype analysis of amniotic fluid puncture by means of sequencing, bioinformatics analysis, and follow-up. Utilizing the ion proton semiconductor sequencing platform, we report a performance evaluation of NIPT-positive results at Third Affiliated Hospital of Zhengzhou University of Henan Province, China, by classifying Z-scores as $3 \leq Z<5$, $5 \leq Z < 9$ and $Z \geq 9$. The findings indicate that positive NIPT results at $Z \geq 9$ have a higher accuracy compared with positive NIPT results at $5 \leq Z < 9$ and $3 \leq Z<5$.

**Conclusions:** The findings show that Z-scores of NIPT results are closely related to the accuracy of non-invasive prenatal testing. However, false-positive NIPT results at $3 \leq Z<5$ may occur due to confined placental mosaicism (CPM).

**Keywords:** Non-invasive prenatal testing (NIPT), False positive, Confined placental mosaicism (CPM), Trisomies

## Background

Non-invasive prenatal testing (NIPT) is frequently being applied to screen for trisomies 13, 18 and 21 for prenatal diagnosis. Due to its simple operation and avoidance of amniocentesis, NIPT, as opposed to invasive procedures (chorionic villus sampling (CVS) or amniotic fluid), is regarded as the first choice when screening is required for fetal assessment in pregnant women. Indeed, NIPT is an attractive option because it is procedurally safe for both mother and fetus, can be conducted as early as 10 weeks of gestation, and is highly accurate [1]. Nonetheless, NIPT performs poorly when compared with invasive testing and thus should not be used to diagnose trisomies [2]. Confined placental mosaicism (CPM), which can occur through a mitotic nondisjunction event or through aneuploidy rescue, has one of the greatest obstacles on NIPT result confirmation [3]. CPM is a phenomenon whereby a cytogenetic abnormality, most often trisomy, is confined to the placenta [4]. False-positive NIPT results can occur due to CPM.

Recent NIPT technologies are predominantly based on next-generation sequencing (NGS) [5]. NGS enables rapid and effective clinical testing such as the IONA® test, which uses the Ion proton semiconductor sequencing platform, has a turnaround time, from the start of sample processing to the result, of 3 days [6]. For most genome-wide methods, the result of NIPT for an individual woman is calculated as a Z-score, where the

* Correspondence: jialiting@sina.com
[1]Department of Clinical Laboratory, The Third Affiliated Hospital of Zhengzhou University, No. 7 Front Kangfu Street, Er'qi District, Zhengzhou 450052, China
Full list of author information is available at the end of the article

individual sample is compared with a control group of normal (diploid) samples. In some research, an a posteriori risk (PPR) calculator is used to more accurately express the true likelihood of carrying a fetus with a trisomy. For an individual woman, a positive NIPT result with a sensitivity and specificity of more than 99% does not necessarily indicate that she actually has more than a 99% chance of carrying a fetus with a trisomy. The true likelihood depends not only on the NIPT result but also on the prevalence of the anomaly in the population to which she belongs [7], which is expressed as an a priori risk. Thus, to properly counsel women about a positive result by cell-free fetal DNA screening, it can be useful to express the result as a personalized PPR, which takes the woman's a priori risk into account. Research shows that PPR is effectively independent under all conditions for Z-scores above 6, and high PPR for low a priori risk can only be reached at Z-scores> 5 [8].

In the present study, we report a performance evaluation of NIPT-positive results in our hospital by classifying Z-scores as $3 \leq Z<5$, $5 \leq Z < 9$ and $Z \geq 9$. The results of our study indicate that positive NIPT results with Z-scores of $Z \geq 9$ have higher accuracy compared with positive NIPT results with Z-scores of $3 \leq Z<5$ and $5 \leq Z < 9$.

## Methods

### Patients

Written informed consent was obtained from each patient. The study was a retrospective analysis of NIPT-positive results in singleton pregnancies from January 2015 to December 2017 at Third Affiliated Hospital of Zhengzhou University of Henan Province, China. Positive NIPT results would be validated through postpartum follow-up of patients, involving the results of karyotype analysis via amniotic fluid puncture, including trisomies 13, 18, and 21 (T21, T18 and T13); 108 cases were validated in this manner.

### Sequencing process

Maternal peripheral blood (5 ml) was collected into an ethylenediaminetetraacetic acid (EDTA) tube at 12 + 0 to 25 + 6 weeks of gestation. The blood samples were stored at 4 °C immediately after collection. Plasma was isolated within 8 h through a two-step centrifugation protocol, after which the samples were stored at − 80 °C. Cell-free DNA extraction, library construction, sequencing, and bioinformatics analysis were performed according to a previous study [6].

### Bioinformatics analysis

Sequencing data were analyzed by using the ion proton semiconductor sequencing platform and software from Capitalbio Corporation. The binary hypothesis Z-score of particular chromosomes in each sample was determined, as reported previously [7]. To assess fetal risk of T21, T18 and T13, sample with a Z-score ≥ 3 for these chromosomes was classified as positive. We classified the positive samples into three groups according to Z-score = 5 and Z = 9 among them. Group 1 contained samples with NIPT results of $3 \leq Z<5$. Group 2 contained samples with NIPT results of $5 \leq Z<9$. Group 3 contained samples with NIPT results of $Z \geq 9$.

### Karyotype analysis and amniotic fluid puncture

For those with positive NIPT results, karyotype analysis and amniotic fluid puncture were recommended for validation. Amniotic fluid puncture was performed as routinely described; karyotype analysis was performed according to the International System for Human Cytogenetic Nomenclature guidelines [9].

### Follow-up

Follow-up for NIPT-positive cases was performed via telephone. The follow-up duration was 56 days after delivery.

## Results

### Patient characteristics

A total of 21,114 pregnant women were tested by NIPT from 2015 to 2017, with 202 having positive results. According to follow-up, cases of induced labor that was not validated through other invasive methods were removed. Overall, 108 NIPT positive women who were validated via karyotype analysis and amniotic fluid puncture, with a mean maternal age of 33.5 (19–48 years), were included in this study. Gestational age was from 12 weeks to 25 + 6 weeks at blood sample collection. Because the fetal DNA fraction in NIPT needs to be higher than 4% for a singleton and 8% for twins, pregnant women tend to accept NIPT at more than 16 weeks to obtain a higher fetal fraction. As cases of NIPT-positive results should be validated through karyotype analysis and amniotic fluid puncture, we would suggest that the patients accept NIPT within 20 weeks. The patient characteristics are listed in Table 1.

### Relationship of NIPT-positive results group 1 with karyotype analysis and amniotic fluid puncture

In total, 18 NIPT-positive cases were included in Group 1 ($3 \leq Z<5$); 15 cases with false-positive results were validated through karyotype analysis and amniotic fluid puncture. Conversely, 3 true-positive cases were validated through karyotype analysis and amniotic fluid puncture, with a positive predictive value (PPV) of only 16.67%. The NIPT-positive cases in Group 1 are listed in Table 2. By analyzing the data of the 3 true-positive NIPT cases, we found that the fetal DNA fraction

**Table 1** Basic Characteristics of 108 NIPT-Positive Patients

| Characteristics | Numbers |
|---|---|
| Maternal age(years) | |
| ≤ 20 | 1 |
| 20–24 | 5 |
| 25–29 | 31 |
| 30–34 | 21 |
| 35–39 | 35 |
| 40–45 | 13 |
| ≥ 45 | 2 |
| Mean | 33.5 |
| Range | 19–48 |
| Gestation at NIPT tests(weeks) | |
| 12–12 + 6 | 4 |
| 13–13 + 6 | 9 |
| 14–14 + 6 | 5 |
| 15–15 + 6 | 8 |
| 16–16 + 6 | 17 |
| 17–17 + 6 | 14 |
| 18–18 + 6 | 14 |
| 19–19 + 6 | 17 |
| 20–20 + 6 | 5 |
| 21–21 + 6 | 6 |
| 22–22 + 6 | 2 |
| 23–23 + 6 | 5 |
| 24–24 + 6 | 0 |
| 25–25 + 6 | 2 |

**Table 2** The 18 NIPT-Positive Cases in Group 1 (3 ≤ Z<5)

| No. | Sample ID | Z-scores | NIPT results | Fetal karyotype |
|---|---|---|---|---|
| 1 | YC150550 | 3.330 | T21 | 46,XN |
| 2 | YC150816 | 4.342 | T13 | 46,XN |
| 3 | YC151439 | 3.643 | T21 | 47,XN + 21 |
| 4 | YC161217 | 4.056 | T13 | 46,XN |
| 5 | YC163341 | 4.778 | T13 | 46,XN |
| 6 | YC164267 | 3.968 | T13 | 46,XN |
| 7 | YC165157 | 3.392 | T21 | 46,XN |
| 8 | YC165602 | 3.362 | T18 | 46,XN |
| 9 | YC167031 | 3.075 | T21 | 46,XN |
| 10 | YC171503 | 3.207 | T21 | 46,XN |
| 11 | YC173711 | 4.951 | T21 | 47,XN + 21 |
| 12 | YC174141 | 3.242 | T21 | 47,XN + 21 |
| 13 | YC175988 | 3.713 | T21 | 46,XN |
| 14 | YC175996 | 4.111 | T18 | 46,XN |
| 15 | YC176477 | 3.351 | T18 | 46,XN |
| 16 | YC176775 | 3.620 | T21 | 46,XN |
| 17 | YC177355 | 3.263 | T21 | 46,XN |
| 18 | YC177383 | 3.697 | T13 | 46,XN |

estimation for samples YC151439 and YC173711 was less than 4%; the fetal DNA fraction estimation for sample YC174141 was 6.4%, which was less than 8%.

## Relationship of NIPT-positive results for group 2 with karyotype analysis and amniotic fluid puncture

A total of 34 NIPT-positive cases were in Group 2 (5 ≤ Z<9). Four cases of false positivity were validated through karyotype analysis and amniotic fluid puncture. In contrast, 30 true-positive results were validated via karyotype analysis and amniotic fluid puncture, with a PPV of 88.24%. Table 3 lists the positive NIPT cases in Group 2.

Based on analysis of the data for the 4 false-positive cases, sample YC167160 was validated as CPM through karyotype analysis and amniotic fluid puncture (Table 3). Sample YC160356 was possibly affected by chromosome duplication from the maternal fragment (Fig. 1). The false-positive NIPT result for samples YC166422 and YC177345 might have resulted from a small region of chromosome duplication (Fig. 2 and Fig. 3).

## Relationship of NIPT-positive results for group 3 with karyotype analysis and amniotic fluid puncture

Group 3 (Z ≥ 9) comprised 56 cases of NIPT positivity. Only one false-positive case was validated by karyotype analysis and amniotic fluid puncture. For sample YC175377, a unique sample with a false-positive result, a unique sample with a false-positive result, the discordant NIPT result was caused by a vanished twin, as revealed by NIPT in the 4 weeks during follow-up. In total, 55 true-positive cases were validated through karyotype analysis and amniotic fluid puncture; the PPV was 98.12%. The positive NIPT cases in Group 3 are listed in Table 4.

Among all of the 21,114 patients accepting NIPT, two cases of false-negative NIPT results were found. However, those with false-negative NIPT results refused to accept further validation of aborted tissue.

## Discussion

NIPT has been widely used in the last few years for prenatal screening of T21, T18 and T13. Although PPR calculation suggests that high PPR for low a priori risk can only be reached at Z-scores> 5 [7], large-scale clinical studies to validate the hypothesis are lacking. The present study including 108 NIPT-positive cases was

**Table 3** The 34 NIPT-Positive Cases in Group 2 (5 ≤ Z<9)

| No. | Sample ID | Z-scores | NIPT results | Fetal karyotype |
|---|---|---|---|---|
| 1 | YC150539 | 5.570 | T21 | 47,XN + 21 |
| 2 | YC150431 | 5.960 | T18 | 47,XN + 18 |
| 3 | YC150725 | 7.463 | T21 | 47,XN + 21 |
| 4 | YC152284 | 8.249 | T21 | 47,XN + 21 |
| 5 | YC153184 | 8.532 | T21 | 47,XN + 21 |
| 6 | YC160356 | 8.830 | T21 | 46,XN |
| 7 | YC161880 | 8.188 | T21 | 47,XN + 21 |
| 8 | YC163276 | 5.467 | T18 | 47,XN + 18 |
| 9 | YC163808 | 6.104 | T21 | 47,XN + 21 |
| 10 | YC164065 | 5.219 | T18 | 47,XN + 18 |
| 11 | YC164811 | 8.489 | T21 | 47,XN + 21 |
| 12 | YC165074 | 6.677 | T21 | 47,XN + 21 |
| 13 | YC165729 | 5.944 | T21 | 47,XN + 21 |
| 14 | YC166180 | 6.150 | T21 | 47,XN + 21 |
| 15 | YC166202 | 6.220 | T18 | 47,XN + 18 |
| 16 | YC166253 | 5.931 | T21 | 46XX + 21, der(14;15)(q10,q10) |
| 17 | YC166422 | 8.945 | T13 | 46,XN |
| 18 | YC167160 | 5.710 | T18 | 46,XX/47,XX + 18(28:2) |
| 19 | YC167331 | 7.790 | T21 | 47,XN + 21 |
| 20 | YC168025 | 6.840 | T21 | 47,XN + 21 |
| 21 | YC170096 | 8.280 | T21 | 47,XN + 21 |
| 22 | YC171234 | 6.119 | T21 | 47,XN + 21 |
| 23 | YC171535 | 7.273 | T21 | 47,XN + 21 |
| 24 | YC171540 | 6.019 | T21 | 47,XN + 21 |
| 25 | YC173331 | 5.330 | T21 | 47,XN + 21 |
| 26 | YC173539 | 7.514 | T21 | 47,XN + 21 |
| 27 | YC173759 | 6.834 | T21 | 47,XN + 21 |
| 28 | YC175051 | 6.908 | T21 | 47,XN + 21 |
| 29 | YC175492 | 8.646 | T18 | 47,XN + 18 |
| 30 | YC175694 | 6.704 | T13 | 47,XN + 13 |
| 31 | YC176740 | 7.803 | T21 | 47,XN + 21 |
| 32 | YC177345 | 5.178 | T21 | 46,XN |
| 33 | YC176881 | 5.566 | T21 | 47,XN + 21 |
| 34 | YC177644 | 8.523 | T21 | 47,XN + 21 |

performed to investigate the relationship between NIPT Z-scores and accuracy of trisomy 13, 18, and 21 diagnosis.

The PPV is much more meaningful to clinicians and patients than the commonly reported measures of sensitivity and specificity [10]. The PPV referred to here is a population-based figure that reports the chance prior to testing that an abnormal test result is actually reflective of the karyotype of the fetus. Except for the PPV, neither sensitivity nor specificity reflects the prevalence of a disorder in the population [10]. Based on the results of the present study, a sample with Z ≥ 9 has higher accuracy than does a sample with 3 ≤ Z<5 or 5 ≤ Z<9. Although the PPV rate in Group 2 (88.24%) was apparently higher that of Group 1 (16.67%), this approach cannot be used for diagnosis because of the relatively high false-positive rate (11.76%). Nonetheless, positive results at Z ≥ 9 are significant for diagnosing trisomies 13, 18 and 21; However, karyotype analysis is necessary for validating trisomies due to the exist of sample YC175377, whose discordant NIPT result may be caused by a vanished twin. There are many biological reasons for discordant results that can be of either fetal or maternal origin. Contributing fetal factors include an insufficient or absent fetal fraction, confined placental mosaicism and the presence of a vanishing twin [11]. For example, Hall AL et al. reported a case that confirmed positive cell-free fetal DNA (cffDNA) testing for trisomy 13, revealing confined placental mosaicism [12]. In addition, Chen C et al. reported a pregnancy with discordant fetal and placental chromosome 18 aneuploidies, as revealed by invasive and noninvasive prenatal diagnoses [13].

CPM is one of the major factors causing false positivity. cffDNA originates from chorionic villi in the placenta, where the constant turnover of cytotrophoblasts induces apoptosis and cffDNA release into the maternal blood. The cytotrophoblast layer of chorionic villi is not always representative of the fetus, as it is derived from the trophoblast of the blastocyst; in contrast, the fetus is derived from the inner cell mass (epiblast) [14]. Postzygotic mitotic division errors in chromosomally normal

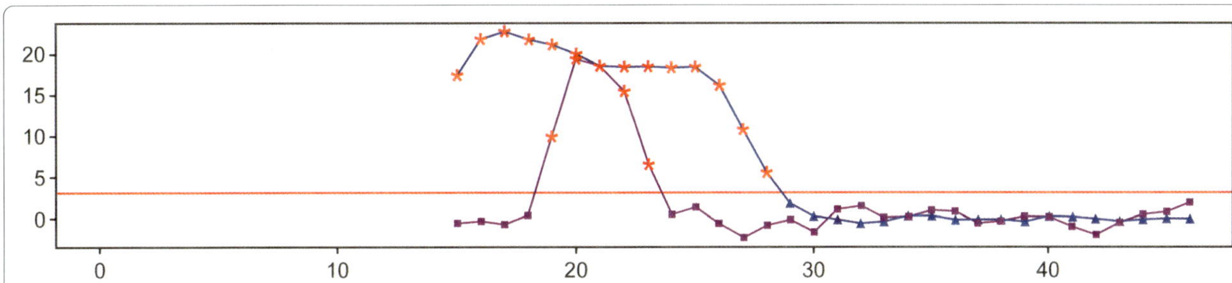


**Fig. 1** The Distribution Curve of Z-scores for Chromosome 21 of Sample YC160356

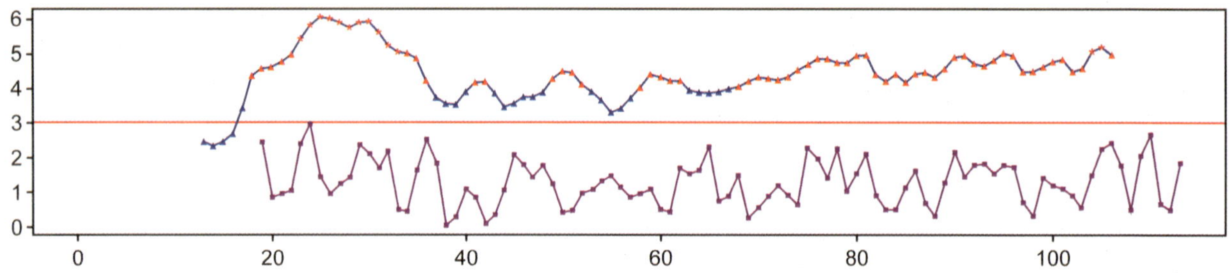

**Fig. 2** The Distribution Curve of Z-scores for Chromosome 13 of Sample YC166422

and abnormal conceptuses will lead to chromosomal mosaicism [15]. Most often, mosaicism is characterized as CPM, in which the abnormal cell line is confined to the cytotrophoblast and/or the mesenchymal core of the chorion villi, whereas the fetus has a normal karyotype [15]. If abnormal cells are restricted to the cytotrophoblast layer and are not present in the mesenchymal core or fetus, such a case is categorized CPM and depending on the extent of mosaicism, will possibly cause a false-positive NIPT result. According to the above, we suggest that the occurrence of CPM may slightly elevate a Z-score for NIPT, higher than 3 but lower than 5.

In addition, estimation of the fetal DNA fraction is important for the accuracy of NIPT results. The definition of the fetal fraction of circulating cell-free DNA in maternal blood is the amount of cffDNA divided by the amount of total cell-free DNA. The circulating cell-free DNA (cfDNA) in a pregnant woman is a mixture of predominant maternal DNA derived from her hematopoietic system and fetal DNA released through apoptosis of cytotrophoblast cells during fetal development [16]. A fetal DNA concentration of less than 4% in a maternal plasma sample would suggest a potential issue present in the quality control (QC) step [17]. Methods for calculating the fetal fraction differ between laboratories. We are aware of six different methods based on methylation [18], single-nucleotide polymorphisms [19], quantitative polymerase chain reaction of the Y-chromosome (only for male fetuses) [20], autosomal regional read counts calculated by SeqFF [21], differences in length between cffDNA and maternal cffDNA [21] and single reads nucleosome-based fetal fraction [22]. The fetal fraction is also related to maternal weight and body mass index. For example, the increased turnover of adipocytes in obese women increases the amount of maternal cell-free DNA and decreases the cffDNA fraction [23]. Furthermore, gestational age influences the fetal fraction. Some research has found that levels of cffDNA increase at 0.1% per week between 10 and 21 weeks of gestation and at 1% per week beyond 21 weeks of gestation [24]. Because the limited amount of fetal DNA molecules to be detected and analyzed may give rise to a false-negative result, we deduce that the Z-scores of samples YC151439, YC173711 and YC174141 were less than 5 because of the estimation of a low fetal DNA fraction.

Regardless, maternally derived chromosomal abnormalities (likely also submicroscopic abnormalities) constitute a rare case of maternal occult malignancy and usually cause false-positive results [25]. Our study validated the hypothesis regarding the false-positive NIPT result for sample YC160356 (Fig. 1).

## Conclusions

NIPT is feasible for prenatal screening of T13, T18 and T21, with higher sensitivity and specificity compared with conventional methods. However, Z-scores of NIPT results are closely related to the accuracy of non-invasive prenatal

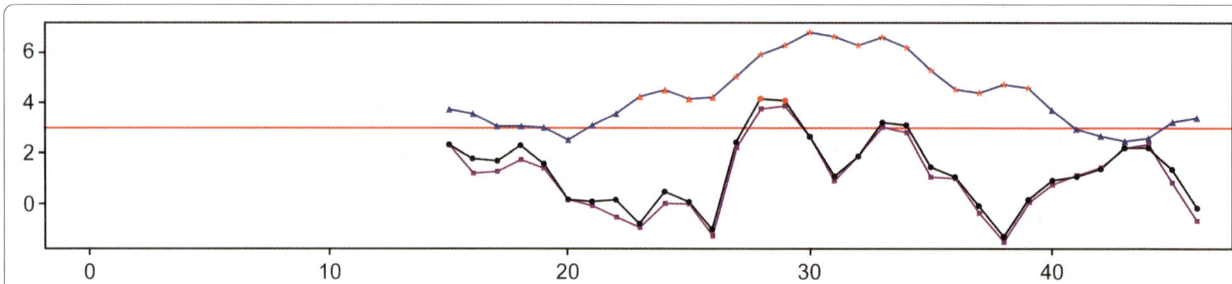

**Fig. 3** The Distribution Curve of Z-scores for Chromosome 21 of Sample YC177345

**Table 4** The 56 NIPT-Positive Cases in Group 2 (Z ≥ 9)

| No. | Sample ID | Z-scores | NIPT results | Fetal karyotype |
|---|---|---|---|---|
| 1 | YC151198 | 11.203 | T21 | 47,XN + 21 |
| 2 | YC151297 | 11.605 | T21 | 47,XN + 21 |
| 3 | YC151374 | 9.306 | T21 | 47,XN + 21 |
| 4 | YC151424 | 19.541 | T21 | 47,XN + 21 |
| 5 | YC151577 | 14.882 | T21 | 47,XN + 21 |
| 6 | YC151725 | 12.367 | T21 | 47,XN + 21 |
| 7 | YC152585 | 18.082 | T21 | 47,XN + 21 |
| 8 | YC153464 | 10.126 | T21 | 47,XN + 21 |
| 9 | YC153533 | 11.864 | T21 | 47,XN + 21 |
| 10 | YC160344 | 14.298 | T21 | 47,XN + 21 |
| 11 | YC161058 | 10.8 | T21 | 47,XN + 21 |
| 12 | YC161066 | 21.457 | T21 | 47,XN + 21 |
| 13 | YC161368 | 13.275 | T21 | 47,XN + 21 |
| 14 | YC162688 | 9.707 | T21 | 47,XN + 21 |
| 15 | YC162822 | 16.21 | T18 | 47,XN + 18 |
| 16 | YC162943 | 11.347 | T21 | 47,XN + 21 |
| 17 | YC163223 | 13.691 | T21 | 47,XN + 21 |
| 18 | YC163261 | 13.627 | T21 | 47,XN + 21 |
| 19 | YC163310 | 13.977 | T18 | 47,XN + 18 |
| 20 | YC163400 | 11.603 | T13 | 47,XN + 13 |
| 21 | YC164204 | 10.546 | T21 | 47,XN + 21 |
| 22 | YC164355 | 11.135 | T21 | 47,XN + 21 |
| 23 | YC164722 | 13.955 | T21 | 47,XN + 21 |
| 24 | YC164999 | 13.661 | T21 | 47,XN + 21 |
| 25 | YC165003 | 11.899 | T18 | 47,XN + 18 |
| 26 | YC165723 | 10.192 | T21 | 47,XN + 21 |
| 27 | YC165823 | 10.346 | T18 | 47,XN + 18 |
| 28 | YC165859 | 11.962 | T18 | 47,XN + 18 |
| 29 | YC166626 | 9.374 | T13 | 47,XN + 13 |
| 30 | YC167544 | 11.253 | T18 | 47,XN + 18 |
| 31 | YC168149 | 11.004 | T21 | 47,XN + 21 |
| 32 | YC170133 | 12.085 | T21 | 47,XN + 21 |
| 33 | YC170411 | 12.536 | T21 | 47,XN + 21 |
| 34 | YC170724 | 10.017 | T21 | 47,XN + 21 |
| 35 | YC170829 | 12.456 | T21 | 47,XN + 21 |
| 36 | YC170974 | 11.555 | T21 | 47,XN + 21 |
| 37 | YC171134 | 9.885 | T21 | 47,XN + 21 |
| 38 | YC171423 | 11.41 | T21 | 47,XN + 21 |
| 39 | YC172015 | 18.693 | T21 | 47,XN + 21 |
| 40 | YC172946 | 20.224 | T21 | 47,XN + 21 |
| 41 | YC173326 | 9.674 | T21 | 47,XN + 21 |
| 42 | YC173370 | 17.431 | T21 | 47,XN + 21 |
| 43 | YC173573 | 26.587 | T21 | 47,XN + 21 |
| 44 | YC173742 | 9.054 | T21 | 47,XN + 21 |
| 45 | YC174011 | 13.767 | T21 | 47,XN + 21 |
| 46 | YC174110 | 11.488 | T21 | 47,XN + 21 |
| 47 | YC174589 | 16.765 | T21 | 47,XN + 21 |
| 48 | YC175377 | 12.367 | T18 | 46,XN |
| 49 | YC175406 | 11.424 | T21 | 47,XN + 21 |
| 50 | YC175583 | 9.772 | T21 | 47,XN + 21 |
| 51 | YC175824 | 13.609 | T21 | 47,XN + 21 |
| 52 | YC175903 | 12.095 | T21 | 47,XN + 21 |
| 53 | YC176469 | 11.443 | T18 | 47,XN + 18 |
| 54 | YC177386 | 25.448 | T18 | 47,XN + 18 |
| 55 | YC176915 | 12.225 | T21 | 47,XN + 21 |
| 56 | YC178093 | 18.509 | T18 | 47,XN + 18 |

testing that employs the ion proton semiconductor sequencing platform. NIPT results with low Z-scores should not be used for diagnosis, which should be performed using invasive testing. However, the relationship between Z-scores of NIPT and CPM lacks validation by clinical trials due to the influence of chorionic villi in the placenta.

#### Abbreviations

cfDNA: Circulating cell-free DNA; CPM: Confined placental mosaicism; EDTA: Ethylenediaminetetraacetic acid; NIPT: Non-invasive prenatal testing; QC: Quality control

#### Author contributions

YT performed the bioinformatics analysis and drafted the manuscript. LZ performed karyotype analysis, amniotic fluid puncture and follow-up. WT recruited the patients, provided blood samples and clinical data for each participant and helped to draft the manuscript. JG performed the NIPT. LJ performed the statistical analysis and helped to draft the manuscript. SC took a plan for the research. All authors read and approved the final manuscript.

#### Funding

National Key Research and Development Program of China,2016YFC1000700,2016YFC1000703.

#### Competing interests

The authors declare that they have no competing interests.

#### Author details

[1]Department of Clinical Laboratory, The Third Affiliated Hospital of Zhengzhou University, No. 7 Front Kangfu Street, Er'qi District, Zhengzhou 450052, China. [2]Department of gynaecology and obstetrics, The Third Affiliated Hospital of Zhengzhou University, No. 7 Front Kangfu Street, Er'qi District, Zhengzhou 450052, China.

#### References

1. Minear MA, Lewis C, Pradhan S, et al. Global perspectives on clinical adoption of NIPT. Prenat Diagn. 2015;35(10):959–67.
2. Lau TK, Cheung SW, Lo PS, et al. Non-invasive prenatal testing for fetal chromosomal abnormalities by low-coverage whole-genome sequencing of maternal plasma DNA: review of 1982 consecutive cases in a single center. Ultrasound Obstet Gynecol. 2014;43(3):254–64.
3. Mardy A, Wapner RJ. Confined placental mosaicism and its impact on confirmation of NIPT results. Am J Med Genet C Semin Med Genet. 2016; 172(2):118–22.

4. Kalousek DK, Vekemans M. Confined placental mosaicism. J Med Genet. 1996;33(7):529–33.
5. Vrachnis N, Vlachadis N, Creatsas G. DNA sequencing versus standard prenatal aneuploidy screening. N Engl J Med. 2014;371(6):578.
6. Papageorghiou AT, Khalil A, Forman M, et al. Clinical evaluation of the IONA test: a non-invasive prenatal screening test for trisomies 21, 18 and 13. Ultrasound Obstet Gynecol. 2016;47(2):188–93.
7. Morain S, Greene MF, Mello MM. A new era in noninvasive prenatal testing. N Engl J Med. 2013;369(6):499–501.
8. Sikkema-Raddatz B, Johansson LF, de Boer EN, et al. NIPTRIC: an online tool for clinical interpretation of non-invasive prenatal testing (NIPT) results. Sci Rep. 2016;6:38359.
9. Gonzalez GJ, Meza-Espinoza JP. Use of the international system for human cytogenetic nomenclature (ISCN). BLOOD. 2006;108(12):3952–3.
10. Meck JM, Kramer DE, Matyakhina L, et al. Noninvasive prenatal screening for aneuploidy: positive predictive values based on cytogenetic findings. Am J Obstet Gynecol. 2015;213(2):211–4.
11. Grati FR. Implications of fetoplacental mosaicism on cell-free DNA testing: a review of a common biological phenomenon. Ultrasound Obstet Gynecol. 2016;48(4):415–23.
12. Hall AL, Drendel HM, Verbrugge JL, et al. Positive cell-free fetal DNA testing for trisomy 13 reveals confined placental mosaicism. GENET MED. 2013; 15(9):729–32.
13. Chen C, Cram DS, Xie F, et al. A pregnancy with discordant fetal and placental chromosome 18 aneuploidies revealed by invasive and noninvasive prenatal diagnosis. Reprod BioMed Online. 2014;29(1):136–9.
14. Bianchi DW, Wilkins-Haug LE, Enders AC, et al. Origin of extraembryonic mesoderm in experimental animals: relevance to chorionic mosaicism in humans. Am J Med Genet. 1993;46(5):542–50.
15. Malvestiti F, Agrati C, Grimi B, et al. Interpreting mosaicism in chorionic villi: results of a monocentric series of 1001 mosaics in chorionic villi with follow-up amniocentesis. Prenat Diagn. 2015;35(11):1117–27.
16. Peng XL, Jiang P. Bioinformatics Approaches for Fetal DNA Fraction Estimation in Noninvasive Prenatal Testing. Int J Mol Sci. 2017:18(2).
17. Canick JA, Palomaki GE, Kloza EM, et al. The impact of maternal plasma DNA fetal fraction on next generation sequencing tests for common fetal aneuploidies. Prenat Diagn. 2013;33(7):667–74.
18. Poon LL, Leung TN, Lau TK, et al. Differential DNA methylation between fetus and mother as a strategy for detecting fetal DNA in maternal plasma. Clin Chem. 2002;48(1):35–41.
19. Dar P, Curnow KJ, Gross SJ, et al. Clinical experience and follow-up with large scale single-nucleotide polymorphism-based noninvasive prenatal aneuploidy testing. Am J Obstet Gynecol. 2014;211(5):521–7.
20. Hudecova I, Sahota D, Heung MM, et al. Maternal plasma fetal DNA fractions in pregnancies with low and high risks for fetal chromosomal aneuploidies. PLoS One. 2014;9(2):e88484.
21. Kim SK, Hannum G, Geis J, et al. Determination of fetal DNA fraction from the plasma of pregnant women using sequence read counts. Prenat Diagn. 2015;35(8):810–5.
22. Straver R, Oudejans CB, Sistermans EA, et al. Calculating the fetal fraction for noninvasive prenatal testing based on genome-wide nucleosome profiles. Prenat Diagn. 2016;36(7):614–21.
23. Haghiac M, Vora NL, Basu S, et al. Increased death of adipose cells, a path to release cell-free DNA into systemic circulation of obese women. Obesity (Silver Spring). 2012;20(11):2213–9.
24. Wang E, Batey A, Struble C, et al. Gestational age and maternal weight effects on fetal cell-free DNA in maternal plasma. Prenat Diagn. 2013; 33(7):662–6.
25. Bianchi DW, Chudova D, Sehnert AJ, et al. Noninvasive prenatal testing and incidental detection of occult maternal malignancies. JAMA. 2015; 314(2):162–9.

6

# The exon junction complex factor Y14 is dynamic in the nucleus of the beetle *Tribolium castaneum* during late oogenesis

Artem M. Kiselev[1,2,3], Irina S. Stepanova[1], Leonid S. Adonin[1], Florina M. Batalova[1^], Vladimir N. Parfenov[1^], Dmitry S. Bogolyubov[1*] and Olga I. Podgornaya[1,4,5*]

**Abstract**

**Background:** The oocyte chromosomes of the red flour beetle, *Tribolium castaneum*, are gathered into a knot, forming a karyosphere at the diplotene stage of meiotic prophase. Chromatin rearrangement, which is a characteristic feature of oocyte maturation, is well documented. The *T. castaneum* karyosphere is surrounded by a complex extrachromosomal structure termed the karyosphere capsule. The capsule contains the vast majority of oocyte RNA. We have previously shown using a BrUTP assay that oocyte chromosomes in *T. castaneum* maintain residual transcription up to the very end of oocyte maturation. Karyosphere transcription requires evidently not only transcription factors but also mRNA processing factors, including the components of the exon junction complex with its core component, the splicing factor Y14. We employed a gene engineering approach with injection of mRNA derived from the Myc-tagged Y14 plasmid-based construct in order to monitor the newly synthesized fusion protein in the oocyte nuclei.

**Results:** Our preliminary data have been presented as a brief correspondence elsewhere. Here, we provide a full-length article including immunoelectron-microscopy localization data on Y14–Myc distribution in the nucleus of previtellogenic and vitellogenic oocytes. The injections of the fusion protein Y14–Myc mRNA into the oocytes showed a dynamic pattern of the protein distribution. At the previtellogenic stage, there are two main locations for the protein: SC35 domains (the analogues of interchromatin granule clusters or nuclear speckles) and the karyosphere capsule. At the vitellogenic stage, SC35 domains were devoid of labels, and Y14–Myc was found in the perichromatin region of the karyosphere, presumably at the places of residual transcription. We show that karyosphere formation is accompanied by the movement of a nuclear protein while the residual transcription occurs during genome inactivation.

**Conclusions:** Our data indicate that the karyosphere capsule, being a destination site for a protein involved in mRNA splicing and export, is not only a specializes part of nuclear matrix separating the karyosphere from the products of chromosome activity, as believed previously, but represents a special nuclear compartment involved in the processes of gene expression in the case the karyosphere retains residual transcription activity.

**Keywords:** *Tribolium castaneum*, Y14 (Tsunagi), Oocyte nucleus, Karyosphere, Karyosphere capsule, Interchromatin granule clusters, Microinjections, Molecular cloning, Gene manipulation, Transcription in vitro

* Correspondence: dbogol@mail.ru; dmitr@incras.ru; opodg@yahoo.com; o.podgornaya@spbu.ru
^Deceased
[1]Laboratory of Cell Morphology, Institute of Cytology, Russian Academy of Sciences, St. Petersburg 194064, Russia
Full list of author information is available at the end of the article

## Background

The red flour beetle, *Tribolium castaneum*, a member of the family Tenebrionidae, is a significant pest wherever processed grain products are in abundance. *Tribolium* has a generation time of 3–8 weeks depending on temperature and can reproduce for a long time [1]. These features make *Tribolium* an ideal lab animal and it thus became an early and important model of classical genetics, in particular population genetics [2].

The *T. castaneum* genome is the first genome of a beetle that has been sequenced [3], and its database is being constantly revised to provide more comprehensive genomic information [4]. At an estimated 160 Mb, the euchromatic genome of *T. castaneum* is about one-third bigger than that of *Drosophila*. Also in terms of gene number, *T. castaneum* currently scores higher, with an estimated about 16 thousands genes [3, 5]. What is more noteworthy is that, by and large, *Tribolium* seems to be 'less derived' than some of other insects for which the genomes have been sequenced, in particular the fruitfly and the mosquito. Overall, *T. castaneum* shares more genes with humans than the dipterans do. *Tribolium* researchers are surely be tempted to use this finding to argue that this organism is 'more ancestral', 'more representative' or simply 'less weird' than *Drosophila* [2]. Now the beetle becomes a model of the developmental biology [6, 7]. The key event of development is gametogenesis, but morphological descriptions of the *T. castaneum* oocyte nucleus (germinal vesicle, GV) were absent in the literature until the beginning of our work [8].

In general, nuclear architecture comprises a number of extrachromosomal structures, nuclear compartments, or domains [9–11]. The great bulk of comprehensive studies that allow deciphering the role of nuclear domains in the support of mRNA during its journey in the nucleus to the nuclear pore are being made on mammalian tissue-culture somatic cells. It is still unclear whether the results of these studies are fully applicable for other cell types, especially for specialized cells such as the oocytes.

In many organisms including beetles, oocyte chromosomes join together in a limited volume of the GV, forming a karyosphere (karyosome) during the diplotene stage of meiotic prophase [12]. Oocyte chromosomes assembled into the karyosphere may be additionally separated from the rest of the nucleoplasm by a complex extrachromosomal structure termed the karyosphere capsule (KC). Similar KC develops in the nucleus of *Tribolium* oocytes. Biological significance of the KC is still unclear. It is generally assumed that the KC represents a specialized component of oocyte nuclear matrix supporting the chromosomes in large GVs [12, 13]. However, immunolocalization studies carried out on the GV of a weevil [14] and the red flour beetle [8] have suggested the KC could also represent a peculiar storage compartment for pre-mRNA processing factors. Our data shows that the perichromatin region (PR), i.e., the space between the KC and condensed chromatin, is rather the place of active residual transcription.

Nuclear speckles, or SC35 domains, also known as interchromatin granule clusters (IGCs) in terms of electron microscopy, are suggested as one of the most universal and evolutionarily conserved nuclear domains [15, 16]. They primarily represent nuclear sites to store pre-mRNA splicing factors [17–20], but extensive studies carried out during the last decades have introduced the idea that IGC functions are broader than those supposed previously, and these domains are involved in many other nuclear processes closely linked to gene expression [16, 21].

Nucleoplasmic transport and export of mRNA are important steps of gene expression, presenting an integral part of mRNA biogenesis [22]. It is now evident that the steps preceding export of mRNA-protein complexes (mRNPs) through nuclear pores make an essential contribution to the efficiency of mRNP export itself [23]. A number of RNA-binding proteins and/or protein complexes playing a role in RNA export bind mRNA before export, forming export-competent mRNPs. Some mRNA export factors are recruited to active genes during transcription [24], whereas other components of mRNA export complexes bind pre-mRNA later, in a splicing-dependent manner [25, 26].

Export of mRNPs is enhanced by evolutionarily conserved multiprotein transcription-export complex (TREX) that is deposited on the pre-mRNA near the 5′-end cap [27]. Also facilitating mRNP export is the exon-exon junction complex (EJC) that shares two proteins, Aly/REF and UAP56, with the TREX. The EJC consists of more than dozen proteins and comprises a constitutive core including proteins Y14–Magoh, eIF4A3 and MLN51 [28]. The EJC assembly in vivo occurs within or around nuclear speckles/IGCs [29, 30], and export-incompetent mRNAs which carry an incomplete or destabilized EJC are retained in the speckles [31].

In the present work, we studied nuclear distribution of the EJC core protein Y14 in the GV of *T. castaneum*. Our preliminary data have been presented as a brief one-page correspondence elsewhere [32]. Here, we provide a full-length article including immunoelectron-microscopy localization data on Y14–Myc distribution in the nucleus of previtellogenic and vitellogenic oocytes. A special attention was paid to possible relations between Y14 and oocyte nuclear domains: the karyosphere, its capsule and nuclear bodies. The plasmids encoding the fusion protein Y14–Myc were constructed. Myc-tagged Y14 mRNA synthesized in vitro was microinjected into the oocytes, and nuclear distribution of Y14–Myc was monitored with the use of immunofluorescent (IF) and immunoelectron microscopy (IEM) and antibodies against the Myc tag.

Nuclear distribution of the newly synthesized Y14–Myc was found to be quite dynamic. The fusion protein was localized in the PR of the karyosphere and in the KC. Y14 was also revealed in IGCs/speckles (SC35 domains) in the GV of previtellogenic but not vitellogenic oocytes. Localization sites of Y14–Myc in the PR of the karyosphere apparently correspond to the places of residual transcription. We suggest that the KC is the protein destination site, while oocyte nuclear bodies (IGCs/SC35 domains) represent transient domains for Y14.

## Methods

### Laboratory insects and tissue preparation

The wild-type strain of *Tribolium castaneum* (Herbst.) (Coleoptera–Polyphaga, Tenebrionidae) was reared at 28 ° C on whole wheat flour containing 5% (*w*/w) brewer's yeast which formed the upper substrate level, and the lower substrate of oatmeal. The larvae used for RNA extraction were kept for 1 day on dry filter paper at normal cultivation temperature. For IF and IEM studies, ovaries of adult females were isolated in the solution for insects (0.75% NaCl, 0.035% KCl, 0.021% $CaCl_2$) or in Ex-Cell™ 420 insect medium (SAFC Biosciences) with 10% fetal bovine serum (Hyclone) [33].

### HEK293 cell line

The HEK293 cell line derived from primary human embryonic kidney cells, transformed with human adenovirus type 5 DNA and prepared with the use of standard techniques [34] was grown in Eagle's minimum essential medium (MEM) supplemented with non-essential amino acids and ~10% calf serum. Transformation of the cells by Y14–Myc (pcDNA 3.1 Myc-His(A) + Y14 vector) was carried out using the calcium technique as described [35]. 3 days after exposure to DNA the cultures were switched to low $Ca^{2+}$ medium [36] and examined periodically for the presence of the colonies of transformed cells. Then, the cells were grown routinely in Eagle's medium containing 10% calf serum.

### Construction with unspliced *T. castaneum* Y14 gene

The *Y14* sequence was selected from the *T. castaneum* genome DNA with the use of primers ## 7, 8 (Table 1; accession NCBI number: NW_001093646.1). The genomic *Y14* sequence was amplified, and then treated with appropriate restrictases (Table 1). The fragment was cloned in the pBMC vector containing the cytomegalovirus promoter (Fig. 1a') [37]. Total RNA was extracted from cells 72 h after transfection, reverse transcription was performed, and the fragment of *T. castaneum Y14* gene was amplified with the same primers. The fragment was cloned and sequenced as described (see below), the result was a plasmid pBMC + genomicY14 (Fig. 1a').

### CDS Y14–Myc construction

Total mRNA was isolated from *T. castaneum* larvae using TRI-REAGENT (Sigma Aldrich) according to the standard acid phenol-guanidinium thiocyanate-chloroform extraction protocol. cDNA was prepared using RevertAid First Strand cDNA Synthesis Kit (Termo Scientific). For routine DNA amplification, Taq polymerase (Termo Scientific) was used according to standard recommendations [38].

Y14 sequence was obtained from NCBI (Gene ID: 656135). Specific primers were constructed, and the 5′ end was modified in order to insert restriction enzyme recognition sites (## 1, 2 in Table 1). These primers were used for routine DNA amplification with Taq polymerase (Termo Scientific) according to standard recommendations [38].

After PCR reaction, a 506 bp fragment (full length without stop codon) was amplified. The fragment was purified from gel using cut gel purification protocols (TermoScientific). Then, the fragment was ligated in PTZ57R/T TA cloning vector (Termo Scientific) according to standard InsTAclone PCR Cloning Kit protocol – TA cloning procedure. The resulting vector was transfected by the standard *E. coli* electroporation method [38]. The clones were examined by PCR. The plasmid was purified with QIAGEN–QIAprep Spin Miniprep Kit and restricted by XhoI and KpnI restriction enzymes (Termo Scientific). The fragment was cut from gel and cloned in pDNA 3.1

**Table 1** List of primers

| ## | Primer Name | Sequence (5′–3′) | Inserted sites |
|---|---|---|---|
| 1 | 006-XhoI-RNA-Forv | TTCTCGAGATGGCAG**ATG**TTTTGGACA | XhoI |
| 2 | 007-KpnI-RNA-Rev | TAGGTACCGTGTCTCCTTGCACGTTTC | Kpn1 |
| 3 | 020-BamH1-RNA-Forv | GAGGATCCATGGCAGATGTTTTGGACA | BamH1 |
| 4 | 011-EcoRI-Stop-Myc-Rev | TCGAATTCTCAATTCAGATCCTCTTC***TGA***GATG | EcoR1, TGA(stop) |
| 5 | M13(-20) Forv | GTAAAACGACGGCCAGT | |
| 6 | M13(-26) Rev | GGAAACAGCTATGACCA | |
| 7 | 001-DnaNheI-Forv | GTGCTAGCCACC**ATG**GCAGATGTTTTGGAC | NheI |
| 8 | 002-DnaNot-Rev | ACGCGGCCGCTCAGTGTCTCCTTGCACG | NotI |

Bold, start codon; bold italic, stop codon

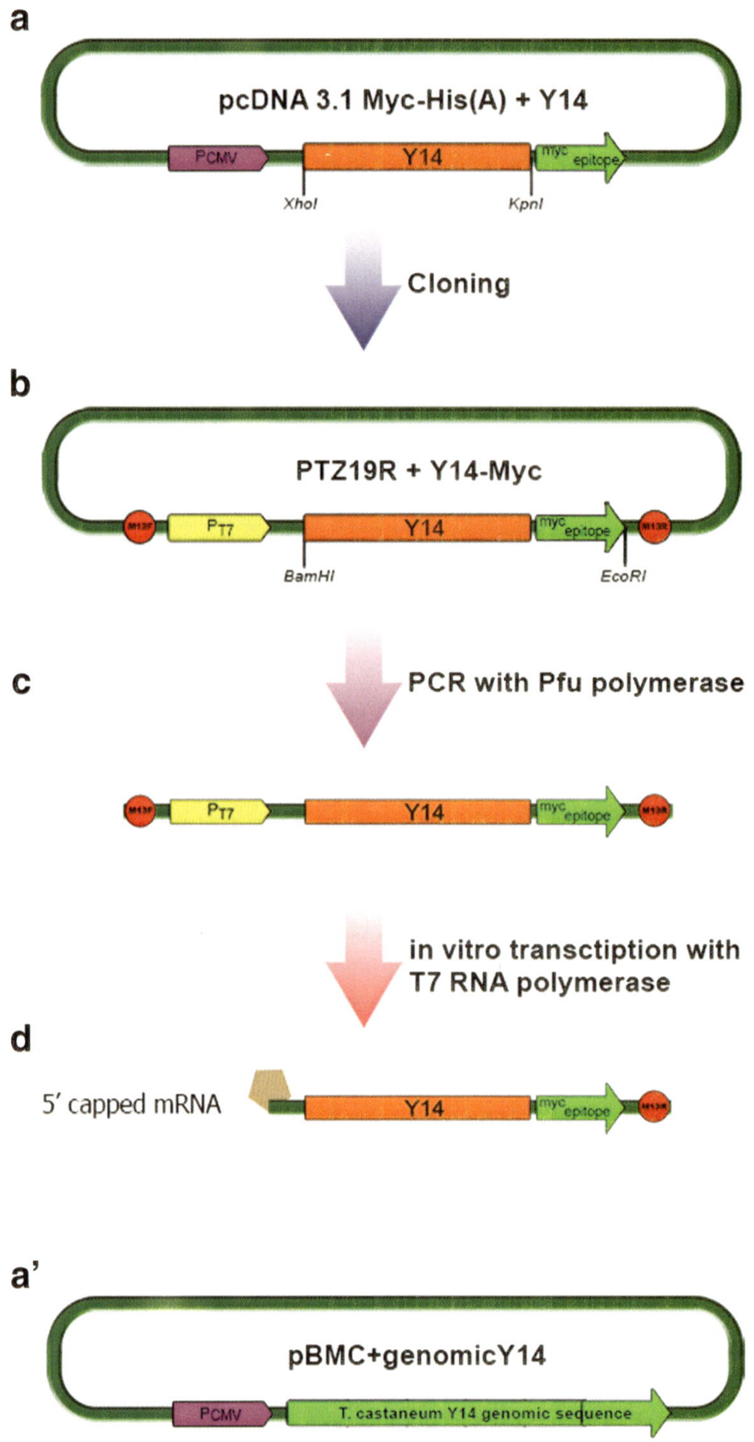


**Fig. 1** The scheme of Y14–Myc mRNA constructing (**a,b,c,d**) and Y14 genomic construction (**c'**). **a**, Y14 (506 bp) cloned in pcDNA 3.1 Myc–His; **b**, Y14 + Myc tag (542 bp) cloned in PTZ19R; **c**, PCR (639 bp) matrix for in vitro transcription; **d**, Y14–Myc mRNA (609 bp) transcribed in vitro. *Yellow*, T7 promoter; *orange*, Y14 coding sequence; *light green*, Myc epitope; *red circles*, M13 primers; *brown*, 5' cap analog; *dark green*, parts of the vector not significant in this case

Myc-His(A) vector (Invitrogen) using the Myc tag and cytomegalovirus promoter (Fig. 1a).

The pairs of primers specific to the full length Y14–Myc (## 3,4 in Table 1) were used in a subsequent PCR to generate 506 bp full length *T. castaneum* Y14 + Myc with downstream stop codon in order to clone this fragment in PTZ19R vector (Termo Scientific) containing T7 promoter for in vitro transcription (Fig. 1b).

Resulting plasmid B was checked for correct assembling with the correspondent pairs of primers by PCR.

The plasmid A design (Fig. 1a) gives the possibility to transfect the cultured cells to check transcription and translation. The plasmid B with the inserted T7 promoter (Fig. 2b) was designed for in vitro transcription of the whole Y14–Myc mRNA.

### mRNA synthesis in vitro

The templates used for mRNA synthesis in vitro were PCR products prepared using Pfu polymerase for error-free amplification (Termo Scientific) and universal M13 forward and reverse primers (## 5,6 in Table 1) to amplify full length fusion Y14–Myc with the T7 promoter located upstream (Fig. 1c). RNA (Fig. 1d) was synthesized on the template using the TranscriptAid™ T7 High Yield Transcription Kit (Termo Scientific) with adding of Ribo $m^7G$ Cap Analog (Promega) for 5′ mRNA capping based on the standard TranscriptAid™ protocol. DNA templates and other reaction components were removed with RNAqueous kit (Ambion). RNA electrophoresis under denaturing conditions with PFA was performed according to the standard protocol [38] (Fig. 2 II, 2;3).

### Microinjections

Separate ovarioles, anatomical units of insect female gonads, were used for microinjections into the oocytes. The injections were carried out by using glass capillaries and an Eppendorf 5242 microinjector equipped with a Narishige micromanipulator. After microinjection, the ovarioles were kept in a moist chamber for 4–6 h, then squashed and prepared for IF or IEM (see below). Approximately 0.1 μl of 50 ng/μl mRNA solution (5 ng RNA per oocyte) was microinjected into the ooplasm [39]. About 30 oocytes were injected. Approximately 15% oocytes were survived the procedure and used for immunostaining experiments.

### Immunofluorescent microscopy

For IF microscopy, squashed preparations of oocyte nuclei were prepared as described [40, 41]. Ovarioles were gently squashed on a siliconized coverslip with a Polysine® microscope slide (Menzel) and frozen in liquid nitrogen. After the coverslip had been removed with a razor blade, the slide was fixed in 2% formaldehyde freshly prepared from paraformaldehyde (Ted Pella) in 96% ethanol for 45 min, rinsed in 70% ethanol and finally in PBS.

Preparations were incubated in 10% fetal calf serum (Gibco) in PBS for 10 min to prevent non-specific antibody binding. The incubation in primary antibody solution was carried out overnight in a moist chamber at 4 °C. After rinsing in PBS, preparations were incubated with secondary antibodies conjugated with Alexa-488 or Alexa-568 (Invitrogen, dilution 1:200) for 1.5 h at room temperature. To visualize DNA, preparations were additionally stained with 1 μg/ml To-Pro-3 dye (Molecular Probes) for 5 min, then rinsed in PBS and mounted in Vectashield® medium (Vector Laboratories) or directly mounted in the medium containing 1 μg/ml DAPI. For simultaneous DNA and RNA visualization, acridine orange staining method [42] was used. The samples were examined with a Leica TCS SP5 confocal laser scanning microscope equipped with Ar-UV diode (405 nm), Ar- (488 nm) and He–Ne- (543 and 633 nm) lasers.

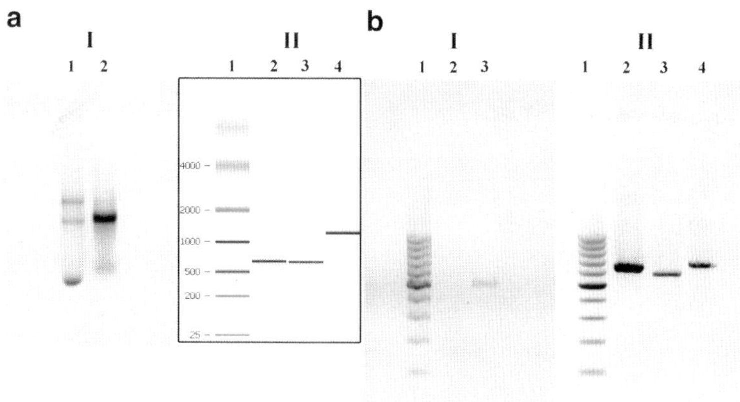


**Fig. 2** Electrophoretic control of the fragments of Y14–Myc construction. **a**, RNA electrophoresis. I — RNA electrophoresis under denaturing conditions; line 1, total RNA from rat liver (for control); line 2, total *T. castaneum* RNA from pupae. II — RNA transcribed in vitro and analyzed with microfluidics-based Agilent 2100 Bioanalyzer; line 1, a ladder (Agilent 2100 Bioanalyzer built-in function); lines 2 and 3, 5'-capped *T. castaneum* Y14-Myc RNA transcribed in vitro, 200 ng and 100 ng, respectively; line 4, mouse GABDH mRNA (for control, 200 ng). **b**, DNA electrophoresis. I — DNA electrophoresis of the reverse transcription PCR products; line 1, DNA ladder (100 bp); line 2, negative control; line 3, PCR with cDNA after RT-PCR with total *T. castaneum* RNA (506 bp), primers ## 1, 2 (see Table 1). II — DNA electrophoresis of PCR products amplified with Pfu polymerase on the PTZ19R + Y14-Myc vector for in vitro transcription (639 bp); line 1, DNA ladder (100 bp); line 2, primers ## 5, 4 (Table 1); line 3, primers ## 3, 6 (Table 1); line 4, primers ## 5, 6 (Table 1)

Confocal images were taken with a 63× objective (NA 1.32). Merged images were obtained using ImageJ 1.47.

#### Immunogold labeling electron microscopy

For IEM, single ovarioles with injected oocytes were prefixed for 2 h in in PBS containing 4% formaldehyde and 0.5% glutaraldehyde at room temperature, and then fixed overnight in 2% formaldehyde at 4 °C. After rinsing in PBS containing 0.05 M $NH_4Cl$ and subsequent dehydration in an ethanol series, ovarioles were embedded in LR White resin (medium grade, Sigma). Ultrathin sections were incubated for 10 min in blocking buffer containing 0.5% fish gelatin (Sigma) and 0.02% Tween-20 in PBS, pH 7.4. After blocking, the sections were incubated overnight in antibody 9E10 solution in a moist chamber at 4 ° C. After rinsing in TBS-Tween (TBST), the sections were incubated in the solution of biotinylated goat anti-mouse antibodies (Vector Laboratories) diluted 1:50 in TBST for 1 h at room temperature. After rinsing in TBST, the sections were incubated in the solution of gold-conjugated (15 nm) streptavidin (Aurion) diluted 1:20 in TBST. The sections were contrasted with uranyl acetate and examined in a Libra 120 electron microscope at 80 kV.

#### Primary antibodies

Primary antibodies used were the following: goat polyclonal antibody C-20 raised against a peptide at the C-terminus of human Y14 (Santa Cruz Biotechnology, Inc.) (IF, dilution 1:50), rabbit polyclonal antibody ab9106 (Abcam) (IF, dilution 1:100) or mouse monoclonal antibody 9E10 against Myc epitope [43] (IEM, culture supernatant), mouse monoclonal antibody against SC35 [44] (IF, 2.5 μg/ml), mouse monoclonal antibody 030 against double-stranded DNA (Chemicon) (IEM, dilution 1:300).

#### Computer based methods

Ugene software and Jalview software were used for the initial search of Y14 in the BeetleBase. Cloning in silico was made with Geneious and Bioedit tools. Primers were selected using Primer 3 plus web-based tool. Protein alignment was made by the Geneious software. The sequence of *Y14* gene was obtained from the NCBI database (Gene ID: 656135).

## Results

### *T. castaneum* Y14 gene

We took the advantage of the wealth of background genetic information with a recently published beetle draft genome [3]. The Y14 proteins extracted from the databases indicated were aligned (Additional file 1: Figure S1). The preliminary analysis shows that *Tribolium* shares more genes with humans than the dipterans do [2], and Y14 alignment confirms this. The alignment showed a high degree of homology, and all the main human protein features are present in the *T. castaneum* protein. Human and beetle Y14 mRNA sequences are similar in general, especially in RRM domain region, but in a NLS/YNS region there is less similarity. The direct (non-degenerate) primers have been designed from the sequence to pick up the beetle gene (Table 1).

#### Y14–Myc construct

The construct was designed for accurate detection of Y14 pathways and its localization in the *T. castaneum* GV [32]. The Myc epitope was chosen as a tag due to its low impact on the structure of the fusion protein. Two constructions were made. The first construct was used to add the Myc epitope sequence to the Y14 coding sequence and for the control of its transcription activity in HEK293 cells (Fig. 1a). The second construct was used for transcription in vitro (Fig. 1b). The principal scheme of the constructing is shown in Fig. 1 (see also Materials and Methods).

Although the strategies are straightforward, a care should be taken to design plasmid constructions that encode protein tags, to generate high-quality mRNA in an RNase-free environment and to control the nonspecific effects of exogenous mRNA. In most vectors, protein expression is driven by the enhancer/promoter cassette of the immediate early gene of human cytomegalovirus. This cassette generates high levels of protein expression in most mammalian cell lines and is suitable for in vitro expression. The human cytomegalovirus major immediate early promoter is commercially available for the expression of various heterologous genes.

#### Plasmid transcription and Y14 mRNA splicing in human HEK293 cells

Prior to Y14–Myc RNA microinjections into *T. castaneum* oocytes we tested the transcription activity of *T. castaneum* Y14 coding sequence in HEK293 cells. The best way to check whether a plasmid was constructed correctly, is obtaining its transcription in the transfected beetle cell line, but such a line is not established yet. So, the human HEK293 cells were transfected with the plasmid A by calcium method. No less than 10% cells were transfected and expressed fused Y14–Myc (Fig. 3a, b). The fusion protein was localized mainly in the cytoplasm rather than in the nucleus (Fig. 3b). Such a behavior might be explained by the differences of NLS in human and beetle genes (Additional file 1: Figure S1).

We also checked whether *T. castaneum* Y14 pre-mRNA splicing is correct in human cells. The sequencing of 10 clones has shown that all the sequences are identical and differ from normally spliced Y14 mRNA (Additional file 2: Figure S2.). The *T. castaneum* Y14 pre-mRNA being processed in HEK293 cells does not lose the first intron (Additional file 2: Figure S2); two redundant GC nucleotides remain at the 3′ end of this intron. Exons 2 and 3 are being removed during splicing, while exon 4 remains. Thus, the plasmid is

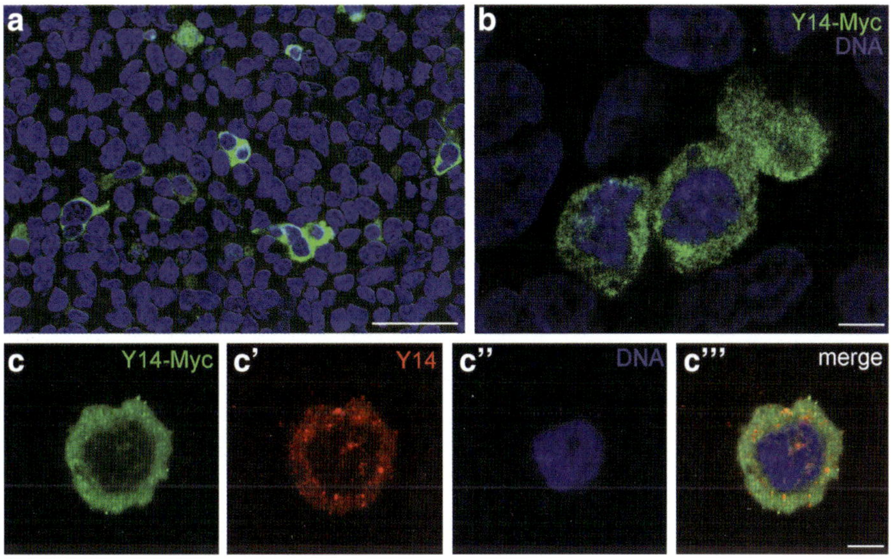


**Fig. 3** Plasmid A expression in HEK293 cells transfected with Myc-His-A with inserted Y14 sequence. Transfected cells at low (**a**) and high (**b**) magnification; anti-Myc staining is *green*, DNA stained with DAPI is *blue*. **c—c'''**, a transfected cell stained with antibodies against the Myc epitope (*green*) and Y14 (*red*); the nucleus is counterstained with DAPI (*blue*). Bars represent 50 μm in A and 5 μm in **b**, **c—c'''**

transcribed successfully, but is not being processed in the heterologous system. The reasons of this require a special study. The abortive splicing of insect pre-mRNA in human cells is in accordance with the data published [45].

Abortive splicing might explain why the location of the fusion protein and the intrinsic Y14 in HEK293 cells were found rather different after double immunostaining with antibodies against the Myc tag and Y14 (Fig. 3c–c'''). The bright foci corresponding Y14 in the vicinity of the nucleus probably represent translation factories that do contain the fusion protein. Nuclear intrinsic Y14 is visible in spots, which probably correspond to speckles. These domains do not include the fusion protein. The fusion protein seems cannot be imported to the nucleus of human cells due to unique NLS (Additional file 1: Figure S1). Nevertheless, the plasmid A is being transcribed successfully in human somatic cells. Still, to ensure the main aim of this study, we have constructed the plasmid B (Fig. 1) in order to synthesize in vitro 5′-capped mRNA and inject this RNA into the oocytes.

### Oocyte stages, karyosphere capsule morphology and the perichromatin region

Initially, we characterized oocyte stages in *T. castaneum* adult females morphologically with special emphasis on the development of the karyosphere and its capsule (KC). *T. castaneum* oocytes develop in typical meroistic telotrophic ovaries. The imago ovaries contain already differentiated oocytes and nurse cells [46]. General morphology of follicles, follicular epithelium and the stages of vitellogenesis studied in *Tenebrio* [47] together with our observations on the morphodynamics of *Tribolium* oocyte nuclear structures including the karyosphere and KC allowed us to propose a nomenclature for the stages of *T. castaneum* oocyte development during the long-term diplotene [8]. In *T. castaneum* oocytes, karyosphere formation begins in the stage IV oocyte, and the KC reaches the highest morphological complexity at the stages V–VII. The stages of *T. castaneum* GVs based on morphological criteria are presented in Fig. 4.

A well-developed KC in *T. castaneum* oocytes (Fig. 5a) was found to consist of three main different structures: (i) an electron-dense "shell" containing F-actin; (ii) fibrillar strands also containing actin and organized into cross-striated bundles; and (iii) lamin B-containing filamentous material consisting of entangled threads. Several nuclear bodies are scattered in the nucleoplasm and some are often seen attached to the KC. Amongst these bodies, coilin- and SC35-containing domains have been identified [8].

During the period of the existence of karyosphere, chromatin condensation is observed in the *T. castaneum* GV, but it is not absolute. Labeling of ultrathin sections of the *T. castaneum* GV with an anti-DNA antibody revealed compact chromatin blocks and loose DNA loops in the space abut to the KC (Fig. 5b). The latter space (the perichromatin region, PR) could be a place for residual transcription.

### RNA amount and residual transcription in the GV

Fluorescent staining of *T. castaneum* GVs with acridine orange showed that all DNA is concentrated in the karyosphere, as expected. At the same time, RNA is unevenly distributed in the nucleoplasm and highly enriches in the KC that contains the vast majority of oocyte RNA (Fig. 6). The nature of this RNA is not known. We would like to establish whether the KC is an RNA storage place or active transcription occurs at the vicinity of the KC.

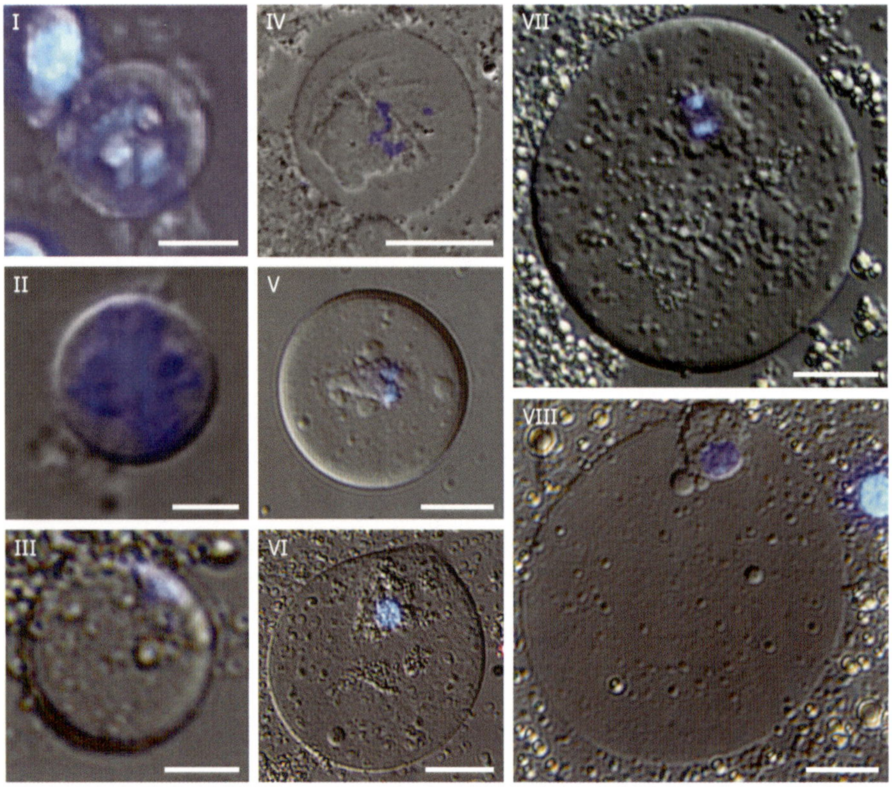


**Fig. 4** Morphology of the *T. castaneum* germinal vesicles at different stages of oocyte growth, squashed preparations of the stage **I** oocyte and the GVs from later stage oocytes. DIC, DAPI staining. Chromatin is dispersed and active transcription occurs at the stages **II-III**, before karyosphere formation that begins at the stage **IV**; **V** — late previtellogenic stage, a karyosphere capsule is formed; **VII** — vitellogenic stage, the capsule is fully developed, reaching its maximal complexity. Bars represent 5 μm for **I—II**; 10 μm for **II**; 20 μm for **III—VIII**

Using BrUTP assay, we found that *T. castaneum* oocyte chromosomes united into the karyosphere maintain residual transcription even in the late stage VII oocytes, predominately in the PR that contains chromatin loops and perichromatin fibrils. The hyperphosphorylated form of RNA polymerase II and basal transcription factors (TFIID and TFIIH) as well as poly(A)$^+$ RNA have also been demonstrable in the PR of the *T. castaneum* karyosphere. The residual transcription in the karyosphere apparently requires not only transcription factors but also RNA processing factors, including the components of the exon junction complex (EJC). The EJC core protein Y14 in the *T. castaneum* KC was revealed with antibodies [8]. In the present study, we employed a gene engineering approach to have a dynamic picture of the distribution of the newly synthesized protein in the GV. The Myc-tagged Y14 plasmid-based construct is the template (Fig. 1c, b) for the capped mRNA to be injected into the oocyte.

### Y14–Myc RNA microinjections in *T. castaneum* oocytes

Injection into insect oocyte is not an easy task by itself and counted as impossible until BrUTP was successfully injected [48]. Here, we used late previtellogenic (stage V) and vitellogenic (stage VII) oocytes with, respectively, partially or fully formed KC in microinjection experiments. 5′-end capped Y14-Myc RNA was synthesized on the template of the 639 bp fragment from the plasmid B (Fig. 2a, II). This RNA was injected into the ooplasm. The karyosphere with the KC and nuclear bodies are well-recognizable using DIC optics (Fig. 7a). During 3–5 h following mRNA injection, translation of the fusion protein actively occurs, and the protein successfully traveled into the GV (Fig. 7b). In the stage V oocyte (late previtellogenesis), Y14–Myc was localized in the KC. Nucleoplasmic nuclear bodies were also found enriched in the fusion protein at this stage (Fig. 7b). In later oocytes (the stage VII, vitellogenesis), the fusion protein was also revealed in the vicinity of condensed chromatin, in the KC, but not in the vast majority of SC35 domains (speckles) (Fig. 8). At higher magnification (Fig. 8b), some DNA is seen to extend from the condensed chromatin in the karyosphere into the PR. Decondensed chromatin in the PR of the karyosphere can be clearly detected at the ultrastructural level with the use of anti-DNA antibody (Fig. 5b). Myc-positive foci were also observed in the nucleoplasm, but they did not coincide with SC35 domains as revealed by double immunostaining with Myc antibodies (Fig. 8).

The IEM study confirmed IF data on the distribution and dynamics of Y14–Myc in the *T. castaneum* GV. In

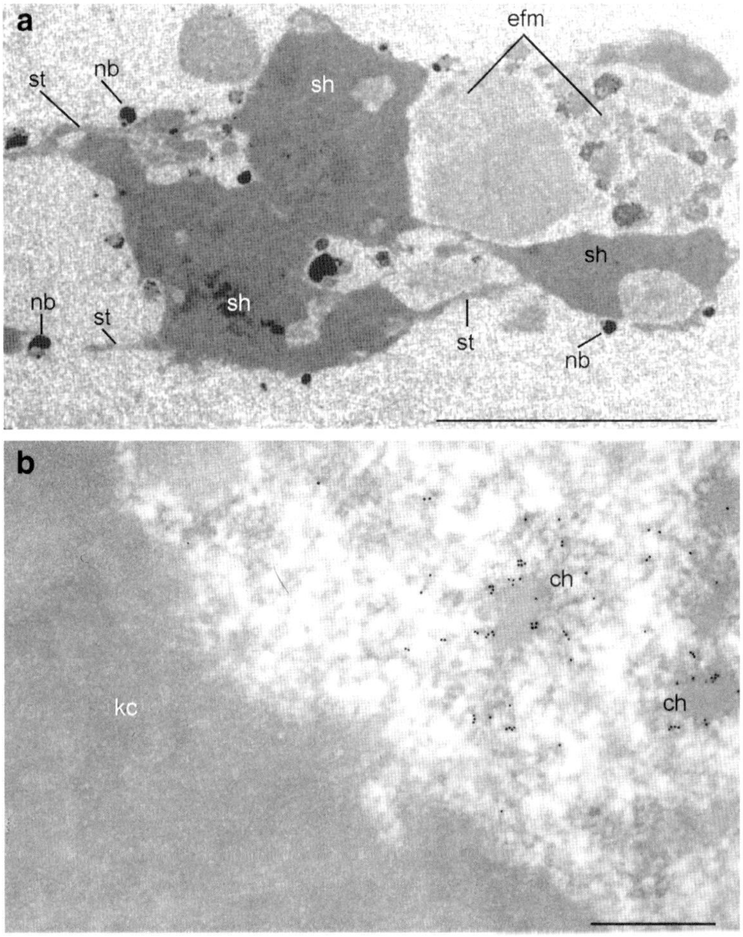


**Fig. 5** Ultrastructure of a fragment of *T. castaneum* karyosphere capsule in the stage 7 oocyte (**a**) and a fragment of karyosphere after immunogold labeling with anti-DNA antibody (**b**). In the karyosphere capsule, electron dense 'the shell material' (sh) and fibrillar 'the strands' (st) as well as the entangled filamentous material (efm) of medium electron density are distinguished; several nuclear bodies (nb) are located in the vicinity of the capsule (**a**). Condensed chromatin clumps (ch) and perichromatin region containing diffuse DNA loops are labeled with anti-DNA antibody; karyosphere capsule (kc) is devoid of the labels (**b**). Bars represent 5 μm in A and 0.5 μm in B

the stage V (late previtellogenic) oocytes microinjected with Y14–Myc mRNA, nucleoplasmic nuclear bodies of the 2nd type according to our nomenclature were labeled with antibody against Myc (Fig. 9a), whereas similar domains were devoid of labels in the stage VII (vitellogenic) oocytes (Fig. 9b). We have previously determined the *T. castaneum* oocyte nuclear bodies of the 2nd type as SC35-containing domains [8]. A complex KC is maintained in the injected oocytes, and some anti-Myc labels were observed in the PR of the karyosphere and in a fibrous material composing the capsule (Fig. 9c, d). The design of our experiments allowed reaching equilibrium between Y14–Myc synthesized in the ooplasm and the protein moving into the nucleus due to its NLS. Some labels masking the fusion protein was localized at the ultrastructural level close to the nuclear envelope (Fig. 9e).

Y14–Myc mRNA injections into oocyte shows the dynamic pattern of the fusion protein distribution. At the previtellogenic stage, there are two main locations for the protein: SC35 domains (IGCs/speckles) and the KC. At the vitellogenic stage, IGCs/speckles were devoid of the labels, and Y14–Myc was found in the PR of the karyosphere. The latter area apparently includes the places of residual transcription.

## Discussion

Here, we performed a gene engineering-based study to localize Y14 protein in oocyte nuclear structures of a model insect, *T. castaneum*. The oocyte nucleus (GV) of this beetle is characterized by the presence of a meiosis-specific structure formed by condensed chromosomes (the karyosphere), and of the extrachromosomal structures including the karyosphere capsule (KC) and various nuclear bodies. Since the *T. castaneum* karyosphere retains residual transcription activity [8], it was not surprising that Y14 involved in the processes of gene expression localizes to the perichromatin region (PR)

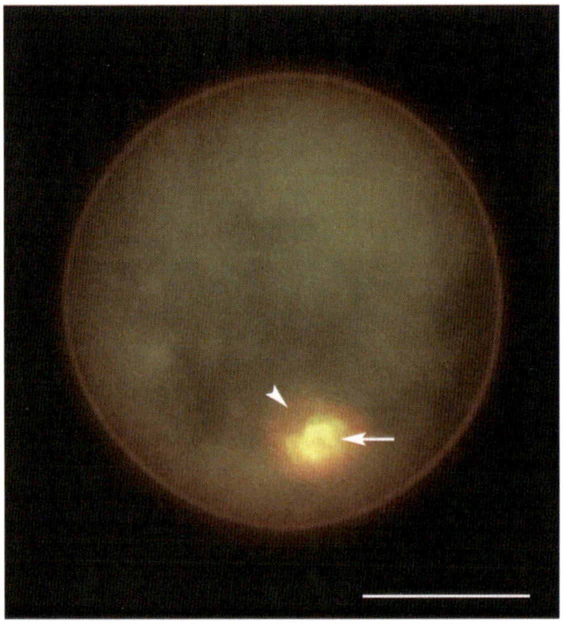

**Fig. 6** *T. castaneum* GV isolated from vitellogenic (stage VII) oocyte and stained with acridine orange. Note that all DNA is concentrated in the karyosphere (arrow); the karyosphere capsule (arrowhead) is highly enriched in RNA which is also unevenly distributed in the nucleoplasm. Bar represents 20 μm

of the karyosphere in all developmental stages studied. Our finding that this protein demonstrates a dynamic pattern of intranuclear distribution in respect of specific structures such as the KC and nuclear bodies is more essential. While in pre-vitellogenic oocytes Y14 localizes to both the KC and SC35-containing bodies analogous to nuclear speckles/IGCs, a destination site for this protein in late vitellogenic oocytes is the KC only. Our results accentuate the specificity of oocyte nuclear structures and suggest that the KC as a peculiar nuclear compartment of oocytes may be involved in nuclear metabolism of RNAs and proteins rather than representing just a passive barrier to separate the condensed chromosomes assembled into a karyosphere from the rest of the nucleoplasm.

### RNA content and residual transcription in the karyosphere

The *T. castaneum* GV staining for total RNA (Fig. 6) has shown that late vitellogenic oocyte GVs contain a significant amount of RNA. The main portion of this RNA accumulates in the area corresponding to the KC. IF and IEM studies unexpectedly revealed that the KC in the oocytes of *T. castaneum* [8] and also of another beetle, *Anthonomus pomorum* [14], is highly enriched in small nuclear (sn) RNPs. In particular, snRNAs revealed in the KC of these species carry the 2,2,7-trimethylguanosine (TMG) cap, characteristic of the 5′ end of many splicing snRNAs that have already completed the cytoplasmic period of their processing [49]. Interestingly, the "Sm-epitope" of snRNPs was detected recently in the KC of frog oocytes [50] (Ilicheva et al., 2016). Even in the species without a well-developed fibrous capsule (e.g., *Tenebrio molitor* or *Panorpa communis*), oocyte chromosomes are tightly associated with a fibrogranular material containing snRNPs and other RNA transcription and processing factors [51–53].

The presence of RNA in the KC is in agreement with the idea that this nuclear domain represents a specialized part of oocyte nuclear matrix [12, 13]. In somatic cells, nuclear matrix in vivo contains RNPs and a set of

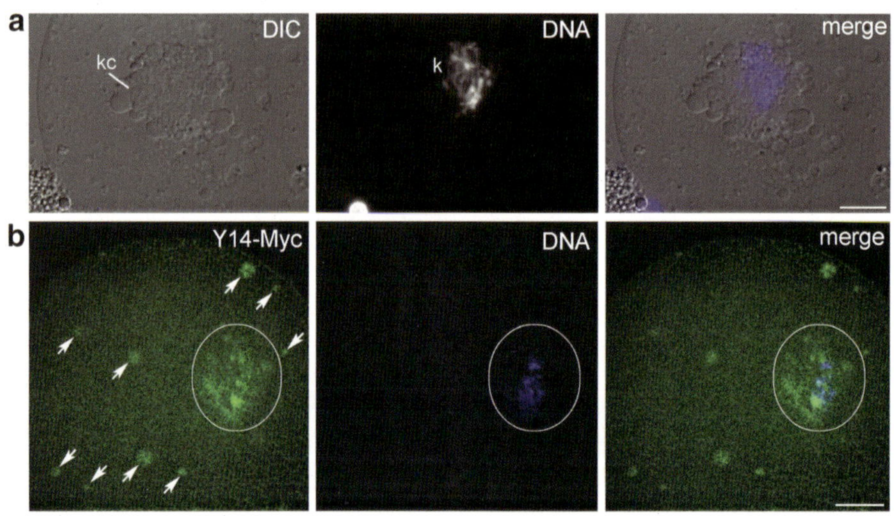


**Fig. 7** Squashed *T. castaneum* GVs (stage V) after microinjections of Y14-Myc mRNA into the ooplasm. **a**, DIC with DAPI staining; karyosphere capsule (kc) and karyosphere (k) are marked. **b**, Staining with anti-Myc AB (*green*) and anti-DNA dye To-Pro-3 (*blue*); nuclear area containing the karyosphere and its capsule is encircled; *arrows* indicate nucleoplasmic nuclear bodies. Bars represent 10 μm

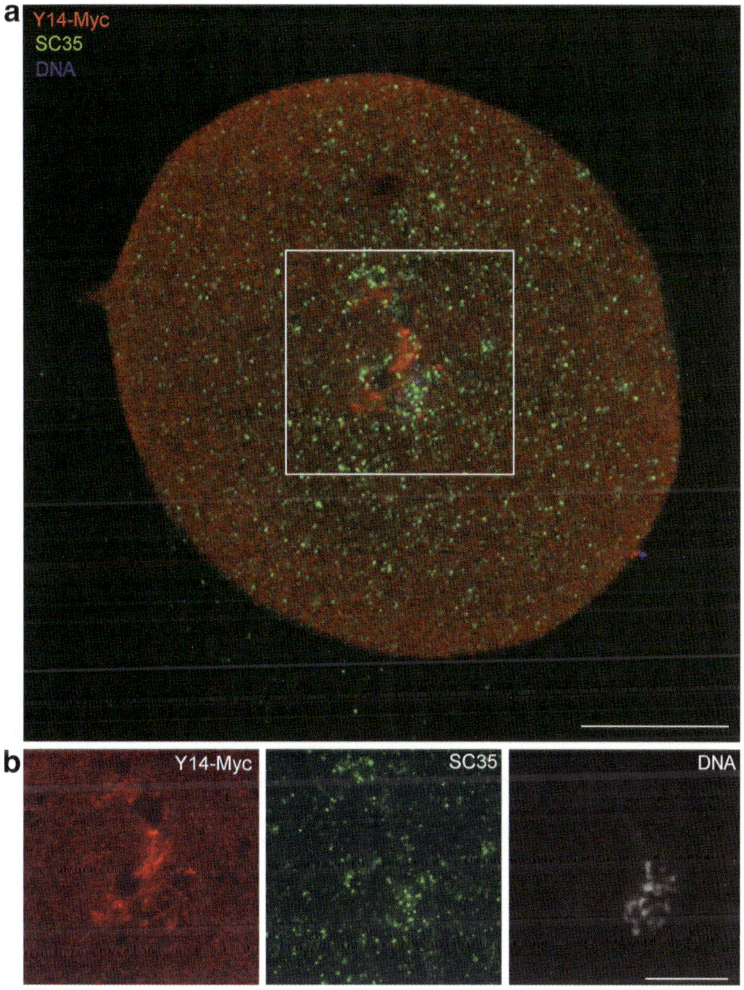


**Fig. 8** *T. castaneum* GV isolated from vitellogenic (stage VII) oocyte microinjected with Y14–Myc mRNA transcribed in vitro. **a**, The merged image of the whole GV. **b**, Localization of Y14–Myc (*red*) in the area outlined in A; SC35 (*green*); DNA was counterstained with To-Pro-3 (grey scale) to reveal the karyosphere. Bars represent 10 μm

proteins associated with RNA together with the structural proteins [54, 55].

Certain structural proteins (F-actin, lamin B) are prominent compounds of the *T. castaneum* KC [8]. F-actin was revealed as a basic component of the KC in several insects [56, 57] and also in frogs [58]. It has been shown that actin plays a crucial role in the maintenance of oocyte nuclear architectonics, and its depolymerization leads to a collapse of nuclear structures [59]. It is likely, that nuclear actin can form complexes with Y14, as well as with mRNA export adapter Aly/REF and export receptor NXF1, as revealed with the use of FRET analysis carried out in mouse early embryos [60]. Also, the active role of nuclear actin in transcription [61, 62] and chromatin remodeling [63] is well-documented for somatic cells.

It cannot be excluded that a KC develops when the karyosphere maintains residual transcriptional activity in late oocytes. In tenebrionid beetles, a karyosphere usually has an external KC [64] with the exception of *Tenebrio* [52, 53]. BrUTP incorporation assay showed that chromatin in the karyosphere devoid of a capsule (the scorpionfly, *Panorpa*, and the yellow mealworm, *Tenebrio*) is transcriptionally silent at the final stages of oocyte growth [48], whereas the transcriptional activity in oocytes with a well-developed KC does not entirely ceased. In such the organisms as the lacewing, *Chrysopa* [65], the darkling beetle, *Blaps* [66], and the grass frog, *Rana temporaria* [67], which possess a KC, residual RNA synthesis in the GV was found. In contrast, incorporation of $^{3}$H–uridine was not registered in a human karyosphere (karyosome) which is devoid of a capsule [68]. The question which RNA is last-synthesized in the oocyte with rather inactivated genome has a principal significance for developmental biology. It could be expected that RNAs deposited in a KC, especially those last-synthesized during oogenesis, might be essential for the organization of future embryo.

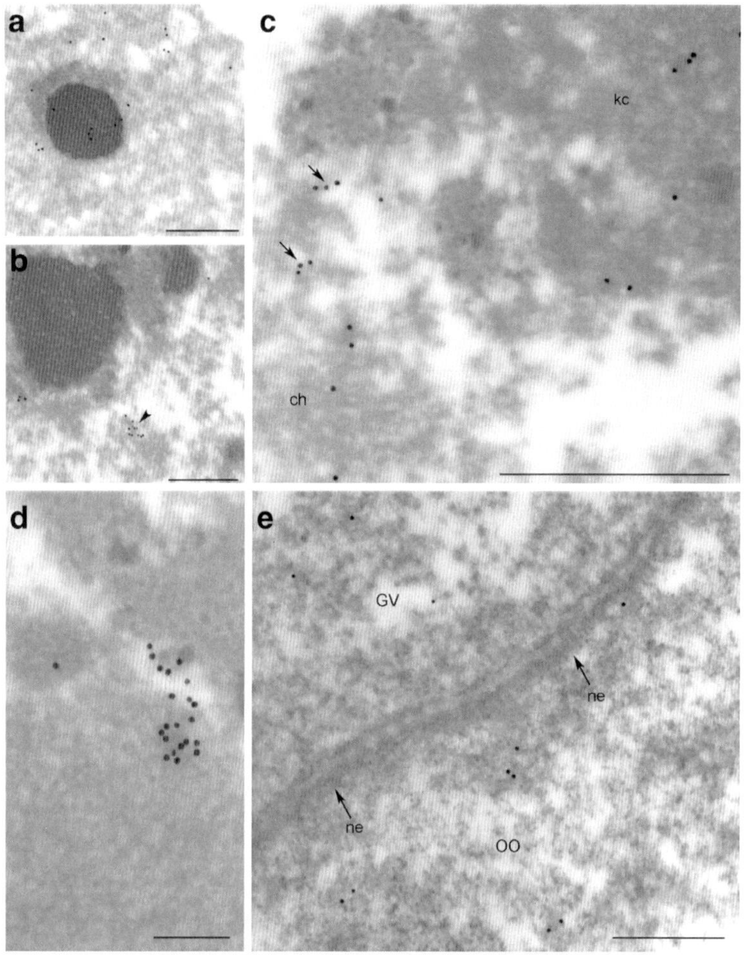


**Fig. 9** Ultrathin sections of *T. castaneum* GVs from oocytes injected with Y14–Myc mRNA after labeling with anti-Myc AB. **a**, Labeled nuclear body (SC35 domain) in the stage V oocyte. **b**, Similar nuclear body devoid of labels in the stage VII oocyte; a patch of labels (*arrowhead*) is visible and does not belong to the body. **c**, An overview of the fragment of karyosphere (ch, chromatin) and its capsule (kc); labels masking the fibrillar material in the perichromatin region are marked by arrows. **d**, The fragment of the karyosphere capsule; a patch of labels does not correspond SC35 domain. **e**, Anti-Y14–Myc labels near the nuclear envelope (ne); GV, germinal vesicle (oocyte nucleus); oo, ooplasm. Bars represent 0.5 μm in **a**—**c**, **e** and 200 nm in **d**

In the *T. castaneum* GV of the stage V–VII oocytes, the sites of residual transcription are clearly defined, representing the PR of the karyosphere. Y14-Myc targeted to this area after microinjection of Myc-tagged Y14 mRNA (Figs. 7b, 8, and 9c). The concept of the PR implies that this area cannot be considered separately from chromatin [69]. It serves not only as the main site of transcribed DNA and nascent pre-mRNAs, but co-transcriptional pre-mRNA processing including splicing, DNA replication and, perhaps, reparation also occur there [70–72]. The KC that separates late transcription in the GV could be a useful model to find out what is the nature of these RNA.

The retention of mRNAs encoding the proteins of the maternal effect is well-documented for the ooplasm and has a significant impact on embryonic development. For instance, Oskar mRNA determines the future primary axes in unfertilized eggs, and Y14–Magoh is responsible to Oskar localization [73]. On the contrary, data on the distribution of different RNA types in the GV are scanty in literature [74, 75]. The organisms with a well-developed KC may be talkative objects in order to solve this issue.

### EJC core protein Y14

The protein to trace in the current work, Y14, is a pre-mRNA splicing factor and EJC core protein. In the eukaryotic cell, mRNA biogenesis intimately depends on the EJC, which had received wide attention due to both its original assembly pathway on mRNAs and the ability to communicate with various mRNA-related cellular machineries [76, 77]. The EJC is loaded onto mRNA by spliceosomes during splicing at a precise point upstream the exon-exon junctions and serves as a binding platform for mRNA export factors [78, 79]. Y14 is one of the best-characterized proteins of the EJC core. This core is able to interact directly with pre-mRNA and is assembled prior to exon ligation [80]. At this stage, Y14 associates with pre-mRNA [81, 82] and accompanies the spliced mRNA until translation in the cytoplasm [83, 84]. A special domain YNS/NLS located near the N-terminus of the Y14 molecule is simultaneously serves as a NLS and also confers Y14 nuclear export [85]. Also, Y14 contains a well-defined RNA recognition motif (RRM, Additional file 1: Figure S1), but it is buried almost entirely at the interface of the Y14–Magoh heterodimer [86–88]. This suggests that Y14 does not bind pre-mRNA directly, and this binding requires one or more intermediary proteins. Nevertheless, Y14 is found associated with both nuclear and newly exported cytoplasmic mRNAs.

The approach based on oocyte microinjections with synthesized in vitro Myc-tagged Y14 mRNA allowed us to trace nuclear dynamics of the newly synthesized protein. We found that this RNA microinjected in oocytes is being translated successfully for 3 h, and the product of translation is imported into the GV. A significant level of fluorescence was registered in the PR of the karyosphere where loose DNA loops are located. Y14 is localized at different oocyte stages in a different way. In the stage V oocytes, at the beginning of KC formation, it is revealed in SC35 domains; however, Y14 enriches a well-formed KC rather than SC35 domains at later stages. It could be supposed that like in somatic cells [16] oocyte SC35-containing nuclear bodies represent transient domains for some proteins involved in mRNA transport and export. It is well-known that somatic extrachromosomal nuclear domains contain not only resident slow-mobile proteins including the proteins of the nuclear matrix. For instance, pre-mRNA splicing factors located in IGCs/speckles are highly dynamic and are being stored in IGCs not longer than in other parts of the nucleoplasm [89] in spite of their 5–10 times higher concentration in IGCs [90]. It is possible that oocyte nuclear bodies may contain other proteins that are included as compounds of the KC at the end of oocyte growth; Myc-Y14 fusion protein is the first which dynamic distribution was confirmed.

Chromatin rearrangement, which is a characteristic feature of oocyte maturation, is well documented; we showed that it accompanied with the movement of a nuclear protein in the case of residual transcription during genome inactivation.

## Conclusion

Our data presented here suggest the KC is not only a specialized part of nuclear matrix supporting the karyosphere (a knot of condensed chromosomes) and separating it from the products of chromosome activity, as believed previously. Using a gene engineering approach with injections of mRNA derived from the Myc-tagged Y14 plasmid-based construct, we showed for the first time that the KC is a destination site for a nuclear protein involved in mRNA splicing and export. Thus, we believe that the KC could represent a special nuclear compartment involved in the processes of gene expression in the case the karyosphere retains residual transcription activity. However, it is still unclear, why the KC appears during oogenesis in some species and does not exist in closely related others, which exhibit the same structural and functional pattern of the ovaries and possess similar biological features. Further comparative studies using a complex of modern approaches, including in vivo studies, are required.

## Additional files

**Additional file 1: Figure S1.** Protein alignment of *Tribolium castaneum* Y14 (XP_967777), *Drosophila melanogaster* Y14 (NP_610454) and *Homo sapiens* Y14 (NP_005096). Y14 RNA binding/recognition domain (RRM/RBM8) indicated with *grey*. Identical amino acids highlighted in *black*, similar in *grey*. Alignment and visualization performed with Geneious 6 Software (TIFF 181 kb)

**Additional file 2: Figure S2.** Differences between Y14 splicing systems in human and *T. castaneum* cells. A, The genome sequence of *T. castaneum* Y14. B, Normally spliced Y14 mRNA of *T. castaneum*. C, Abnormal splicing of *T. castaneum* Y14 mRNA in human HEK293 cells (TIFF 204 kb) Green, exons; blue, introns.

### Abbreviations

EJC: Exon-exon junction complex; GV: Germinal vesicle (oocyte nucleus); IEM: Immunoelectron microscopy; IF: Immunofluorescence; IGC: Interchromatin granule cluster; KC: Karyosphere capsule; PR: Perichromatin region

### Acknowledgements

We are indebted to J.G. Gall (Carnegie Institution of Washington) for providing antibodies 9E10 and anti-SC35. The authors thank B.V. Murashev, L.L. Krukovskaya, E.B. Akulova and A.P. Kozlov for their assistance in the molecular biology and cell culture parts of the work.

### Funding

This work was supported by the Government of Russian Federation grant № 074-U01, the granting program 'Molecular and Cell Biology' of the Russian Academy of Sciences grant № 01201457147, Russian Science Foundation grant № 15-15-20,026, Russian Foundation for Basic Research grant № 15-04-01857.

### Authors' contributions

AMK carried out gene engineering experiments, including molecular cloning, gene manipulation and transcription in vitro. ISS performed microinjection experiments. LSA participated in molecular genetic and cytochemical studies. FMB completed electron microscopy analysis, including immunoelectron microscopy. VNP initiated the project and designed all the experiments. DSB participated in immunofluorescent and electron microscopy experiments. DSB and OIP coordinated the works, drafted the manuscript and are responsible for the manuscript preparation. All the authors, with except of FMB and VNP who suddenly died, read and approved the final manuscript.

**Competing interests**

The authors declare that they have no competing interests.

**Author details**

[1]Laboratory of Cell Morphology, Institute of Cytology, Russian Academy of Sciences, St. Petersburg 194064, Russia. [2]Federal Almazov North-West Medical Research Centre, St. Petersburg 197341, Russia. [3]ITMO University, Institute of Translational Medicine, St. Petersburg 197101, Russia. [4]Department of Cytology and Histology, Faculty of Biology, St. Petersburg State University, St. Petersburg 199034, Russia. [5]Far Eastern Federal University, School of Biomedicine, Vladivostok 690950, Russia.

**References**

1. Sokoloff A. The biology of *Tribolium*: with special emphasis on genetic aspects. Oxford: Clarendon Press; 1972.
2. Maderspacher F. Genomics: an inordinate fondness for beetles. Curr Biol. 2008;18:R466–8. doi:10.1016/j.cub.2008.04.068.
3. Richards S, Gibbs RA, Weinstock GM, Brown SJ, Denell R, Beeman RW, et al. The genome of the model beetle and pest *Tribolium castaneum*. Nature. 2008;452:949–55. doi:10.1038/nature06784.
4. Kim HS, Murphy T, Xia J, Caragea D, Park Y, Beeman RW, et al. BeetleBase in 2010: revisions to provide comprehensive genomic information for *Tribolium castaneum*. Nucleic Acids Res. 2010;38:437–42. doi: 10.1093/nar/gkp807.
5. Adams MD, Celniker SE, Holt RA, Evans CA, Gocayne JD, Amanatides PG, et al. The genome sequence of *Drosophila melanogaster*. Science. 2000;287:2185–95. doi:10.1126/science.287.5461.2185.
6. Nunes da Fonseca R, von Levetzow C, Kalscheuer P, Basal A, van der Zee M, Roth S. Self-regulatory circuits in dorsoventral axis formation of the short-germ beetle *Tribolium castaneum*. Dev Cell. 2008;14:605–15. doi:10.1016/j.devcel.2008.02.011.
7. Benton MA, Akam M, Pavlopoulos A. Cell and tissue dynamics during *Tribolium* embryogenesis revealed by versatile fluorescence labeling approaches. Development. 2013;140:3210–20. doi:10.1242/dev.096271.
8. Bogolyubov DS, Batalova FM, Kiselyov AM, Stepanova IS. Nuclear structures in *Tribolium castaneum* oocytes. Cell Biol Int. 2013;37:1061–79. doi:10.1002/cbin.10135.
9. Kumaran RI, Thakar R, Spector DL. Chromatin dynamics and gene positioning. Cell. 2008;132:929–34. doi:10.1016/j.cell.2008.03.004.
10. Mao YO, Sunwoo H, Zhang B, Spector DL. Direct visualization of the co-transcriptional assembly of a nuclear body by noncoding RNAs. Nat Cell Biol. 2010;13:95–101. doi:10.1038/ncb2140.
11. Dundr M. Nuclear bodies: multifunctional companions of the genome. Curr Opin Cell Biol. 2012;24:415–22. doi:10.1016/j.ceb.2012.03.010.
12. Gruzova MN, Parfenov VN. Karyosphere in oogenesis and intranuclear morphogenesis. Int Rev Cytol. 1993;144:1–52.
13. Gruzova MN. The nucleus during oogenesis with special reference to extrachromosomal structures. In: Dettlaff TA, Vassetzky SG, editors. Oocyte growth and maturation. New York: Consultants Bureau; 1988. p. 77–163.
14. Świątek P, Jaglarz MK. SnRNPs are present in the karyosome capsule in the weevil germinal vesicle. Tissue Cell. 2004;36:253 62. doi:10.1016/j.tice.2004.04.001.
15. Bogolyubov D, Stepanova I, Parfenov V. Universal nuclear domains of somatic and germ cells: some lessons from oocyte interchromatin granule cluster and Cajal body structure and molecular composition. BioEssays. 2009;31:400–9. doi:10.1002/bies.200800100.
16. Spector DL, Lamond AI. Nuclear speckles. Cold Spring Harb Perspect Biol. 2011;3:a000646. doi:10.1101/cshperspect.a000646.
17. Spector DL. Macromolecular domains within the cell nucleus. Annu Rev Cell Biol USA. 1993;9:265–315. doi:10.1146/annurev.cb.09.110193.001405.
18. Misteli T, Spector DL. The cellular organization of gene expression. Curr Opin Cell Biol. 1998;10:323–31. doi:10.1016/S0955-0674(98)80007-0.
19. Misteli T. Cell biology of transcription and pre-mRNA splicing: nuclear architecture meets nuclear function. J Cell Sci. 2000;113:1841–9. 10806095
20. Dundr M, Misteli T. Functional architecture in the cell nucleus. Biochem J. 2001;356:297–310.
21. Hall LL, Smith KP, Byron M, Lawrence JB. Molecular anatomy of a speckle. Anat Rec A Discov Mol Cell Evol Biol. 2006;288:664–75. doi:10.1002/ar.a.20336.
22. Björk P, Wieslander L. Nucleocytoplasmic mRNP export is an integral part of mRNP biogenesis. Chromosoma. 2011;120:23–38. doi:10.1007/s00412-010-0298-1.
23. Rodríguez-Navarro S, Hurt E. Linking gene regulation to mRNA production and export. Curr Opin Cell Biol. 2011;23:302–9. doi:10.1016/j.ceb.2010.12.002.
24. Lei EP, Krebber H, Silver PA. Messenger RNAs are recruited for nuclear export during transcription. Genes Dev. 2001;15:1771–82. doi:10.1101/gad.892401.
25. Reed R. Coupling transcription, splicing and mRNA export. Curr Opin Cell Biol. 2003;15:326–31. doi:10.1016/S0955-0674(03)00048-6.
26. Reed R, Hurt E. A conserved mRNA export machinery coupled to pre-mRNA splicing. Cell. 2002;108:523–31. doi:10.1016/S0092-8674(02)00627-X.
27. Cheng H, Dufu K, Lee C-S, Hsu JL, Dias A, Reed R. Human mRNA export machinery recruited to the 5' end of mRNA. Cell. 2006;127:1389–400. doi:10.1016/j.cell.2006.10.044.
28. Le Hir H, Andersen GR. Structural insights into the exon junction complex. Curr Opin Struct Biol. 2008;18:112–9. https://doi.org/10.1016/j.sbi.2007.11.002.
29. Schmidt U, Richter K, Berger AB, Lichter P. *In vivo* BiFC analysis of Y14 and NXF1 mRNA export complexes: preferential localization within and around SC35 domains. J Cell Biol. 2006;172:373–81. doi:10.1083/jcb.200503061.
30. Daguenet E, Baguet A, Degot S, Schmidt U, Alpy F, Wendling C, et al. Perispeckles are major assembly sites for the exon junction core complex. Mol Biol Cell. 2012;23:1765–82. doi:10.1091/mbc.E12-01-0040.
31. Schmidt U, Im K-B, Benzing C, Janjetovic S, Rippe K, Lichter P, Wachsmuth M. Assembly and mobility of exon-exon junction complexes in living cells. RNA. 2009;15:862–76. doi:10.1261/rna.1387009.
32. Kiselev A, Stepanova I, Adonin L, Batalova F, Parfenov V, Bogolyubov D, Podgornaya O. Characterization of *Tribolium castaneum* oocyte nuclear structures using microinjection of a fusion nuclear protein mRNA. Mol Reprod Dev. 2015;82:628–9. doi:10.1002/mrd.22514.
33. Goodman CL, Stanley D, Ringbauer JA, Beeman RW, Silver K, Park Y. A cell line derived from the red flour beetle *Tribolium castaneum* (Coleoptera: Tenebrionidae). In Vitro Cell Dev Biol Anim. 2012;48:426–33. doi:10.1007/s11626-012-9524-x.
34. Graham FL, Smiley J, Russell WC, Nairn R. Characteristics of a human cell line transformed by DNA from human adenovirus type 5. J Gen Virol. 1977;36:59–74. doi:10.1099/0022-1317-36-1-59.
35. Graham FL, van der Eb AJ. Transformation of rat cells by DNA of human adenovirus 5. Virology. 1973;54:536–9.
36. Freeman AE, Black PH, Vanderpool EA, Henry PH, Austin JB, Huebner RJ. Transformation of primary rat embryo cells by adenovirus type 2. Proc Natl Acad Sci U S A. 1967;58:1205–12.
37. Murashev B, Kazennova E, Kozlov A, Murasheva I, Dukhovlinova E, Galachyants Y, et al. Immunogenicity of candidate DNA vaccine based on subtype a of human immunodeficiency virus type 1 predominant in Russia. Biotechnol J. 2007;2:871–8. doi:10.1002/biot.200700024.
38. Sambrook J, Russell DW. Molecular cloning – a laboratory manual. 3rd ed. New York: Cold Spring Harbor Laboratory Press; 2001.
39. Sible JC, Wroble BN. Expression of exogenous mRNA in *Xenopus laevis* embryos for the study of cell cycle regulation. Methods Mol Biol. 2009;518:1–15. doi:10.1007/978-1-59745-202-1_1.
40. Hulsebos T, Hackstein J, Henning W. Lampbrush loop-specific protein of *Drosophila hydei*. Proc Natl Acad Sci U S A. 1984;81:3404–8. 6587357
41. Liu J-L, Buszczak M, Gall JG. Nuclear bodies in the *Drosophila* germinal vesicle. Chromosom Res. 2006;14:465–75. doi:10.1007/s10577-006-1062-5.
42. Dart LH Jr, Turner TR. Fluorescence microscopy in exfoliative cytology. Report of acridine orange examination of 5491 cases, with comparison by the Papanicolaou technic. Lab Investig. 1959;8:1513–22. 13814155
43. Evan GI, Lewis GK, Ramsay G, Bishop JM. Isolation of monoclonal antibodies specific for human c-myc proto-oncogene product. Mol Cell Biol. 1985;5:3610–6.
44. X-D F, Maniatis T. Factor required for mammalian spliceosome assembly is localized to discrete regions in the nucleus. Nature. 1990;343:437–41. doi:10.1038/343437a0.
45. Sekelsky JJ, Brodsky MH, Rubin GM, Hawley RS. *Drosophila* and human RecQ5 exist in different isoforms generated by alternative splicing. Nucleic Acids Res. 1999;27:3762–9.
46. Trauner J, Büning J. Germ-cell cluster formation in the telotrophic meroistic ovary of *Tribolium castaneum* (Coleoptera, Polyphaga, Tenebrionidae) and

its implication on insect phylogeny. Dev Genes Evol. 2007;217:13–27. doi:10.1007/s00427-006-0114-3.
47. Ullmann SL. Oogenesis in *Tenebrio molitor*: histological and autoradiographical observations on pupal and adult ovaries. J Embryol Exp Morphol. 1973;30:179–217. 4729945
48. Bogolyubov D. Localization of RNA transcription sites in insect oocytes using microinjections of 5-bromouridine 5′-triphosphate. Folia Histochem Cytobiol. 2007;45:129–34. 17597027
49. Will CL, Lührmann R. Spliceosomal UsnRNP biogenesis, structure and function. Curr Opin Cell Biol. 2001;13:290–301. doi:10.1016/S0955-0674(00)00211-8.
50. Ilicheva NV, Kiryushina DY, Baskakov AV, Podgornaya OI, Pochukalina GN. The karyosphere capsule in oocytes of hibernating frogs *Rana temporaria* contains actin, lamins, and snRNP. Cell Tissue Biol. 2016;10:422–9. doi:10.1134/S1990519X16050059.
51. Batalova F, Stepanova I, Skovorodkin I, Bogolyubov D, Parfenov V. Identification and dynamics of Cajal bodies in relation to karyosphere formation in scorpionfly oocytes. Chromosoma. 2005;113:428–39. doi:10.1007/s00412-004-0328-y.
52. Bogolyubov D, Alexandrova O, Tsvetkov A, Parfenov V. An immunoelectron study of karyosphere and nuclear bodies in oocytes of mealworm beetle, *Tenebrio molitor* (Coleoptera: Polyphaga). Chromosoma. 2000;109:415–25. doi:10.1007/s004120000090.
53. Bogolyubov D, Parfenov V. Immunogold localization of RNA polymerase II and pre-mRNA splicing factors in *Tenebrio molitor* oocyte nuclei with special emphasis on karyosphere development. Tissue Cell. 2001;33:549–61. doi:10.1054/tice.2001.0210.
54. Podgornaya OI, Voronin AP, Enukashvily NI, Matveev IV, Lobov IB. Structure-specific DNA-binding proteins as the foundation for three-dimensional chromatin organization. Int Rev Cytol. 2003;224:227–96.
55. Malyavantham KS, Bhattacharya S, Barbeitos M, Mukherjee L, Xu J, Fackelmayer FO, Berezney R. Identifying functional neighborhoods within the cell nucleus: proximity analysis of early S-phase replicating chromatin domains to sites of transcription, RNA polymerase II, HP1γ, matrin 3 and SAF-A. J Cell Biochem. 2008;105:391–403. doi:10.1002/jcb.21834.
56. Świątek P. Formation of the karyosome in developing oocytes of weevils (Coleoptera, Curculionidae). Tissue Cell. 1999;31:587–93. doi:10.1054/tice.1999.0073.
57. Rübsam R, Büning J. F-actin is a component of the karyosome in neuropteran oocyte nuclei. Arthr Struct Dev. 2001;30:125–33. doi:10.1016/S1467-8039(01)00026-3.
58. Parfenov VN, Davis DS, Pochukalina GN, Sample CE, Bugaeva EA, Murti KG. Nuclear actin filaments and their topological changes in frog oocytes. Exp Cell Res. 1995;217:385–94. doi:10.1006/excr.1995.1101.
59. Maslova A, Krasikova A. Nuclear actin depolymerization in transcriptionally active avian and amphibian oocytes leads to collapse of intranuclear structures. Nucleus. 2012;3:300–11. doi:10.4161/nucl.20393.
60. Bogolyubova I, Stein G, Bogolyubov D. FRET analysis of interactions between actin and exon-exon-junction complex proteins in early mouse embryos. Cell Tissue Res. 2013;352:277–85. doi:10.1007/s00441-012-1545-y.
61. Kukalev A, Nord Y, Palmberg C, Bergman T, Percipalle P. Actin and hnRNP U cooperate for productive transcription by RNA polymerase II. Nat Struct Mol Biol. 2005;12:238–44. doi:10.1038/nsmb904.
62. Grosse R, Vartiainen MK. To be or not to be assembled: progressing into nuclear actin filaments. Nat Rev Mol Cell Biol. 2013;14:693–7. doi:10.1038/nrm3681.
63. Kapoor P, Shen X. Mechanisms of nuclear actin in chromatin-remodeling complexes. Trends Cell Biol. 2014;24:238–46. doi:10.1016/j.tcb.2013.10.007.
64. Gruzova MN. Ultrastructure of the karyosphere in darkling beetles (Tenebrionidae Coleoptera Polyphaga). Monit Zool Ital. 1982;16:231–46. doi:10.1080/00269786.1982.10736402.
65. Gruzova MN, Zaichikova ZP, Sokolov II. Functional organization of the nucleus in the oogenesis of *Chrysopa perla* L. (Insecta, Neuroptera). Chromosoma. 1972;37:353–85. doi:10.1007/BF00284886.
66. Gruzova MN, Batalova FM. Nuclear structures in the telotrophic ovarioles of nocturnal ground beetles (Tenebrionidae, Polyphaga). II. The oocyte nucleus of *Blaps lethifera* and *Gnaptor spinimanus*. Light optical data. Ontogenez. 1979;10:323–31. 481847
67. Parfenov VN, Gruzova MN. Nuclear structures at late stages of *Rana temporaria* oogenesis. II. Autoradiographic data. Tsitologiia. 1975;17:1263–8. 1084064
68. Parfenov V, Potchukalina G, Dudina L, Kostyuchek D, Gruzova M. Human antral follicles: oocyte nucleus and the karyosphere formation (electron microscopic and autoradigraphic data). Gamete Res. 1989;22:219–31. doi:10.1002/mrd.1120220209.
69. Albiez H, Cremer M, Tiberi C, Vecchio L, Schermelleh L, Dittrich S, et al. Chromatin domains and the interchromatin compartment form structurally defined and functionally interacting nuclear networks. Chromosom Res. 2006;14:707–33. doi:10.1007/s10577-006-1086-x.
70. Fakan S, van Driel R. The perichromatin region: a functional compartment in the nucleus that determines large-scale chromatin folding. Semin Cell Dev Biol. 2007;18:676–81. https://doi.org/10.1016/j.semcdb.2007.08.010.
71. Markaki Y, Gunkel M, Schermelleh L, Beichmanis S, Neumann J, Heidemann M, et al. Functional nuclear organization of transcription and DNA replication: a topographical marriage between chromatin domains and the interchromatin compartment. Cold Spring Harb Symp Quant Biol. 2011;75:475–92. doi:10.1101/sqb.2010.75.042.
72. Niedojadło J, Perret-Vivancos C, Kalland K-H, Cmarko D, Cremer T, van Driel R, Fakan S, Transcribed DNA. Is preferentially located in the perichromatin region of mammalian cell nuclei. Exp Cell Res. 2011;317:433–344. doi:10.1016/j.yexcr.2010.10.026.
73. Mohr SE, Dillon ST, Boswell RE. The RNA-binding protein Tsunagi interacts with Mago Nashi to establish polarity and localize *oskar* mRNA during *Drosophila* oogenesis. Genes Dev. 2001;15:2886–99. doi:10.1101/gad.927001.
74. Edström J-E. Composition of ribonucleic acid from various parts of spider oocytes. J Biophys Biochem Cytol. 1960;8:47–51.
75. Fadloun A, Le Gras S, Jost B, Ziegler-Birling C, Takahashi H, Gorab E, et al. Chromatin signatures and retrotransposon profiling in mouse embryos reveal regulation of LINE-1 by RNA. Nat Struct Mol Biol. 2013;20:332–8. doi:10.1038/nsmb.2495.
76. Tange TØ, Nott A, Moore MJ. The ever-increasing complexities of the exon junction complex. Curr Opin Cell Biol. 2004;16:279–84. doi:10.1016/j.ceb.2004.03.012.
77. Giorgi C, Moore MJ. The nuclear nurture and cytoplasmic nature of localized mRNPs. Semin Cell Dev Biol. 2007;18:186–93. doi:10.1016/j.semcdb.2007.01.002.
78. Le Hir H, Izaurralde E, Maquat LE, Moore MJ. The spliceosome deposits multiple proteins 20–24 nucleotides upstream of mRNA exon–exon junctions. EMBO J. 2000;19:6860–9. doi:10.1093/emboj/19.24.6860.
79. Le Hir H, Gatfield D, Izaurralde E, Moore MJ. The exon–exon junction complex provides a binding platform for factors involved in mRNA export and nonsense-mediated mRNA decay. EMBO J. 2001;20:4987–97. doi:10.1093/emboj/20.17.4987.
80. Bono F, Gehring NH. Assembly, disassembly and recycling: the dynamics of exon junction complexes. RNA Biol. 2011;8:24–9. doi:10.4161/rna.8.1.13618.
81. Jurica MS, Moore MJ. Pre-mRNA splicing. awash in a sea of proteins Mol Cell. 2003;12:5–14. doi:10.1016/S1097-2765(03)00270-3.
82. Reichert VL, Le Hir H, Jurica MS, Moore MJ. 5′ exon interactions within the human spliceosome establish a framework for exon junction complex structure and assembly. Genes Dev. 2002;16:2778–91. doi:10.1101/gad.1030602.
83. Dostie J, Dreyfuss G. Translation is required to remove Y14 from mRNAs in the cytoplasm. Curr Biol. 2002;12:1060–7. doi:10.1016/S0960-9822(02)00902-8.
84. Lejeune F, Ishigaki Y, Li X, Maquat LE. The exon junction complex is detected on CBP80-bound but not eIF4E-bound mRNA in mammalian cells: dynamics of mRNP remodeling. EMBO J. 2002;21:3536–45. doi:10.1093/emboj/cdf345.
85. Kataoka N, Diem MD, Yoshida M, Hatai C, Dobashi I, Dreyfuss G, et al. Specific Y14 domains mediate its nucleo-cytoplasmic shuttling and association with spliced mRNA. Sci Rep. 2011;1:92. doi:10.1038/srep00092.
86. Fribourg S, Gatfield D, Izaurralde E, Conti E. A novel mode of RBD-protein recognition in the Y14-Mago Complex. Nat Struct Biol. 2003;10:433–9. doi:10.1038/nsb926.
87. Lau CK, Diem MD, Dreyfuss G, Van Duyne GD. Structure of the Y14-Magoh core of the exon junction complex. Curr Biol. 2003;13:933–41. doi:10.1016/S0960-9822(03)00328-2.
88. Shi H, Xu R-M. Crystal structure of the *Drosophila* Mago Nashi-Y14 complex. Genes Dev. 2003;17:971–6. doi:10.1101/gad.260403.
89. Phair RD, Misteli T. High mobility of proteins in the mammalian cell nucleus. Nature. 2000;404:604–9. doi:10.1038/35007077.
90. Wei X, Somanathan S, Samarabandu J, Berezney R. Three-dimensional visualization of transcription sites and their association with splicing factor-rich nuclear speckles. J Cell Biol. 1999;146:543–58.

7

# Distinct subtypes of genomic *PTEN* deletion size influence the landscape of aneuploidy and outcome in prostate cancer

Thiago Vidotto[1], Daniel Guimarães Tiezzi[2] and Jeremy A. Squire[1,3,4*]

**Abstract**

**Background:** Inactivation of the *PTEN* tumor suppressor gene by deletion occurs in 20–30% of prostate cancer tumors and loss strongly correlates with a worse outcome. PTEN loss of function not only leads to activation of the PI3K/AKT pathway, but is also thought to affect genome stability and increase levels of tumor aneuploidy. We performed an in silico integrative genomic and transcriptomic analysis of 491 TCGA prostate cancer tumors. These data were used to map the genomic sizes of *PTEN* gene deletions and to characterize levels of instability and patterns of aneuploidy acquisition.

**Results:** *PTEN* homozygous deletions had a significant increase in aneuploidy compared to *PTEN* tumors without an apparent deletion, and hemizygous deletions showed an intermediate aneuploidy profile. A supervised clustering of somatic copy number alterations (SCNA) demonstrated that the size of *PTEN* deletions was not random, but comprised five distinct subtypes: (1) "Small Interstitial" (70 bp-789Kb); (2) "Large Interstitial" (1-7 MB); (3) "Large Proximal" (3-65 MB); (4) "Large Terminal" (8-64 MB), and (5) "Extensive" (71-132 MB). Many of the deleted fragments in each subtype were flanked by low copy repetitive (LCR) sequences. SCNAs such as gain at 3q21.1-3q29 and deletions at 8p, *RB1*, *TP53* and *TMPRSS2-ERG* were variably present in all subtypes. Other SCNAs appeared to be recurrent in some deletion subtypes, but absent from others. To determine how the aneuploidy influenced global levels of gene expression, we performed a comparative transcriptome analysis. One deletion subtype (Large Interstitial) was characterized by gene expression changes associated with angiogenesis and cell adhesion, structure, and metabolism. Logistic regression demonstrated that this deletion subtype was associated with a high Gleason score (HR = 2.386; 95% C.I. 1.245–4.572), extraprostatic extension (HR = 2.423, 95% C.I. 1.157–5.075), and metastasis (HR = 7.135; 95% C.I. 1.540–33.044). Univariate and multivariate Cox Regression showed that presence of this deletion subtype was also strongly predictive of disease recurrence.

**Conclusions:** Our findings indicate that genomic deletions of *PTEN* fall into five different size distributions, with breakpoints that often occur close LCR regions, and that each subtype is associated with a characteristic aneuploidy signature. The Large Interstitial deletion had a distinct gene expression signature that was related to cancer progression and was also predictive of a worse prognosis.

**Keywords:** TCGA, Prostate cancer, Genomic instability, PTEN, Chromosome 10

* Correspondence: jsquireinsp@gmail.com
[1]Department of Genetics, Ribeirão Preto Medical School, University of São Paulo, Ribeirão Preto, Brazil
[3]Department of Pathology and Legal Medicine, Ribeirão Preto Medical School, University of São Paulo, 3900 Bandeirantes Avenue, Monte Alegre, Ribeirão Preto, São Paulo 14040-900, Brazil
Full list of author information is available at the end of the article

## Background

Prostate Cancer is the most frequent solid tumor in men and is the third most common cancer type in the world [1]. Genomic deletion of the *PTEN* tumor suppressor gene occurs in 20–30% of prostate cancer tumors, and presence of this aberration strongly correlates with a worse outcome [2–5]. There is therefore increasing interest in the use of loss of the *PTEN* gene and its protein as a predictive biomarker of outcome [5–7]. Moreover, PTEN loss is associated with increased levels of chromosomal instability [8] and the accumulation of high levels of aneuploidy in tumors [9].

The occurrence of aneuploidy, arising as a consequence of genomic instability, is one of the most prominent features of human cancers [10]. Through clonal expansion, tumors often acquire high levels of sequence mutations together with numerical and structural chromosomal rearrangements due to loss of integrity in the DNA repair machinery. In this way, these defects in the genome and chromosome maintenance may also provide a selectively advantageous progression for the malignant cells [11].

The *PTEN* gene is located at 10q23.31 and mapping studies have shown that *PTEN* genomic deletions in prostate cancer vary in size from a few hundred kb of DNA to several Mb. Interestingly, *PTEN* deletions often appear to have breakpoints that initiate close to low copy repeat (LCR) regions [12]. The LCR repetitive elements (also known as segmental duplications) are unstable DNA sequences that are represented two or more times in the genome with high sequence identity, but not arising by retrotransposition [13]. On chromosome 10 there is one LCR hotspots 400 kb centromeric of *PTEN* that may facilitate the inter- and intragenomic alterations leading to *PTEN* loss [14, 15]. LCRs can promote the occurrence of somatic copy number alterations (SCNAs) through non-allelic homologous recombination (NAHR), non-homologous end-joining (NHEJ), and fork stalling and template switching (FoSTeS) [16–19]. To date, *PTEN* gene deletions have been extensively analyzed through FISH assays [4, 5, 20, 21], but a detailed mapping of chromosome 10 deletions that span *PTEN* and their impact on SCNAs and levels of aneuploidy in prostate cancer outcome have not been investigated in detail [22, 23].

This study was designed to determine whether the observed variations in the size of *PTEN* genomic deletions has an impact on overall levels of genomic instability and the acquisition of aneuploidy in the prostate cancer genome. Our study design also addresses whether the initiation of deletion events is influenced by the proximity of LCR elements along chromosome 10 and whether deletion size correlates with any clinical features associated with prostate cancer progression.

## Results

### Impact of homozygous and Hemizygous *PTEN* deletions on genomic instability and aneuploidy

We identified homozygous or hemizygous *PTEN* gene deletions in 118/491 (24.1%) of the prostate tumors and the regions of genomic loss varied in length from 70 bp to 132 MB. Overall we found that 44/491 (9%) had homozygous *PTEN* deletions and 74/491 (15.1%) had hemizygous deletions. Since about 5% of prostate cancers inactivate a *PTEN* allele by a somatic point mutation (frameshift deletions and insertions, in-frame deletions, missense mutations, or splice-site mutation) [24] and not by a large genomic deletion, it was necessary to consider the effect of any mutation caused by sequence alterations. We found that 66% of tumors with hemizygous genomic deletions also harbored somatic mutations in the remaining *PTEN* allele. Such tumors would be expected to express no PTEN protein. In contrast, when there is a hemizygous deletion but the remaining *PTEN* gene appears to be undeleted (*PTEN* intact), the protein expression levels may be reduced so that functional haploinsufficiency may occur (discussed below).

To evaluate the impact of homozygous vs. hemizygous *PTEN* deletions on genomic instability and aneuploidy, we performed a Kruskal-Wallis test considering the total number of SCNAs, the percentage of genome altered, the total number of mutations, and the MATH tumor heterogeneity score. Tumors with *PTEN* homozygous deletions had a higher number of SCNA ($P$-value < 0.0001), increased aneuploidy (percentage of genome altered, $P$-value < 0.0001), and an increased number of mutations ($P$-value = 0.015). The loss of one copy of the *PTEN* gene was sufficient to affect levels of instability since hemizygous deletions demonstrated significant differences when compared to *PTEN* intact (Additional file 1).

### The different sizes of *PTEN* genomic deletions influence the SCNA landscape and pattern of aneuploidy in prostate cancer

To determine whether the deletions had non-random size distributions along chromosome 10, we performed a supervised clustering of all the SCNA leading to *PTEN* deletion. This analysis demonstrated that there were five distinct deletion subtypes classified as: (1) Small Interstitial (size range 70 bp-789Kb); (2) Large Interstitial (1-7 MB); (3) Large Proximal (3-65 MB); (4) Large Terminal (8-64 MB), and (5) Extensive (71-132 MB) (Fig. 1). The deletion subtypes presented similar proportions of hemi- and homozygous deletions (Additional file 2). The list of all genes present in the regions of chromosome 10 loss for each deletion subtype is shown in Additional file 3.

Many of the deletions breakpoints occurred close to genomic regions containing LCRs (see Fig. 1).

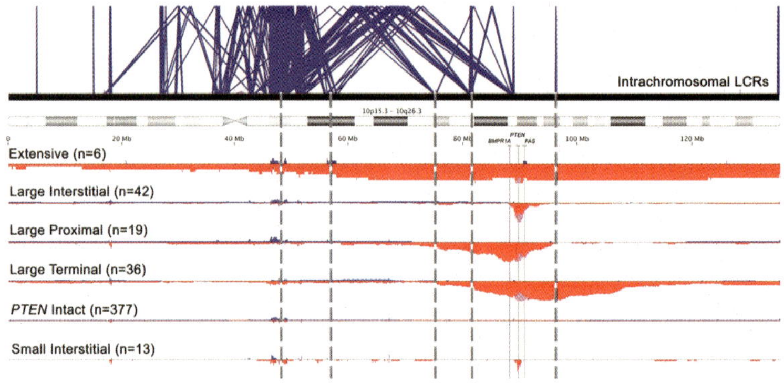


**Fig. 1** Chromosome 10 characterization and LCR mapping of the different *PTEN* deletion subtypes in prostate cancer. The panel below the schematic map of chromosome 10 demonstrates the different deletion subtypes and their frequency for each group. The genome is displayed horizontally, and the frequency of somatic copy number alterations (SCNA) at any given location are displayed on the y-axis. Red, pink and blue indicate the frequencies as a percentage of hemizygous deletions, homozygous deletions, and gains, respectively. The three thin continuous vertical lines show the precise location of the genes *BMPR1A, PTEN,* and *FAS* genes. The number of deletions for each subtype is shown in parentheses. The tumors that have *PTEN* intact are also shown. The panel above shows the intrachromosomal LCR regions along chromosome 10 with related regions of homology linked by thin blue lines. The five grey vertical dashed lines identify clusters of LCRs that map to the vicinity of *PTEN* deletion breakpoints defined by copy number transitions. Many deletions appear to originate at the small LCR cluster in between *PTEN* and *BMPR1A*. Mapping was performed using data from the Segmental Duplication database (http://humanparalogy.gs.washington.edu) for sequences with more or equal to 5Kb and showing equal or more similarity in 90% of the duplicated sequence

Additionally, the breakpoint regions of all deletion subtypes showed a high number of flanking LCRs having >1Kb and 90–99% similarity levels in both upper and lower extremities of the deleted fragments (manuscript in preparation).

To determine if the five *PTEN* deletion subtypes had distinct patterns of aneuploidy, we compared their SCNA landscapes to overall levels of copy number change in tumors without an apparent *PTEN* gene loss (Fig. 2). Some of the imbalances such as gain at 3q21.1-3q29 and deletions at 8p, *RB1, TP53,* and *TMPRSS2* were found with varying incidences in all five subtypes. The 3q21.1-3q29 region has eight cancer-related genes: *PIK3CA, ZNF9, FOXL2, ATR, WWTR1, GMPS, MLF1,* and *TBLIXR1.* Other SCNAs appeared to be enriched in some subtypes and not in others. For example, both the Small and Large Interstitial deletion subtypes were characterized by having gains of chromosome 7. The Large Terminal, Proximal and Extensive had losses of chromosome 6. The Small Interstitial deletion was the only subtype to have extensive gains of chromosome 11. The Extensive deletions had the largest region of copy number loss and were characterized by concurrent deletions of chromosome 12p, 18q, whole chr13, and gains at 5p11 (Fig. 2).

### The effect of the different *PTEN* deletion subtypes on genomic instability and the somatic mutation rate in prostate cancer

When comparing the five *PTEN* deletion subtypes to the tumors without apparent PTEN loss, the Large Terminal and Large Interstitial deletion subtypes exhibited a significant increase in the total number of SCNAs. Moreover, we observed that Large Proximal and Large Interstitial demonstrated increased levels of mutations and that all deletion subtypes except Small Interstitial exhibited a significant increase in the percentage of genome altered (Fig. 3).

We then investigated whether tumors with concomitant *PTEN* hemizygous deletion and a somatic mutation in the remaining allele would lead to a more significant impact in aneuploidy. We observed that patients with both hemizygous deletions and somatic mutations demonstrated high levels of aneuploidy (percentage of genome altered, $P$-value = 0.008), total number of SCNAs ($P$-value < 0.0001), and total number of mutations ($P$-value = 0.05) when compared to *PTEN* intact and tumors with both alleles present with a somatic mutation in one of the alleles (Additional file 4).

MutSigCV analysis presented the 19 most differentially mutated genes across the cases: *CDKN1B, FBXO46, FRG1, GAST, KIAA1257, LCE1F, MLF2, PTEN, SNRNP27, SPOP, TMEM211, YWHAQ, TP53, FOXA1, ZMYM3, KDM6A, RYBP, SMARCA1,* and *ZFHX3.* To determine whether *PTEN* hemi- and homozygous deletions impact the mutational signatures of the 19 genes, a chi-square was performed. Differences in *TP53, SPOP,* and *PTEN* gene mutations ($P$-value < 0.001) were observed. *TP53* mutations were present in 16% and 27% in tumors with hemi- and homozygous deletions of *PTEN*, respectively. *SPOP* mutations were present in 3% of hemi- and 3% of homozygous deletion tumors and in 94% of *PTEN* intact tumors.

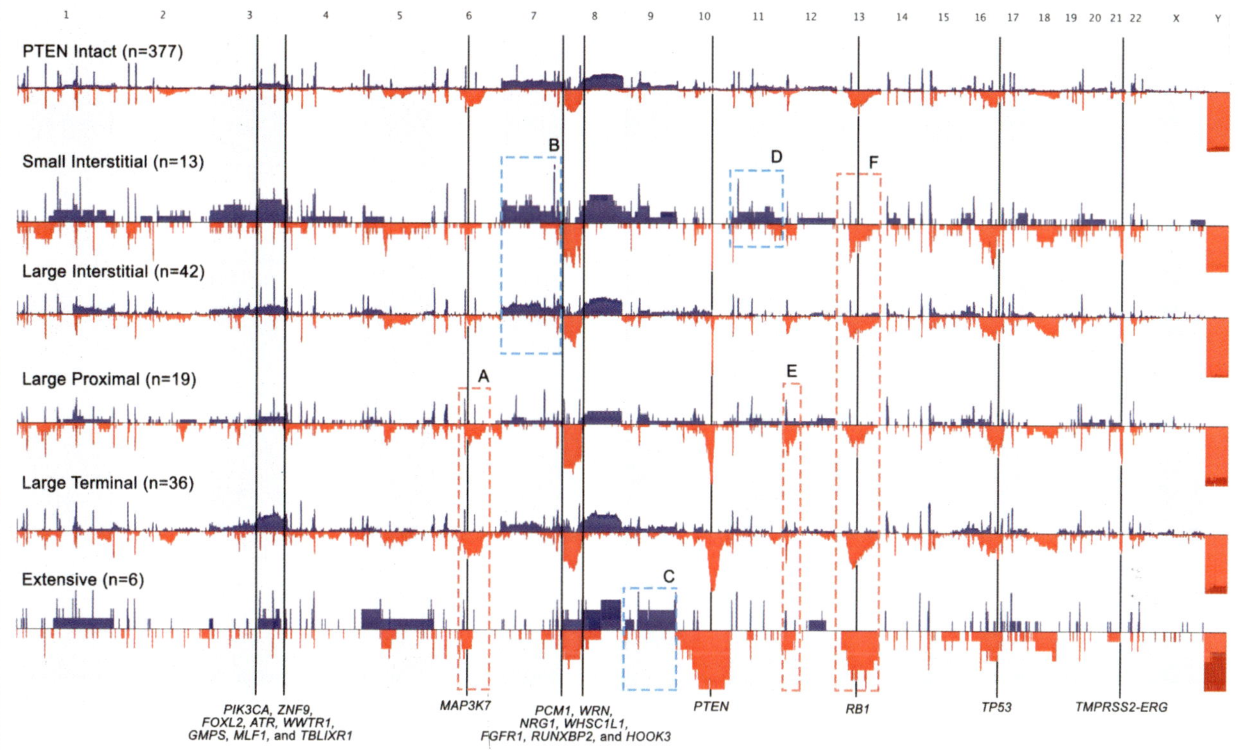


**Fig. 2** Whole genome snapshot of varying levels of aneuploidy in the different *PTEN* deletion subtypes. The genome is displayed horizontally, and the frequency of SCNAs at any given location are displayed on the y-axis. Red and blue indicate losses and gains, respectively. The black vertical continuous lines identify the chromosomal regions common to all subtypes that have marked differential copy numbers in comparison to *PTEN* intact. Chromosomes 3, 8, 13, and 21 were the most affected regions common to all subtypes. The red and blue dashed boxes identify regions that presented a high frequency of deletions and gains, respectively. Box A identifies the three deletion subtypes with a high frequency of losses of chromosome 6. Box B shows that the Large Proximal and Large Interstitial subtypes both have high levels of aneuploidy of chromosome 7. Box C shows high rates of gains at chromosome 9 in the Extensive deletions. Box D demonstrates a high number of gains of chromosome 11 in the Small Interstitial subtype. Box E highlights the gains of chromosome 12p in three subtypes: Large Proximal, Large Terminal and Extensive. Box F shows a progressive increase of chromosome 13 deletions with whole chromosome losses in Extensive deletion type. Files obtained in Nexus Copy Number v8.0 (Biodiscovery)

When we compared the frequency of mutation in the 19 genes across the *PTEN* deletion subtypes to the frequency in the *PTEN* intact tumors, we identified significant differences for *TP53* (*P*-value = 0.0001), *SPOP* (*P*-value = 0.013), and *YWHAQ* (*P*-value = 0.0001) genes. In addition, the Large Interstitial type presented the higher number of mutations in *TP53* (20%) when compared to the other deletion subtypes.

### Effects of *PTEN* deletion subtypes on differential gene expression

Initially, we checked the RNAseq dataset to confirm that when the *PTEN* gene was deleted the PTEN transcript level was decreased as expected. These analyses showed that *PTEN* homozygous deletions presented the lowest PTEN mRNA expression value, followed by *PTEN* hemizygous deletions (*P*-value < 0.0001) (Additional file 5a). In comparison to *PTEN* intact tumors, the average for PTEN mRNA expression was significantly decreased for all *PTEN* deletion subtypes (*P*-value < 0.0001), but there were no differences in the relative levels of PTEN mRNA expression across the five deletion subtypes (Additional file 5b).

To determine how the different genomic sizes of the *PTEN* deletions can affect global levels of gene expression levels, we performed a group transcriptome comparison of all five subtypes to the expression observed in the tumors without a *PTEN* deletion. The Large Interstitial deletion subtype was the most different, with 1073 differentially expressed genes in comparison to *PTEN* intact tumors. The Large Proximal and Large Terminal deletions presented with 197 and 248 differentially expressed genes, respectively. Extensive and Small Interstitial losses had less marked differences with 50 and just seven differentially expressed genes.

Enrichment analysis of the differentially expressed genes from all *PTEN* deletion subtypes showed that only Large Interstitial and Large Proximal deletions significantly demonstrate alterations of cancer-related pathways (Fig. 4). We observed that Large Interstitial deletions influence the gene expression profile of

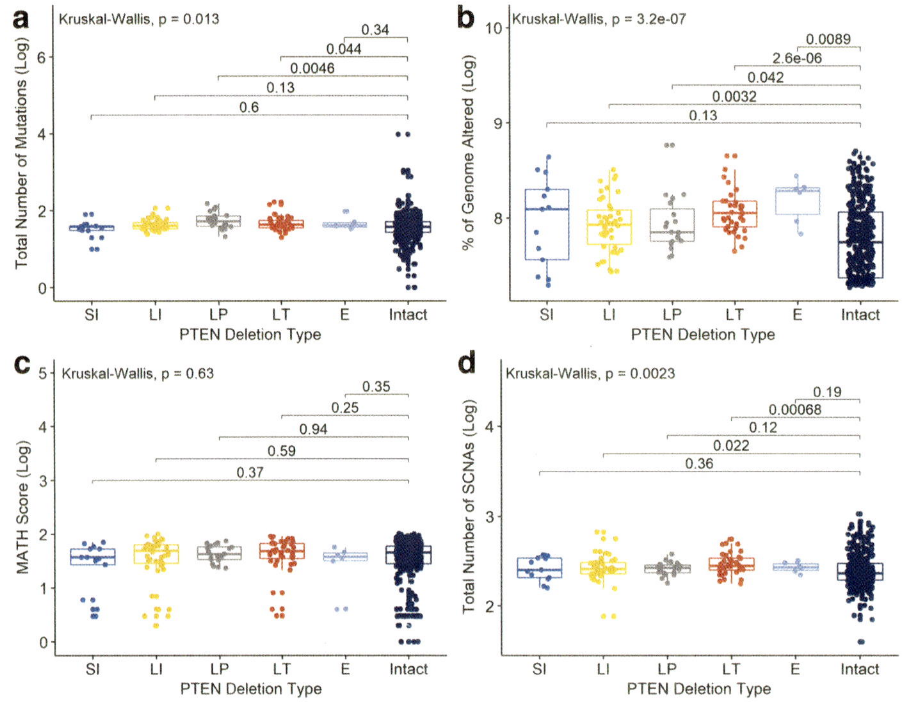


**Fig. 3** Variation of mutation, tumor heterogeneity, aneuploidy, and genomic instability in *PTEN* deletion subtypes in prostate cancer. The boxplots show **a** - the total number of mutations, **b** – aneuploidy, as percentage of genome altered, **c** - Mutant-Allele Tumor Heterogeneity (MATH) score, and **d** - total number of SCNAs. The different deletion subtypes show increased heterogeneity for all evaluated parameters. *PTEN* intact tumors also show increased heterogeneity, with a significant number of outliers. SCNA – somatic copy number alteration, SI – Small Interstitial, LI – Large Interstitial, LP – Large Proximal, LT – Large Terminal, E – Extensive

proteins associated with angiogenesis (e.g., *VEGF, SAT1, EMCN, CAV1, HTATIP2, NRP1, CSPG4, PDE3B, ANPEP,* and *TNFSF12*), and cell metabolism (e.g., *POLR1B, AMPD3, PGM2, POLD4, PDE2A, NUDT9, NT5M*), adhesion (*MCAM, JAM3, COMP, NOV, ICAM1, ITGA11, ADAM17,* and *ADAM9*) migration (e.g., PRKD1, LAMC2, SEMA3B, PDGFD, TRIP6, LAMB1, and F2R) and structure (e.g., *KCNC2, CTNNAL1, SLC44A1, ADCY1, SLC22A18, EFNA3, UTRN, CSPG4, SLC7A8, KIAA1324,* and *LPAR3*). Moreover, Large Proximal deletions show influence on the expression of genes related to cell metabolism (e.g., *OVGP1, UGDH, GAA, GLO1,* and *GLB1*) and structure (e.g., *FZD8, ACER3, FAM198B, RAB43, GNPTAB,* and *CLSTN3*) (Fig. 4).

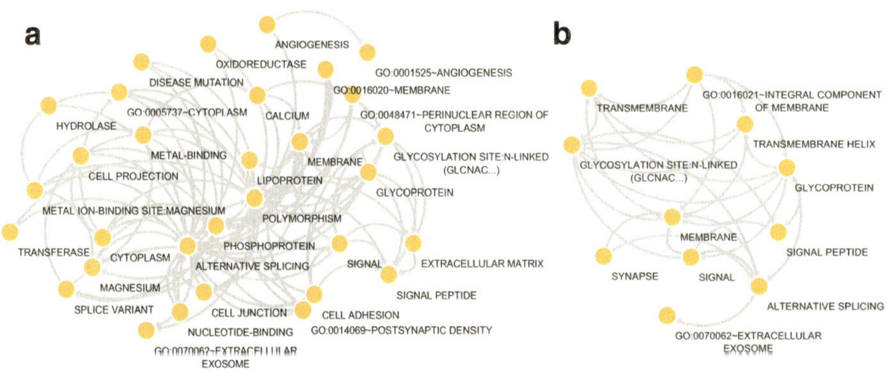


**Fig. 4** Enrichment analysis of gene expression in deletion subtypes with extensive aneuploidy. Two *PTEN* deletion subtypes had distinctive patterns of aneuploidy and were significantly enriched for pathways related to cancer progression. The Large Interstitial subtype (**a**) was enriched for metabolism, cell structural adhesion and also angiogenesis. The Large Proximal deletions (**b**) showed effects in pathways associated with cell metabolism and structure. Enrichment analysis was performed through DAVID database and nodes were generated through Enrichment Map (Cytoscape)

**Large interstitial deletions of chromosome 10 that harbor *PTEN* gene predicts worse outcome in prostate cancer**

In order to identify the effect of the different *PTEN* deletion subtypes on clinical and pathological features of prostate cancer, we performed a Chi-square test for race, Gleason score, presence of extraprostatic extension, lymph node invasion, pathologic grade, presence of metastasis, and disease recurrence. *PTEN* hemi- and homozygous deletions showed significant effects on all investigated clinical parameters (data not shown). For the different deletion subtypes, we observed differences for lymph node invasion (*P*-value < 0.0001), presence of seminal vesicle invasion (*P*-value = 0.003), presence of extraprostatic extension (*P*-value – 0.002), race (*P*-value < 0.0001), and a trend for pathological M (*P*-value = 0.08) (Additional file 6). Among the deletion subtypes, Large Interstitial deletions showed the higher rates of extraprostatic extension (36%), seminal vesicle invasion (41%), lymph node invasion (36%), metastasis (75%), and disease recurrence (46%) (Additional file 6). We did not observe any differences in time to disease recurrence (*P*-value = 0.69) and age at diagnosis (*P*-value = 0.10) for the *PTEN* deletion subtypes, but there was a trend towards men of African-American ancestry having a lower overall incidence of *PTEN* deletions (*P*-value <0.0001).

We then performed a univariate logistic regression analysis to investigate whether deletion subtype could significantly predict the occurrence of tumors with high Gleason score (≥8), extraprostatic extension, metastasis, and disease recurrence. We observed that Large Interstitial deletions (*P*-value = 0.009; HR = 2.386; C.I. 95% 1.245–4.572) significantly predict higher Gleason scores (Table 1). In addition, Large Interstitial (*P*-value = 0.019; HR = 2.423; C.I. 95% 1.157–5.075) and Large Proximal deletions (*P*-value = 0.014; HR = 6.436; C.I. 95% 1.466–28.260) predict the occurrence of extraprostatic extension in patient samples. Similarly, Small Interstitial (*P*-value = 0.03; HR = 3.431; C.I. 95% 1.119–10.412), Large Interstitial (*P*-value = 0.001; HR = 2.660; C.I. 95% 1.389–5.091), and Large Proximal deletions (*P*-value = 0.04; HR = 2.633; C.I. 95% 1.038–6.677) predict the occurrence of seminal vesicle invasion. Large Interstitial deletions also predict the occurrence of metastasis (*P*-value = 0.01; HR = 7.135; C.I. 95% 1.540–33.044) (Table 1).

Kaplan Meyer and log-rank analysis showed a significant difference between tumors with *PTEN* homozygous deletions, *PTEN* hemizygous deletions, and *PTEN* intact for the prediction of earlier disease recurrence events (*P*-value = 0.002) (Additional file 7a). In addition, Kaplan Meyer curves and log-rank analysis were performed for disease recurrence and demonstrated no significance in the curve for the different *PTEN* deletion subtypes (*P*-value = 0.11) (Additional file 7b). Univariate Cox Regression analysis showed that Large Interstitial deletions are significantly associated with increased chance of disease recurrence (*P*-value = 0.04; HR = 1.845; C.I. 95% 1.012–3.367) (Table 2).

We then investigated the influence of genomic instability parameters on the likelihood of disease recurrence through univariate Cox Regression. We only found Significant associations were observed for the percentage of genome altered, showing that increased levels of aneuploidy may predict prostate cancer disease

**Table 1** Univariate logistic regression results for clinical parameters considering the five *PTEN* deletion subtypes. *PTEN* intact was set as a baseline in the model. Large Interstitial deletions are reliable predictors of high Gleason scores, extraprostatic extension, and metastasis. The model represents the occurrence of each event analyzed. High Gleason score was obtained through dichotomization: Gleason scores ≤7 were considered as low, and ≥8 were considered as high. *Significant *P*-value < 0.05

| Clinical Feature | *P*-value | Odds Ratio | 95% C.I. | |
|---|---|---|---|---|
| | | | Lower | Upper |
| High Gleason Score | | | | |
| Small Interstitial | 0.26 | 1.893 | 0.624 | 5.744 |
| Large Interstitial | 0.009* | 2.386 | 1.245 | 4.572 |
| Large Proximal | 0.91 | 0.946 | 0.364 | 2.460 |
| Large Terminal | 0.45 | 1.298 | 0.651 | 2.587 |
| Extensive | 0.057 | 8.112 | 0.938 | 70.137 |
| *PTEN* Intact | 0.00 | 0.616 | . | . |
| Extraprostatic Extension | | | | |
| Small Interstitial | 0.16 | 2.524 | 0.683 | 9.322 |
| Large Interstitial | 0.01* | 2.423 | 1.157 | 5.075 |
| Large Proximal | 0.01* | 6.436 | 1.466 | 28.260 |
| Large Terminal | 0.31 | 1.451 | 0.701 | 3.005 |
| Extensive | 0.99 | . | 0.000 | . |
| *PTEN* Intact | 0.00 | 1.321 | . | . |
| Metastasis | | | | |
| Small Interstitial | . | . | . | . |
| Large Interstitial | 0.01* | 7.135 | 1.540 | 33.044 |
| Large Proximal | . | . | . | . |
| Large Terminal | 0.38 | 2.650 | 0.288 | 24.364 |
| Extensive | . | . | . | . |
| *PTEN* Intact | 0.00 | 0.011 | . | . |
| Seminal Vesicle Invasion | | | | |
| Small Interstitial | 0.03* | 3.431 | 1.119 | 10.412 |
| Large Interstitial | 0.001* | 2.660 | 1.389 | 5.091 |
| Large Proximal | 0.04* | 2.633 | 1.038 | 6.677 |
| Large Terminal | 0.98 | 1.013 | 0.458 | 2.239 |
| Extensive | 0.19 | 2.926 | 0.580 | 14.744 |
| *PTEN* Intact | 0.00 | 0.342 | . | . |

**Table 2** Univariate and multivariate Cox Regression analysis for disease recurrence considering the five *PTEN* deletion subtypes. Multivariate analysis exhibits age-adjusted results. PTEN intact was set as the baseline for the model. *Significant *P*-value < 0.05

| Univariate | | | | | Multivariate | | | | |
|---|---|---|---|---|---|---|---|---|---|
| | *P* | HR | 95% C.I. | | | *P* | HR | 95% C.I. | |
| | | | Lower | Upper | | | | Lower | Upper |
| Small Interstitial | 0.32 | 0.373 | 0.052 | 2.694 | Small Interstitial | 0.38 | 0.419 | 0.058 | 3.039 |
| Large Interstitial | 0.04* | 1.845 | 1.012 | 3.367 | Large Interstitial | 0.04* | 1.844 | 1.007 | 3.377 |
| Large Proximal | 0.72 | 1.239 | 0.387 | 3.960 | Large Proximal | 0.74 | 1.213 | 0.379 | 3.881 |
| Large Terminal | 0.13 | 1.705 | 0.845 | 3.440 | Large Terminal | 0.19 | 1.587 | 0.785 | 3.208 |
| Extensive | 0.13 | 2.955 | 0.719 | 12.153 | Extensive | 0.22 | 2.448 | 0.584 | 10.258 |
| *PTEN* Intact | 0.26 | . | . | . | *PTEN* Intact | 0.38 | . | . | . |
| Age | 0.15 | 1.024 | 0.991 | 1.057 | Age | 0.18 | 1.022 | 0.990 | 1.055 |
| Percentage of genome altered | 0.009* | 1.745 | 1.147 | 2.654 | Percentage of genome altered | 0.02* | 1.629 | 1.065 | 2.491 |

*PTEN* intact was set as a baseline in the model. Percentage of genome altered was dichotomized in high (>average) and low (≤average)

recurrence (*P*-value = 0.009; HR = 1.745; CI 95% 1.147–2.654). Finally, age-adjusted Cox Regression models showed that the presence of the Large Interstitial deletion subtype and an increased percentage of genome altered together were predictive of disease recurrence (Table 2).

## Discussion

To date, *PTEN* gene and protein have been widely investigated as biomarkers of prognosis in prostate cancer [5, 12, 25, 26]. However, since *PTEN* deletions may also influence the stability of the genome, it is important to determine how *PTEN* loss influences SCNAs and affects aneuploidy levels in tumors.

The mechanism of *PTEN* genomic deletion is poorly understood. Chromosome 10 presents a large number of LCRs that increase the chances that intra- or interchromosomal rearrangements may occur. Moreover, many of these LCRs cluster both proximal and distal to the *PTEN* gene at 10q23.31, and these unstable regions may facilitate the genomic rearrangements leading to deletion events [12]. In this study, we observed five deletion subtype distributions that are flanked by many LCR hotspots, which may initiate of the chromosomal rearrangements leading to gains, losses and the recombination events of chromosome 10 [27, 28].

In prostate cancer, whole genome mate-pair sequencing has shown that the 10q23.31 region has many complex intrachromosomal and interchromosomal rearrangements [22]. Our comparative SCNA analysis showed that large chromosome 10 deletions (Extensive deletions) are linked to increased aneuploidy levels in prostate cancer. Whole chromosome aberrations may occur through defects on mitosis checkpoints, centromere overduplication, and cohesion defects in sister chromatids that may lead to missegregation during mitosis and resulting in an altered SCNA landscape of tumor samples [29]. In addition, the presence of whole chromosome alterations may trigger secondary chromosomal aberrations during tumor progression due to improper cytokinesis, which leads to frequent DNA double-strand breaks that are incorrectly repaired by non-homologous end joining (NHEJ) repair machinery [11, 16, 29]. Concomitantly, the whole chromosome 10 deletion may also independently initiate the dysregulation of the cell cycle, centromere stability and DNA double-strand repair maintained by PTEN [30, 31].

In the cytoplasm, PTEN acts dephosphorylating PIP3, which leads to decreased cell survival, growth and proliferation through the AKT/mTOR axis. Furthermore, in the nucleus, PTEN can downregulate MAPK (ERK-P), promoting the G0-G1 arrest due to cyclin D1 regulation [32], and also upregulate RAD51 expression, which promotes double-stranded-break repair [30]. The PTEN protein can also interact with CENP-C to enhance centromere stability and overall genomic stability [30]. Conversely, *PTEN* deletions and protein loss are associated with increased copy number alterations and higher levels of aneuploidy in prostate cancer [9]. Taken together, these data demonstrate that PTEN influences cell proliferation and survival, in addition to having a role in the maintenance of genomic and chromosomal stability.

Genomic instability has a critical role in the creation of variants within tumor cell populations, leading to clonal evolution, inter- and intratumoral heterogeneity and therapeutic resistance [11]. By considering genomic instability parameters, we observed that *PTEN* homozygous deletions demonstrated a significant increase in the total number of SCNA, increased aneuploidy, and total number of mutations when compared to *PTEN* intact samples. Additionally, *PTEN* hemizygous deletions showed an intermediate aneuploidy profile. For the *PTEN* deletion subtypes, we only found that Large Terminal deletions presented an increased total number of SCNA and higher aneuploidy levels when compared to *PTEN* intact tumors.

It has been proposed that the haploinsufficiency of tumor suppressor genes can increase cell proliferation rates that consequently could promote the accumulation of mutations and increased aneuploidy in the genome [33]. Furthermore, hemizygous deletions that harbor proliferation inhibitory genes are thought to be preferentially selected during tumor development [34]. This would be in keeping with mouse studies, which have shown that hemizygous deletion of the Pten C-terminal domain promotes genomic instability and leads to preferential rearrangements at fragile sites [35]. Thus, when both *PTEN* alleles are lost, the genome of prostate cancer may be significantly impacted due to the complete absence of cell cycle regulation, double-strand break repair, centromere stability, as well as increased cell proliferation rates mediated by the AKT/PI3K/mTOR and NF-κB signaling pathways [30, 31, 36, 37].

In this study, the Large Interstitial deletion subtype showed the most significant influence on prostate cancer outcome compared to other deletion subtypes. This deletion type presented a distinct profile in most of the investigated parameters. Large Interstitial deletions influence pathways associated with angiogenesis, cell structure, metabolism, adhesion, and migration. Altered cell adhesion is strongly related to tumorigenesis and tumor differentiation [38], increased invasive and metastatic potential [39] and associated with tumor cell stemness [40]. Moreover, Large Interstitial deletions exhibit altered cell structure, being concordant with the observation that these cells might be less differentiated [10]. Such mechanisms are in agreement with our finding that tumors with Large Interstitial deletions showed increased invasive non-organ confined disease, defined by high rates of extraprostatic extension and seminal vesicle invasion. Additionally, altered angiogenesis may promote an increased tumorigenic potential in these tumors [10], since these changes will affect the tumor microenvironment, which could in turn influence the immune cell infiltration profile and extracellular matrix remodelation [41].

Remarkably, the tumors with Large Interstitial deletions also had high rates of *TP53* mutations. *Pten/Tp53* null murine models of prostate cancer have reduced AR-dependent gene expression and altered cell metabolism [42]. Similarly, for human *TP53* mutated prostate tumors, there is a strong association with poor outcome [43]. However, *TP53* inactivation alone does not lead to genomic instability in physiological conditions [44]. Perhaps collectively the haploinsufficiency of *PTEN*, together with the other flanking genes present in Large Interstitial deletions, and with *TP53* inactivation, may result in reduced apoptosis rates and senescence escape in a replicative stress condition [45, 46].

The haploinsufficiency of the genes located in Large Interstitial deletions are also related to cancer development and progression. *KLLN*, which shares a promoter region with *PTEN*, promotes cell cycle arrest and apoptosis. In addition, *KLLN* gene deletions are linked to high risk for thyroid [47] and breast cancer [48]. *FAS* gene loss of function is also associated with dysregulated apoptosis in vitro [49]. In this way, we suggest that the haploinsufficiency of the genes present in Large Interstitial deletions may drive *TP53* inactivation and consequently an acquisition of a greater level of aneuploidy.

Interestingly, we observed that men of African-America ancestry might have a lower overall incidence of *PTEN* deletions. However, due to the predominantly Caucasian representation in the TCGA cohort, a detailed investigation of deletion size in the context of racial origins could not be conducted. This type of study could be performed on a cohort with more mixed racial origins. It has recently been shown that primary prostate tumors arising in African-Americans have reduced rates of *PTEN* loss when compared to tumors of European-American patients [50–52]. Moreover, the association between *PTEN* loss and poor prognosis appears to be in dependent of racial ancestry [52].

## Conclusion

These findings allow us to hypothesize on both the order of genomic events and the impact on aneuploidy when *PTEN* becomes deleted in prostate cancer. It is possible that the acquisition of the initial hemizygous *PTEN* deletions or mutations may increase levels of genomic instability because of protein haploinsufficiency. The presence of clusters of microhomology at LCR regions along chromosome 10 may then facilitate second genomic deletion events that remove the remaining functional *PTEN* allele in the five characteristic size distributions that we observed. The Large Interstitial deletion subtype appears to have a distinct pattern of aneuploidy and gene expression changes that confer more aggressive disease. Collectively, *PTEN* genomic deletions may thus not only lead to activation of the PI3K/AKT pathway, but the size of the deletion events themselves may influence gene expression and the levels of acquired aneuploidy.

## Methods

### Cohort and data description

The TCGA provisional cohort comprises 499 prostate cancer samples. In this study, we evaluated the genomic and transcriptomic profiles of 491 prostate cancer specimens. The TCGA cohort is composed by tumor samples obtained from different centers located in the United States (85.3%), Germany (11%), Australia (1.8%), United Kingdom (1.4%), and Brazil (0.4%). We downloaded level

3 RNA sequencing (RNAseq), array Comparative Genomic Hybridization (aCGH), and single nucleotide variation (SNV), and clinical data from the TCGA data portal (https://portal.gdc.cancer.gov/). Data normalization and segmentation were carried out in Nexus Copy Number 8.0 and Nexus Expression 3.0 (Biodiscovery, Santa Clara). SNV data was analyzed in R v3.4.2. Statistical analyses were carried out in R v3.4.2.

#### Classification of *PTEN* deletions

We first evaluated the presence or absence of *PTEN* deletions through analysis of aCGH data. In this analysis, samples were classified according to the presence of loss of one copy of *PTEN* gene (hemizygous) or loss of both copies of the *PTEN* gene (homozygous). Each deletion was considered separately in all tumors with homozygous deletions. We performed a supervised SCNA classification using Nexus Copy Number 8.0 to visualize and map the respective sizes of each *PTEN* deletion based on the distance between the positions of the copy number transitions along chromosome 10. In this analysis, we considered the largest deletion size when there was both a hemi- and a homozygous *PTEN* deletions with divergent lengths in the same tumor. A supervised SCNA classification was then performed using Nexus Copy Number 8.0 to visualize and map the respective sizes of each *PTEN* deletion based on the distance between the positions of the copy number transitions along chromosome 10. The five deletion subtypes were defined by the clustering of their respective size distributions along chromosome 10.

To investigate the presence of LCRs around the breakpoint regions, we searched the genomic position of the chromosome 10 deletion of each patient using the segmental duplication track of UCSC genome browser (http://genome.ucsc.edu browser; Human Genome Build 37). The analysis was carried out by using known LCRs (segmental duplication >1 kb of non-repeat masked sequence with over 90% similarity) through Galaxy platform (https://usegalaxy.org/) [53, 54]. Further, the number of LCRs with high similarity (>90%) and in the same orientation were counted for the upper and lower breakpoints of each sample.

#### Genomic and chromosomal instability analysis

We evaluated the effect of the different *PTEN* deletions on chromosomal and genomic instability. Chromosomal instability parameters were obtained from Nexus Copy Number 8.0. We evaluated the percentage of genome altered (ratio of the total length of all gain and loss calls by the length of the genome) and the total number of SCNAs (number of gains and losses events) for each tumor sample. No loss of heterozygosity or allelic imbalances were considered for the calculation of the percentage of genome altered and the total number of SCNAs. The genomic instability parameters were obtained through analysis of single nucleotide variants (SNVs). We performed an analysis of the total number of mutations in the genome, which included frameshift deletions and insertions, in-frame deletions, missense mutations, and splice-site. We also performed the analysis of the most significantly mutated genes through the MutSigCV algorithm [55]. Tumor heterogeneity levels were accessed through the mutant-allele tumor heterogeneity (MATH), which is the ratio of the width to the center of distribution of mutant-allele fractions among tumor-specific mutated loci [56].

#### SCNA and transcriptome analysis

Significant genomic changes were assessed by comparing the SCNA landscape of each group of *PTEN* deletion type through Nexus Copy Number 8.0. Differential SCNA calls between the compared groups were observed through the application of Fisher Exact Test with $P$-value = 0.05 and alteration threshold percentage equal to 25%. To access the genes associated with cancer pathways that were in regions of loss or gain, we analyzed the Cancer Gene Census feature from Nexus Copy Number 8.0. This feature generates a list of cancer-related genes for each SCNA call.

For identification of differentially expressed genes between different *PTEN* deletion subtypes, matched RNA-seq and aCGH data were analyzed. From 20,532 RNAseq probes, low variance probes (<0.2) were filtered, resulting in 6081 probes. We then evaluated the expression of the 6081 genes and compared their expression profiles between each group of *PTEN* deletion subtypes with *PTEN* intact samples. Differentially expressed genes were obtained through Fisher Exact test through a log-ratio threshold of 0.1 and multiple test correction (FDR - Benjamini Hochberg, $Q < 0.01$).

Further, we conducted an enrichment analysis of all differentially expressed genes obtained by comparing each deletion type with *PTEN* intact tumors. Pathway analysis was conducted through Database for Annotation, Visualization, and Integrated Discovery (DAVID, http://www.david.niaid.nih.gov) (version 6.8). The gene list for each deletion was imputed in DAVID, and Functional Annotation Charts were downloaded and analyzed through Cytoscape 3.0 (http://www.cytoscape.org). Enrichment node construction was performed through Enrichment Map plugin (http://apps.cytoscape.org/apps/enrichmentmap) for Cytoscape 3.0 using default options.

#### Effect of the deletion subtypes in clinical parameters

Analysis of the effect of the different *PTEN* deletion subtypes on clinical parameters was carried out in R v3.4.2. We performed Chi-square tests for categorical data and Kruskal-Wallis tests for continuous clinical data. When significant associations were found by Chi-square analysis, we conducted univariate logistic regression analysis for the particular variable. We investigated the effect of each deletion type in the prediction of extraprostatic extension, seminal vesicle invasion, disease recurrence (defined the presence of at least one of the following events after radical prostatectomy: distant metastasis, local metastasis, biochemical recurrence, or new primary tumor), Gleason score, pathological T and N, age at diagnosis, time to disease recurrence, and race. Additionally, log-rank test and Kaplan Meier curves were applied with disease recurrence as the endpoint. We also conducted univariate and multivariate Cox Regression models (Survival package) for the evaluated parameters. The comparisons were considered significantly different when *P*-value was ≤0.05.

## Additional files

**Additional file 1:** Effect of the copy number variation of *PTEN* gene in the chromosomal and genomic instability parameters. The boxplots show A - the total number of mutations, B - percentage of genome altered, C - MATH score, and D - total number of SCNAs. *PTEN* homozygous deletions show an apparent effect on the SCNA and mutational landscapes, observed by an increased percentage of genome altered, total number of SCNAs, and total number of mutations. *Kruskal-Wallis test, *P*-value <0.05. (PNG 91 kb)

**Additional file 2:** Incidence of hemi- and homozygous deletions of *PTEN* per deletion subtype. (DOCX 12 kb)

**Additional file 3:** List of the genes in the deleted regions from chr10 for each deletion subtype. (DOCX 18 kb)

**Additional file 4:** Effect of *PTEN* inactivation in the aneuploidy and mutational landscapes in prostate cancer. Tumors with one allele inactive exhibit either a point mutation or one allele deletion (hemizygous deletion) of *PTEN* gene, resulting in reduced protein. Tumors with both alleles inactive exhibit either both copies of *PTEN* deleted (homozygous deletion) or one allele loss (hemizygous deletion) plus a point mutation in the remaining allele, resulting in an expected total loss of protein. From the 491 tumors, 367 were *PTEN* intact, 6 exhibited both copies of *PTEN* plus a point mutation, 62 presented hemizygous deletion of *PTEN,* 12 presented hemizygous deletion and one point mutation in the remaining *PTEN* allele, and 44 presented homozygous deletions of *PTEN*. SCNA – somatic copy number alteration. (PNG 84 kb)

**Additional file 5:** Boxplot showing the differences in PTEN mRNA expression for *PTEN* deletions. Kruskal-Wallis test was applied to identify significant differences in PTEN mRNA expression between the groups. (A) *PTEN* homozygous deletions showed the lowest levels of *PTEN* mRNA expression. (B) All *PTEN* deletion subtypes presented a significant decline in PTEN mRNA expression when compared to *PTEN* intact tumors. We did not observe any significant differences in PTEN mRNA expression levels within the subtype group. SI – Small Interstitial, LI – Large Interstitial, LP – Large Proximal, LT – Large Terminal, E – Extensive. (PNG 66 kb)

**Additional file 6:** Clinical and pathological characterization for each deletion type. (DOCX 16 kb)

**Additional file 7:** Kaplan Meier plots and log-rank analysis of disease recurrence for tumors with distinct *PTEN* deletions in prostate cancer. (A) Log-rank test showed a significant difference between tumors with *PTEN* deletions and *PTEN* intact. (B) We did not observe a significant difference between the deletion subtypes through log-rank analysis. (PNG 978 kb)

### Abbreviations

FISH: Fluorescence in situ hybridization; FoSTeS: Fork stalling and template switching; LCR: Low copy repeat; NAHR: Non-allelic homologous recombination; NHEJ: Non-homologous end-joining (NHEJ); PTEN: Phosphatase and tensin homolog; SCNA: Somatic copy number alterations

### Funding

JAS was supported by São Paulo Research Funding Agency (FAPESP) grant no. 2015/09111-5 and CNPq Bolsa Produtividade em Pesquisa - Nível: PQ-1B grant no. 306864/2014-2. TV and DGT are funded by FAPESP grants no. 2015/22785-5 and 2016/02730-4, respectively.

### Authors' contributions

TV conducted all bioinformatics and statistical analyses, interpreted all data, and wrote the manuscript; DGT performed MutSig and MATH score analyses; JAS supervised the study. All authors read and approved the final manuscript.

### Competing interests

The authors declare that they have no competing interests.

### Author details

[1]Department of Genetics, Ribeirão Preto Medical School, University of São Paulo, Ribeirão Preto, Brazil. [2]Deparment of Gynecology and Obstetrics, Clinical Hospital of Ribeirão Preto, Ribeirão Preto, Brazil. [3]Department of Pathology and Legal Medicine, Ribeirão Preto Medical School, University of São Paulo, 3900 Bandeirantes Avenue, Monte Alegre, Ribeirão Preto, São Paulo 14040-900, Brazil. [4]Department of Pathology and Molecular Medicine, Queen's University, Kingston, Canada.

### References

1. Howlader N, Noone AM, Krapcho M, Miller D, Bishop K, Kosary CL et al. SEER Cancer Statistics Review, 1975–2014, National Cancer Institute 2017.
2. Verhagen P, van Duijn P, Hermans K, Looijenga L, van Gurp R, Stoop H, et al. The PTEN gene in locally progressive prostate cancer is preferentially inactivated by bi-allelic gene deletion. J Pathol. 2006;208:699–707.
3. Mithal P, Allott E, Gerber L, Reid J, Welbourn W, Tikishvili E, et al. PTEN loss in biopsy tissue predicts poor clinical outcomes in prostate cancer. Int J Urol. 2014;21:1209–14.
4. Troyer DA, Jamaspishvili T, Wei W, Feng Z, Good J, Hawley S, et al. A multicenter study shows PTEN deletion is strongly associated with seminal vesicle involvement and extracapsular extension in localized prostate cancer. Prostate. 2015;75:1206–15.
5. Picanço-Albuquerque CG, Morais CL, Carvalho FLF, Peskoe SB, Hicks JL, Ludkovski O, et al. In prostate cancer needle biopsies, detections of PTEN loss by fluorescence in situ hybridization (FISH) and by immunohistochemistry (IHC) are concordant and show consistent association with upgrading. Virchows Arch. 2016;468:607–17.
6. Fontugne J, Lee D, Cantaloni C, Barbieri CE, Caffo O, Hanspeter E, et al. Recurrent prostate cancer genomic alterations predict response to brachytherapy treatment. Cancer Epidemiol Biomark Prev. 2014;23:594–600.
7. Silva MP, Barros-Silva JD, Ersvær E, Kildal W, Hveem TS, Pradhan M, et al. Cancer prognosis defined by the combined analysis of 8q, PTEN and ERG. Transl Oncol. 2016;9:575–82.
8. Hou S-Q, Ouyang M, Brandmaier A, Hao H, Shen WH. PTEN In the maintenance of genome integrity: from DNA replication to chromosome segregation. BioEssays. 2017;39:1700082.
9. Williams JL, Greer PA, Squire JA. Recurrent copy number alterations in prostate cancer: an in silico meta-analysis of publicly available genomic data. Cancer Genet Elsevier Inc. 2014;207:474–88.
10. Hanahan D, Weinberg RA. Hallmarks of cancer: the next generation. Cell. 2011;144:646–74.
11. Tapia-Laliena MA, Korzeniewski N, Hohenfellner M, Duensing S. High-risk prostate cancer: a disease of genomic instability. Urol Oncol Semin Orig Investig. 2014;32:1101–7.

12. Yoshimoto M, Ludkovski O, Degrace D, Williams JL, Evans A, Sircar K, et al. PTEN genomic deletions that characterize aggressive prostate cancer originate close to segmental duplications. Genes Chromosom Cancer. 2012; 51:149–60.
13. Biscotti MA, Olmo E, Heslop-Harrison JSP, Repetitive DNA. In eukaryotic genomes. Chromosom Res. 2015;23:415–20.
14. Deloukas P, Matthews LH, Ashurst J, Burton J, Gilbert JGR, Jones M, et al. The DNA sequence and comparative analysis of human chromosome 20. Nature. 2001;414:865–71.
15. Stankiewicz P, Kulkarni S, Dharmadhikari AV, Sampath S, Bhatt SS, Shaikh TH, et al. Recurrent deletions and reciprocal duplications of 10q11.21q11.23 including CHAT and SLC18A3 are likely mediated by complex low-copy repeats. Hum Mutat. 2012;33:165–79.
16. Kloosterman WP, Guryev V, van Roosmalen M, Duran KJ, de Bruijn E, Bakker SCM, et al. Chromothripsis as a mechanism driving complex de novo structural rearrangements in the germline. Hum Mol Genet. 2011;20:1916–24.
17. Kass EM, Moynahan ME, Jasin M. When genome maintenance goes badly awry. Mol Cell. 2016;62:777–87.
18. Bishop AJ, Schiestl RH, et al. Hum Mol Genet. 2000;9:2427–334.
19. Hastings PJ, Lupski JR, Rosenberg SM, Ira G. Mechanisms of change in gene copy number. Nat Rev Genet. 2009;10:551–64.
20. Yoshimoto M, Cunha IW, Coudry RA, Fonseca FP, Torres CH, Soares FA, et al. FISH analysis of 107 prostate cancers shows that PTEN genomic deletion is associated with poor clinical outcome. Br J Cancer. 2007;97:678–85.
21. Choucair K, Ejdelman J, Brimo F, Aprikian A, Chevalier S, Lapointe JPTEN. Genomic deletion predicts prostate cancer recurrence and is associated with low AR expression and transcriptional activity. BMC Cancer. 2012;12: 543–51.
22. Murphy SJ, Karnes RJ, Kosari F, Castellar BERP, Kipp BR, Johnson SH, et al. Integrated analysis of the genomic instability of PTEN in clinically insignificant and significant prostate cancer. Mod Pathol. 2016;29:143–56.
23. Fraser M, Sabelnykova VY, Yamaguchi TN, Heisler LE, Livingstone J, Huang V, et al. Genomic hallmarks of localized, non-indolent prostate cancer. Nature. 2017;541:359–64.
24. Abeshouse A, Ahn J, Akbani R, Ally A, Amin S, Andry CD, et al. The molecular taxonomy of primary prostate cancer. Cell. 2015;163:1011–25.
25. Lotan TL, Wei W, Ludkovski O, Morais CL, Guedes LB, Jamaspishvili T, et al. Analytic validation of a clinical-grade PTEN immunohistochemistry assay in prostate cancer by comparison with PTEN FISH. Mod Pathol. 2016;29:904–14.
26. Cuzick J, Yang ZH, Fisher G, Tikishvili E, Stone S, Lanchbury JS, et al. Prognostic value of PTEN loss in men with conservatively managed localised prostate cancer. Br J Cancer. 2013;108:2582–9.
27. Chaisson MJP, Wilson RK, Eichler EE. Genetic variation and the de novo assembly of human genomes. Nat Rev Genet. 2015;16:627–40.
28. de Smith AJ, Walters RG, Coin LJM, Steinfeld I, Yakhini Z, Sladek R, et al. Small deletion variants have stable breakpoints commonly associated with alu elements. PLoS One. 2008;3:1–11.
29. Duijf PHG, Benezra R. The cancer biology of whole-chromosome instability. Oncogene. 2013;32:4727–36.
30. Shen WH, Balajee AS, Wang J, Wu H, Eng C, Pandolfi PP, et al. Essential role for nuclear PTEN in maintaining chromosomal integrity. Cell. 2007;128:157–70.
31. Bassi C, Ho J, Srikumar T, Dowling RJO, Gorrini C, Miller SJ, et al. Nuclear PTEN controls DNA repair and sensitivity to genotoxic stress. Science. 2013; 341:395–9.
32. Kurfurstova D, Bartkova J, Vrtel R, Mickova A, Burdova A, Majera D, et al. DNA damage signalling barrier, oxidative stress and treatment-relevant DNA repair factor alterations during progression of human prostate cancer. Mol Oncol. 2016;10:879–94.
33. Davoli T, AW X, Mengwasser KE, Sack LM, Yoon JC, Park PJ, et al. Cumulative haploinsufficiency and triplosensitivity drive aneuploidy patterns and shape the cancer genome. Cell. 2013;155:948–62.
34. Solimini NL, Xu Q, Mermel CH, Liang AC, Schlabach MR, Luo J, et al. Recurrent hemizygous deletions in cancers may optimize proliferative potential. Science. 2012;337:104–9.
35. Sun Z, Huang C, He J, Lamb KL, Kang X, Gu T, et al. PTEN C-terminal deletion causes genomic instability and tumor development. Cell Rep. 2014;6:844–54.
36. Hopkins BD, Hodakoski C, Barrows D, Mense SM, Parsons REPTEN. Function: the long and the short of it. Trends Biochem Sci. 2015;39:183–90.
37. Zhao D, Lu X, Wang G, Lan Z, Liao W, Li J, et al. Synthetic essentiality of chromatin remodelling factor CHD1 in PTEN-deficient cancer. Nature. 2017; 542:484 8.
38. Isaacs WB, Carter BS, Debruyne FMJ, Schalken JA. Expression of the cellular adhesion molecule E-Cadherin is reduced or absent in high-grade prostate cancer. Cancer Res. 1992;52:5104–9.
39. Ni J, Cozzi P, Hao J, Beretov J, Chang L, Duan W, et al. Epithelial cell adhesion molecule (EpCAM) is associated with prostate cancer metastasis and chemo/radioresistance via the PI3K/Akt/mTOR signaling pathway. Int J Biochem Cell Biol. 2013;45:2736–48.
40. Seguin L, Desgrosellier JS, Weis SM, Cheresh DA. Integrins and cancer: regulators of cancer stemness, metastasis, and drug resistance. Trends Cell Biol. 2015;25:234–40.
41. Zhang Q, Liu S, Zhang Q, Xiong Z, Wang AR, Myers L, et al. Interleukin-17 promotes development of castration-resistant prostate cancer potentially through creating an immunotolerant and pro-angiogenic tumor microenvironment. Prostate. 2014;74:869–79.
42. Martin PL, Yin J-J, Seng V, Casey O, Corey E, Morrissey C, et al. Androgen deprivation leads to increased carbohydrate metabolism and hexokinase 2-mediated survival in Pten/Tp53-deficient prostate cancer. Oncogene. 2017; 36:525–33.
43. Robles AI, Harris CC. Clinical outcomes and correlates of TP53 mutations and cancer. Cold Spring Harb Perspect Biol. 2010;2:1–15.
44. Bunz F, Kinzler KW, Vogelstein B, Lengauer C, Vogelstein B, Fauth C, et al. Targeted inactivation of p53 in human cells does not result in aneuploidy. Cancer Res. 2002;62:1129–33.
45. Macheret M, Halazonetis TD. DNA replication stress as a Hallmark of cancer. Annu Rev Pathol Mech Dis. 2015;10:425–48.
46. Nikolaev SI, Sotiriou SK, Pateras IS, Santoni F, Sougioultzis S, Edgren H, et al. A single-nucleotide substitution mutator phenotype revealed by exome sequencing of human colon adenomas. Cancer Res. 2012;72: 6279–89.
47. Ngeow J, Mester J, Rybicki LA, Ni Y, Milas M, Eng C. Incidence and clinical characteristics of thyroid cancer in prospective series of individuals with cowden and cowden-like syndrome characterized by germline PTEN, SDH, or KLLN alterations. J Clin Endocrinol Metab. 2011;96:2063–71.
48. Nizialek EA, Peterson C, Mester JL, Downes-Kelly E, Eng C. Germline and somatic KLLN alterations in breast cancer dysregulate G2 arrest. Hum Mol Genet. 2013;22:2451–61.
49. Kuehn HS, Caminha I, Niemela JE, Rao VK, Davis J, Fleisher TA, et al. FAS Haploinsufficiency is a common disease mechanism in the human autoimmune Lymphoproliferative syndrome. J Immunol. 2011;186:6035–43.
50. Khani F, Mosquera JM, Park K, Blattner M, O'Reilly C, MacDonald TY, et al. Evidence for molecular differences in prostate cancer between african American and Caucasian men. Clin Cancer Res. 2014;20:4925–34.
51. Lindquist KJ, Paris PL, Hoffmann TJ, Cardin NJ, Kazma R, Mefford JA, et al. Mutational landscape of aggressive prostate tumors in African American men. Cancer Res. 2016;76:1860–8.
52. Tosoian JJ, Almutairi F, Morais CL, Glavaris S, Hicks J, Sundi D, et al. Prevalence and prognostic significance of PTEN loss in African-American and European-American men undergoing radical prostatectomy. Eur Urol. European association of. Urology. 2017;71:697–700.
53. Shinawi M, Liu P, Kang SHL, Shen J, Belmont JW, Scott D, et al. Recurrent reciprocal 16p11.2 rearrangements associated with global developmental delay, behavioural problems, dysmorphism, epilepsy, and abnormal head size. J Med Genet. 2010;47:332–41.
54. Leite AJC, Pinto IP, Da Cruz E, Cunha DM, Ribeiro CL, Da Silva CC, et al. The identification of microdeletion and reciprocal microduplication in 22q11.2 using high-resolution CMA technology. Biomed Res Int. 2016;2016:1–9.
55. Lawrence MS, Stojanov P, Polak P, Kryukov GV, Cibulskis K, Sivachenko A, et al. Mutational heterogeneity in cancer and the search for new cancer-associated genes. Nature. 2013;499:214–8.
56. Mroz EA, Rocco JW. MATH, A novel measure of intratumor genetic heterogeneity, is high in poor-outcome classes of head and neck squamous cell carcinoma. Oral Oncol. 2013;49:211–5.

8

# Limited survivability of unbalanced progeny of carriers of a unique t(4;19)(p15.32;p13.3): a study in multiple generations

Darinka Šumanović-Glamuzina[1], Bernarda Lozić[2], Piotr S. Iwanowski[3], Tatijana Zemunik[4], Zeljka Bilinovac[1], Beata Stasiewicz-Jarocka[3], Barbara Panasiuk[3] and Alina T. Midro[3*]

## Abstract

**Background:** Carriership of a reciprocal chromosomal translocation (RCT) involving the short arm of chromosome 4 (4p) may result in birth of a child with Wolf-Hirschhorn syndrome (WHS) due to monosomy 4p, a priori modified by the impact of the partner chromosome imbalance. Familial transmission studies of RCT enable obtaining empirical risk figures that are essential for genetic counseling. In this study, pedigree data from carriers of a unique t(4;19)(p15.32;p13.3), ascertained by two children with WHS phenotype, were collected through five generations and empirical risk for different pregnancy outcomes was assessed. In addition, the phenotype-karyotype correlation was studied in two unbalanced children against the phenotypes of children (literature data) with pure monosomy 4p15.32 → pter and pure trisomy 19p13.3 → pter, accordingly. The phenotype analysis was conducted using the catalogue of traits according to the Munich Dysmorphology Database. Pedigree segregation analysis was conducted by the direct method according to Stengel- Rutkowski et al.

**Results:** A double segment imbalance, trisomy 19p13.3 → pter with monosomy 4p15.32 → pter, was diagnosed in WHS progeny at birth. No essential modification of WHS phenotype by the additional trisomy 19p was observed, except for a limited survivability (death in infancy). Pedigree segregation analysis covered 39 relatives showed the probability rate for liveborn with unbalanced karyotype of 3.7 ± 3.6% (1/27), for stillbirth/neonatal death at 7.4 ± 5.0% (2/27), for miscarriage at 22.2 ± 8.0% (6/27), for the chance of having a baby without unbalanced karyotype was estimated at 66.7 ± 9.1% (18/27). In addition, the value of 7.4% for genetic counseling for any carrier of RCT at risk for single segment 19p13.3 → pter imbalance at birth was evaluated as such value have not been estimated so far.

**Conclusion:** Carriership of a t(4;19)(p15.32;p13.3) is at low risk for an unbalanced child at birth and for stillbirth/neonatal death but high for miscarriages. The chance of having a baby without unbalanced karyotype was estimated to be high. Monosomy 4p15.32 → pter together with trisomy 19p13.3 → pter as a double segment imbalance in children with WHS may be connected with a limited survivability in infancy.

**Keywords:** Estimation of recurrence probability, Miscarriages, Monosomy 4p15.32 → pter, Morphological phenotype, Stillbirth, Trisomy 19p13.3 → pter, t(4;19)(p15.32;p13.3), Wolf-Hirschhorn syndrome

* Correspondence: alinamidro@gmail.com; midro@umb.edu.pl
[3]Department of Clinical Genetics, Medical University of Bialystok, Waszyngtona St. 13, PO Box 22, 15-089 Białystok, Poland
Full list of author information is available at the end of the article

## Background

Partial chromosome 4p monosomy results in a well recognizable morphological and behavioral phenotype, known as Wolf-Hirschhorn Syndrome (WHS) (MIM: #194190). That phenotype is defined by characteristic somatic, neurological and behavioral features including prenatal/postnatal growth retardation, microcephaly, seizures, muscular hypotonia, facial dysmorphism, skeletal anomalies, congenital heart defects, antibody deficiencies, urinary tract malformations, and others. The facial gestalt includes prominent and broad nose ridge continuing to forehead, prominent glabella, ocular hypertelorism, epicanthus, highly arched eyebrows, short philtrum, downturned mouth, micrognathia, and poorly formed ears with pits/tags [1–4].

Apart from the essential underlying chromosome aberration, monosomy 4p, WHS may also be due to a double segment imbalance with monosomy 4p included, resulting from meiotic malsegregation of a parental reciprocal chromosome translocation (RCT). In such cases the imbalance of the partner chromosome segment may impact the phenotype, so the clinical diagnosis of WHS may be "biased" by that effect [2, 5].

In this paper we present two children with WHS due to monosomy 4p15.32 → pter together with trisomy 19p13.3 → pter. To our knowledge only one report of WHS due to unbalanced t(4;19) is available in literature, from a family study including a maternal carrier of a subtle t(4;19)(p16.3;p13.3) ascertained by a girl with WHS [6]. In addition, clinical data on pure chromosome 19p trisomy are scanty, too, due to its rarity. To date, only two children with pure 19p13.3 → pter trisomy have been reported [7, 8].

Following this study of familial transmission of the unique translocation t(4;19)(p15.32;p13.3) across five generations including follow-up of families with different pregnancy outcomes we are able to propose the empirical risk figures for genetic counseling. In addition, thanks to extensive pedigree data collected, we propose the use of obtained figures for prediction of probability rates for 19p13.3 → pter single segment imbalance in progeny of any carrier of RCT involving that segment.

### Clinical report

#### *Child 1*

Our proband (V:2, Fig. 1a-d, Additional file 1: Table S1) was a boy born at 39th week of gestation as the second child of young (mother/father: 24/30 years old) and healthy parents (IV:2; IV:3). During pregnancy intrauterine growth retardation (IUGR) was observed. His birth weight was 1880 g (<3rd ct.), length 45 cm (<3rd ct.), and head circumference 29 cm (<3rd ct.). Apgar scores were 8 and 9 points. As a newborn he was small for gestational age and he was transferred to an intensive care unit (ICU) where he developed respiratory distress syndrome, early sepsis, meningitis, renal failure with mineral imbalance, glucose intolerance, seizures, and muscular hypotonia. Feeding difficulties and failure to thrive were observed in course of further hospitalization. Because of his facial gestalt suggestive of WHS, echocardiography, abdominal and cerebral ultrasonography, and clinical laboratory analysis were performed shortly after birth looking for malformations and other clinical abnormalities. Heart defect (atrial septal defect, ASD), mild-brain ventriculomegaly and agenesis of left kidney were found. He was hospitalized several times during infancy due to prolonged seizures. He died at the age of 12 months in course of severe bronchopneumonia, renal failure and drug resistant epileptic status.

#### *Child 2*

A boy (V:10 Fig. 1e-h, Additional file 1: Table S1) was born at 39th week of third pregnancy of young parents (mother/father: 34/36 years old) (IV: 7; IV: 8). His birth weight was 1690 g (<3rd ct.), length 34 cm (<3rd ct.) and head circumference (<3.ct.). Apgar scores were 9 and 10 points. WHS was diagnosed based on his morphological and clinical features. He was treated several times at a pediatric department due to congenital abnormalities, seizures and severe anemia. Radiology examinations showed heart defect (ASD, pulmonary stenosis and persistent ductus arteriosus), agenesis of left kidney, right side inguinal hernia, and left hip dislocation. He died at the age of 11 months during an episode of bronchopneumonia and persistent seizures.

## Methods

### Morphologic and clinical phenotype analysis

A detailed analysis was performed using the catalogue of morphologic and clinical traits by the Munich Dysmorphology Database (MDDB) [9]. Its outcome was used for comparison with the phenotypes of three children with pure monosomy 4p15.32 → pter at corresponding age published by us earlier [2] and to literature data on phenotypes of two children with pure trisomy 19p13.3 → pter [7, 8]. Facial trait characteristics were supplemented by re-examination of photographs according to the catalogue of traits by MDDB.

### Cytogenetic studies

Cytogenetic analysis was performed on chromosomes from lymphocyte cultures of peripheral blood according to standard procedures. GTG and RBG banding techniques were used. FISH studies using WHSCR probe (4p16.3) (D4S 166-D4S3327) and the 19pter subtelomere specific probe (Cytocell) were done for confirmation of cytogenetic diagnosis and to differentiate terminal and subterminal breakpoint positions on derivative chromosome

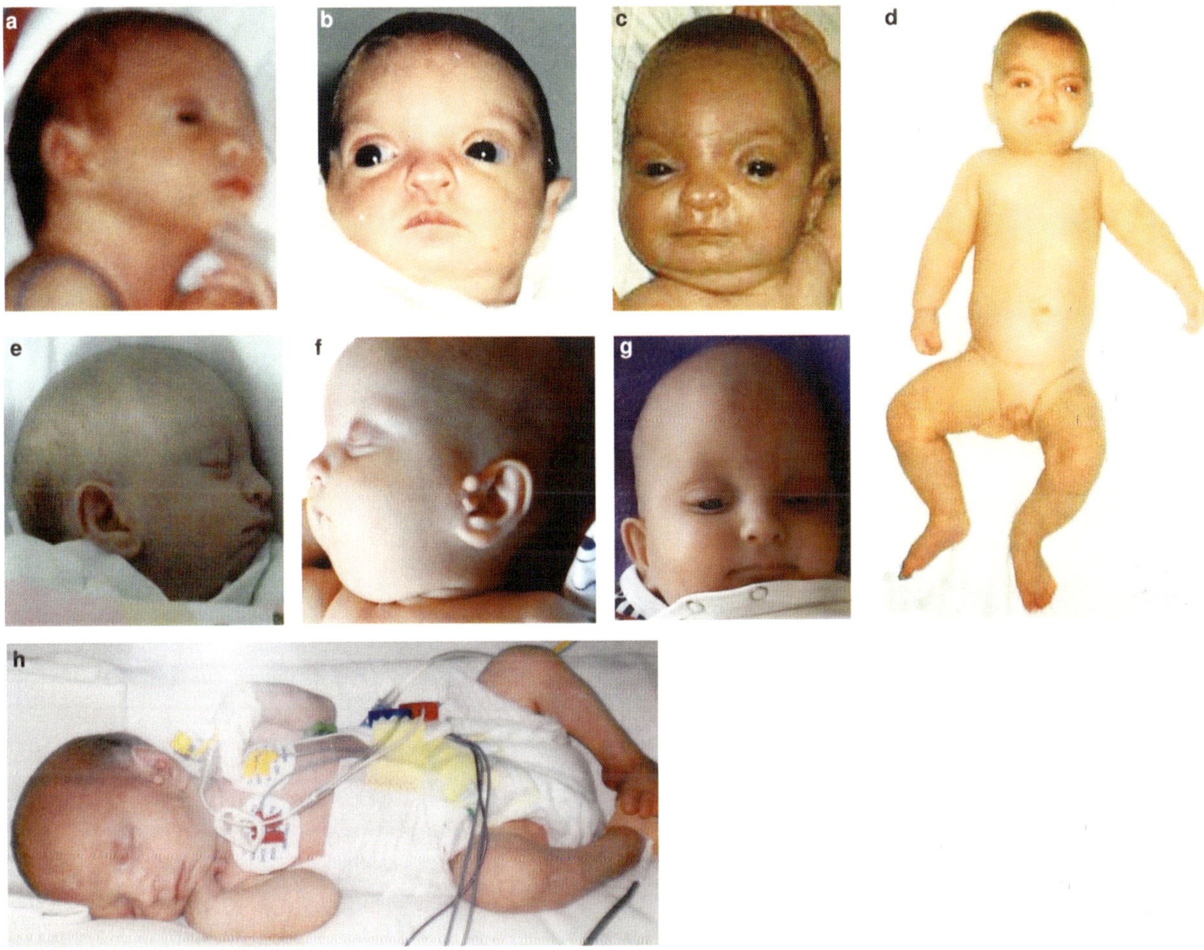

**Fig. 1** Phenotype of children: Child 1 (V:2) at the age of: **a** 7 days. **b** 40 days. **c** 3 months. **d** 10 months. Child 2 (V:10) at the age of: **e** 20 days. **f,g** 3 months. **h** 7 days

19. The interpretation of breakpoint positions of RCT was done according to the ISCN 2013 nomenclature [10].

**Probability rate estimation for different pregnancy outcomes**

***Analysis of meiotic malsegregation of parental chromosomes and prediction of survivality till birth of progeny***

Different forms of possible chromosome imbalance following meiotic disjunction and segregation were considered for the meiotic quadrivalent of t(4;19)(p15.32;p13.3). Prediction of survivality till birth was done by empirical data from the pedigree analyzed in conjunction with the published data [2, 11–17].

***Direct method for pedigree segregation analysis***

Pedigree segregation analysis was performed according to Stengel-Rutkowski et al. (1988) [16]. Empirical probability rates were calculated separately for each category of pregnancy outcomes: liveborn with unbalanced karyotype, stillbirth, miscarriage, and child without unbalanced karyotype- further referred to as child with normal phenotype. Ascertainment correction (i. e., elimination of the proband, their parents and relatives in direct line of ascent) was made as per Stene and Stengel-Rutkowski (1988) [18]. Each unfavorable pregnancy outcomes following ascertainment correction was counted and compared to the total number of pregnancies.

The following formulas were used:

$p = \frac{a}{n} \pm S$ $S = \sqrt{\frac{a(n-a)}{n^3}}$ and when a = 0 $p_{\max} = 1\text{–}e^{-\frac{1}{2n}}$.

p: probability (risk) value for different pregnancy outcomes.

a: number of unfavorable pregnancies after ascertainment correction.

n: number of all pregnancies after ascertainment correction.

S: standard deviation.

$p_{\max}$: maximum risk value.

e: 2.71828 (base number for natural logarithms).

## Results

### Phenotype analyses

Analysis of morphological and clinical traits of children 1 and 2 with partial monosomy 4p15.32 → pter and trisomy 19p13.3 → pter is presented in Additional file 1: Table S1, along with traits present in three children with pure monosomy 4p15.32 → pter (own analysis previously published [2]) and two patients with pure trisomy 19p13.3 → pter reported by Andries et al. (2002) and Ishikawa et al. (2013) [7, 8].

### Cytogenetic study

Cytogenetic analysis (University Hospital, Split, Croatia) by GTG technique in child 1 (proband) revealed a male karyotype with derivative chromosome 4. Parental chromosome studies showed a maternal balanced RCT between chromosomes 4 and 19, i.e. 46,XX,t(4;19)(p15.32;p13.3), confirmed by RBG technique (Medical University of Bialystok, Poland) (Fig. 3a). The following karyotype of the proband was concluded: 46,XY,der(4)t(4;19)(p15.32;p13.3)mat. Hence, monosomy 4p15.32 → pter with trisomy 19p13.3 → pter resulted from a 2:2 disjunction and adjacent-1 meiotic segregation.

A FISH study (in V:1 carrier) showed the breakpoint position proximal to WHSCR on der(4) and subterminal on der(19) (Fig. 3b). Therefore this RCT was classified at risk for a double segment imbalance in progeny.

### Family studies (Fig. 2)

The familial t(4;19)(p15.32;p13.3) was ascertained by a newborn with WHS phenotype (proband V:2, child 1) with an unbalanced RCT der(4)t(4;19)(p15.32;p13.3)mat. Subsequently another child with WHS (V:10, child 2) was born to a relative (IV:7,8). The unbalanced karyotype also was found in two stillbirths following amniocentesis (V:6; V:8). In all children and stillbirths with unbalanced karyotype the same form of imbalance was observed, i.e. monosomy 4p15.32 → pter with trisomy 19p13.3 → pter. Family studies revealed 10 carriers of t(4;19)(p15.32;p13.3) (V:1; IV:3–5,8; III:1,8; II:6,8; I:1 or I:2). Five pregnancies resulted in miscarriage including three in proband's parents (V:3–5) and two in a cousin of proband's mother (V:9,11).

### Recurrence risks estimation for different pregnancy outcomes

#### *Analysis of the possible form of imbalance produced by meiotic malsegregation of parental chromosomes in progeny at birth (Fig. 3c, d)*

The imbalance in form of monosomy 4p15.32 → pter with trisomy 19p13.3 → pter, resulting from a 2:2 disjunction

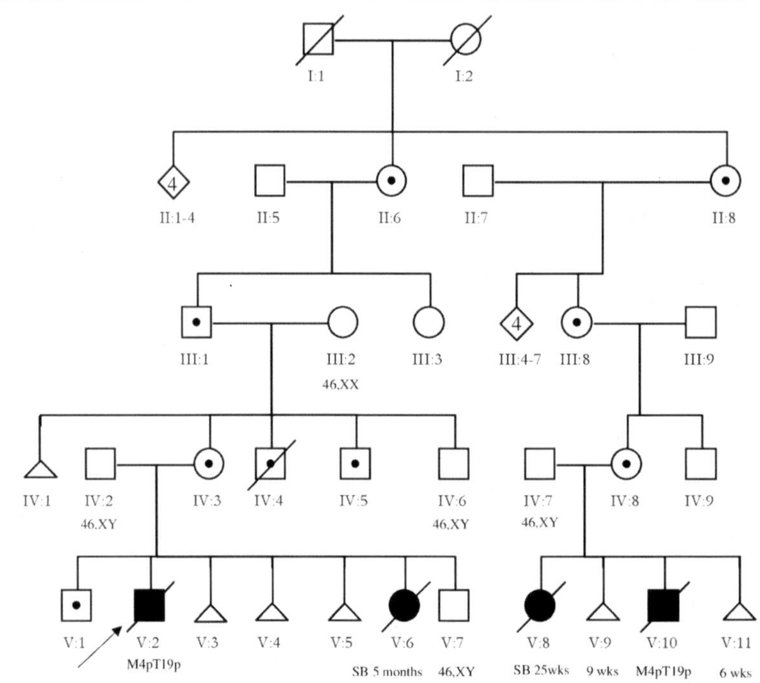


**Fig. 2** Pedigree data with indication of ascertainment (pedigree was drawn according to Bennett et al. (2008) [34]). Symbols and abbreviations: P proband, female, male carriers of translocation, number of siblings, miscarriage, dead of child with M4p15.32 → pter/T19p13.3 → pter, SB stillbirth

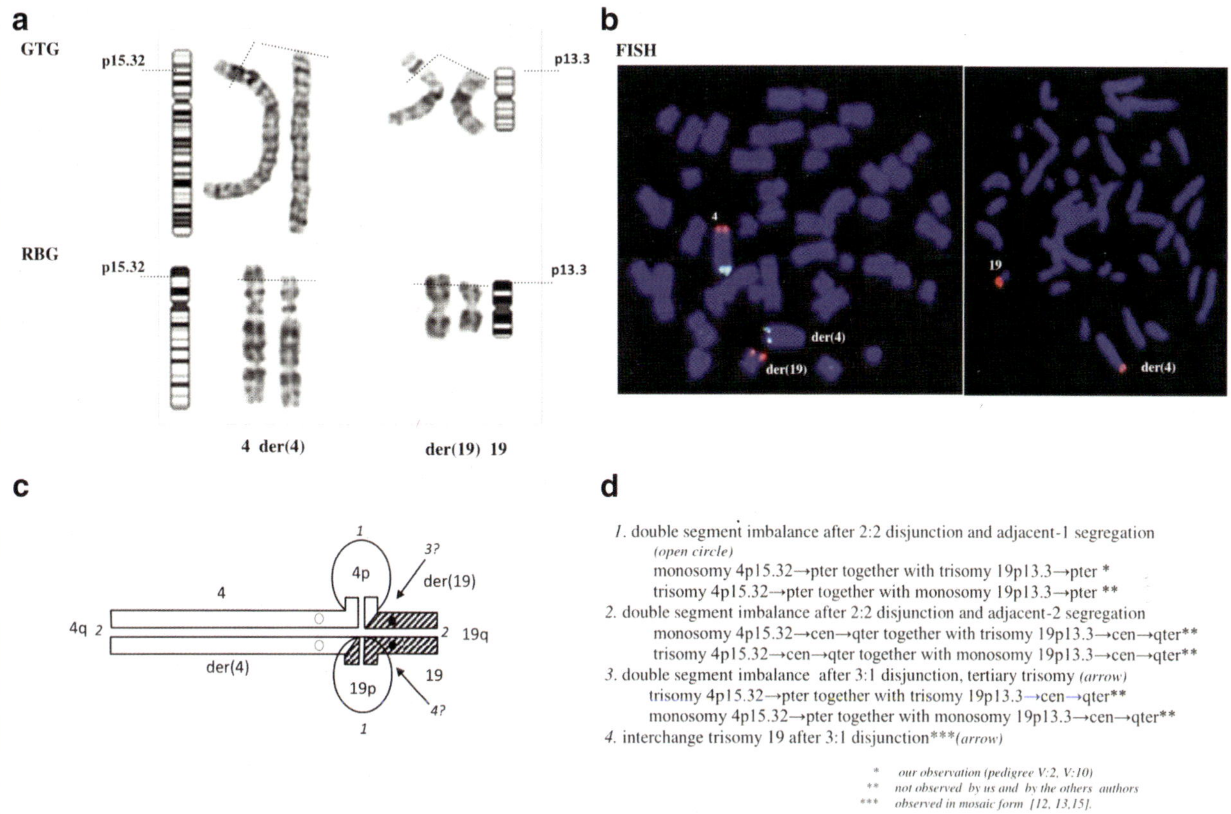


**Fig. 3** Cytogenetic studies and scheme of meiotic quadrivalent of t(4;19)(p15.32;p13.3). **a** Partial karyotype of t(4;19)(p15.32;p13.3) carrier (V;1) studied by GTG (*upper line*) and RBG (*lower line*) techniques with indication of the breakpoint position on chromosomes and ideograms. **b** FISH studies on metaphase chromosomes of t(4;19)(p15.32;p13.3) carrier (V;1), *left:* WHSCR probe (red) and control probe 4qter (green): one red hybridization signal seen on normal chromosome 4 and second one on der(19)t(4;19)(p15.32;p13.3) indicating the breakpoint position on der(4) proximally to WHSCR; two green signals are seen: one on normal chromosome 4 and second one on der(4)t(4;19)(p15.32;p13.3); *right:* 19pter subtelomere specific probe (red): one hybridization signal is seen on normal chromosome 19 and second one on der(4)t(4;19)(p15.32;p13.3) indicating breakpoint position on der(19) proximally to 19pter subtelomere specific probe. **c** Scheme of meiotic quadrivalent of t(4;19)(p15.32;p13.3) carrier with possible forms of imbalance following meiotic disjunction and segregation. **d** Analysis of survival data in progeny till birth with possible forms of imbalance produced following meiosis in a t(4;19)(p15.32;p13.3) carrier

and adjacent-1 segregation, is compatible with survival, as directly observed in the pedigree.

The alternative product of imbalance in liveborn, trisomy 4p15.32 → pter with monosomy 19p13.3 → pter was not found in that family; however it might be compatible with survival with regards to available reports on children with trisomy 4p15.3, as a part of a double segment imbalance, as well as monosomy 19p13.3 → pter [11, 17].

Progeny with imbalance of longer segments of chromosome 4 (monosomy 4p15.32 → cen → qter or trisomy 4p15.32 → cen → qter) following 2:2 disjunction and adjacent-2 segregation is expectedly lethal and was never observed so far.

Tertiary trisomy 19 or interchange trisomy 19 after 3:1 disjunction were not so far reported in liveborn progeny. However, the survival might be possible for children with trisomy 19 in mosaic form as children with supernumerary r(19) in mosaic forms and pure trisomy 19 were described by others [12, 13, 15].

### *Direct pedigree segregation analysis for different pregnancy outcomes (Table 1)*

Following 31 pregnancies of 7 carriers of RCT two children with unbalanced karyotype, two stillbirths with unbalanced karyotype, six miscarriages, and 21 children with normal phenotype were observed. Four individuals, namely the male proband (V:2), his mother (IV:3), grandfather (III;1) and great-grandmother (II;6) were omitted from estimation due to the ascertainment correction. Hence, 27 pregnancies were used for calculation

**Table 1** Results of a direct segregation analysis of pedigree showing the probability of recurrence estimates obtained separately for: liveborn with unbalanced karyotype, stillbirth/early neonatal death, miscarriage, and child with normal phenotype

| Carrier | Parental sex | Liveborn with unbalanced karyotype | | Stillbirth | | Miscarriage | | Child with normal phenotype | | Pregnancies | | Rate | | | |
|---|---|---|---|---|---|---|---|---|---|---|---|---|---|---|---|
| | | U | u | S | s | M | m | N | n | P | p | u/p | s/p | m/p | n/p |
| | | 1 | 0 | 1 | 1 | 3 | 3 | 2 | 2 | 7 | 6 | 0/6 | 1/6 | 3/6 | 2/6 |
| III:1 | PAT | - | - | - | - | 1 | 1 | 4 | 3 | 5 | 4 | –/4 | –/4 | 1/4 | 3/4 |
| II:6 | MAT | - | - | - | - | - | - | 2 | 1 | 2 | 1 | –/1 | –/1 | –/1 | 1/1 |
| IV:8 | MAT | 1 | 1 | 1 | 1 | 2 | 2 | - | - | 4 | 4 | 1/4 | 1/4 | 2/4 | –/4 |
| III:8 | MAT | - | - | - | - | - | - | 2 | 2 | 2 | 2 | –/2 | –/2 | –/2 | 2/2 |
| II:8 | MAT | - | - | - | - | - | - | 5 | 5 | 5 | 5 | –/5 | –/5 | –/5 | 5/5 |
| I:1;I:2 | MAT? PAT? | - | - | | | - | - | 6 | 5 | 6 | 5 | –/5 | –/5 | –/5 | 5/5 |
| | Total | 2 | 1 | 2 | 2 | 6 | 6 | 21 | 18 | 31 | 27 | 1/27 | 2/27 | 6/27 | 18/27 |
| | | | | | | | | | Probability | | (%) | 3.7±3.6 | 7.4±5.0 | 22.2±8.0 | 66.7±9.1 |

*U* number of children with unbalanced karyotype, *u* number of children with unbalanced karyotype after ascertainment correction, *S* number of stillbirth, *s* number of stillbirth after ascertainment correction, *M* number of miscarriages, *m* number of miscarriages after ascertainment correction, *N* number of children with normal phenotype, *n* number of children with normal phenotype after ascertainment correction, *P* total number of pregnancies, *p* total number of pregnancies after ascertainment correction

of the probability rates of different categories of pregnancy outcomes.

The probability rate for having a liveborn child with unbalanced karyotype was estimated as 1/27, i.e. 3.7 ±3.6% and classified as low (<5%). The probability rate for a child with normal phenotype was 18/27, i.e. 66.7 ±9.1% (high probability, >10%). Risk value for stillbirth was 2/27, i.e. 7.4 ±5.0% (medium risk, 5 to 10%) and for miscarriage 6/27, i.e. 22.2 ±8.0% (high risk).

### Probability rate prediction for carriers of RCT at risk for a single segment imbalance of 19p13.3 → pter at birth

No empiric data is available so far for the single segment 19p13.3 → pter imbalance. Therefore on the basis of obtained individual probability rate for imbalance at birth for carriers of t(4;19)(p15.32;p13.3) (direct method) we calculate the probability rate for child with unbalanced karyotype for the single segment 19p13.3 → pter imbalance by doubling of value 3.7% obtained in this study according to Stene and Stengel–Rutkowski (1988) [18]. Hence this value is 7.4%.

## Discussion

### Phenotype of monosomy 4p15.32 → pter with trisomy 19p13.3 → pter due to a unique t(4;19)(p15.32;p13.3)

The current report is the second family study on chromosome 19 partnering chromosome 4 in a unique rearrangement resulting in WHS phenotype. A similar RCT t(4;19)(p16.3;p13.3) was first described by Altherr et al. (1991) [6]. In that report, a smaller segment of chromosome 4 was deleted compared to RCT from this report whereas the 19p13.3 → pter imbalance was presumably comparable. Both children reported here had a number of features in common with those reported by Altherr et al. (1991) [6] including IUGR, microcephaly, hyperterlorism, downward eye slant, low set ears, and heart defect, each of those reflecting the WHS phenotype. The following traits were though found in either child reported here but not explicitly reported by Altherr et al. (1991) [6]: weak fetal movements, newborn feeding difficulties and hypotonia, renal agenesis/ectopic kidney with urinary tract anomalies, seizures or abnormal EEG record, cerebral malformation, prominent glabella, hypomimia, long palpebral fissures, laterally descending eyebrows, downturned mouth angles, microgenia, broad ears, broad neck, and inguinal hernia. However, the clinical and morphological report by Altherr et al. (1991) [6] was rather scanty and apparently not based on a systematic analysis of features. Moreover, most of the latter features are compatible with WHS phenotype, too. Therefore no binding conclusion can be drawn which features, if at all, observed in addition in both children with monosomy 4p15.32 → pter with trisomy 19p13.3 → pter are possibly due to a larger 4p deletion.

The phenotype of single segment 4p15.32 → pter monosomy had been delineated by Iwanowski et al. (2011) [2] through a systematic phenotypic analyses based on the same catalogue of traits (MDDB) (see Additional file 1: Table S1). The traits present in both children reported by us but not in patients by Iwanowski et al. (2011) [2] include: reduced birth length, asymmetric skull, high forehead, downward eye slant, short nose ridge, microgenia, inguinal hernia, and urinary tract anomalies. Of them, reduced birth length, high forehead, downward eye slant, short nose ridge, and microgenia were reported in at least one of the only two patients with a pure 19p13.3 → pter trisomy reported so far [7, 8]. It is therefore likely that those latter few features are associated with the 19p trisomy and add to the otherwise dominating features of the WHS (monosomy 4p) phenotype.

Either child reported here showed an early onset of seizures with fatal outcome within the first year of life. We can assume that beside the monosomy 4p15.32 → pter, also the trisomy 19p13.3 → pter contributes to seizure phenotype with an unfavorable outcome. Quigley et al. (2004) [19] who described a RCT t(9;19)(q34.3;p13.3) observed microcephaly, alopecia and autoimmune abnormalities supposedly linked with trisomy 19p. Both our patients died in infancy, had microcephaly and were hospitalized several times because of prolonged seizures and died in status epilepticus after severe bronchopneumonia. Seizures in infancy were also described in cases of microduplication of 19p13.3 region, probably overlapping the trisomic region of both children reported here [8, 20–22]. However, Battaglia et al. (2008) [23] in their study of 87 patients with WHS observed a high percentage (93%) of seizure disorder, generally with a favorable outcome [23]. Shannon et al. (2001) in their WHS study showed that there is relationship between the 4p deletion size, severity phenotype and life expectancy [24]. Although they also observed that survival is poorer in RCTs than in de novo deletions, the difference was not statistically significant.

To date only two patients with pure trisomy of 19p13.3 → pter segment have been reported by Andries et al. (2001) [7] and Ishikawa et al. (2013) [8]. Those reports include multiple malformations i.e. heart defect, developmental delay, and distinctive facial appearance [7, 8]. Other six published reports are on interstitial partial duplications of 19p13.3 [20–22, 25]. There are five further reports of partial trisomy 19p13.3 but with partial monosomy of another chromosome involved (13q, 16p, 9q, 1p) [19, 26–29], in addition to the report on chromosome 4p monosomy discussed above [6]. In all those RCTs, monosomy for the partner chromosome segment most likely contributes to, or even dominates, the ultimate hybrid phenotype.

### *Probability rate estimation for different pregnancy outcomes*

In our analysis, the probability rate for birth of a child with unbalanced karyotype, namely monosomy 4p15.32 → pter with trisomy 19p13.3 → pter, was classified as low and it was medium for stillbirth. Those risks are markedly lower compared to a single segment imbalance of RCT at risk for monosomy 4p15.32 → pter at birth estimated at a rate of about 30% [14, 16]. The reason for that difference might be the segment imbalance of the partner chromosome 19 involved in t(4;19). The terminal part of chromosome 19 is known as a gene density region [30]. Our data confirm the general rule saying that the probability rate for viable unbalanced child from carriers of a double segment imbalance is generally lower compared to the rates for carriers of a single segment imbalance [18, 31]. That is because the other forms of imbalance presumably lead to miscarriages. Unfortunately, miscarriage material had not been karyotyped in the families reported.

The analysis of the possible forms of imbalance produced by meiotic malsegregation of parental chromosomes indicates that trisomy 4p15.32 → pter and monosomy 19p13.3 → pter after 2:2 adjacent-1 segregation might also be compatible with survival as either single segment imbalance has been described in liveborn progeny [11, 17]. In addition, survival of children with tertiary trisomy 19 and interchange trisomy could be considered by indirect evidence from published data on mosaic form of trisomy 19 and supernumerary r(19) [12, 13, 15]. Collection of further empirical and cytogenetic data from RCT carrier pedigrees is needed [18, 31].

The frequencies of particular forms of unbalanced gametes produced by carriers of a balanced RCT are contingent on several factors including the size of chromosomal segments involved, their genetic content, sex of RCT carrier, and location of chromosome breakpoints. Survival of progeny with particular imbalances plus possibly other factors influence the risk estimation for the individual RCT carrier [5, 32, 33]. Therefore each empirical study is useful for genetic counseling.

## Conclusions

The evaluation of a phenotype – karyotype correlation did not show any essential modification of WHS phenotype by the additional trisomy 19p13.3 → pter, except for limited survivability. The limited survival (death in infancy of both children reported) is presumably due to additional trisomy 19p13.3 → pter.

Segregation analysis of a large (five-generation) pedigree of t(4;9)(p15.32;p13.3) carriers allowed estimation of probability rates for different pregnancy outcomes for genetic counseling. Carriership of t(4;19)(p15.32;p13.3) is at low risk for an unbalanced child at birth and for stillbirth/neonatal death but high for miscarriages. The chance of having a baby without unbalanced karyotype was estimated to be high. Our pedigree and cytogenetic data collected allowed for calculation, by the indirect method, of a risk value for carriers of RCT at risk for progeny with trisomic, single segment imbalance of 19p13.3 → pter; it is 7.4%.

**Acknowledgements**

We thank families for their interest and cooperation. Special thanks for parents of children with WHS for kind cooperation.

**Funding**

This work was supported by Polish grants of Medical University of Bialystok (No. 113-06825 L, No. N/ST/ZB/16/001/1106).

**Authors' contributions**

ATM, DSG - study concepts. DSG, BL, PSI, TZ, ZB, BSJ, BP, ATM - phenotype, cytogenetic data analyzes and interpretation. ATM, DSG, BSJ, BP, PSI - manuscript preparation. All authors read and approved the final manuscript.

**Competing interests**

The authors declare that they have no competing interest.

**Author details**

[1]Department of Pediatrics, University Hospital Mostar, Mostar, Bosnia and Herzegovina. [2]Department of Pediatrics, University Hospital Centre Split, Split, Croatia. [3]Department of Clinical Genetics, Medical University of Bialystok, Waszyngtona St. 13, PO Box 22, 15-089 Białystok, Poland. [4]Department of Medical Biology, School of Medicine Split, University of Split, Split, Croatia.

**References**

1. Battaglia A, Carey JC, South ST. Wolf-Hirschhorn syndrome: a review and update. Am J Med Genet C Semin Med Genet. 2015;169(3):216–23.
2. Iwanowski P, Panasiuk B, Van Buggenhout G, Murdolo M, Myśliwiec M, Maas N, Lattante S, Korniszewski L, Posmyk R, Pilch J, Zajączek S, Fryns JP, Zollino M, Midro AT. Wolf-Hirschhorn Sydrome due to pure and translocation form of Monosomy 4p16.1→pter. Am J Med Genet A. 2011;155:1833–47.
3. Maas NM, Van Buggenhout G, Hannes F, Thienpont B, Sanlaville D, Kok K, Midro A, Andrieux J, Anderlid BM, Schoumans J, Hordijk R, Devriendt K, Fryns JP, Vermeesch JR. Genotype-phenotype correlation in 21 patients with wolf-Hirschhorn syndrome using high resolution array comparative genome hybridisation (CGH). J Med Genet. 2008;45(2):71–80.
4. Zollino M, Murdolo M, Marangi G, Pecile V, Galasso C, Mazzanti L, Neri G. On the nosology and pathogenesis of wolf-Hirschhorn syndrome: genotype-phenotype correlation analysis of 80 patients and literature review. Am J Med Genet C Semin Med Genet. 2008;148C(4):257–69.
5. Midro AT, Zollino M, Wiland E, Panasiuk B, Iwanowski PS, Murdolo M, Śmigiel R, Sąsiadek M, Pilch J, Kurpisz M. Meiotic and pedigree segregation analyses in carriers of t(4;8)(p16;p23.1) differing in localization of breakpoint positions at 4p subband 4p16.3 and 4p16.1. J Assist Reprod Genet. 2016;33(2):189–97.
6. Altherr MR, Bengtsson U, Elder FF, Ledbetter DH, Wasmuth JJ, McDonald ME, Gusella JF, Greenberg F. Molecular confirmation of wolf-Hirschhorn syndrome with a subtle translocation of chromosome 4. Am J Hum Genet. 1991;49:1235–42.
7. Andries S, Sartenaer D, Rack K, Rombout S, Tuerlinckx D, Gillerot Y, Van Maldergem L. Pure terminal duplication of the short arm of chromosome 19 in a boy with mild microcephaly. J Med Genet. 2002;39(10):E60.
8. Ishikawa A, Enomoto K, Tominaga M, Saito T, Nagai J, Furuya N, Ueno K, Ueda H, Masuno M, Kurosawa K. Pure duplication of 19p13.3. Am J Med Genet A. 2013;161A(9):2300–4.
9. Gierl L, Stengel-Rutkowski S. Integrating consultation and semi-automatic knowledge acquisition in a prototype based architecture. Experiences with dysmorphic syndromes. Artif Intell Med. 1994;6:29–49.
10. ISCN. In: Shaffer LG, McGowan-Jordan J, Schmid M, editors. International system for human cytogenetic nomenclature. Basel: S. Karger; 2013.
11. Archer HL, Gupta S, Enoch S, Thompson P, Rowbottom A, Chua I, Warren S, Johnson D, Ledbetter DH, Lese-Martin C, Williams P, Pilz DT. Distinct phenotype associated with a cryptic subtelomeric deletion of 19p13.3-pter. Am J Med Genet A. 2005;136(1):38–44.
12. Faucz FR, Souza J, Bonalumi Filho A, Sotomaior VS, Frantz E, Antoniuk S, Rosenfeld JA, Raskin S. Mosaic partial trisomy 19p12-q13.11 due to a small supernumerary marker chromosome: a locus associated with Asperger syndrome? Am J Med Genet A. 2011;155:2308–10.
13. Novelli A, Ceccarini C, Bernardini L, Zuccarello D, Digilio MC, Mingarelli R, Dallapiccola B. Pure trisomy 19p syndrome in an infant with an extra ring chromosome. Cytogenet Genome Res. 2005;111:182–5.
14. Panasiuk B, Leśniewicz R, Spółczyńska A, Myśliwiec M, de Die Smulders C, Sawicka A, Midro AT. Translocation form of wolf-Hirschhorn syndrome - assessment of recurrence rate probability. Adv Med Sci. 2007;52(Suppl 1):166–70.
15. Rethoré MO, Debray P, Guesne MC, Amédée-Manesme O, Iris L, Lejeune J. A case of trisomy 19 mosaicism (author's transl). Ann Genet. 1981;24(1):34–6.
16. Stengel-Rutkowski S, Stene S, Gallano P. Risk estimates in balanced parental reciprocal translocations. Monographie des Annales de Génétique, Expansion Scientifique Francaise; 1988. p. 147.
17. Stumm M, Reuter M, Mandon U, Brückner R, Wieacker P. Trisomy 4p as result of a maternal translocation t(4;8)(q11;p23). Klin Padiatr. 1999;211:35–93.
18. Stene J, Stengel-Rutkowski S. Genetic risks of familial reciprocal and robertsonian translocation carriers. In: Daniel A, editor. Cytogenetics of mammalian Autosomal rearrangements. New York: Alan R. Liss Inc; 1988. p. 1–54.
19. Quigley DI, Kaiser-Rogers K, Aylsworth AS, Rao KW. Submicroscopic deletion 9(q34.3) and duplication 19(p13.3): identified by subtelomere specific FISH probes. Am J Med Genet A. 2004;15:125A(1):67-72.
20. Lybaek H, Ørstavik KH, Prescott T, Hovland R, Breilid H, Stansberg C, Steen VM, Houge G. An 8.9 Mb 19p13 duplication associated with precocious puberty and a sporadic 3.9 Mb 2q23.3q24.1 deletion containing NR4A2 in mentally retarded members of a family with an intrachromosomal 19p-into-19q between-arm insertion. Eur J Hum Genet. 2009;17(7):904–10.
21. Orellana C, Roselló M, Monfort S, Mayo S, Oltra S, Martínez F. Pure duplication of 19p13.3 in three members of a family with intellectual disability and literature review. Definition of a new microduplication syndrome. Am J Med Genet A. 2015;167(7):1614–20.
22. Siggberg L, Olsén P, Näntö-Salonen K, Knuutila S. 19p13.3 aberrations are associated with dysmorphic features and deviant psychomotor development. Cytogenet Genome Res. 2011;132(1–2):8–15.
23. Battaglia A, Filippi T, Carey JC. Update on the clinical features and natural history of wolf-Hirschhorn (4p-) syndrome: experience with 87 patients and recommendations for routine health supervision. Am J Med Genet C Semin Med Genet. 2008;15:148C(4):246-51.
24. Shannon NL, Maltby EL, Rgby AS, Quarrell OW. An epidemiological study of wolf-Hirschhorn syndrome: life expectancy and cause of mortality. J Med Genet. 2001;38(10):674–9.
25. Stratton RF, DuPont BR, Olsen AS, Fertitta A, Hoyer M, Moore CM. 1995. Interstitial duplication 19p. Am J Med Genet. 1995;17:57(4):562-4.
26. Byrne JLB, Korn GA, Dev VG, Bunch GM, Brooks K, Friedman JM, Harrod MJE. Partial trisomy 19p. Am J Hum Genet. 1980;32:A64.
27. Brown J, Horsley SW, Jung C, Saracoglu K, Janssen B, Brough M, Daschner M, Beedgen B, Kerkhoffs G, Eils R, Harris PC, Jauch A, Kearney L. Identification ofa subtle t(16;19)(p13.3;p13.3) in an infant with multiple congenital abnormalities using a 12-colour multiplex FISH telomere assay, M-TEL. Eur J Hum Genet. 2000;8(12):903–10.
28. Descartes M, Mikhail FM, Franklin JC, McGrath TM, Bebin M. Monosomy1p36.3 and trisomy 19p13.3 in a child with periventricular nodular heterotopia. Pediatr Neurol. 2011;45(4):274–8.
29. Puvabanditsin S, Garrow E, Brandsma E, Savla J, Kunjumon B, Gadi I. Partial trisomy 19p13.3 and partial monosomy 1p36.3: clinical report and a literature review. Am J Med Genet A. 2009;149A(8):1782–5.
30. Deloukas P, Schuler GD, Gyapay G, Beasley EM, Soderlund C, Rodriguez-Tomé P, Hui L, Matise TC, McKusick KB, Beckmann JS, Bentolila S, Bihoreau M, Birren BB, Browne J, Butler A, Castle AB, Chiannilkulchai N, Clee C, Day PJ, Dehejia A, Dibling T, Drouot N, Duprat S, Fizames C, Fox S, Gelling S, Green L, Harrison P, Hocking R, Holloway E, Hunt S, Keil S, Lijnzaad P, Louis-Dit-Sully C, Ma J, Mendis A, Miller J, Morissette J, Muselet D, Nusbaum HC, Peck A, Rozen S, Simon D, Slonim DK, Staples R, Stein LD, Stewart EA, Suchard MA, Thangarajah T, Vega-Czarny N, Webber C, Wu X, Hudson J, Auffray C, Nomura N, Sikela JM, Polymeropoulos MH, James MR, Lander ES, Hudson TJ, Myers RM, Cox DR, Weissenbach J, Boguski MS, Bentley DR. A physical map of 30,000 human genes. Science. 1998;23:282(5389):744-6.
31. Midro AT, Panasiuk B, Stasiewicz-Jarocka B, Iwanowski PS, Fauth C, Speicher MR, Lesniewicz R. Risk estimates for carriers of chromosome reciprocal translocation t(4;9)(p15.2;p13). Clin Genet. 2000;58(2):153–5.
32. Midro AT, Wiland E, Panasiuk B, Leśniewicz R, Kurpisz M. Risk evaluation of carriers with chromosome reciprocal translocation t(7;13)(q34;q13) and concomitant meiotic segregation analyzed by FISH on ejaculated spermatozoa. Am J Med Genet A. 2006;1:140(3):245-56.
33. Midro AT, Panasiuk B, Stasiewicz-Jarocka B, Olszewska M, Wiland E, Myśliwiec M, Kurpisz M, Shaffer LG, Gajecka M. Recurrence risks for different pregnancy outcomes and meiotic segregation analysis of spermatozoa in carriers of t(1;11)(p36.22;q12.2). J Hum Genet. 2014;59(12):667–74.
34. Bennett RL, French KS, Resta RG, Doyle DL. Standardized human pedigree nomenclature: update and assessment of the recommendations of the National Society of genetic counselors. J Genet Couns. 2008;17:424–33.

# 9

# Importance of biomarkers in glioblastomas patients receiving local BCNU wafer chemotherapy

Steffi Urbschat[1], Christoph Sippl[1], Jana Engelhardt[1], Kai Kammers[2], Joachim Oertel[1] and Ralf Ketter[1*]

**Abstract**

**Background:** To assess the influence of molecular markers with potential prognostic value to groups of patients with newly diagnosed glioblastoma patients were examined: group A with 36 patients (surgical resection plus standard combined chemoradiotherapy) and group B with 36 patients (surgical resection, standard combined chemoradiotherapy plus carmustine wafer implantation).

Our aim was to determine chromosomal alterations, methylation status of MGMT, p15, and p16 (CDKN2A) in order to analyse the influence on patient survival time as well as radio- and chemotherapy responses. Promoter hypermethylation of MGMT, p16, and p15 genes were determined by MS-PCR. Comparative genomic hybridisation (CGH) analyses were performed with isolated, labelled DNA of each tumor to detect genetic alterations.

**Results:** Age of onset of the disease showed a significant effect on overall survival (OS) ($p < 0.0001$). Additional treatment with carmustine wafer (group B) compared to the control group (group A) did not result in improved OS ($p = 0.562$). Patients with a methylated MGMT promotor showed a significant longer OS compared to those patients with unmethylated MGMT promotor ($p = 0.041$). Subgroup analyses revealed that patients with methylated p15 showed a significant shorter OS when administered to group B rather than in group A ($p = 0.0332$). In patients additionally treated with carmustine wafer an amplification of 4q12 showed a significant impact on a reduced OS ($p = 0.00835$). In group B, a loss of 13q was significantly associated with a longer OS ($p = 0.0364$). If a loss of chromosome 10 occurred, patients in group B showed a significantly longer OS ($p = 0.0123$).

**Conclusion:** A clinical benefit for the widespread use of additional carmustine wafer implantation could not be found. However, carmustine wafer implantation shows a significantly improved overall survival if parts of chromosome 10 or chromosome 13 are deleted. In cases of 4q12 amplification and in cases of a methylated p15 promotor, the use of carmustine wafers is especially not recommended.

The MGMT promoter methylation is a strong prognostic Biomarker for benefit from temozolomide and BCNU chemotherapy.

**Keywords:** Glioblastoma, CGH, Carmustin wafer, Prognostic factors, Standard combined radiochemotherapy

## Background

Glioblastoma multiforme (GBM) is the most aggressive and most common form of primary brain cancer [1]. At an incidence of 3 to 4 in 100,000 and a slight male predominance of 1.2–1.9:1 it can strike all ages [2–4]. The gold standard treatment for GBM is a grand total resection combined with radiochemotherapy consisting of 60 Gy radiation and temozolomide (TMZ) according to Stupp et al. [5]. Another option in the treatment of GBM is, in addition to the Stupp-regime, the implantation of carmustin (BCNU) eluted wafer into the resection cave. Hence a higher concentration of anti-neoplastic agents can be released to the tissue adjacent to the tumor. This strategy minimizes the systemic effects and maximizes the anti-neoplastic effect by bypassing the blood brain barrier [6]. Despite this theoretical

* Correspondence: ralf.ketter@uks.eu
[1]Department of Neurosurgery, Saarland University, 66421 Homburg/Saar, Germany
Full list of author information is available at the end of the article

**Table 1** Primer for MS-PCR

| | |
|---|---|
| p15 [22]:<br>(methylated, 148 bp, 60 °C)<br>forward:<br>5'-GCGTTCGTATTTT<br>GCGGTT-3'<br>reverse:<br>5'-CGTACAATAACC<br>GAACGACCGA-3'<br>(unmethylated,<br>154 bp, 60 °C)<br>forward:<br>5'-TGTGATGTGTTTG<br>TATTTTGTGGTT-3'<br>reverse:<br>5'-CCATACAATAACC<br>AAACAACCAA-3' | p16 [23]:<br>(methylated 150 bp, 65 °C)<br>forward:<br>5'-TTATTAGAGGGTGGG<br>GCGGATCGC-3'<br>reverse:<br>5'-GACCCCGAACC<br>GCGACCGTAA-3'<br>(unmethylated 151 bp, 65 °C)<br>forward:<br>5'-TTATTAGAGGG<br>TGGGGTGGATTGT-3'<br>reverse:<br>5'-CAACCCCAAACCAC<br>AACCATAA-3' |
| MGMT [21]:<br>(methylated, 122 bp, 54 °C)<br>forward:<br>5'-GTTTTTAGAACGTT<br>TTGCGTTTCGAC-3'<br>reverse:<br>5'-CACCGTCCCGAAA<br>AAAAACTCCG-3'<br>(unmethylated, 129 bp, 56 °C)<br>forward:<br>5'-TGTGTTTTTAGAATG<br>TTTTGTGTTTTGAT-3'<br>reverse:<br>5'-CTACCACCATCCCA<br>AAAAAAAACTCCA-3' | |

advantage, the clinical benefit remains in dispute. Some authors showed a benefit regarding overall survival (OS) when carmustin wafers were implanted postresectionally [7, 8]. In contrast Pallud et al. could not show a long-term benefit in (OS) at a cohort of 354 patients [9]. However, some adverse effects like cerebral edema and postoperative wound infection can be increased [10]. Therefore, it would be eligible to predict the response characteristics of a carmustin wafer therapy. Whether carmustine wafer implantation is recommendable or not could depend on patients' individual (genetic) characteristics.

A marker, which is known to predict chemotherapy response in GBM, is the promotor methylation status of O6-methyl-guanine-methyl transferase (MGMT), a DNA repair enzyme. This protein repairs alkylating DNA damage induced by TMZ in tumor cells and hereby promotes tumor progression of GBM [11]. Several clinical studies showed that low MGMT expression was significantly related to ameliorated TMZ therapy response [12–19]. Carmustine as the active drug in carmustine wafer is also a DNA alkylating agent, which can be counteracted by MGMT [20]. Another potential marker for the clinical course of GBM is a hypermethylation status of p15 that was shown to be associated with a shorter OS [21].

Furthermore, chromosomal alterations like gains on chromosome 7 and losses of parts of chromosome 10 and of/parts of the short arm of chromosome 9 are common phenomenon in glial tumors. Especially losses on chromosome 9p and 10q are often associated with a poor prognosis for patients with GBM [22]. Losses of chromosome 9 affects p16, a cell cycle controlling protein located on 9p21.3.

The aim of this experimental trial was to find new markers for treatment response in GBM on genetic and also epigenetic levels and to investigate the effects of additional carmustine wafer therapy on known markers. In particular, we focused on genes regulating cell cycle, e.g., p15, p16, and the DNA repair enzyme MGMT. For further stratification and subgroup analyses, we also incorporated two different treatment modalities: one patient cohort treated according to Stupp et al. and the other patient cohort received carmustine wafer implantation after resection in addition the Stupp et al. regime [5].

## Methods

### Patients

In this trial, we enclosed 72 patients with newly diagnosed GBM who underwent surgery between 2005 and

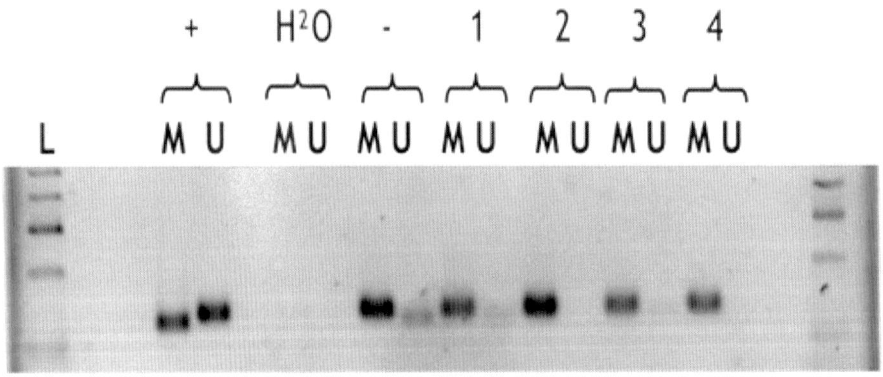


**Fig. 1** Methylation specific PCR of MGMT promotor in GBMs. L = Molecular size marker; U = unmethylated DNA; M = methylated DNA; + = positive control; – = negative control; $H_2O$ = blank value; 1 = case 1442/08; 2 = case 1510/10; 3 = case 1219/19; 4 = case 288/08

**Table 2** Clinical, epigenetic and CGH results (univariates Coxmodel)

| | HR | 1/HR | lover.95 | upper.95 | *p* value |
|---|---|---|---|---|---|
| Clinical data | | | | | |
| groupe | 1.1561 | 0.8649 | 0.7079 | 1.8880 | $p = 0.5620$ |
| age | 1.0479 | 0.9542 | 1.0242 | 1.0721 | $p = 0.6081$ |
| gender | 1.1889 | 0.8410 | 0.7151 | 1.9767 | $p = 0.5046$ |
| Methylation | | | | | |
| MGMT | 0.5929 | 1.6866 | 0.3590 | 0.9789 | $p = 0.041$ |
| p15 | 0.7883 | 1.2684 | 0.4065 | 1.5287 | $p = 0.4816$ |
| p16 | 1.5724 | 0.6359 | 0.6735 | 3.6711 | $p = 0.2954$ |
| Comparative genetic hybridization [CGH) | | | | | |
| 1q | 2.1684 | 0.4611 | 0.6683 | 7.0355 | $p = 0.1974$ |
| amp4q12 | 2.3050 | 0.4338 | 1.1815 | 4.4965 | $p = 0.01431$ |
| 7 | 1.5579 | 0.6418 | 0.7591 | 3.1973 | $p = 0.2267$ |
| amp7p12 | 1.4766 | 0.6771 | 0.8132 | 2.6813 | $p = 0.2002$ |
| 9p | 1.0812 | 0.9248 | 0.6633 | 1.7626 | $p = 0.7538$ |
| 10 | 1.0692 | 0.9352 | 0.6536 | 1.7490 | $p = 0.7897$ |
| 10q | 0.8369 | 1.1948 | 0.4945 | 1.4162 | $p = 0.5071$ |
| 12q | 1.0097 | 0.9903 | 0.5659 | 1.8015 | $p = 0.9737$ |
| 13 | 0.6853 | 1.4591 | 0.4169 | 1.1264 | $p = 0.1361$ |
| 17 | 1.0081 | 0.9919 | 0.5704 | 1.7816 | $p = 0.9778$ |
| 20 | 1.4714 | 0.6796 | 0.8380 | 2.5835 | $p = 0.1787$ |
| 22 | 1.0570 | 0.9459 | 0.5908 | 1.8912 | $p = 0.8515$ |

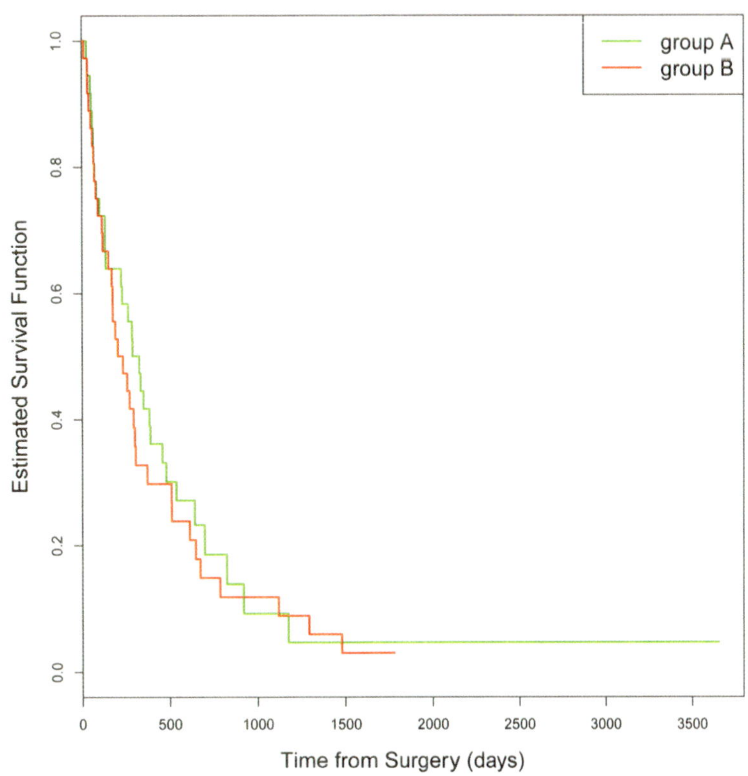


**Fig. 2** OS in group A (standard Stupp regime) and group B (standard Stupp regime + carmustine wafer)

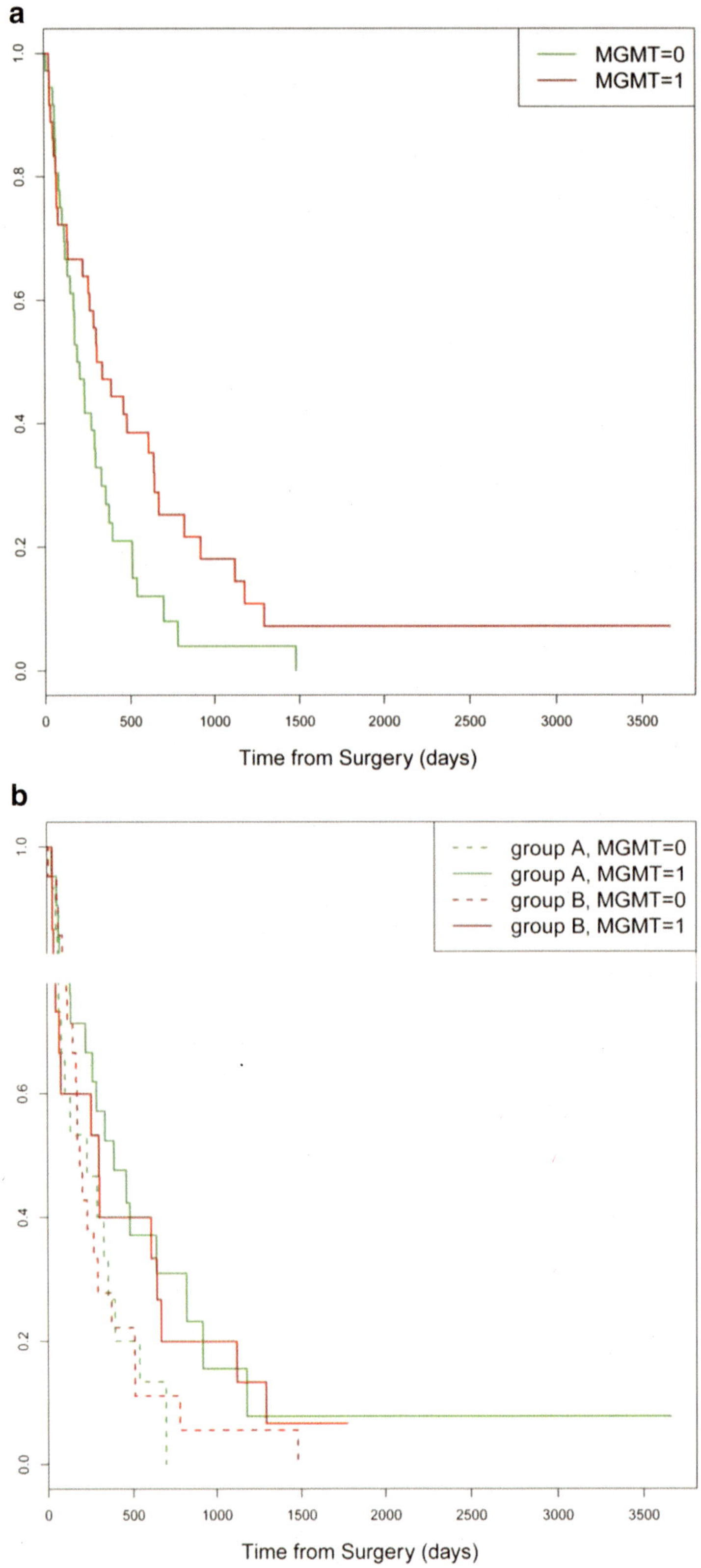


**Fig. 3 a** OS depending on MGMT methylation status. *Green*: no methylation of MGMT promoter. *Red*: methylation of MGMT promoter. **b**: OS in group A and B depending on MGMT methylation status. 0: no methylation of MGMT promoter. 1: methylation of MGMT promoter

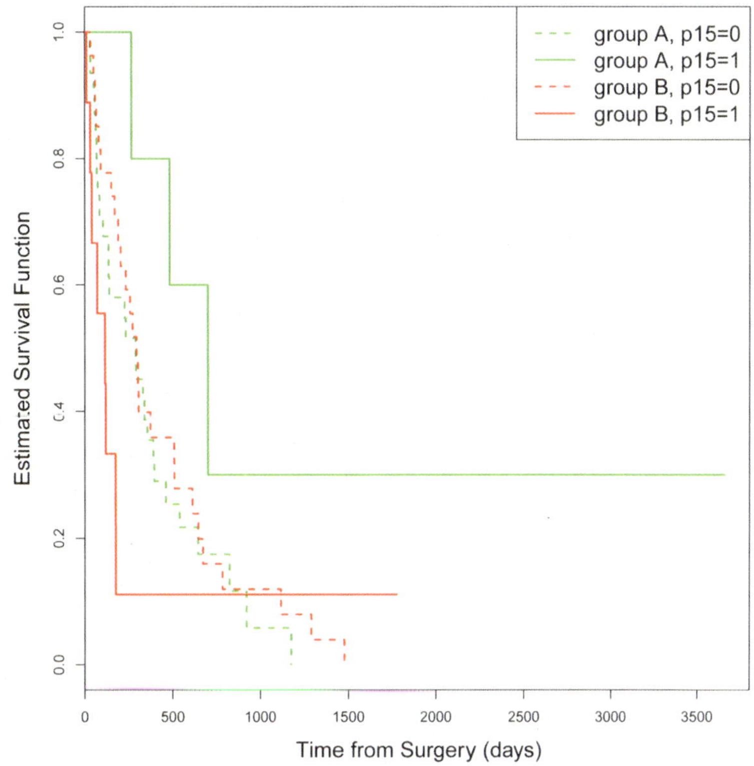


**Fig. 4** OS in group A and B depending on p15 methylation status. *Green*: group A (Stupp regime). *Red*: group B (Stupp regime + carmustine wafer)

2012 at the department of neurosurgery at the university medical center Homburg/Saar, divided into two matched pair groups with 36 patients each. After tumor resection one group was treated according to the standard Stupp regime (group A), whereas the other cohort was treated according to the standard Stupp regime with carmustine wafer implantation (group B).

Tumor tissue was collected at the time of surgery, if clinically indicated. All tissue samples were frozen immediately after the tumor was resected using liquid nitrogen and stored in our tumor bank at −80 °C. This study was approved by the local ethic board of Saarland and written informed consent was obtained from all patients.

## Methylation analysis

DNA isolation was performed using DNA isolation kit (Qiagen, QIAamp DNA Mini Kit 50). The methylation status of promoter regions of the genes p15, p16 and MGMT were determined by methylation specific polymerase chain reaction (MS-PCR). Therefore, 500 ng DNA of each tumor specimen, as well as appropriate control samples were bisulfite-treated (ZYMO RESEARCH, EZ DNA Methylation-Gold Kit 200) [23]. In summary, thus unmethylated cytosine is converted to uracil, whereas methylated cytosine remained unchanged. The modified DNA was recovered by ethanol precipitation and dissolved in water. For the analysis of the methylation status the primer sequences listed in Table 1 were used.

PCR was performed with a 25 μl reaction volume and 38 PCR cycles. All PCR products were separated by electrophoresis on a 2% agarose gel. As methylated and unmethylated control we used Universal Methylated Human DNA (ZYMO RESEARCH). As blank value we added water in place of DNA [Fig. 1].

## CGH analysis

Comparative genomic hybridisation (CGH) was used to screen the tumors for chromosomal imbalances. Metaphasic preparation was acquired via short term lymphocytic culture. CGH was performed as described previously [24].

## Statistics

Comparisons of survival times between groups defined by clinical variables, methylation status and parts of chromosome deletions were performed by Kaplan-Meier curves and with two-sided log rank tests. Methylation index was defined as percentage of patients with promotor methylation of the total cohort in percent. Univariate Cox regression [25] analysis was performed to identify significant predictors for overall survival (OS). Effects of individual predictors on OS in all models were

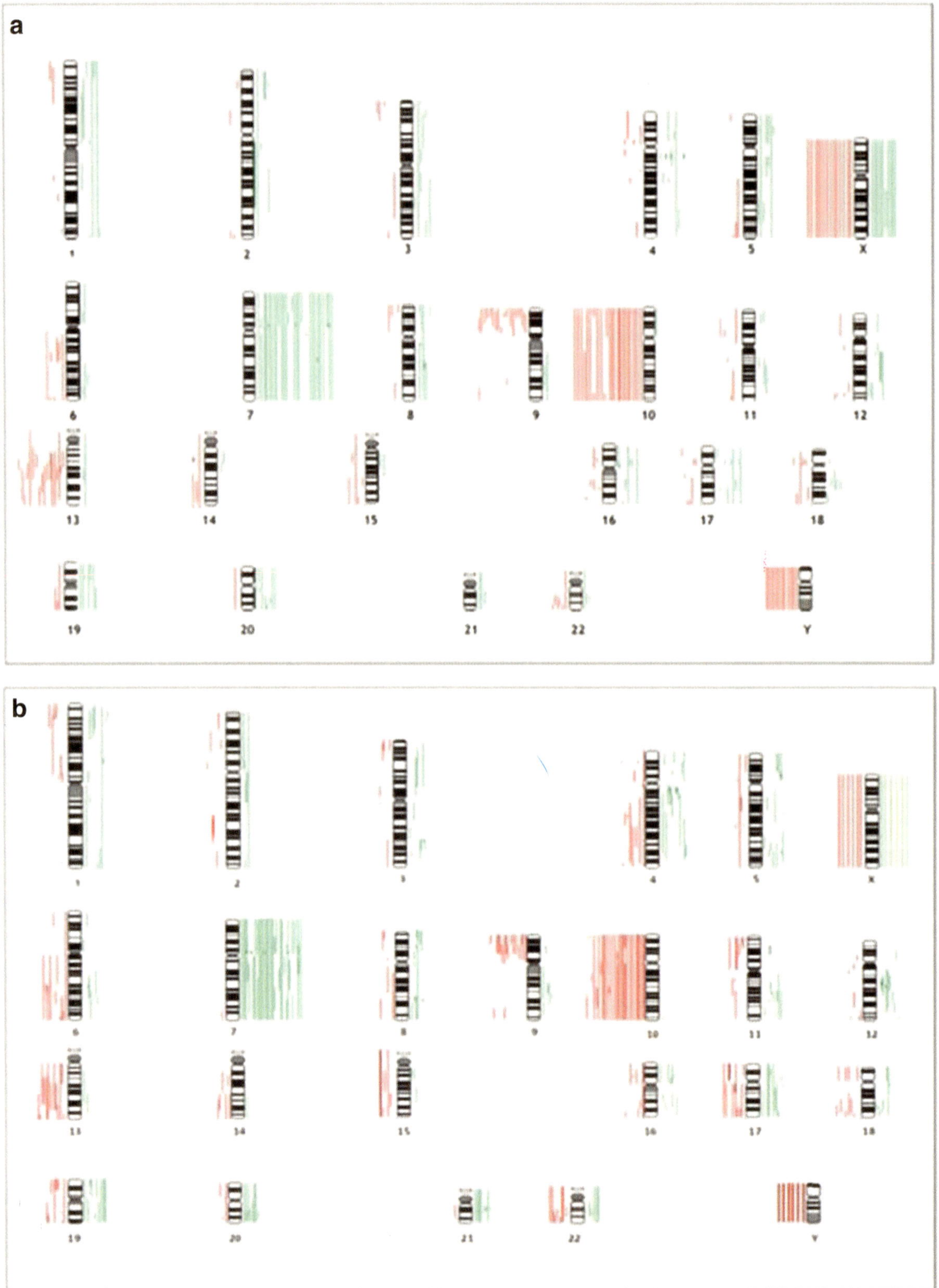


**Fig. 5 a** Overview of genetic imbalances of the Carmustin-group. Lines on the left represent losses, and lines on the right represent gains; amplifications are in bold. **b**: Overview of genetic imbalances of the conventionally treated-group. Lines on the left represent losses, and lines on the right represent gains; amplifications are in bold

**Table 3** Clinical chacteristics and CGH results of the Carmustin group

**Table 3** Clinical chacteristics and CGH results of the Carmustin group *(Continued)*

| Cases | Histology | Ages/ gender | CGH - results |
|---|---|---|---|
| 2065/ 08 | pGBM | 80/f | +X, +7, −9p, −10, −14q24qter, −17p12pter, −22q11.2q13.2 |
| 270/ 10 | pGBM | 80/m | −4, −6, +7, −8q21.1qter, +9q12q34.1, −10, −11p14pter, −16, −17q, −18p11.2pter, +19, +20, +21 |
| 1526/ 07 | pGBM | 75/m | -X, +1p33pter, −1p11p22.1, amp4q12, +6p12p21.3, +7, −9p13pter, −10, +11q23.3q25, +15q11.2q14, +16p, +17p12pter, +20q12q13.2 |
| 220/ 10 | pGBM | 72/f | +X, −6q25.3qter, +7p, amp7p12, +7q11.1q31.1, −9p23pter, −10, −11p15.3pter, −13q33qter, +17, −18q22qter, +21, −22 |
| 479/ 09 | pGBM | 69/f | +5q23.3q32, +7q21.1q36 |
| 740/ 10 | pGBM | 69/f | −2p16p21, −3p24.1pter, −3p12p13, −3q24qter, −4q13.3q33, +7q11.2, −9p21p23, −11p14p15.3, −15q21.3q25, −16q13q22, +17, −18q12.3q22 |
| 1442/ 08 | pGBM | 52/f | +4q13.1q32, +7q, -10, +12q13.3.q15, −19, −22 |
| 1578/ 10 | pGBM | 52/f | +1q, +4p15.3pter, +5q12q14, −6q23.1qter, +6p22.3pter, +7, −8p11.1p12, −8q12q21.3, −9p21pter, −10, +11p14p15.3, −12q24.1qter, +15q11.1q15, +17p12p13, −17q25qter, +19p13.3pter, +19q, +20, +21, +22q11.1q13.1 |
| 1966/ 11 | pGBM | 40/f | -X, +3q21q24, amp7p12, +7q22qter, −17q25qter, +22q12.1q13.1 |
| 2404/ 11 | pGBM | 75/m | −2p23pter, −4p15.3p16, +7, +9p21p23, −10p13pter, −10q, +12q13.1q21.2, amp12q14, −12q24.3qter, −16p11.2p13.2, −19q13.3qter, −22q12.1q13.1 |
| 1210/ 09 | pGBM | 71/m | −4q28q32, −8p21.1pter, −9p21pter, −11p, −13, −15q12q21.3, −15q26.1qter, +16q11.2q21, −18p, −18q12.1qter, +19p, −20 |
| 1510/ 10 | pGBM | 69/m | +1p32.3p36.1, −3p24.1pter, +3q26.1q26.3, +4q24q34, −5p14pter, +5q31.1q32, +6q16.1q22.3, amp6q21, −6q27, +7, −9p22pter, −10, −11p, −11q14.1qter, +12q12q23, amp12q14q15, −13q23qter, −15q25qter, −16p12p13.1, +16q21q22, −18p, −18q23qter, +19q13.3, +20q11.2q12.3, +21, +22 |
| 1370/ 07 | pGBM | 63/m | +1p11p22.1, +2p11.1p33, +7, amp 7p12, −3p21.3p25, −9p13p23, −9q31qter, −10, −17, −19p13.2pter, −20q13.1q13.2, −21q22.1q22.2, −22q13.1qter |
| 1663/ 07 | pGBM | 58/m | -X, +1p34.1pter, −1p21p31.1, −2q24.1q32.3, −4p11p15.1, −4q11q28, −5q21q22, +5q32qter, −6q11q21, +7, +8q24.1qter, −9p21pter, −10, −12p11.2p12.3, −12q11q12, +12q15q22, −13q14.3q31, −14q12q21, +17, +20q, +22 |
| 1219/ 09 | pGBM | 58/m | −1p13.1p13.2, −6q22.2q24, +7, amp7p12, +11q14.3q22.3, −12q24.3qter, +18q21.3q22, −19p13.2pter, +21p11.2p21 |
| 1809/ 11 | pGBM | 55/m | −1p26.1pter, +3p12p22, amp4q12, +5p14pter, +5q11.2q21, -6p22.3pter, +6q22.2qter, +7, +8p11.2p21.1, +8q11.2, +8q22.3q23, −9p, +9q21.3q22.3, −9q34.1qter, −10p11.1p12.3, −10q, +11p14p15.3, +11q13.2q14.3, +12q12q23, −13q11q32, -14q22qter, −15 |
| 1362/ 07 | pGBM | 52/m | −1p34.3pter, −5q12q14, +7, −9p11p22, −10, +18q21.3qter, +19p |
| 288/ 08 | pGBM | 52/m | amp7p12, +7q31.3q35, +9q21.2q32, −10, −11q12q13.2, -13q12.3q31, −17q11.1q21.1 |
| 1350/ 06 | sGBM | 46/m | +1q12q23, amp4q12, +4q12q22, +8q23qter, −1p21p36.1, -4q28qter, −6q, −13q14.3q33, −18q12.3q23, −19q13.1q13.3, -22q12.3qter |
| 1455/ 08 | pGBM | 46/m | +4p14p15.1, amp4q12, +7p, +8p21.2p22, +11q14.1q22.3 |
| 768/ 09 | pGBM | 44/m | −6q25.1qter, +7q21.2q32, +12q13.2q21.1, −18p, −19 |
| P.E. | pGBM | 44/m | +1q43qter, +2p11.1p13, +2q13q22, +2q37.1qter, +3p13p33, +4p15.3pter, +5p14pter, +5q31.1qter, +6q23.1q22.3, +7, +9q22.3q31, −10q22.1q22.3, +11q23.3, +12q15q21.3, −13, +16q23q24, +17q12q24, +18q22 |
| 1741/ 08 | pGBM | 54/f | −9p21pter, −10, −17q, +18q12.3q22 |
| 1701/ 07 | pGBM | 67/m | amp 4q12, +7, +17q, −4q21.3q34, −5, −10, −11q12q21, -13q14.1qter, −17p, −19p11pter |
| 1935/ 08 | pGBM | 70/m | amp4q12, +7q11q21.3, −9p21pter, −10, −18q22qter, −20p11.2pter |
| 1618/ 09 | pGBM | 54/f | −2q24.1q34, −3p11.1p14.1, −3q11.1q13.1, -4q24q26, −5p11p12, -6p11p12, amp7p12, +7q34qter, −10q11.1q21.1, +10q26.2qter, -13q14.1q31, −14q12q22, +16p, +17q24qter, +19q, +22 |
| A.W. | pGBM | 75/m | +3q24q27, +4p, +5p, amp5p13.1p14, +5q32, +7, amp7p12, −9p21pter, −10, −12q12q13.1, −13q21.3q33, +14q23qter, +15q21.1q24, +17p11.2p12, +19, +20, +21q11.2q21 |
| 1934/ 11 | pGBM | 69/f | +X, +3q24q26.1, +4q13.1q32, +6q15q22.3, +7q21.1q32, −9q13q21.1, +11q14.1q22.3, +12q21.3q24.1, −16p, −17p, −19q13.2qter, −22 |
| 1381/ 06 | pGBM | 44/m | -X, −Y, +1q32.2qter, −2p15p23, +2q11.1q21.3, −4q24q28, −6q21q22.3, +7p, +7q33qter, +8, amp 8p23.1pter, −10q22.1q25.1, −11p, +11q, −13q11q31, −14q22q31, −21q11.1q22.1, −22 |
| 1080/ 10 | pGBM | 73/m | +X, −1p34.1pter, +4p14p16, +6q23.1q24, +7p, +8p22pter, −9q34qter, −10, +12p11.2p13.1, +16p11.2p12,-16q24qter, −17q, +18p11.2pter |

**Table 3** Clinical chacteristics and CGH results of the Carmustin group *(Continued)*

| | | | |
|---|---|---|---|
| 725/ 12 | pGBM | 50/m | -X, +1, +2, +3p13p25, +3q24, +4p, +4q26q34, +5p13.1p13.3, +5q14q15, +5q23.1q34, −6q, +7, +8p21.1pter, +8q23, -10q21.1q21.3, +11q14.1qter, −13q33qter, −14q24.2qter, +16p, +16q11.2q22, +18, +19, +20, +21 |
| 778/ 10 | pGBM | 70/m | +1p36.1, −4q34qter, amp7p12, +7q11.1q22, -10p15pter,+12q24.3qter, −13q23.1qter, +17p11.1p11.2, +18p11.1p11.2, +19,+20q12q13.2 |
| 563/ 12 | pGBM | 60/m | −7q36qter |
| 904/ 11 | pGBM | 65/m | -X, +1p36.1p36.3, −4p16, −9p23pter, +16p12p13.1 |
| 1346/ 06 | pGBM | 50/f | −5q21q23.1, −8q23qter, −10q23.2qter, −15, −17 |
| 175/ 12 | pGBM | 45/m | -X, +1p31.1p32.3,-2p11.2p13, +3q24q26.1, +4q31.3q34, +7, +8q23q24.1, +16q12.2qter, +16p12p13.2, −19q, +21q11.2q22.1 |

quantified by estimated hazard ratios (HR) estimates with corresponding 95% confidence intervals.

## Results

### Clinical data

Overall median survival was 267 days (95% CI = [176, 372]) with 309 days in group A (95% CI = [138, 481]) and 219 days in group B (95% CI = [151, 372]).

Univariate Cox models of clinical covariates revealed that age of onset of the disease had a statistically significant effect on OS (HR = 1.048, 95% CI = [1.024, 1.072], $p < 0.0001$). The average age of onset was 60.1 years in group A and 60.2 years in group B. Gender did not show a significant effect on OS (HR =1.19, 95% CI = [0.715–1.977], $p = 0.504$) (see Table 2).

A statistically significant effect of additional treatment with carmustine wafer (group B) in comparison to the standard Stupp regime (group A) on OS could not be detected (HR = 1.15, 95% CI = [0.708, 1.888], $p = 0.562$) [Fig. 2].

### Methylation analysis

We found a MGMT methylation index (MI) of 58% (21/36) in group A and a methylation index of 42% (15/36) in group B. At the p15 promotor we found a MI of 14% (5/36) in group A and 25% (9/36) in group B, respectively. The methylation index in p16 showed 8% (3/36) in both groups.

Patients with an unmethylated MGMT showed a median OS of 6.6 months. If MGMT was methylated the median OS was 10.7 months. A univariate Cox model with MGMT as predictor results in MGMT has a statistically significant effect on OS (HR = 0.593, 95% CI = 0.359 – 0.979, $p = 0.041$). If stratified for treatment group there was neither in group A nor in group B a significant correlation between OS and MGMT methylation (group A: $p = 0.0635$, group B: $p = 0.319$) [Fig. 3a/b].

Subgroup analyses revealed that patients with a p15 methylation showed a significant shorter OS when administered to group B (median OS: 115 days) than in group A (median OS: 481 days) ($p = 0.0332$). A promotor methylation of p16 had no significant impact on any group [Fig. 4].

Within the whole population in this study ($N = 72$) 3 patients showed an OS longer than 36 months, 2 of them were in group B, one in group A. All three cases showed a methylated MGMT promotor whereas p15 and p16 were not methylated.

### CGH

In total, each tumor showed on average 11 aberrations and a total number of 754 aberrations could be detected. The distribution of alterations in both groups showed in general no differences [Fig. 5 a/b]. We found different chromosomal alterations in all the analyzed tumor specimens. One of the most frequent alterations were gains on chromosome 7 in 85% (61/72), chromosome 16 in 33% (24/72), chromosome 4 in 22% (16/72), chromosome 5 in 21% (15/72), chromosome 12 in 19% (14/72) and chromosome 20 in 22% (16/72).

In contrast losses were prevalently detected on the short arm of chromosome 9 in 47% (34/72), chromosome 10 in 67% (48/72), the long arm of chromosome 13 in 47% (34/72), on chromosome 6 in 25% (18/72), on the long arm of chromosome 22 in 22% (16/72), of the long arm of chromosome 4 in 19% (14/72) and on the long arm of chromosome 17 in 18% (13/72) [Fig. 5 a/b].

We also found amplifications at 4q12 in 15% (11/72), at 7p12 in 19% (14/72) and in the region of 12q in 4% (3/72). In one case an amplification of 6q21 and in another case of 8p23.1pter were found (Tables 3, 4 and 5).

Patients in group B whose tumors showed an amplification of 4q12 had a statistically significant reduced OS (log-rank test, $p = 0.00835$). An amplification of 4q12 for patients of group A did not show this worsening effect on OS. In contrast if a loss of chromosome 10 occurred in tumor samples, patients in group B, who additionally received carmustine wafer implantation, showed a significantly longer OS ($p = 0.0123$). This effect could not be observed in group A.

A loss of 13q in group B was significantly associated with a longer OS ($p = 0.0364$). Again, this effect could not be observed in group A.

No further significant correlations regarding clinical, chromosomal and epigenetic data could be observed.

## Discussion

The focus of this study was to find new molecular markers for treatment response in GBM. Only a few

**Table 4** Clinical characteristics and CGH results of the Controll group

| Cases | Histology | Ages/ gender | CGH-results |
|---|---|---|---|
| 1553/ 07 | pGBM | 82/f | +2q12q33, +3p24.2p25, +3q22q24, amp4q12, +7, −9p13p24, −10, +11q13.2q14.1, −13q12.1q14.3,-15q21.3q23, +16p, +17p12pter, +18q23qter |
| 1042/ 12 | pGBM | 83/f | −2p23p24, −4p12p15.1, −4q21.2q22, amp7p12, +7q, −10, −13q14.1q21.1, −16q13q21, −18q12.3q22 |
| 1117/ 05 | pGBM | 71/m | +3, +7, −9p21pter, −10, −13, −14, +16p11.2p13 |
| 139/ 10 | pGBM | 73/f | +1p13.1p33, +1q21.1q31, +2, +3p12p14.1, +3p25pter, +3q13.1q21, +4q22q24, +5p14, +7, +8p23.1pter, +8q11.2qter, +9p23pter, +9q22.1q33, −10, +13q14.1q21.3, +14q12q21, −16p12p13.1, +16q23qter, −17p11.1p11.2, −18p11.2p11.3, −19, −22 |
| 1588/ 09 | pGBM | 70/f | +X, +1p21p36.1, +3p14.1p24.1, −3q11.1q26.1, +5q23.2q32, +7, amp 7p12, −9p22pter, −10, +12q21.3q24.3, −17p11.1p11.2, +17q21.3q22, −18p11.1p11.3, +19, +20 |
| 1191/ 08 | pGBM | 68/f | +1p36.1pter, −1q42.2q43, amp4q12, +7, −10, -13q14.1q21.3, +16q11.2q21, −17q12qter, +18p11.1p11.2 |
| 1355/ 08 | pGBM | 52/f | -X, −1q31, +6q24q26, +7, −8p21.1pter, −9p22pter, −10, +11p15.1p15.4, +12q21.3qter, −13q12.2qter, +15q11.1q15, +16, −18, −19q13.2qter, +20p, +20q11.1q12, +21, −22q13.2qter |
| 922/ 12 | pGBM | 54/m | +1p13.1p13.3, +1q43qter, +2q12q14.1, -2q37.1qter, +4p13pter, +4q24q25, +5, +7, +8p12pter, +8q12q13, -10, +11p15.1pter, +11q13.1q23.3, -13q12.1q21.3, +16p12p13.1, +17p11.1p12, +19q13.1q13.2, +22 |
| 881/ 10 | pGBM | 40/f | +1, +2p21pter, −5q14qter, −6q14q21, −9p24pter, −9q31q33, −10, −11p, −12q12q13.1, −12q24.1q24.3, -13q14.1q21.2, +16p11.2p13.1, +17q21.1qter, +22q11.2q12.3 |
| 1229/ 08 | pGBM | 72/m | −1p31.2p36.1, −1q23q24, +3q26.1qter, amp4q12, +4q11q21.2, −4q33qter, −6q13q21, +7, −9p23p24, −10, −11q14.1qter, −13q14.1qter, −14q22q32.1, +16, +17p11.1p12, −22q13.1q13.2 |
| 375/ 10 | pGBM | 72/m | +1p36.1pter, +2p21pter, −4p11p12, +6p12p21.3, −9p13p21, −13q21.1q31, +15q13q21.3, +17, +20q12qter |
| 1988/ 09 | pGBM | 68/m | amp7p12, −10p, +11q13.5q23.3, −12p, +20q31.1qter, +22q12.3q13.1 |
| 838/ 12 | sGBM | 70/m | +7, −9p, −10, +19 |
| 926/ 09 | pGBM | 58/m | −3q27qter, −6q26qter, +7, amp7p12, −8p23.1pter, −9p13pter, −10, −16p, +16q11.2q21, −18q21.3qter, +19, +20q12q13.2, −22q12.3qter |
| 983/ 04 | pGBM | 54/m | −3p24.3pter, −4q23q25, −6q16.3q21, −8q24.1qter, −10, −11q23.3qter, −13q22qter, −17q25qter |
| 837/ 12 | pGBM | 54/f | +7, −8p22pter, −9p13p24, −10, +17q21.2q22, +18q12.1q12.3, +19p |
| 1078/ 09 | pGBM | 54/m | +Xp, +Xq11.1q21.3, +1, −3p21.3pter, +3q13.2qter, −4p14pter, +4q28q34, +5p, +5q11.2q13.2, −5q33.1qter, +6p, +6q21qter, +7, +8, −9p23pter, +12p, +12q11q13.1, −13, −14q21qter, amp 14q11.2q12, +17, +19, −20, +21 |
| 776/ 05 | pGBM | 50/m | +3p23p24.3, +5q23.3q31.1, +7p14p22 |
| 1861/ 03 | pGBM | 43/m | +2p23p24, +2q22q34, +6q22.3q24, +7, −8p, −9p23pter, −10, amp12q13.12q21.3, +13, −15q12q14, +18q12.1q21.2, −22q11.2q13.1 |
| 1216/ 11 | pGBM | 50/m | +7p11.1pter, amp7p12, −9p21pter, −10q21qter, +11q21q22.3, +12q13.1qter, −13q14.1q21.3, −22q13.3qter |
| 1110/ 05 | pGBM | 41/m | +7p |
| 1457/ 03 | pGBM | 37/m | −5q34qter, +8q21.3qter, +10p11.2pter, −12q24.1q24.3, −13q33qter, +18q12.2q21.1 |
| 378/ 12 | pGBM | 59/f | +1q42.2qter, −4p11p13, −4q11q13.1, +5p14p15.2, -6q, +7, amp7p12, +8p22pter, −9p13pter, −10, −11p12p14, −13q14.3q33, +14q11.1q13, −16q23q24, −17p13pter, −18p11.1p11.3, +19q, +20, +21q11.1q22.1 |
| 1583/ 08 | pGBM | 68/f | −2p23p24, −5q21q31.1, +5q33.1qter, −6q12q14, +7, +8p23.1pter, −8p11.1p12, −9q22.3qter, −10, −13q33qter, +16p11.2p13.1, +17p11.1p12, +19p13.1p13.3, +20, +21q11.2q22.1, −22q11.2qter |
| 655/ 09 | pGBM | 71/f | −6q12qter, +7, −9p21pter, −10, −12q21.3q23, −13q12.3qter, +20 |
| 291/ 09 | pGBM | 51/f | +4p14, −6q26qter, +7p13pter, +18q11.1q21.1, +Xq21.2q27 |
| 156/ 12 | sGBM | 76/f | -1p34.2pter, +5, +7, +9q13qter, −15q21.3qter, −16q11.2q13, −17q11.2q21.1 |
| 1286/ 08 | pGBM | 65/m | +7, −10q25.1qter, +16p12 |
| 1458/ 10 | pGBM | 49/f | +7q11.2, −13q12.3q14.1, −15q26.1qter |
| 1431/ 05 | pGBM | 69/f | −2p12p15, −2q37.1qter, −3p24.1pter, amp4q12, −5p15.3pter, +7, −9p13p23, −9q33qter, −10, −11p12p15.3, −12q24.1qter, −13q13q21.1, −16q23q24 |
| T 6929 | pGBM | 50/m | +1p21p31.2, +3q12q13.2, +3q25.3qter, −4p16pter, +6q12q13, +7, −9p21p23, −9q13q23.1, −10, −11q23.1q23.3, −12q22qter, −13q12.3qter, −17, −18p11.1p11.3, −20, +Xq13q23 |
| 338/ 12 | pGBM | 72/m | -X, +7, −9p21pter, −11q12q13.2, +17p11.2p12, +20 |
| 791/ 08 | pGBM | 56/m | No aberrrations |
| 663/ 12 | pGBM | 65/f | +4, +7, −10p14pter, −10q25.2qter, +12q13.1q13.3, −15 |
| 754/ 12 | pGBM | 56/m | +5p, +5q11.2q14, +7, −10, −13q11q21.1, −17q24qter, −19q |

**Table 4** Clinical characteristics and CGH results of the Controll group *(Continued)*

| | | | |
|---|---|---|---|
| 2512/11 | pGBM | 42/m | -Xp, +4q, amp4q12, −5q13.3qter, −7p14pter, +7q, +8p, −9q34.1qter, −10q22.3qter, −11p, −11q24qter, −12p, −12q14q23, −13, −18p11.2pter, −18q22qter, −21 |

previous retrospective and prospective studies have analyzed the combination of carmustine wafer implantation with the combined standard chemoradiation protocol for the treatment of newly diagnosed glioblastoma [26–35].

We report here the impact of carmustin wafer implantation together with the combined standard chemoradiation protocol in newly diagnosed supratentorial glioblastoma in adults. To overcome the limitations inherent to retrospective observational studies, we performed a confirmatory case matched analysis ($N = 72$). The data from our study confirmed previous trials suggesting that MGMT is a predictive marker for TMZ therapy response [11, 14–19]. We also found a significant correlation between MGMT methylation status and OS in our total collective. This significance vanished when the patients were stratified for treatment group A or B. This may result from the limited number per treatment cohort. Losses of chromosome 10 are among the most frequent in GBM [36–38]. Patients with additional carmustine wafer treatment and a loss of chromosome 10 showed a significantly longer OS than patients without that chromosomal loss. An explanation for this could be the MGMT gene locus on 10q21. A loss of this region results in a loss of MGMT expression and therefore ameliorate the treatment response of both TMZ and the local carmustin therapy. Wemmert et al. could show a similar effect regarding TMZ therapy alone [38]. In our trial this effect occurred only in patients receiving both TMZ/RT → TMZ regime and carmustin wafer implantation, but not in patients who received TMZ/RT → TMZ regime alone. Possibly other so far unknown gene loci might also play an important role.

**Table 5** Overview of the chromosomal alterations

| Alteration | Group B frequency | Group A frequency |
|---|---|---|
| amplification 4q12 | 6/36 (17%) | 5/36 (14%) |
| gain on chromosome 7 | 30/36 (83%) | 31/36 (86%) |
| amplification on 7p12 | 8/36 (22%) | 6/36 (17%) |
| loss on 9p | 16/36 (44%) | 18/36 (50%) |
| loss on 10q | 23/36 (64%) | 25/36 (69%) |
| gain on 12q | 9/36 (25%) | 6/36 (17%) |
| loss of chromosome 13 | 13/36 (36%) | 21/36 (58%) |
| loss of chromosome 20 | 8/36 (22%) | 9/36 (25%) |
| loss of chromosome 22 | 8/36 (22%) | 7/36 (19%) |

Mutations and deletions of p15 and p16 are frequent genetic alterations in glial tumors [39–43]. p15 and p16 inhibits CDK4 and CDK6, therefore p15 and p16 act as tumor suppressors and lead to cell cycle arrest in the late G1 phase [33]. Previous studies indicated that a loss of expression, resulting from deletion, mutations or methylation of p15 and p16 is associated with a significantly worse prognosis for survival in glioblastoma [21, 38, 44, 45]. Our data supports this point of view, at least regarding p15. Interestingly patients administered to group B with methylated p15 showed significantly the shortest OS of all subgroups within our trial. The low number of only six p16 methylated tumors shows that p16 is not of significant impact on our collective. Considering the findings of the literature this is not surprising [21, 38, 44–46].

Another important finding of our study is the amplification of the region 4q12 as a prognostic marker in patients additionally treated with carmustine wafer. Patients in group B whose tumor showed this amplification had a significantly shortened OS. PDGFRα, a tyrosine kinase, is located in the region of 4q12. PDGFRα is known to play a major role in tumor angiogenesis by stimulation of cell growth [47, 48]. The exact mechanism of PDGFRα in vasculogenesis and tumor angiogenesis is yet unknown, but an overexpression of PDGFRα caused by gene amplification may result in more aggressive tumor growth.

This effect was not observable in group A. Maybe PDGFRα is not the only determinant gene influencing OS and due to the described tumor heterogeneity in GBM it did not reach a statistical significant level [24, 49, 50].

We also detected a better prognosis in group B if chromosome 13 or parts of chromosome 13 were lost. This is concordant with previous findings where a survival benefit in patients treated with alkylating agents was found, if chromosome 13 was lost [38]. A further genetic hotspot is the RB1 gene, which is located on 13q14.2. Maybe a loss of this gene influences the oncological behavior of tumor cells in such a manner that additional carmustine wafer therapy shows an improved impact on the clinical course. This effect could not be shown in the standard therapy group treated with Stupp regime. Hence a loss of chromosome 13 is maybe a prognostic marker for an ameliorated clinical course which would recommend the implantation of carmustine wafers.

Besides to the molecular findings described above, we found no significant survival benefit between group A and B in general. We think it is not recommendable to use additional carmustine wafer implantation in every single case. This is conclusive with the data of other clinical studies and the widespread use of carmustine wafers is highly controversial due to its debatable clinical impact. Pallud et al. could e.g., not show a long-term benefit regarding overall survival (OS) in a cohort of 354 patients [9]. This controversy is even more understandable if the clinical side effects of carmustine wafer implantation is taken into account. Especially operative wound infection and cerebral edema can be increased [10].

Therapy with carmustine wafers should be individually assessed for each patient. This also represents the current opinion in treatment guidelines, in general.

Overall, our findings suggest that carmustin wafer implantation in combination with maximal safe resection, followed by combined standard chemoradiation protocols, is a promising treatment option for patients with supratentorial glioblastoma harboring MGMT promoter methylation.

## Conclusion

A clinical benefit for the widespread use of additional carmustine wafer implantation could not be found. However, carmustine wafer implantation shows a significantly improved overall survival if chromosome 10 and particularly 10q or chromosome13 are deleted. In cases of 4q12 amplification and in cases of a methylated p15 promotor, the use of carmustine wafers is especially not recommended.

The MGMT promoter methylation is a strong prognostic Biomarker for benefit from temozolomide and BCNU chemotherapy

Therefore we propose to use BCNU wafers in a second line therapy, when the chromosomal and epigenetic data from the primary tumor are available. However, owing to the small number of patients these findings would need to be corroborated in lager patients cohorts.

### Abbreviations

CGH: Comparative genomic hybridization; TMZ: Temozolomide; WHO: World Health Organization

### Acknowledgments

We thank Cornelia Lerner, Silke Wemmert and Ulrike Bechtel for expert technical assistance and helpful discussions.

### Funding

This work was supported by Archimedes GmbH (L204150209).

### Authors' contributions

US carried out the comparative genetic hybridization and wrote the manuscript, SC and EJ carried out the methylation analysis, KK performed the statistical analysis, OJ and RK did surgery of the patients and participated in its design. All authors read and approved the final manuscript.

### Competing interests

Ketter R. had done speaking engagements (including travel and accommodation) and is consultant for Kyowa Kirin GmbH.
All other authors declare they have no competing interests.

### Author details

[1]Department of Neurosurgery, Saarland University, 66421 Homburg/Saar, Germany. [2]Division of Biostatistics and Bioinformatics, Department of Oncology, Sidney Kimmel Comprehensive Cancer Center, Johns Hopkins University School of Medicine, Baltimore, MD, USA.

### References

1. Louis DN. Molecular pathology of malignant gliomas. Annu Rev Pathol. 2006;1:97–117.
2. Dolecek TA, Propp JM, Stroup NE, Kruchko C. CBTRUS statistical report: primary brain and central nervous system tumors diagnosed in the United States in 2005–2009. Neuro-Oncology. 2012;14 Suppl 5:1–49.
3. Wen PY, Kesari S. Malignant gliomas in adults. N Engl J Med. 2008;359(5):492–507.
4. Clarke J, Butowski N, Chang S. Recent advances in therapy for glioblastoma. Arch Neurol. 2010;67(3):279–83.
5. Stupp R, Mason WP, van den Bent MJ, Weller M, Fisher B, Taphoorn MJ, et al. Radiotherapy plus concomitant and adjuvant temozolomide for glioblastoma. N Engl J Med. 2005;352:987–96.
6. WU MP, Tamada JA, Brem H, Langer R. In vitro degradation of controlled release polymers for intracranial surgical therapy. J Biomed Mater Res. 1994;28(3):387-95.
7. De Bonis P, Anile C, Pompucci A, et al. Safety and efficacy of Gliadel wafers for newly diagnosed and recurrent glioblastoma. Acta Neurochir. 2012;154:1371–8.
8. Westphal M, Hilt DC, Bortey E, Delavault P, Olivares R, Warnke PC, Whittle IR, Jääskeläinen J, Ram Z. A phase 3 trial of local chemotherapy with biodegradable carmustine (BCNU) wafers (Gliadel wafers) in patients with primary malignant glioma. Neuro-Oncology. 2003;4:79–88.
9. Pallud J, Audureau E, Noel G, Corns R, Lechapt-Zalcman E, et al. Long-term results of carmustine wafer implantation for newly diagnosed glioblastomas: a controlled propensity-matched analysis of a French multicenter cohort. Neuro-Oncology. 2015;17(12):1609–19.
10. Weber EL, Goebel EA. Cerebral edema associated with gliadel wafers: two case studies. Neuro-Oncology. 2005;7:84–9.
11. Hegi ME, Liu L, Herman JG, et al. Correlation of O6-methylguanine methyltransferase (MGMT) promoter methylation with clinical outcomes in glioblastoma and clinical strategies to modulate MGMT activity. J Clin Oncol. 2008;26(25):4189–99.
12. Hegi ME, Diserens AC, Gorlia T, et al. MGMT gene silencing and benefit from temozolomide in glioblastoma. N Engl J Med. 2005;352(10):997–1003.
13. Zhang W, Zhang J, Hoadley K, Kushwaha D, Ramakrishnan V, et al. miR-181d: a predictive glioblastoma biomarker that downregulates MGMT expression. Neuro-Oncology. 2012;14(6):712–9.
14. Weller M, Stupp R, Reifenberger G, Brandes AA, van den Bent MJ, Wick W, et al. MGMT promotor methylation in malignant gliomas; ready for personalized medicine? Nat Rev Neurol. 2010;6:39–51.
15. Wick W, Hartmann C, Engel C, Stoffels M, Felsberg J, Stockhammer F, et al. NOA-04 randomized phase III trial of sequential radiochemotherapy of anaplastic glioma with procarbazine, lomustine, and vincristine or temozolomide. J Clin Oncol. 2009;27:5874–80.
16. van den Bent MJ, Dubbink HJ, Sanson M, van der Lee-Haarloo CR, Hegi M, Jeuken JW, et al. MGMT promotor methylation is prognostic but not predictive for outcome to adjuvant PCV chemotherapy in anaplastic oligodendroglial tumours: a report from EORTC Brain Tumour Group Study 26951. J Clin Oncol. 2009;27:5881–6.
17. Bady P, Sciuscio D, Diserens AC, Bloch J, van den Bent MJ, Marosi C, et al. MGMT methylation analysis of glioblastoma on the Infinium methylationBeadChip identifies two distinct CpG regions associated with gene silencing and outcome, yielding a prediction model for comparison across datasets, tumor grades, and CIMP status. Acta Neuropathol. 2012;124:547–60.
18. Wick W, Meisner C, Hentschel B, Platten M, Schilling A, Wiestler B, et al. Prognostic or predictive value of MGMT promotor methylation in gliomas depends on IDH1 mutation. Neurology. 2013;81:1515–22.
19. Tolcher AW, Gerson SL, Denis I, Geyer C, Hammond LA, Patnaik A, et al. Marked inactivation of O6-alkylguanine-DNA alkyltransferase activity with protracted temozolomide schedules. Br J Cancer. 2003;88:1004–11.
20. Wait SD, Prabhu RS, Burri SH, Atkins TG, Asher AL. Polymeric drug delivery for the treatment of glioblastoma. Neuro-Oncology. 2015;7(S2):9–23.
21. Wemmert S, Bettscheider M, Alt S, Ketter R, Kammers K, Feiden W, et al. p15 promoter methylation - a novel prognostic marker in glioblastoma patients. Int J Oncol. 2009;34(6):1743–8.

22. Tada K, Shiraishi S, Kamiryo T, Nakamura H, Hirano H, Kuratsu J, et al. Analysis of loss of heterozygosity on chromosome 10 in patients with malignant astrocytic tumors: correlation with patient age and survival. J Neurosurg. 2001;95(4):651–9.
23. Herman JG, Graff JR, Myohanen S, et al. Methylation-specific PCR: a novel PCR assay for methylation status of CpG islands. Proc Natl Acad Sci U S A. 1996;93: 9821–6.
24. Jung V, Romeike BFM, Henn W, Feiden W, Moringlane JR, Zang KD, Urbschat SM. Heterogeneity of gliomas revealed by microdissection dop-pcr and comparative genomic hybridization. J Neuropathol Exp Neurol. 1999;58:993–9.
25. Cox DR. Regression models and life tables (with discussion). JR Stat Soc B. 1972;34(2):187–220.
26. Mcgirt MJ, Than KD, Weingart JD, et al. Gliadel (BCNU) wafer plus concomitant temozolomide therapy after primary re of glioblastoma multiforme. J Neurosurg. 2009;110(3):583–8.
27. Duntze J, Litré CF, Eap C, et al. Implanted carmustin wafers followed by concomitant radiochemotherapy to treat newly diagnosed malignant gliomas; prospective, observational. Multicentre study on 92 cases. Ann Surg Oncol. 2012;20(6):2065–72.
28. Affronti ML, Heery CR, Herndon JE, et al. Overall survival of newly diagnosed glioblastoma patients receiving carmustine wafers followed by radiation and concurrent temozolomide plus rotational multiagent chemotherapy. Cancer. 2009;115(15):3501–11.
29. Menei P, Metellus P, Parot-Schinkel E, et al. Biodegradable carmustin wafers (Gliadel) alone or in combination with chemoradiotherapy: the French experience. Ann Surg Oncol. 2010;17(7):1740–6.
30. La Rocca RV, Mehdorn HM. Localized BCNU chemotherapy and the multimodal management of malignant glioma. Curr Med Res Opin. 2009;25(1):149–60.
31. Pan E, Mitchell SB, Tsai JS. A retrospective study of the safety of BCNU wafers with concurrent temozolomide and radiotherapy and adjuvant temozolomide for newly diagnosed glioblastoma patients. J Neuroonkol. 2008;88(3):353–7.
32. Pavlov V, Page P, Abi-Lahoud G et al. Combining intraoperative carmustine wafers and Stupp regimen in multimodal first-line treatment of primary glioblastomas. Br J Neurosurgery. 2015. doi: 10.3109/02688697.2015.1012051
33. Bock HC, Puchner MJA, Lohmann F, et al. First-line treatment of malignant glioma with carmustine implants followed by concomitant radiochemotherapy: a multicentre experience. Neurosurg Rev. 2010;33(4):441–9.
34. Noel G, Schott R, Froelich S, et al. Retrospective comparison of chemoradiotherapy followed by adjuvant chemotherapy, with or without prior gliadel implantation (carmustine) after initial surgery in patients with newly diagnosed high-grade gliomas. Int J Radiat Oncol Biol Phys. 2012;82(2):749–55.
35. Miglierini P, Bouchekoua M, Rousseau B, et al. Impact of the per-operatory application of GLIADEL wafers (BCNU, carmustine) in combination with temozolomide and radiotherapy in patients with glioblastoma multiforme: efficacy and toxicity. Clin Neurol Neurosurg. 2012;114(9):1222–5.
36. Karlbom AE, James CD, Boethius J, Cavenee WK, Collins VP, Nordenskjöld M, Larsson C. Loss of heterozygosity in malignant gliomas involves at least three distinct regions on chromosome 10. Human genetics. 1993;92(2):169–74.
37. Kimmelman AC, Ross DA, Liang BC. Loss of heterozygosity of chromosome 10p in human gliomas. Genomics. 1996;34(2):250–4. doi:10.1006/geno.1996.0277.
38. Wemmert S, Ketter R, Rahnenführer J, Beerenwinkel N, Strowitzki M, Feiden W, et al. Patients with high-grade gliomas harboring deletions of chromosomes 9p and 10q benefit from temozolomide treatment. Neoplasia. 2005;7(10):883–93.
39. Jen J, Harper JW, Bigner SH, et al. Deletion of p16 and p15 genes in brain tumors. Cancer Res. 1994;54:6353–8.
40. Schmidt EE, Ichimura K, Reifenberger G, Collins VP. CDKN2 (p16/MTS1) gene deletion or CDK4 amplification occurs in the majority of glioblastomas. Cancer Res. 1994;54:6321–4.
41. Simon M, Köster G, Menon AG, Schramm J. Functional evidence for a role of combined CDKN2A [p16/p14(arf)]/CDKN2B (p15) gene inactivation in malignant gliomas. Acta Neuropathol. 1999;98:444–52.
42. Rasheed A, Herndon JE, Stenzel TT, et al. Molecular markers of prognosis in astrocytic tumors. Cancer. 2002;94:2688–97.
43. Wemmert S, Romeike BF, Ketter R, Steudel WI, Zang KD, Urbschat S. Intratumoral genetic heterogeneity in pilocytic astrocytomas revealed by CGH-analysis of microdissected tumor cells and FISH on tumor tissue sections. Int J Oncol. 2006;28(2):353–60.
44. Gil J, Peters G. Regulation of the INK4b-ARF-INK4a tumour suppressor locus: all for one or one for all. Nat Rev Mol Cell Biol. 2006;7:667–77.
45. Kamiryo T, Tada K, Shiraishi S, et al. Analysis of homo- zygous deletion of the p16 gene and correlation with survival in patients with glioblastoma multiforme. J Neurosurg. 2002;96:815–22.
46. Wong IH, Lo YM, Yeo W, Lau WY, Johnson PJ. Frequent p15 promoter methylation in tumor and peripheral blood from hepatocellular carcinoma patients. Clin Cancer Res. 2000;6(9):3516–21.
47. Shih AH, Holland EC. Platelet-derived growth factor (PDGF) and glial tumorigenesis. Cancer Lett. 2006;232(2):139–47. doi:10.1016/j.canlet.2005.02.002.
48. Varela M, Ranuncolo SM, Morand A, Lastiri J, De Kier J, Elisa B, Puricelli LI, Pallotta MG. EGF-R and PDGF-R, but not bcl-2, overexpression predict overall survival in patients with low-grade astrocytomas. J Surg Oncol. 2004; 86(1):34–40. doi:10.1002/jso.20036.
49. Cui XL, Zhao ZG, Ren XH, Sui DL, Chu JS, Tang K, et al. Characteristics of combining loss of heterozygosity of 1p/19q in glioma. Zhonghua wai ke za zhi [Chinese journal of surgery]. 2010;48(11):852–5.
50. Cairncross JG, Ueki K, Zlatescu MC, Lisle DK, Finkelstein DM, Hammond RR, et al. Specific genetic predictors of chemotherapeutic response and survival in patients with anaplastic oligodendrogliomas. J Natl Cancer Inst. 1998; 90(19):1473–9.

# 10

# Familial intellectual disability as a result of a derivative chromosome 22 originating from a balanced translocation (3;22) in a four generation family

Kaihui Zhang[1†], Yan Huang[2†], Rui Dong[1†], Yali Yang[2], Ying Wang[1], Haiyan Zhang[1], Yufeng Zhang[1], Zhongtao Gai[1*] and Yi Liu[1*]

**Abstract**

**Background:** Balanced reciprocal translocation is usually an exchange of two terminal segments from different chromosomes without phenotypic effect on the carrier while leading to increased risk of generating unbalanced gametes. Here we describe a four-generation family in Shandong province of China with at least three patients sharing severe intellectual disability and developmental delay resulting from a derivative chromosome 22 originating from a balanced translocation (3;22) involving chromosomes 3q28q29 and 22q13.3.

**Methods:** The proband and his relatives were detected by using karyotyping, chromosome microarray analysis, fluorescent in situ hybridization and real-time qPCR.

**Results:** The proband, a 17 month-old boy, presented with severe intellectual disability, developmental delay, specific facial features and special posture of hands. Pedigree analysis showed that there were at least three affected patients. The proband and other two living patients manifested similar phenotypes and were identified to have identically abnormal cytogenetic result with an unbalanced translocation of 9.0 Mb duplication at 3q28q29 and a 1.7Mb microdeletion at 22q13.3 by karyotyping and chromosome microarray analysis. His father and other five relatives had a balanced translocation of 3q and 22q. Fluorescence in situ hybridization and real-time qPCR definitely validated the results.

**Conclusions:** The abnormal phenotypes of the proband and his two living members in four generations of the family confirmed the 3q duplication and 22q13.3 deletion inherited from familial balanced translocation. This is the first report of familial balanced reciprocal translocation involving chromosomes 3q28q29 and 22q13.3 segregating through four generations.

**Keywords:** 3q duplication syndrome, 22q13.3 microdeletion syndrome, Balanced translocation

## Background

Balanced reciprocal translocation, the most common chromosomal rearrangement in humans, is usually an exchange of two terminal segments from different chromosomes without genetic material loss which occur in 0.16%–0.20% (1/625–1/500) of live births [1–3]. Almost all balanced translocation have no phenotypic effect on the carrier but lead to increased risk of generating unbalanced gametes. Of the significant hazards is unfavorable pregnancy outcomes such as recurrent miscarriages, still births, early newborn deaths, or the offspring with birth defects due to the different forms of the unbalanced gametes produced during the meiotic segregation of chromosomes. Meiotic segregation of reciprocal translocation produces gametes with a variety of combinations of normal and translocated chromosomes. The partial chromosome complement of 32 possible zygotes could be

* Correspondence: gaizhongtao@sina.com; y.liu99@yahoo.com
†Equal contributors
[1]Pediatric Research Institute, Qilu Children's Hospital of Shandong University, 23976 Jingshi Road, Jinan, Shandong 250022, China
Full list of author information is available at the end of the article

produced by the union of gametes from a translocation carrier parent and a non-carrier parent [4].

Here, we describe a four-generation Chinese family with six individuals carrying a karyotypically balanced chromosomal translocation t(3;22)(q28;q13) manifesting normal phenotype, while there are three patients with severe intellectual disability and developmental delay carrying 3q28q29 duplication and 22q13.33 deletion. The conventional cytogenetic analysis combined with chromosome microarray identified the submicroscopic imbalances deciphering the etiology of such patients in the family. We reviewed the literature of partial trisomy 3q associated with 3q duplication syndrome [5] and 22q13.3 microdeletion syndrome [6], and discussed the genotype-phenotype correlation related to this case.

## Methods

### Clinical description

The proband, 17 month-old boy, is the first child of a couple of unrelated healthy parents. His mother had one time of active abortion before (see Fig. 1 for the pedigree chart of the family) without obviously inducing factors. The boy's gestation period was normal.

The boy was born at 40 weeks of gestation with weight of 3.2 kg and length of 50 cm. His head circumference was 34 cm and Apgar score was 10. His audition test was normal. The boy showed normal development at birth. From 6 month-old, he gradually displayed developmental retardation. At age of 17 month, his mental and motor development was significantly delayed. He was 12 kg mass and 80 cm tall, the head circumference was 44 cm. He showed facial dysmorphism with protruding forehead, bushy eyebrows, big eyes, hypertelorism, big cup ears, low nasal bridge, downturned corners of the mouth, pointed jaw, and apathia, and special posture of hands including both hands ulnar deviation at the state of relation, middle finger straight while other fingers bending, strong proximal belly-finger, and grasping only with his thumb and middle finger. His development was tested with Gesell Developmental Observation-Revised (GDO-R) demonstrating extremely severe developmental delay for adaptability (score: 22 points), moderate delay for gross motor (score: 41 points) and fine motor (score: 51 points), severe delay for language (score: 38 points) and personal-social interaction (score: 36 points). Now, He could mumbled "mama, baba" in occasional unconsciousness, but neither walked nor followed instructions. He manifested less eye contact with casual eye tracking. Other examinations including magnetic resonance imaging of brain, electroencephalogram (EEG), cardiac and abdominal ultrasound were all normal.

A total of 22 family members in four generations were investigated in the family. Additional two family members (III:3 and III:7) were found to manifest the same phenotypes as the proband. The oldest living patient (III:7) was a 21-year-old male presenting severe intellectual disability, speech disorder, motor retardation, specific facial features and special posture of hands.

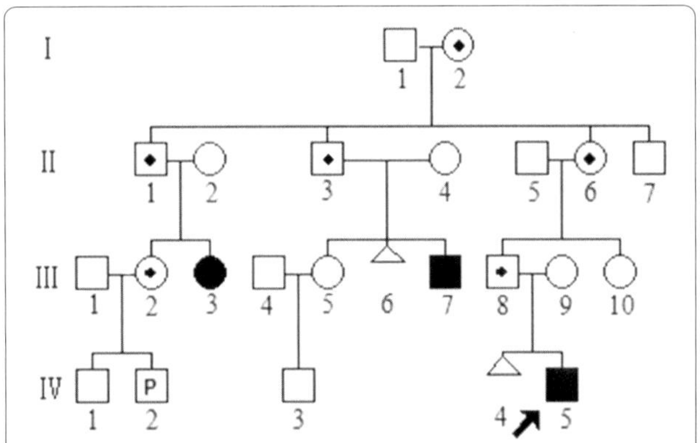


**Fig. 1** The pedigree chart of the family. The pedigree chart of the family. The proband and additional two relatives are affected patients. His father and five members are obligate carriers. His mother is normal. □ healthy male; ○ healthy female; ■/●male/female patient; ⊡/⊙male/female obligate carrier; ↗ proband; / dead; △ abortion; P pregnancy; ⊡ ⊙ not detected

### G-banding karyotyping

Peripheral blood leukocytes from the proband and other family members were stimulated by phytohemagglutinin. Routine cytogenetic analysis by G-banding techniques at the 400 bands of resolution was performed using imaging software for humans according to the International System for Human Cytogenetic Nomenclature (ISCN, 2016).

### Fluorescence in situ hybridization (FISH) analysis

To verify the balanced translocation found in karyotyping and to validate the obligate carriers in the family, subtelomeric FISH studies were performed using Agilent SureFISH probes (Agilent, Beijing, China) for 3p26.2 (SureFISH 3p26.2 CNTN4 RD, Orange Red) and 3q29 (SureFISH, 3q29 WDR53 211 kb, Green), 22q13.33 (SureFISH 22q13.33 SHANK3, Green) and 22CEP (SureFISH 22CEP, Orange Red) according to manufacturer's procedure. Selected subtelomeric probes were used for carriers and healthy family members to identify balanced carriers. The 22CEP probe is not a centromere specific but a locus specific centromere-near probe at 22q11.

### Chromosome microarray analysis (CMA)

Chromosome microarray was performed for the proband using Affymetrix CytoScan HD array (Affymetrix, Santa Clara, CA), and data were analyzed with the software of

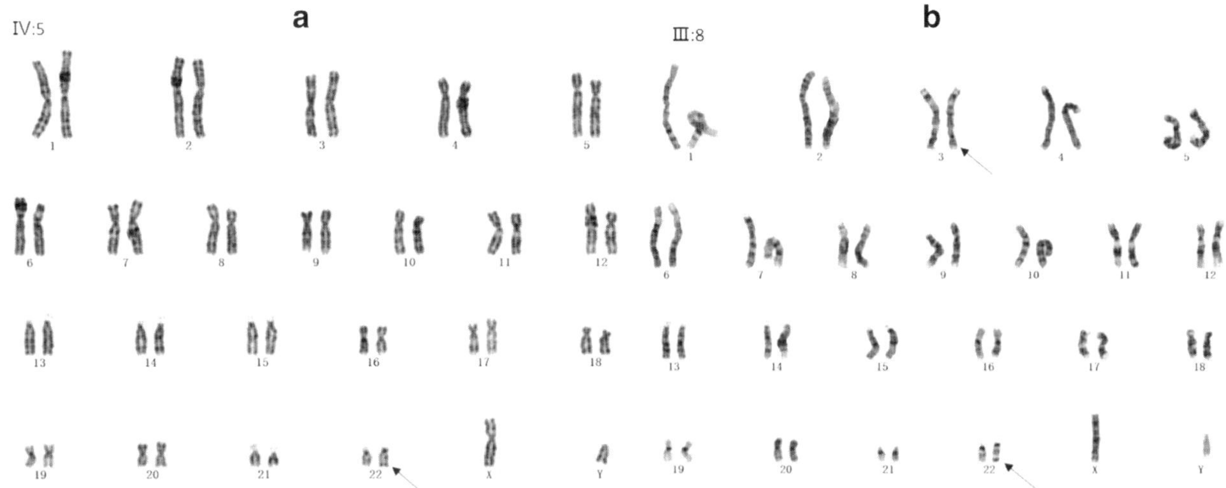


**Fig. 2** Representative G-banding karyotyping results. **a** Representative karyotype of the patient (proband IV:5) showing der(22)t(3;22). **b** Representative karyotype of obligate carriers (the proband's father, III:8) showing t(3;22)(q28;q13)

Chromosome Analysis Suite (ChAS) (Affymetrix, Santa Clara, CA) using the following filtering criteria: deletions > 5 kb (a minimum of five markers) and duplications > 10 kb (a minimum of 10 markers). DNA digestion, ligation, fragmentation, labeling, hybridization, staining and scanning were performed following the Affymetrix's protocol. The Database of Genomic Variants (GRCh37/hg19) and OMIM, DECIPHER, ISCA were used to evaluated the array data and analyze genotype-phenotype correlation.

### Real-time quantitative PCR validation

To verify the chr22q13.3 microdeletions in the patients of the family, a pair of primers were designed to target the deleted gene SHANK3 (chr22:50674415-50733298) using an online primer designing tool-Primer 3 (http://primer3.ut.ee/) and synthesized by Shanghai Invitrogen Biotechnology Company (Shanghai, China). Assays were carried out in accordance with manufacturer recommendations on the 7500 Real-Time PCR system (Applied Biosystems, Foster city, California). The copy number variations were determined based on the ratio of deletion fragment copies to reference gene (GAPDH) copies in samples. Both genomic DNA samples from the normal male and female individuals were used simultaneously as two control samples. Each qPCR was carried out in triplicate with the SYBR Premix Ex Taq II PCR reagent kit (TakaRa Bio, Dalian, China) according to the manufacturer's protocol.

## Results

### Karyotyping

Fifty metaphase cells were examined for the proband and other family members. An apparently abnormal karyotype was identified in proband (IV:5) and two living relatives (III:3 and III:7) as der(22)t(3;22) (q28;q13.3).

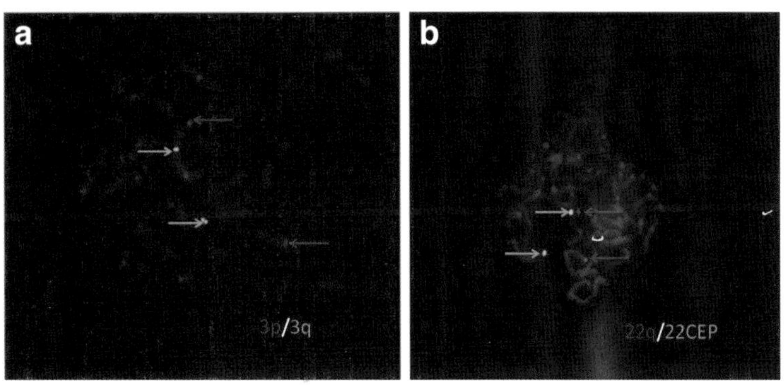


**Fig. 3 a** Representative results from the carrier (proband's father III:8) showing 3q29 signal (Green) separated from 3p26 signal (Red); **b** Representative results from the carrier (proband's father III:8) showing 22q13.3 signal (Red) separated from 22 CEP (a locus specific centromere-near probe) signal

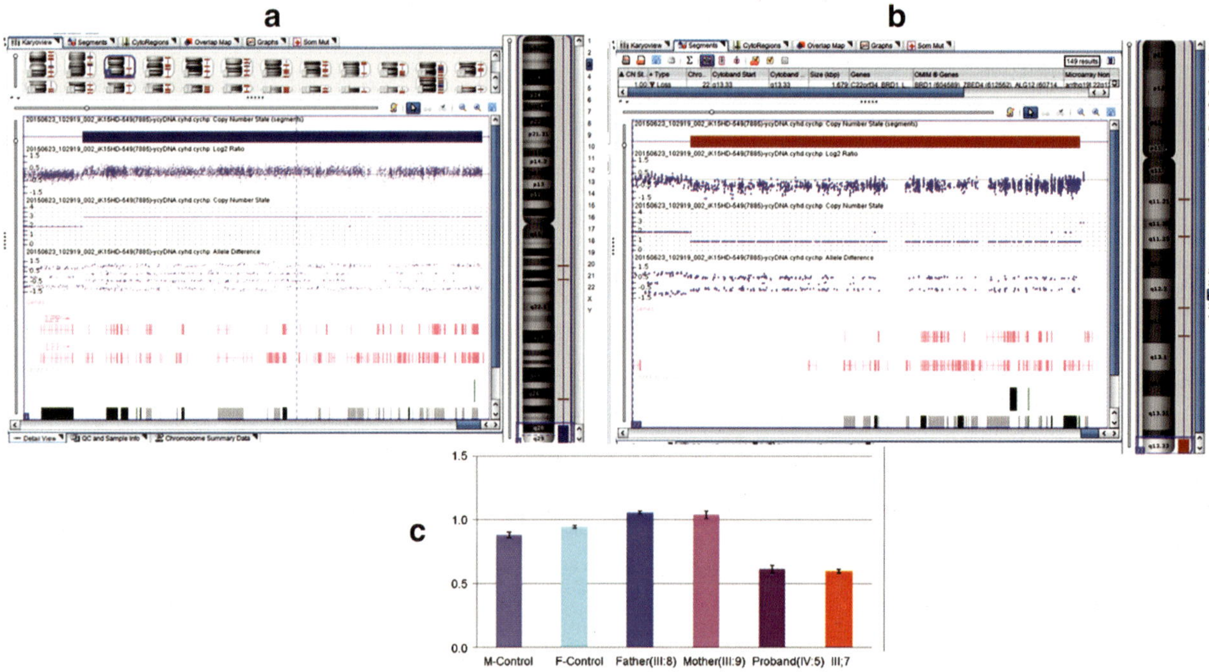


**Fig. 4** CMA and real-time qPCR results. Whole-genome Chromosome microarray analysis for the proband(IV:5) was arr[GRCh37]. 3q28q29(188823885–197,851,986) × 3,22q13.33(49,505,152–51,183,871) × 1 pat. **a** CMA showing a 9.0-Mb duplication at 3q28q29; **b** CMA showing a 1.7-Mb deletion at 22q13.33. **c** Real-time qPCR showing the proband(IV:5) and the living patient (III:7) had the deletion of *SHANK3* gene in 22q13.33, but the proband parents (III:8, III:9) were normal as control

The derivative chromosome in proband (IV:5) was paternally (III:8) inherited, whereas his mother (III:9) showed a normal karyotype. In other family members, the apparently balanced t(3;22) (q28;q13.3) translocation was present in six living persons of I:2, II:1, II:3, II:6, III:2 and III:8. The representative results are shown in Fig. 2a, b.

### FISH

FISH was performed for predicted carriers and healthy members of the family. The results showed that 22q13.33 signal (Red) separated from 22CEP signal and translocated into 3q in proband's father (III:8) and other five members of I:2, II:1, II:3, II:6 and III:2, indicating that the six family members were obligate carriers of balanced translocation of 3q and 22q (Fig. 3a, b). The abnormal unbalanced translocation in proband was inherited from his balanced translocation carrier father.

### CMA

To detect the microdeletion in 22q13.33 and identify exact variation of genes involved in the abnormal chromosome of the patients. CMA was carried out and two abnormal copy number variants were identified as follows: arr[GRCh37] 3q28q29(188823885-197851986)× 3,22q13.33(49,505,152-51,183,871) × 1 pat. It included a 3q terminal duplication (9.0 Mb) and a 22q terminal deletion (1.7 Mb) (Fig. 4a, b). Terminal 3q duplication contains lots of genes, the important OMIM genes like CLDN1 and CLDN16, are partially overlapped with a previously described region related to 3q duplication syndrome. Terminal 22q deletion contains 38 RefSeq genes (having 27 OMIM genes and a critical SHANK3 gene) associated with 22q13.3 microdeletion syndrome (Phelan-McDermid syndrome, PMS, OMIM: 606230).

### Real-time quantitative PCR

Real-time quantitative PCR performed on the family and two control samples (both male and female healthy individuals) showed that the proband and the living patient (III:7) had the deletion of SHANK3 gene in 22q13.33 and the proband's parents were same as controls (Fig. 4c).

## Discussion

Intellectual disability (ID) is a common, variable and heterogeneous manifestation of central nervous system dysfunctions affecting 1–3% of the population [6]. Unfortunately only less than one-half of ID could be identified the specific etiologies [7, 8]. In this study, we described a familial balanced reciprocal translocation involving chromosomes 3q and 22q segregating through four generations in which six family members (I:2, II:1, II:3, II:6, III:2 and III:8) carrying the balanced translocation. The proband was firstly referred to our hospital for his severe physical and mental retardation, and then at least three patients with the same phenotypes were found in his four-generation family by means of the pedigree investigation which highlighted the potential chromosomal abnormalities in the family. By using the G-banding karyotyping analysis, an abnormal long arm of charomosome 22 was found in the proband. To study the etiology of the proband, CMA was applied and showed the derivative chromosome 22 with 9.0 Mb duplication of 3q28q29 and 1.7 Mb microdeletion of the 22q13.33.

It is known that the subtelomeric regions among the gene rich regions of the genome, are particularly prone to recombination and therefore often involved in chromosomal rearrangements, in which subtle rearrangements at the telomere regions may cause unexplained ID [9], and many of these subtelomeric deletions or duplications are now recognized as clinically recognizable phenotypes [9, 10]. According to the literature, the 3q26.3-3q29 duplications being the minimal critical region could cause 3q duplication syndrome [11], and the 22q13.33 microdeletion was associated with 22q13.3 deletion syndrome (Phelan-McDermid syndrome, PMS) [12].

Arıkan et al. [13] summarized the most common abnormal features of 3q duplication syndrome, such as facial dysmorphism (hypertrichosis, prominent eyelashes, bushy eyebrows, broad nose with anteverted nares and depressed nasal bridge hypertelorism, epicanthic folds, long philtrum, micrognathia, low anterior hairline, malformed auricles), limb anomalies (rhizomelic shortening of the limbs, hypoplasia of the phalanges, camptodactyly and clinodactyly), congenital heart defects (septal defects), renal malformations (polycystic kidneys or dysplasia), seizures, brain malformations, and so on. However, partial trisomy 3q cases with duplication of different segments showed significant differences from each other. Approximately 60–75% cases with 3q distal duplication have a concomitant deletion of another chromosomal segment carrying unbalanced translocation, and the deletion of the chromosomal segment could contribute to the phenotype as the present case [14, 15]. Our case has characteristic features of the 3q duplication syndrome such as facial features (protruding forehead, bushy eyebrows, hypertrichosis, low nasal bridge, and malformed auricles), special posture of hands (camptodactyly and clinodactyly) and the severe development delay (mental, motor, and language).

It has been reported that the EPHB3, CLDN1 and CLDN16 located at 3q26.31–q29 were important to 3q duplication syndrome [11]. Our case has a 9.0-Mb duplication of 3q28q29 encompassing CLDN1 and CLDN16. CLDN1 (OMIM 603718) and CLDN16 (OMIM 603959) locating at 3q28 encode Claudin 1 and Claudin 16, respectively, which are epithelial or endothelial cell-to-cell adhesion tight junction proteins. Loss of Claudin 1 function mutations could result in neonatal ichthyosis-sclerosing cholangitis syndrome [16, 17], while the gene mutations in CLDN16 could cause familial hypomagnesemia with hypercalciuria and nephrocalcinosis (FHHNC) which is a rare autosomal recessive renal disease [18]. The detailed mechanism of how haploinsufficiency of CLDN1 and CLDN16 causing disorders remains to be elucidated. It has been known that the fragment duplication of 3q28 encompassing CLDN16 was associated with multiple congenital abnormalities including coarctation of the aorta, atrial septal defect (ASD) and ventrical septal defect (VSD), hypertrichosis and umbilical hernia/omphalocele [19], while our patients presented the phenotype of hypertrichosis in which CLDN16 might play an important role.

In addition, the present case was identified to have a 1.7 Mb 22q subtelomeric deletion associated with 22q13.3 deletion syndrome also known as Phelan-McDermid syndrome (PMS) [20]. PMS is characterized by developmental delay, absent or impaired speech, neonatal hypotonia, autistic traits and mild dysmorphic features. Shank3 encoding by SHANK3 gene (also known as PROSAP2, OMIM: 606230) is a postsynaptic scaffolding protein with the key role in spine shape/maturation, localization of glutamate receptors, and growth cone motility [21]. The mutations of SHANK3 gene have been considered to be responsible for the neurological features of the PMS phenotype [22]. The association between deletion size and phenotypes expanded the genomic region of interest in PMS, in which small deletion size is mainly related to autism spectrum disorders, but large deletion size is prone to severe phenotypes. In the DECIPHER database, all deletions referred to PMS ranging in size from 100 kb to over 9 Mb contain SHANK3, and 75% PMS cases carried the simple terminal deletions while approximately 25% cases were comprised of translocations in the 22q13 region, ring chromosome 22 and mosaics [23, 24]. Our case had a 1.7 Mb deletion including 38 RefSeq genes and his family patients were accompanied by PMS phenotypes: severe developmental delay, hypotonia, speech/language delay, facial dysmorphism. We deduced that the variations of large fragment and genes referring to unbalanced translocation of 3q and 22q contributed to the severe phenotypes.

## Conclusions

In this study, we presented the molecular cytogenetic characterization of 3q28q29 duplication and 22q13.33 microdeletion in a proband with severe intellectual disability and developmental delay. This is the first report of a familial reciprocal translocation t(3,22)(q28;q13.3) segregating through four generations. Three patients carrying an unbalanced condition with der(22)t(3:22) were found, It was reported that a cross-like quadrivalent configuration in gametocytes of reciprocal translocation carriers was usually observed [3, 25]. The meiotic segregation patterns of the quadrivalent are alternate, adjacent-1, adjacent-2 and 3:1. We deduced the unbalanced state in the patients was likely from an adjacent-1 segregation, in which der(22)t(3:22) was rearranged. Perhaps, there is another possibility that the chromosomal pairs 3 and 22 were arranged in bivalents instead of quadrivalents (as usual for a translocation) in meiosis. However, homologous chromosomes for up to 9.0 Mb of 3q Subtelomere failed to pair together during meiosis, which is a great hazard for the long unmatched fragment in meiosis. Meanwhile, most researches showed that the actual proportion of normal and balanced translocation zygotes for the offspring of reciprocal translocation carriers was much higher than the theory of 2:32. Also the interesting fact that up to now only male carriers of the balanced translocation produced an offspring with der (22) in the family. All of the above need to be further validated by the pairing configurations occurred in pachytene substage. We reviewed the literature of 3q duplication syndrome and 22q13.3 microdeletion syndrome, and discussed the genotype–phenotype correlation in this case, suggesting that prevention of recurrent intellectual disability in this family can be achieved through carrier screening and prenatal genetic diagnosis.

#### Abbreviations

ASD: Atrial septal defect; CMA: Chromosome microarray; FHHNC: Familial hypomagnesemia with hypercalciuria and nephrocalcinosis;
FISH: Fluorescence in situ hybridization; ID: Intellectual disability;
PMS: Phelan-McDermid syndrome; VSD: Ventrical septal defect

#### Acknowledgements

The authors are grateful to the patient and his family members for their contribution to the study, and would like to thank Dr.Haiming Yuan (Guangzhou Kingmed Center for Clinical Laboratory Co.) for technical supports of CMA and FISH.

#### Funding

This work was financially supported by Development Project of Science and Technology in Shandong Province (2013GSF11829) and Natural Science Training Foundation of Shandong Province (ZR2014HP051). The funders had no role in the design of the study and collection, analysis, and interpretation of data and in writing the manuscript.

#### Authors' contributions

KZ, YL and ZG participated in the study design. YH and YY made clinical diagnosis. KZ and YZ carried out karyotyping analysis. YW, HZ, RD and YL performed the molecular genetic studies. KZ, YL and ZG contributed reagents, materials and analysis tools. KZ, RD and YL drafted the manuscript. All authors read and approved the final manuscript.

#### Competing interests

The authors declare that they have no competing interests.

#### Author details

[1]Pediatric Research Institute, Qilu Children's Hospital of Shandong University, 23976 Jingshi Road, Jinan, Shandong 250022, China. [2]Rehabilitation Center, Qilu Children's Hospital of Shandong University, 23976 Jingshi Road, Jinan, Shandong 250022, China.

#### References

1. Ferfouri F, Bernicot I, Schneider A, Haquet E, Hédon B, Anahory T. Is the resulting phenotype of an embryo with balanced X-autosome translocation, obtained by means of preimplantation genetic diagnosis, linked to the X inactivation pattern? Fertil Steril. 2016;105(4):1035–46.
2. Jacobs PA, Browne C, Gregson N, Joyce C, White H. Estimates of the frequency of chromosome abnormalities detectable in unselected newborns using moderate levels of banding. J Med Genet. 1992;29:103–8.
3. Gardner RJM, Sutherland GR. Autosomal reciprocal translocations. In: Gardner RJM, Sutherland GR, eds. Chromosome abnormalities and genetic counseling. 2nd ed. New York: Oxford University Press; 1996. p. 59–94.
4. Scriven PN, Handyside AH, Ogilvie CM. Chromosome translocations: segregation modes and strategies for preimplantation genetic diagnosis. Prenat Diagn. 1998;18(13):1437–49.
5. Abreu-González M, García-Delgado C, Cervantes A, Aparicio-Onofre A, Guevara-Yáñez R, Sánchez-Urbina R, et al. Clinical, cytogenetic, and biochemical analyses of a family with a t(3;13)(q26.2;p11.2): further delineation of 3q duplication syndrome. Case Rep Genet. 2013;2013:895259.
6. Battaglia A, Hoyme HE, Dallapiccola B, Zackai E, Hudgins L, McDonald-McGinn D, et al. Further delineation of deletion 1p36 syndrome in 60 patients: a recognizable phenotype and common cause of developmental delay and mental retardation. Pediatrics. 2008;121(2):404–10.
7. Vissers LE, de Vries BB, Veltman JA. Genomic microarrays in mental retardation: from copy number variation to gene, from research to diagnosis. J Med Genet. 2010;47(5):288–97.
8. Mohamed AM, Kamel A, Mahmoud W, Abdelraouf E, Meguid N. Intellectual disability secondary to a 16p13 duplication in a 1;16 translocation. Extended phenotype in a four-generation family. Am J Med Genet A. 2015;167A(1):128–36.
9. Ambrosini A, Paul S, Hu S, Riethman H. Human subtelomeric duplicon structure and organization. Genome Biol. 2007;8(7):R151.
10. Holinski-Feder E, Reyniers E, Uhrig S, Golla A, Wauters J, Kroisel P, et al. Familial mental retardation syndrome ATR-16 due to an inherited cryptic subtelomeric translocation, t(3;16)(q29;p13.3). Am J Hum Genet. 2000;66(1):16–25.
11. Chen CP, Lin CJ, Chen YY, Wang LK, Chern SR, Wu PS, et al. 3q26.31-q29 duplication and 9q34.3 microdeletion associated with omphalocele, ventricular septal defect, abnormal first-trimester maternal serum screening and increased nuchal translucency: prenatal diagnosis and aCGH characterization. Gene. 2013;532(1):80–6.
12. Sarasua SM, Dwivedi A, Boccuto L, Rollins JD, Chen CF, Rogers RC, et al. Association between deletion size and important phenotypes expands the genomic region of interest in Phelan-McDermid syndrome (22q13 deletion syndrome). J Med Genet. 2011;48(11):761–6.
13. Arıkan DC, Coşkun A, Arıkan I, Kıran G, Ceylaner G. Prenatally diagnosed partial trisomy 3q case with an omphalocele and less severe phenotype. J Turk Ger Gynecol Assoc. 2010;11(4):228–32.
14. Meins M, Hagh JK, Gerresheim F, Einhoff E, Olschewski H, Strehl H, et al. Novel case of dup(3q) syndrome due to a de novo interstitial duplication 3q24-q26.31 with minimal overlap to the dup(3q) critical region. Am J Med Genet A. 2005;132A(1):84–9.
15. Aqua MS, Rizzu P, Lindsay EA, Shaffer LG, Zackai EH, Overhauser J, et al. Duplication 3q syndrome: molecular delineation of the critical region. Am J Med Genet. 1995;55(1):33–7.
16. Katoh M, Katoh M. CLDN23 gene, frequently down-regulated in intestinal-type gastric cancer, is a novel member of CLAUDIN gene family. Int J Mol Med. 2003;11(6):683–9.
17. Kirchmeier P, Sayar E, Hotz A, Hausser I, Islek A, Yilmaz A, et al. Novel mutation in the CLDN1 gene in a Turkish family with neonatal ichthyosis sclerosing cholangitis (NISCH) syndrome. Br J Dermatol. 2014;170(4):976–8.
18. Deeb A, Abood SA, Simon J, Dastoor H, Pearce SH, Sayer JA. A novel CLDN16 mutation in a large family with familial hypomagnesaemia with hypercalciuria and nephrocalcinosis. BMC Res Notes. 2013;6:527.

19. Türkmen M, Kasap B, Soylu A, Böber E, Konrad M, Kavukçu S. Paracellin-1 gene mutation with multiple congenital abnormalities. Pediatr Nephrol. 2006;21(11):1776–8.
20. Phelan K, McDermid HE. The 22q13.3 deletion syndrome (Phelan-McDermid syndrome). Mol Syndromol. 2012;2(3–5):186–201.
21. Speed HE, Kouser M, Xuan Z, Reimers JM, Ochoa CF, Gupta N, et al. Autism-associated insertion mutation (InsG) of Shank3 exon 21 causes impaired synaptic transmission and behavioral deficits. J Neurosci. 2015;35(26):9648–65.
22. Sarasua SM, Dwivedi A, Boccuto L, Chen CF, Sharp JL, Rollins JD, et al. 22q13.2q13.32 genomic regions associated with severity of speech delay, developmental delay, and physical features in Phelan-McDermid syndrome. Genet Med. 2014;16(4):318–28.
23. Bonaglia MC, Giorda R, Beri S, De Agostini C, Novara F, Fichera M, et al. Molecular mechanisms generating and stabilizing terminal 22q13 deletions in 44 subjects with Phelan/McDermid syndrome. PLoS Genet. 2011;7(7): e1002173.
24. Costales JL, Kolevzon A. Phelan-McDermid syndrome and SHANK3: implications for treatment. Neurotherapeutics. 2015;12(3):620–30.
25. Kociucka B, Szczerbal I, Bugaj S, Orsztynowicz M, Switonski M. A high incidence of adjacent-1 meiotic segregation pattern, revealed by multicolor sperm FISH, in a carrier boar of a new reciprocal translocation t(6;16)(p13; q23). Cytogenet Genome Res. 2014;142(1):21–7.

# Parental origin of deletions and duplications – about the necessity to check for cryptic inversions

Thomas Liehr[1*], Isolde Schreyer[1,2], Alma Kuechler[3], Emmanouil Manolakos[4], Sylke Singer[5], Andreas Dufke[5], Kathleen Wilhelm[1], Tereza Jančušková[6], Radek Čmejla[6], Moneeb A. K. Othman[1], Ahmed H. Al-Rikabi[1], Kristin Mrasek[1], Monika Ziegler[1], Stefanie Kankel[1], Katharina Kreskowski[1] and Anja Weise[1]

**Abstract**

**Background:** Copy number variants (CNVs) are the genetic bases for microdeletion/ microduplication syndromes (MMSs). Couples with an affected child and desire to have further children are routinely tested for a potential parental origin of a specific CNV either by molecular karyotyping or by two color fluorescence in situ hybridization (FISH), yet. In the latter case a critical region probe (CRP) is combined with a control probe for identification of the chromosome in question. However, CNVs can arise also due to other reasons, like a recombination-event based on a submicroscopic, cryptic inversion in one of the parents.

**Results:** Seventy-four patients with different MMSs and overall 81 CNVs were studied here by a novel three color FISH approach. The way how three locus-specific probes are selected (one is the CRP and two are flanking it in a distance of 5-10 Mb) enables to detect or exclude two possible parental conditions as origins of the CNV seen in the index: (i) direct parental origin of the CNV (deletion or duplication) or (ii) a parental cryptic inversion. Thus, for overall 51/81 CNVs (63%) a parental origin could be determined. 36/51 (70.5%) inherited the CNV directly from one of the parents, but 15/51 (29.5%) were due to an exclusively by three color FISH detectable parental inversion. A 2:1 ratio of maternal versus paternal inheritance was found. Also almost two times more male than female were among the index patients.

**Conclusion:** The new, here suggested three color FISH approach is suited for more comprehensive parental studies of patients with MMS. The detection rate for parental origin was increased by 140% in this study. Still, for 30/81 cases (37%) no reason for the 'de novo' MMS in the affected index patient could be found by the here suggested FISH-probe set.

**Keywords:** Copy number variants (CNVs), Microdeletion/microduplication syndromes (MMSs), Three color fluorescence in situ hybridization (FISH), Inversion, Deletion, Duplication

## Background

Copy number variants (CNVs) are a topic of highest interest in research and diagnostics [1]. Gain or loss of submicroscopic regions can either lead to clinical signs and symptoms [1, 2], suspected to be associated with diseases [1–3] or, according to present knowledge, just be variations without any significant meaning for the individual carrier [1, 4].

However, the way how CNVs change their size if they are passed from one generation to the next, i.e. how specific DNA-regions are lost or amplified within a CNV, is not completely understood, yet. Unequal crossing over events in low copy repeat regions [1, 5, 6], or complicated repair mechanisms after DNA-break and/or replication stress, like non allelic homologous recombination (NAHR), microhomology-mediated break-induced replication (MMBIR), or even chromothripsis are discussed [1, 6–8]. Another idea for CNV-formation related to MMBIR is based on the fact that regions involved in microdeletion/microduplication syndromes (MMSs) [2] can be

* Correspondence: Thomas.Liehr@med.uni-jena.de
[1]Jena University Hospital, Institute of Human Genetics, Friedrich Schiller University, Postfach D-07740, Jena, Germany
Full list of author information is available at the end of the article

flanked by repetitive elements being identical to each other, as first described by Jim Lupskis group for a ~ 1.4 Mb region in 17p12 including the *PMP22* gene [9]. Such a genetic environment may cause unequal crossing over during meiosis (or even mitosis [10, 11]), and thus deletion or duplication; i.e. a de novo CNV may arise in gametes or somatic cells. Recently, evidence was provided that at least in a subset of MMSs their corresponding critical regions (CRs) are flanked by DNA-stretches with sequence identity of 10-200 kb in size [12]. Besides, it has been shown that these CRs can be 'inverted' in one of the parents of a patient (e.g. [13, 14]), making a deletion or duplication more likely due to inversion loop formation [15]. Surprisingly, fathers or mothers of an MMS-patient may also be carrier of the identical deletion or duplication as the index patient, but without showing any, or only minimal symptoms of the corresponding syndrome [2]. This has been explained by the so-called two-hit model, suggesting a second large CNV only present in the patient and not in the parent [12, 16], or by a disease causing mutation in the not-deleted, corresponding relevant gene copy [17].

Here we analyzed parents of 74 index patients with different MMSs. A novel molecular cytogenetic approach was applied to detect or exclude two possible parental conditions as origins of the disease, as seen in the index: (i) direct parental origin of the CNV (deletion or duplication) or (ii) a parental cryptic inversion. Therefore we applied one locus-specific probe directly from the affected region (critical region probe = CRP) and flanked it with two probes, located between 5 and 10 Mb proximal and distal to the CRP. The analysis was done using a three color-fluorescence in situ hybridization (FISH) approach (Fig. 1). As 74 families and 81 CNVs were studied overall (Table 1 and Additional file 1: Table S1), a first approximation could be achieved on the frequencies of parental origin versus 'de novo' formation of an MMS. However, cases considered as formed 'de novo' still may be due to NAHRs or inversions, which are too small to be detected by the here suggested FISH-probe set, like listed [4] and discussed elsewhere [18, 19].

## Methods

### Samples

Parents of 74 index patients as summarized in Table 1 and Additional file 1: Table S1 were studied. All index patients suffered from developmental delay and or/dysmorphic features, and each of them had one up to two microdeletions and/or microduplications (Table 1 and Additional file 1: Table S1), as characterized by molecular karyotyping and/or standard GTG-banding

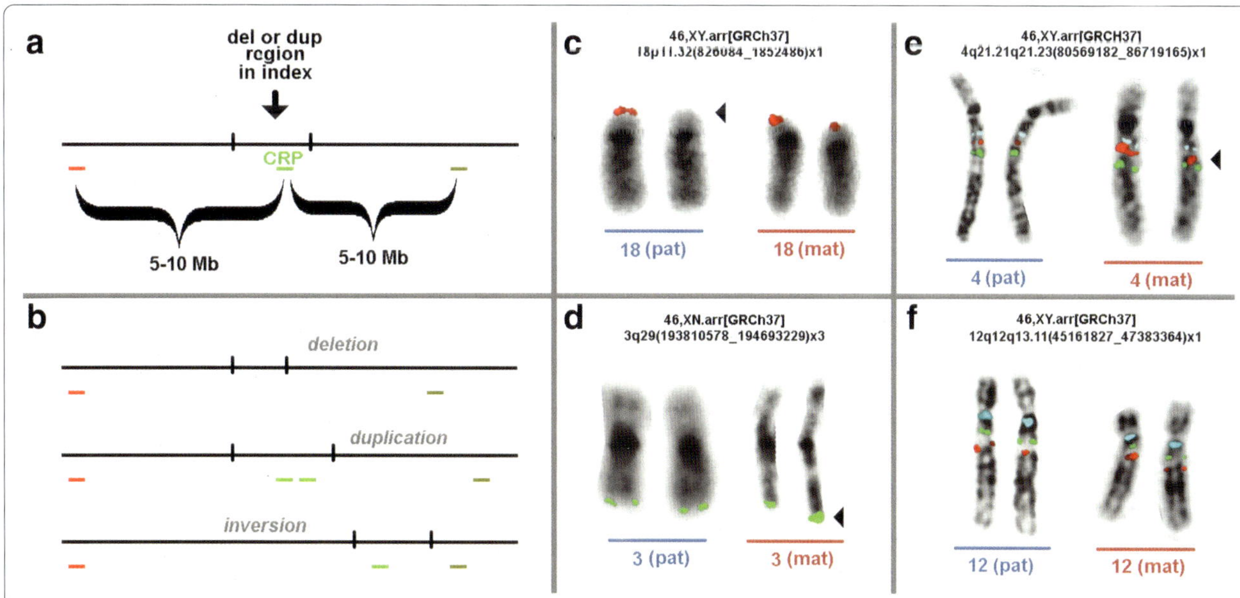


**Fig. 1 a** Scheme of the probe design to detect deletions, duplications or inversions in the parents of an index patient with submicroscopic deletions or duplications. Abbreviations: CRP = critical region probe; Mb = megabasepair. **b** Schematic depiction of expected results. **c-f** Examples of parents of the index patients cases 18, 23, 32 and 54. The corresponding array-CGH results of the index patients are given in the figures; for the applied locus-specific probes see Additional file 1: Table S1. In Figs. **c** and **d** only the probe for the critical regions are depicted. Aberrant chromosomes are highlighted by arrowheads. **c** Case 18 had paternally derived deletion, as clearly visible. **d** Case 23 had a maternally derived duplication; the size of the duplication is too small to lead to two separated signals on the derivative chromosome 3, however, the signal-size and –intensity is clearly doubled compared to signal on the homologous. **e** A cryptic maternal inversion is depicted for case 32, as visible by the shift of the signal of the critical region probe. **f** No alterations could be detected in the parents of case 54; thus a 'de novo' formation of the copy number variant (CNV) in the index patient is suggested; as outlined in the text 'de novo' stands here for real de novo cases and such which may be based other (smaller) cryptic rearrangements not detectable by the here applied probe set

**Table 1** Seventy-four families with affected children having deletion or duplication in one or two chromosomal regions included in this study are listed here. Overall 81 copy number variations (CNVs) distributed on all human chromosomes apart from #11 and Y-chromosome were studied. Cases with two CNVs were numbered as A and B, i.e. cases 11, 13, 14, 17, 19 and 46. For the index patient the chromosomal region affected, the mode of inheritance of the CNV (origin) and the gender are given here; for more details see Additional file 1: Table S1

| Case number | Chromosomal region affected | Origin | Gender carrier | Case number | Chromosomal region affected | Origin | Gender carrier |
|---|---|---|---|---|---|---|---|
| 1 | 2q21.1q21.3 | del(mat/pat)cons. | n.a. | 37 | 7p12.3p14.1 | inv(mat) | m |
| 2 | 12q15q21.2 | del(mat) | f | 38 | 4q13.3q22.1 | inv(mat) | f |
| 3 | 15q11.2 | del(mat) | f | 39 | 16p11.2 | inv(mat) | f |
| 4 | 6q14.3q15 | del(mat) | f | 40 | 17q21.31q21.31 | inv(mat)mos | n.a. |
| 5 | 6q22.33 | del(mat) | m | 41 | 2q23.1q23.2 | inv(mat)mos | m |
| 6 | Xp22.33 | del(mat) | m | 42 | 7q32.3q33 | inv(pat) | n.a. |
| 7 | 12p12.3p12.3 | del(mat) | m | 43 | 7q31.32q32.2 | inv(pat) | m |
| 8a | 4q13.2q21.21 | del(mat) | m | 44 | 6q21q22.31 | inv(pat) | m |
| 9 | 16p11.2 | del(mat) | m | 45 | 15q26.1q26.3 | inv(pat) | m |
| 10 | 2p16.3 | del(mat) | f | 46a | 2p14 | inv(pat) | m |
| 11a | 16p13.11 | del(mat) | n.a. | 47 | 15q13.2-q13.3 | de novo | n.a. |
| 11b | 16p13.11 | del(mat) | n.a. | 48 | 8q24.3q24.3 | de novo | n.a. |
| 12 | 1q43q44 | del(mat) | n.a. | 49 | 19p13.2p13.3 | de novo | m |
| 13a | 16p12.2 | del(mat) | m | 50 | 1p32.1p31.1 | de novo | f |
| 14a | 14q12 | del(mat)mos | n.a. | 51 | 7q31.1q31.1 | de novo | f |
| 14b | 15q11.2 | del(mat)mos | n.a. | 52 | 14q12 | de novo | n.a. |
| 15 | 7q11.23q21.11 | del(pat) | f | 53 | 16p11.2 | de novo | n.a. |
| 16 | 1q21.1 | del(pat) | m | 19b | 15q11.2q13.1 | de novo | f |
| 17a | 16p13.11 | del(pat) | n.a. | 54 | 12q12q13.11 | de novo | m |
| 17b | 16p11.2 | del(pat) | n.a. | 55 | 13q22.2q31.1 | de novo | f |
| 18 | 18p11.32 | del(pat) | m | 56 | 10q22.3q23.2 | de novo | n.a. |
| 19a | 2q13 | del(pat)mos | f | 57 | 7p15.3p15.2 | de novo | m |
| 20 | 7q22.1 | del(pat)mos | m | 58 | 6q13q15 | de novo | n.a. |
| 21 | 15q11.2 | dup(mat) | n.a. | 59 | 4q21.22q22.1 | de novo | f |
| 22 | 5q11.1q11.2 | dup(mat) | n.a. | 60 | 4q35.2 | de novo | n.a. |
| 8b | 22q12.3q13.2 | dup(mat) | m | 61 | 3q26.3q27.3 | de novo | n.a. |
| 23 | 3q29 | dup(mat) | n.a. | 62 | 6q21q22.33 | de novo | m |
| 24 | 3q29 | dup(mat) | n.a. | 63 | 3p14.1p12.3 | de novo | n.a. |
| 25 | 19p13.3p13.3 | dup(mat) | m | 64 | 12q15q21.1 | de novo | f |
| 26 | 22q11.21 | dup(mat)mos | m | 65 | 16q24.1q24.2 | de novo | n.a. |
| 27 | 7q34q36.3 | dup(mat)mos | n.a. | 66 | 7p15.3 | de novo | n.a. |
| 28 | 4q13.1 | dup(pat) | n.a. | 67 | 9q22.31q22.33 | de novo | n.a. |
| 29 | 7q31.31q31.33 | dup(pat) | f | 68 | 16q24.1q24.3 | de novo | n.a. |
| 30 | 4q25 | dup(pat) | n.a. | 69 | 2q31.1 | de novo | n.a. |
| 31 | 13q12.13 | dup(pat) | n.a. | 70 | 21q22.12q22.2 | de novo | n.a. |
| 13b | 8p23.1p22 | dup(pat) | m | 71 | 5q35.2q35.3 | de novo | n.a. |
| 32 | 4q21.21q21.23 | inv(mat) | m | 72 | 4q21.1q21.21 | de novo | n.a. |
| 33 | 20p12.3 | inv(mat) | n.a. | 73 | 10q11.22q11.23 | de novo | n.a. |
| 34 | 1p36.13p16.11 | inv(mat) | n.a. | 46b | 2q31.2q31.3 | de novo | m |
| 35 | 17q12 | inv(mat) | m | 74 | 7q32.3q33 | de novo | n.a. |
| 36 | 17q21.31q21.31 | inv(mat) | m | | | | |

*cons* consanguineous, *del* deletion, *dup* duplication, *inv.* inversion, *mat* maternal, *mos* mosaic, *pat* paternal

elsewhere. Parents were clinically and cytogenetically normal. Chromosomes were prepared from cultured peripheral T-lymphocytes according to standard procedures [20]. Slides for metaphases FISH (see below) were produced following the air-drying protocol [21].

### Molecular cytogenetics

FISH was done according to standard procedures in a three color-FISH variant [22]. To straightforwardly identify the chromosomes of interest a corresponding whole chromosome painting or centromeric probe may be added in a fourth color. The principle scheme how the three color-FISH probe sets were constructed is shown in Fig. 1a. The expected results in case of deletion, duplication and inversion are depicted in Fig. 1b. Bacterial artificial chromosome (BAC) probes serving as CRP should not include regions of known CNVs, like e.g. used in studies detecting parental origin of chromosomes by FISH [23].

The probes as applied for each case are listed in Additional file 1: Table S1. Locus-specific BAC-probes were commercially available from BACPAC Resources Program (bacpac.chori.org) or available to the authors (via Synlab, Czech Republic). Probe labelling was done as previously reported [24]. Ten to Twenty metaphases were analyzed per case. Typical examples for FISH results are depicted in Fig. 1b-f.

## Results

In this study the parental origin of 81 CNVs in 74 index patients was determined by a new three-color FISH approach (Fig. 1a and b). Therefore, one locus-specific probe mapped to the in the index patient affected region (critical region probe = CRP) was flanked by two probes, located between 5 and 10 Mb proximal and distal to the CRP. It could be convincingly shown that such kind of probe set enables simultaneous detection of deletions (Fig. 1c) or duplications (Fig. 1d), as well as cryptic, and in GTG-banding submicroscopic, parental inversions (Fig. 1e); the latter are visible as altered distances of the three probes to each other in the affected chromosome. Overall, the parental origin of potentially disease causing CNVs could be determined in 51 of 81 of the studied cases (63% - see Fig. 2). Also, there remained 37% of non-informative, here denominated as 'de novo' cases (Figs. 1f and 2).

Among the parentally derived cases there was one (case 1) with partial nullisomy 2q21.1 to 2q21.3 in the index patient. This was most likely due to consanguinity of the parents and heterozygosity of both for this CNV. The remainder 50 CNVs could be clearly attributed to be of maternal (33/50 cases = 66%) or paternal inheritance (17/50 cases = 34% - see Fig. 2). The obtained data is broken down more specifically in Fig. 3 for parental

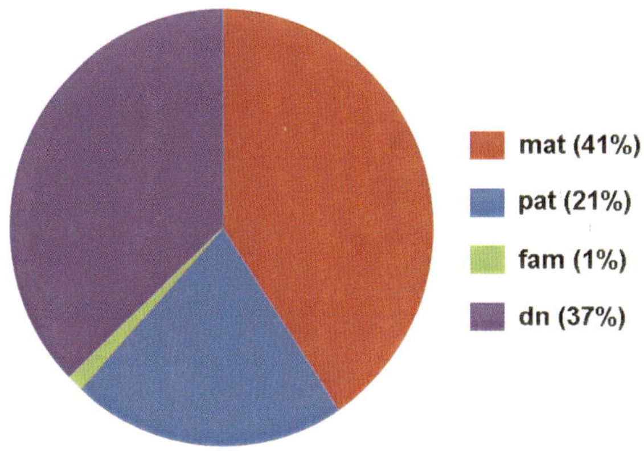


**Fig. 2** Parental origin of the 81 here studied copy number variants (CNVs). Abbreviations: dn = de novo; fam = familial; mat = maternal; pat = paternal

deletions, duplications or inversions. As shown in Table 1, four cases with deletion, and two cases each with duplication and inversion were mosaic in the transmitting parent.

The gender of the index patient was only available in 32 of the 74 cases. Thus, it could be evaluated for 43 CNVs studied here. Interestingly, overall the male to female ratio of the index was 28 to 15; considering only 'de novo' cases the ratio was 1:1, and in inherited cases the ratio was 1.8 to 1 (Fig. 4).

An analysis for the chromosomal origin of the CNVs (Fig. 5) revealed that they derived from practically all chromosomes. 15/81 CNVs were due to parental inversions (18.5%) and those were detected on 6/24 chromosomes (25%). However, 3/11 CNVs studied for chromosome 7, and 3/3 CNVs studied for chromosome 17 were due to parental inversions. Finally, CNVs resulting from detectable parental inversions were between 545,601 bp (case 39) and 17,223,229 bp (case 38) in size. As the corresponding inversions may provide just only one of their breakpoints to the resulting CNV, the underlying inversions may have been larger or smaller.

## Discussion

CNVs may arise by different mechanisms as outlined above [1]. To provide information for affected families about the repetition risk in a following pregnancy, yet the only routinely offered studies for a possible parental origin of a CNV are either molecular karyotyping [25] or two-color-FISH using one CRP and one control probe; the latter is applied to identify the chromosome of interest [10]. Thus, yet only parentally derived deletions or duplications may be detected, but no structural changes. Even though single studies showed that it is necessary in MMS like Angelman/Prader-Willi [13] Williams-Beuren [14] and Sprintzen velocardiofacial syndrome [26] also to check for potentially, in the offspring disease causing

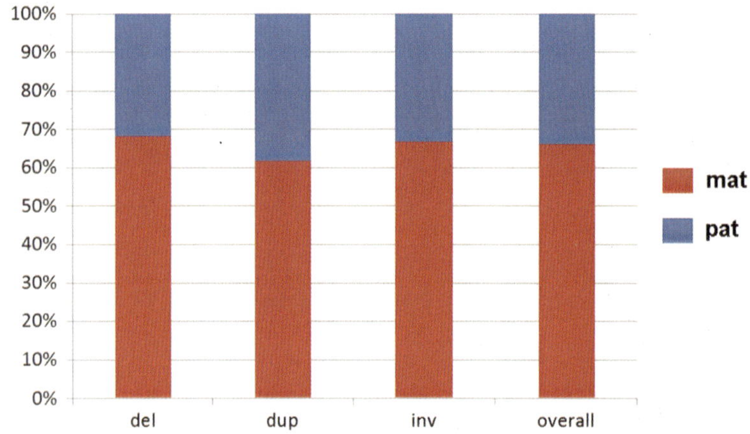


**Fig. 3** Parental derived CNVs of cases 2 to 46a were analyzed here for their maternal and paternal origin; 62 to 68% of the cases were maternally derived. Interestingly, in 8 cases mosaics of normal cells and cells with either maternal or paternal deletion, maternal duplication or maternal inversion were detected in the peripheral blood the tested parents (see Additional file 1: Table S1). Abbreviations: del = deletion; dup = duplication; inv. = inversion; mat = maternal; pat = paternal

inversions, no systematic studies in other MMSs were undertaken, yet. This gap was closed by the present study using a simple three-color-FISH probe set, as suggested here in Fig. 1a, which may be applied in each individual MMS case, as long as a CRP and flanking probes are available.

Thus, the detection rate of a proven parental origin for an MMS can be drastically enhanced. Traditionally, only using FISH with a CRP and a control probe or molecular karyotyping, parental origin of the deletion or duplication would have been solved in the present cohort for only 36/81 CNVs (44%). With the new, here presented approach 15 additional CNVs could be attributed to a parental origin (i.e. an inversion) raising the detection rate up to 63%. The remainder 30 cases, denominated here as 'de novo', could not be resolved with this probe set. They still may be due to NAHR, i.e. processes during gametogenesis like observed in Charcot-Marie-Tooth disease type 1A (CMT1A) [9, 10], or also be based on smaller inversions not detectable by this kind of metaphase-FISH directed probe set, but rather by interphase-FISH [14]. Interestingly, for all three groups (deletion, duplication and inversion) examples were found, which were present only in mosaic state in the transmitting parent. This suggests most likely a postzygotic origin of the rearrangement in the parent; still, also reversion could be considered. Cases like that are already reported e.g. for CMT1A and have been shown to go together with a less severe symptomatic [10], which goes together well with the fact that all parents in this study were considered as asymptomatic. Furthermore, mosaic conditions are known to be variable in

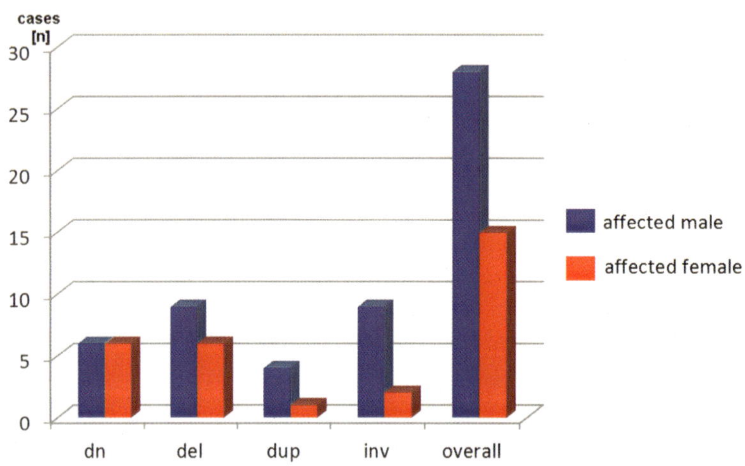


**Fig. 4** In 43 cases the gender of the affected index patient was available. Interestingly, overall more male than female were affected, if the CNV was inherited from one of the parents. Abbreviations: dn = de novo; del = deletion; dup = duplication; inv. = inversion

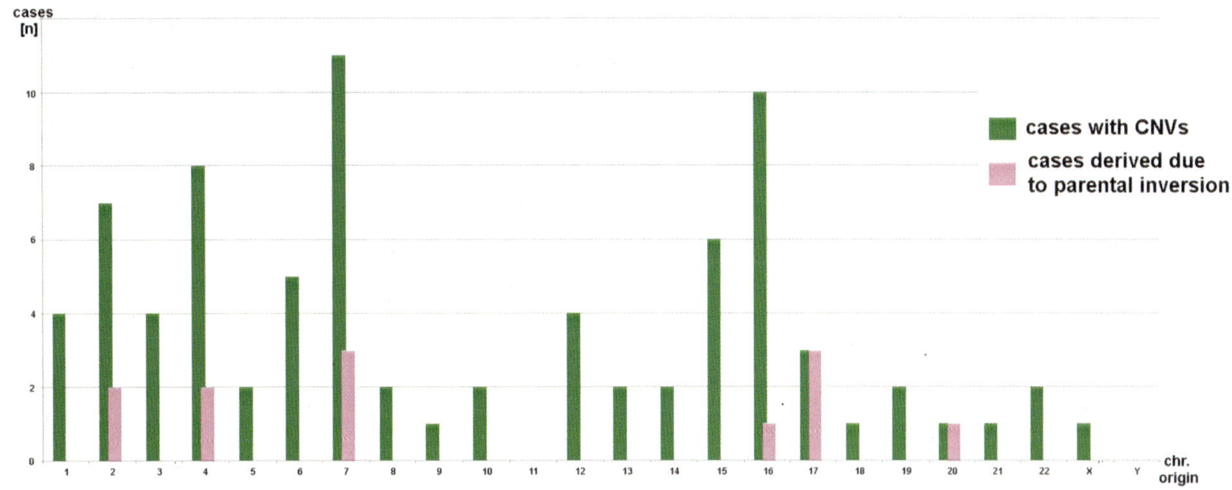


**Fig. 5** The 81 here studied copy number variants (CNVs) sotted according to their chromosomal origin; cases which are due to a parental submicroscopic inversion are highlighted in pink. Abbreviations: CNVs = copy number variants

different tissues of the body [27]; thus, for all parental tests presently available it has always to be considered that gonadal mosaicism can never be excluded [28, 29].

The observed partial nullisomy 2q21.1 to 2q21.3 in the index patient of case 1, which is most likely due to consanguinity and partial monosomy in both of the parents, also reminds of the possibility that in rare cases a uniparental disomy (UPD) may lead to an MMS with nullisomy or partial tetrasomy [30, 31]. For case 1 a UPD(2) was not excluded, as a biparental origin is here much more likely.

Interestingly, the parental origin of the CNVs showed the same 2:1 (maternal: paternal) ratio (Fig. 3) as e.g. known for the inheritance of small supernumerary marker chromosomes [32]. This normally is explained by higher tolerance of the female gamete producing system towards mistakes in the oocytes, than the testes have towards genetically defective sperm [32–34]. However, the gender ratio of the offspring of cases with parental origin of the CNV of 1:1.8 (female: male) (Fig. 4) is not as easy to explain. Besides a possible bias due to small numbers, it may reflect the fact that CNVs in female are better compensated than in male. Such effects are e.g. observed for patients with 'large CNVs', like in trisomy 13 or 18 [35]. Lion hypotheses and the female mosaic condition of the X-chromosome-inactivation of paternal and maternal copy are discussed to be involved here [36].

Finally, it is known that CNVs seem to be present more or less equally distributed over all human chromosomes [4]; for sure, when looking closer there are hot spots for them, as also reflected by different recombination rates of DNA-stretches with and without CNVs [15]. The chromosomal origin of the CNVs in this study provides no surprise here (Fig. 5). If the relative high rates of CNVs due to inversions in chromosomes 7 and 17 are meaningful or not, has to be ruled out by future studies. Interestingly for chromosome 17 an inversion polymorphism was reported recently [37].

## Conclusions

Overall, the here suggested new three-color-FISH approach is straightforward and can be universally applied for more comprehensive parental studies of patients with MMS. The detection rate can be increased by 140% as now also inversions and not only parental deletions and duplications can be detected, which might provide implications for genetic counselling, risk calculation for close relatives, as well as an option for prenatal testing. Still the here applied BAC-probesets are only suited for metaphase-FISH; for interphase-FISH distances of 2-5 Mb between CRP and flanking probes would be indicated [14], and BAC-probes not leading to background and cross-hybridization problems. Nonetheless, the here presented FISH probe set would also be able to detect the elsewhere reported but rare parental insertional balanced translocations as reason of CNV in the offspring [38].

### Abbreviations

BAC: Bacterial artificial chromosome; CMT1A: Charcot-Marie-Tooth disease type 1A; CNVs: Copy number variants; CR: Critical region; CRP: Critical region probe; FISH: Fluorescence in situ hybridization; GTG: G-bands by trypsin using Giemsa; MMBIR: Microhomology-mediated break-induced replication;

MMSs: Microdeletion/microduplication syndromes; NAHR: Nonallelic homologous recombination; UPD: Uniparental disomy

**Acknowledgements**
We thank for providing cases for this study the following colleagues: Dr. Bartels (Göttingen, Germany), PD Dr. Beger (Bielefeld, Germany), Dr. Coci (Braunschweig and Bochum, Germany), Dr. Belitz (Berlin, Germany), Dr. Dahlum (Ulm, Germany), Dr. Ebner (Regensburg, Germany), Dr. Hehr (Regensburg, Germany), Dr. Huhle (Zwickau, Germany), Dr. Louis (Mannheim, Germany) Dr. Ovens-Räder (Munich, Germany), Dr. Pauli (Göttingen, Germany), Dr. Shoukier (Munich, Germany), Dr. Schulze (Hannover, Germany), Prof. Steinberger (Frankfurt am Main, Germany).

**Funding**
Supported in parts by the VDI/VDE-IT (16KN054624).

**Authors' contributions**
TL designed the study and drafted the manuscript, supervised the experiments. IS, AK, SS, AD, KW, AW and KM provided the clinical cases and data; AW, TJ and RC provided locus specific BAC probes for this study. MZ, SK and KK did the FISH-tests. MAKO and AHA-R did the probe amplification and labelling. All authors edited and approved the manuscript.

**Competing interests**
The authors declare that they have no competing interests.

**Author details**
[1]Jena University Hospital, Institute of Human Genetics, Friedrich Schiller University, Postfach D-07740, Jena, Germany. [2]Center for Ambulant Medicine, Jena University Hospital, Jena, Germany. [3]Institut für Humangenetik, Universitätsklinikum Essen, Essen, Germany. [4]Access to Genome, ATG Labs, Athens, Greece. [5]Institut für Medizinische Genetik und angewandte Genomik, Tübingen, Germany. [6]Synlab czech s.r.o., synlab genetics s.r.o, Praha, Czech Republic.

**References**

1. Liehr T. Benign & pathological chromosomal imbalances, 1st edition microscopic and submicroscopic copy number variations (CNVs) in genetics and counseling. New York: Academic Press; 2014.
2. Weise A, Mrasek K, Klein E, Mulatinho M, Llerena JC Jr, Hardekopf D, et al. Microdeletion and microduplication syndromes. J Histochem Cytochem. 2012;60:346–58.
3. Priest JR, Girirajan S, Vu TH, Olson A, Eichler EE, Portman MA. Rare copy number variants in isolated sporadic and syndromic atrioventricular septal defects. Am J Med Genet A. 2012;158A:1279–84.
4. Database of genomic variants. http://dgv.tcag.ca/dgv/app/home. Assessed 18 Dec 2017.
5. Girirajan S, Dennis MY, Baker C, Malig M, Coe BP, Campbell CD, et al. Refinement and discovery of new hotspots of copy-number variation associated with autism spectrum disorder. Am J Hum Genet. 2013;92:221–37.
6. Levinson G, Gutman GA. Slipped-strand mispairing: a major mechanism for DNA sequence evolution. Mol Biol Evol. 1987;4:203–21.
7. Liu P, Carvalho CM, Hastings PJ, Lupski JR. Mechanisms for recurrent and complex human genomic rearrangements. Curr Opin Genet Dev. 2012;22:211–20.
8. Arlt MF, Wilson TE, Glover TW. Replication stress and mechanisms of CNV formation. Curr Opin Genet Dev. 2012;22:204 10.
9. Murakami T, Garcia CA, Reiter LT, Lupski JR. Charcot-Marie-Tooth disease and related inherited neuropathies. Medicine (Baltimore). 1996;75:233–50.
10. Liehr T, Rautenstrauss B, Grehl H, Bathke KD, Ekici A, Rauch A, et al. Mosaicism for the Charcot-Marie-Tooth disease type 1A duplication suggests somatic reversion. Hum Genet. 1996;98:22–8.
11. Mkrtchyan H, Gross M, Hinreiner S, Polytiko A, Manvelyan M, Mrasek K, Kosyakova N, Ewers E, Nelle H, Liehr T, Bhatt S, Thoma K, Gebhart E, Wilhelm S, Fahsold R, Volleth M, Weise A. The human genome puzzle - the role of copy number variation in somatic mosaicism. Curr Genomics. 2010 Sep; 11(6):426–31.
12. Girirajan S, Rosenfeld JA, Cooper GM, Antonacci F, Siswara P, Itsara A, et al. A recurrent 16p12.1 microdeletion supports a two-hit model for severe developmental delay. Nat Genet. 2010;42:203–9.
13. Gimelli G, Pujana MA, Patricelli MG, Russo S, Giardino D, Larizza L, et al. Genomic inversions of human chromosome 15q11-q13 in mothers of Angelman syndrome patients with class II (BP2/3) deletions. Hum Mol Genet. 2003;12:849–58.
14. Morris CA, Mervis CB, Osborne LR. Frequency of the 7q11.23 inversion polymorphism in transmitting parents of children with Williams syndrome and in the general population does not differ between North America and Europe. Mol Cytogenet. 2011;4:7.
15. Bhatt SS, Manvelyan M, Moradkhani K, Hunstig F, Mrasek K, Puechberty J, et al. Inverted segment size and the presence of recombination hot spot clusters matter in sperm segregation analysis. Cytogenet Genome Res. 2014; 142:145–9.
16. Jensen M, Kooy RF, Simon TJ, Reyniers E, Girirajan S, Tassone F. A higher rare CNV burden in the genetic background potentially contributes to intellectual disability phenotypes in 22q11.2 deletion syndrome. Eur J Med Genet. https://doi.org/10.1016/j.ejmg.2017.11.016.
17. Tan L, Bi B, Zhao P, Cai X, Wan C, Shao J, et al. Severe congenital microcephaly with 16p13.11 microdeletion combined with NDE1 mutation, a case report and literature review. BMC Med Genet. 2017;18:141.
18. Aguado C, Gayà-Vidal M, Villatoro S, Oliva M, Izquierdo D, Giner-Delgado C, Montalvo V, García-González J, Martínez-Fundichely A, Capilla L, Ruiz-Herrera A, Estivill X, Puig M, Cáceres M. Validation and genotyping of multiple human polymorphic inversions mediated by inverted repeats reveals a high degree of recurrence. PLoS Genet. 2014;10(3):e1004208.
19. Vicente-Salvador D, Puig M, Gayà-Vidal M, Pacheco S, Giner-Delgado C, Noguera I, Izquierdo D, Martínez-Fundichely A, Ruiz-Herrera A, Estivill X, Aguado C, Lucas-Lledó JI, Cáceres M. Detailed analysis of inversions predicted between two human genomes: errors, real polymorphisms, and their origin and population distribution. Hum Mol Genet. 2017;26(3):567–81.
20. Claussen U, Michel S, Mühlig P, Westermann M, Grummt UW, Kromeyer-Hauschild K, et al. Demystifying chromosome preparation and the implications for the concept of chromosome condensation during mitosis. Cytogenet Genome Res. 2002;98:136–46.
21. Weise A, Liehr T. Pre- and postnatal diagnostics and research on peripheral blood, bone marrow chorion, amniocytes, and fibroblasts. In: Liehr T, editor. Fluorescence in situ hybridization (FISH) – application guide. 2nd ed. Berlin: Springer; 2017. p. 171–80.
22. Liehr T. Two- to three-color FISH. In: Liehr T, editor. Fluorescence in situ hybridization (FISH) – application guide. 2nd ed. Berlin: Springer; 2017. p. 227–32.
23. Weise A, Gross M, Hinreiner S, Witthuhn V, Mkrtchyan H, Liehr T. POD-FISH: a new technique for parental origin determination based on copy number variation polymorphism. Methods Mol Biol. 2010;659:291–8.
24. Liehr T. Homemade locus-specific FISH probes: bacterial artificial chromosomes. In: Liehr T, editor. Fluorescence in situ hybridization (FISH) – application guide. 2nd ed. Berlin: Springer; 2017. p. 101–6.
25. Manolakos E, Vetro A, Kefalas K, Rapti SM, Louizou E, Garas A, et al. The use of array-CGH in a cohort of Greek children with developmental delay. Mol Cytogenet. 2010;3:22.
26. Demaerel W, Hestand MS, Vergaelen E, Swillen A, López-Sánchez M, Pérez-Jurado LA, et al. Nested inversion polymorphisms predispose chromosome 22q11.2 to meiotic rearrangements. Am J Hum Genet. 2017 Oct 5;101(4):616–22.

27. Fickelscher I, Starke H, Schulze E, Ernst G, Kosyakova N, Mkrtchyan H, MacDermont K, Sebire N, Liehr T. A further case with a small supernumerary marker chromosome (sSMC) derived from chromosome 1–evidence for high variability in mosaicism in different tissues of sSMC carriers. Prenat Diagn. 2007;27:783–5.
28. Kuroda Y, Ohashi I, Saito T, Nagai J, Ida K, Naruto T, Wada T, Kurosawa K. Deletion of UBE3A in brothers with Angelman syndrome at the breakpoint with an inversion at 15q11.2. Am J Med Genet A. 2014;164A:2873–8.
29. Reiss R, Ahern D, Sandstrom M, Wilkins-Haug L. Recurrent enlarged nuchal translucency: first trimester presentation of a familial 15q26→qter deletion. Am J Med Genet A. 2015;167A:612–6.
30. Ting JC, Roberson ED, Miller ND, Lysholm-Bernacchi A, Stephan DA, Capone GT, et al. Visualization of uniparental inheritance, Mendelian inconsistencies, deletions, and parent of origin effects in single nucleotide polymorphism trio data with SNPtrio. Hum Mutat. 2007;28:1225–35.
31. Liehr T. Cytogenetic contribution to uniparental disomy (UPD). Mol Cytogenet. 2010;3:8.
32. Liehr T. Familial small supernumerary marker chromosomes are predominantly inherited via the maternal line. Genet Med. 2006;8:459–62.
33. De Braekeleer M, Dao TN. Cytogenetic studies in male infertility: a review. Hum Reprod. 1991;6:245–50.
34. Morel F, Douet-Guilbert N, Le Bris MJ, Herry A, Amice V, Amice J, De Braekeleer M. Meiotic segregation of translocations during male gametogenesis. Int J Androl. 2004;27:200–12.
35. Huether CA, Martin RL, Stoppelman SM, D'Souza S, Bishop JK, Torfs CP, Lorey F, May KM, Hanna JS, Baird PA, Kelly JC. Sex ratios in fetuses and liveborn infants with autosomal aneuploidy. Am J Med Genet. 1996;63:492–500.
36. Rinčić M, Iourov IY, Liehr T. Thoughts about SLC16A2, TSIX and XIST gene like sites in the human genome and a potential role in cellular chromosome counting. Mol Cytogenet. 2016;9:56.
37. Alves JM, Lima AC, Pais IA, Amir N, Celestino R, Piras G, et al. Reassessing the evolutionary history of the 17q21 inversion polymorphism. Genome Biol Evol. 2015;7:3239–48.
38. Nowakowska BA, de Leeuw N, Ruivenkamp CA, Sikkema-Raddatz B, Crolla JA, Thoelen R, Koopmans M, den Hollander N, van Haeringen A, van der Kevie-Kersemaekers AM, Pfundt R, Mieloo H, van Essen T, de Vries BB, Green A, Reardon W, Fryns JP, Vermeesch JR. Parental insertional balanced translocations are an important cause of apparently de novo CNVs in patients with developmental anomalies. Eur J Hum Genet. 2012;20:166–70.

12

# Application of high-resolution genomic profiling in the differential diagnosis of liposarcoma

Magdalena Koczkowska[1*], Beata Stefania Lipska-Ziętkiewicz[1], Mariola Iliszko[1], Janusz Ryś[2], Markku Miettinen[3], Jerzy Lasota[3], Wojciech Biernat[4], Agnieszka Harazin-Lechowska[2], Anna Kruczak[2] and Janusz Limon[1]

## Abstract

**Background:** Rarity and heterogeneity of liposarcomas (LPS) make their diagnosis difficult even for sarcoma-experts pathologists. The molecular mechanism underlying the development and progression of liposarcomas (LPS) remains only partially known. In order to identify and compare the genomic profiles, we analyzed array-based comparative genomic hybridization (array-CGH) profiles of 66 liposarcomas, including well-differentiated (WDLPS), dedifferentiated (DDLPS) and myxoid (MLPS) subtypes.

**Results:** Copy number aberrations (CNAs) were identified in 98% of WDLPS and DDLPS and in 95% of MLPS cases. The minimal common region of amplification at 12q14.1q21.1 was observed in 96% of WDLPS and DDLPS cases. Four regions of CNAs, including losses of chromosome 6, 11 and 13 and gains of chromosome 14 were classified as recurrent in DDLPS; at least one was identified in 74% of DDLPS tumors. The DDLPS-associated losses were much more common in tumors with increased genomic complexity. In MLPS, the most frequent CNAs were losses of chromosome 6 (40%) and gains of chromosome 1 (30%), with the minimal overlapping regions 6q14.1q22.31 and 1q25.1q32.2, respectively.

**Conclusions:** Our findings show that the application of array-CGH allows to delineate clearly the genomic profiles of WDLPS, DDLPS and MLPS that reflect biological differences between these tumors. Although CNAs varied widely, the subtypes of tumors have characteristic genomic profiles that could facilitate the differential diagnosis of LPS subtypes, especially between WDLPS and DDLPS.

**Keywords:** Liposarcoma, Array-based comparative genomic hybridization (array-CGH), Copy number aberrations, Genomic profiling, Genomic imbalances

## Background

Liposarcomas (LPS), the most common soft tissue sarcomas accounting for less than 1% of all human cancer cases, display remarkable clinical and pathological heterogeneity. Morphologically, liposarcomas are divided into four main subtypes: well-differentiated (WDLPS), dedifferentiated (DDLPS), myxoid/round cell (MLPS/MRLPS) and pleomorphic liposarcomas (PLPS). WDLPS represents 40–50% of LPS, followed by MLPS (30–35%) [1, 2].

Somatic copy number aberrations (CNAs) occur commonly in human cancer and evaluation of their characteristic patterns may be used as a diagnostic tool, especially in soft tissue sarcomas [3]. Knowledge of alterations in genome structure could also facilitate identification of corresponding oncogenes or tumor suppressor genes associated with the pathogenesis or progression of the disease. So far, CNAs in LPS were mostly evaluated using classical cytogenetic and targeted FISH approaches. It allowed identification of supernumerary ring giant chromosomes and double-minute chromosomes (dmin) in WDLPS and DDLS. These chromosomes contain amplified segments from the 12q13q15 region, including *MDM2, CDK4* and *HMGA2* oncogenes. Consequently,

* Correspondence: magda.koczkowska@gumed.edu.pl
[1]Department of Biology and Genetics, Medical University of Gdansk, 1 Debinki Street, 80-211 Gdansk, Poland
Full list of author information is available at the end of the article

evaluation of 12q13q15 amplification has been applied clinically as it allows for distinguishing WDLPS/DDLPS from benign adipocytic tumors [4, 5]. However, the differential diagnosis between WDLPS and DDLPS is much more challenging, because about 10% of DDLPS are the recurrences of WDLPS as a non-lipogenic sarcoma of variable histological grade. Little is known about the molecular mechanism of dedifferentiation and no genetic alteration has been identified as contributing to this process yet. Recently, it has been suggested that the number of dedifferentiation events in LPS could be underestimated and that actually DDLPS might be the most common histological subtype [6]. MLPS, the third subtype of LPS, is distinguished by the presence of a specific translocation t(12;16) [7] or t(12;22) [8] that is the key genetic aberration, extremely helpful in differential diagnosis between MLPS and myxofibrosarcomas [5]. These unique chromosomal translocations, detected in more than 95% of cases, result from a fusion of the segments of the *DDIT3* gene (12q13) and the *FUS* gene (16p11) or the *EWSR1* gene (22q12) [1, 9].

In recent years, the application of high-resolution methods, such as array-CGH, results in a significant progress in the whole-genome analysis. A few studies published so far have evaluated application of array-CGH and/or whole exome sequencing (WES) techniques in the cohort of patients with LPS [9–11]. Tap et al. (2011) have reported gains in 1p32 with *JUN* amplification and 6q23 as frequent areas of interest in WDLPS and DDLPS, whereas the loss of 19q13 is thought to be associated with the poorer prognosis [10]. Up to now, no detailed genomic profiles of MLPS using high - resolution array-CGH method have been published.

In this study, we performed array-based comparative genomic hybridization (array-CGH) analyses on 69 LPS tumors aimed at identification of specific patterns of chromosomal aberrations that reflect biological differences between these tumors. Accordingly, the diagnostic value of combining morphology with genetic testing was estimated in the group of patients with LPS.

## Methods

### Tumor specimens

In total, 69 fresh-frozen tissue samples from 53 patients diagnosed with liposarcomas were included in this study: 23 WDLPS (from 18 patients), 23 DDLPS (from 16 patients) and 23 MLPS (from 19 patients). All tissue samples have been stored in the archives of the Department of Biology and Genetics, Medical University of Gdansk. The histological subtypes and tumor tissue content of each sample were evaluated independently by two sarcoma-expert pathologists. The clinicopathological data (patients' gender and age, tumor type and its site of development) are presented in Additional file 1: Table S1. Briefly, the studied group consisted of 28 primary tumors, 31 local recurrences and ten metastases. The median age at initial diagnosis was 50 years (range 32–82). The retroperitoneum (39%, 27/69) was the most prevalent location followed by the extremities (33%, 23/69).

### DNA extraction

Genomic DNA, after verification of neoplastic cell content as exceeding 70%, was extracted from a fresh-frozen tumor tissue sample according to salting-out protocol [12]. Array-CGH analyses were performed on archival material. In most cases peripheral blood from patients was not available, therefore a pool of female DNA, isolated by using QIAamp DNA Blood Midi Kit (Qiagen, Hilden, Germany), was used as the reference DNA.

### Array-CGH analysis

Array-CGH was performed at resolution of 10 kbp using Human CGH 2.1M Whole-Genome Tilling Array (NimbleGen, Roche, Basel, Switzerland) following the instructions provided by manufacturer with modification as previously described [13]. Arrays were scanned at 2 μm with MS200 Microarray Scanner (NimbleGen, Roche, Basel, Switzerland) and analyzed with Deva v1.0.2 and Nexus Copy Number 7.5 softwares (NimbleGen, Roche, Basel, Switzerland and BioDiscovery, El Segundo, CA, USA, respectively). Extracted arrays with a DRL spread <0.3 were included in the analysis (average DRLs = 0.15). A minimum of five consecutive probes were required to define a region as a CNA. All identified genomic imbalances were verified in the in-house database, containing >1000 benign copy number variations (CNVs), identified in local populations as well as in online database of genomic variants (DGV; http://dgv.tcag.ca) [14]. Numbering of map positions was based on hg18 (NCBI36 reference sequence).

### Karyotyping and FISH

Cytogenetic studies were performed using conventional GTG-banding of tumor cells metaphase chromosomes at a 550 band level following standard protocol after the digestion with collagenase [15]. In each analysis from 5 to 30 metaphases were evaluated. In MLPS cases where chromosomal translocation t(12;16) or t(12;22) was not noted by karyotype studies, FISH using Vysis LSI DDIT3 (CHOP) Dual Color, Break Apart Rearrangement Probe (Abbott Molecular Inc, Des Plaines, IL, USA) was performed.

### Quantitative real-time PCR

Small deletions (<300 kbp) were validated by quantitative real-time PCR (qPCR) performed on Light Cycler 480 System (Roche, Basel, Switzerland) using specific FAM pre-labelled probes from Universal Probe Library (Roche, Basel, Switzerland). Target genes within the deleted or duplicated regions were assessed against a control sequence at Xq28 and two reference genes: *GPR15* (3q11.2) and *ERMP1* (9p24.1). All samples were run in triplicates. The dosage of target genes relative to reference genes normalized to control DNA was assessed.

### Statistical analysis

For univariate analysis, Fisher's exact test and Mann-Whitney test or Kruskal-Wallis test were used to compare categorical and continuous variables, respectively. Analyses were performed with the STATISTICA 10 software (StatSoft Inc, Tulsa, OK, USA).

## Results

### General overview

Normal karyotype established by classical karyotyping was observed in 11.6% (8/69) of tumors. Ninety-six percent (66/69) of tumors were successfully profiled by array-CGH. The remaining three samples failed the analysis because of high degree of DNA degradation and were excluded from further analyses. The detailed list of all aberrations detected in each tumor by classic and molecular cytogenetics is presented in Additional file 2: Table S2.

Genomic imbalances were revealed in 97% of the tumors (Fig. 1), including 98% (45/46) of WDLPS and DDLPS and 95% (19/20) of MLPS. CNAs affected on average 9.8% of the genome in DDLPS (range: 0.4–29.2%) vs. 1.9% (range: 0–10.3%) and 3.8% (range: 0–13.3%) in WDLPS and MLPS, respectively; the difference being statistically significant ($p < 0.001$; Kruskal-Wallis test). The losses were much more common in DDLPS than in WDLPS ($p < 0.001$ OR = 0.02 95% CI [0.002–0.146]), while no statistically significant difference in number of gains was observed. No amplification region was observed in MLPS. The comparison of all tumors, irrespective of the histological subtype, demonstrated that losses of chromosome 6 and gains of chromosome 5 were found more common in recurrences and metastases than in the primary tumors ($p = 0.009$ and $p = 0.042$, respectively). Besides, the most complex genomic profiles were observed in recurrences (6.8%; range: 0.1–29.2%), followed by metastases and primary tumors (5.3%; range: 0.7–11.9% and 3.5%; range: 0–24.1%, respectively).

### WDLPS/DDLPS

The most frequently affected chromosomal region in WDLPS and DDLPS was 12q, gained in 44/46 of both LPS subtypes, with the minimal common region at 12q14.1q21.1. The three peaks of amplification in this region were localized in the vicinity of *CDK4*, *HMGA2* and *MDM2* loci (Fig. 2). These genes were amplified in 95.7, 91.3, 95.7% of WDLPS and 91.3, 87, 91.3% of DDLPS, respectively.

Besides, the commonly involved chromosomal regions in WDLPS were gains of short arms of chromosome 5 (9/23; 39%) and 19 (6/23; 26%) (Fig. 3a). The gain of chromosome 19p with the minimal overlapping region of 18 Mbp at 19p13.3p13.11, encompassing a total number of 586

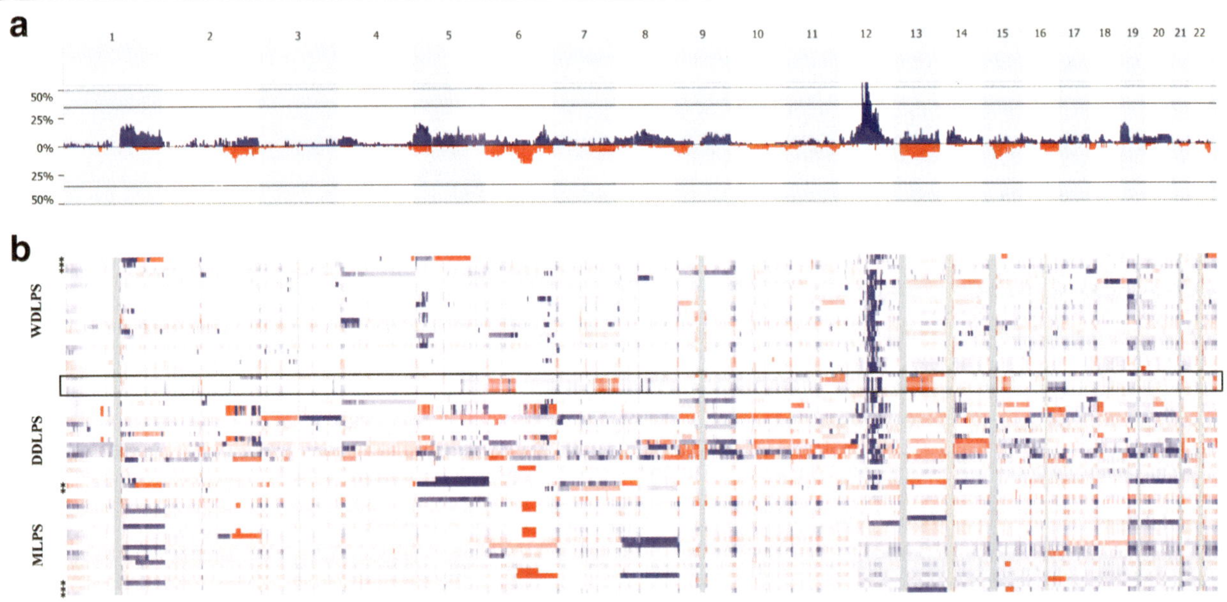


**Fig. 1** Copy number aberrations (CNAs) identified by array-CGH in 66 LPS samples. **a** Frequency plot of CNAs in all LPS samples. **b** Heat map of the CNAs of 66 LPS tumor samples grouped by histological subtypes. *Red* and *blue bars* depict percentage of tumors with losses and gains, respectively in the corresponding region of chromosome. X-axis shows the consecutive chromosome numbers. Color intensity on heat map corresponds to the normalized fluorescence log2 ratio from array-CGH experiments. *Asterisks* (*) indicate samples with the normal genome profile established by conventional karyotyping. Samples denoted by the *black* frame represent tumors with diagnosis refinement based on array-CGH results

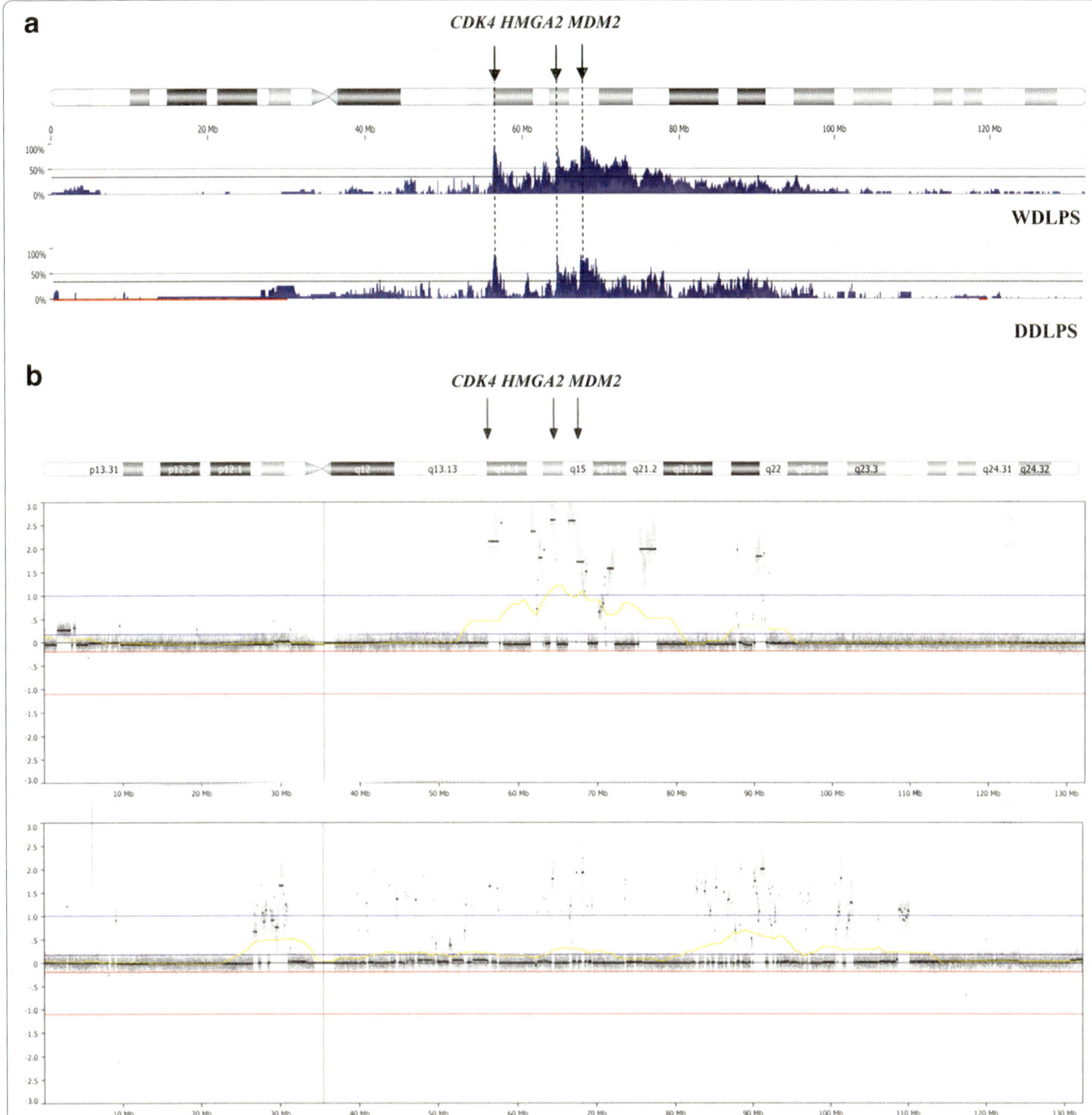


**Fig. 2** Array-CGH profile of chromosome 12 in WDLPS and DDLPS tumors. **a** Penetrance plots of copy number aberrations (CNAs) in 46 cases of WDLPS and DDLPS. **b** Examples of genomic imbalances on chromosome 12 detected by array-CGH. *Blue bars* indicate the percentage of tumors with an amplification in the corresponding region of the chromosome 12. *Black arrows* depict three peaks of amplification in this region with *CDK4, HMGA2* and *MDM2* loci. Increased resolution of array-CGH technique allowed for the establishing the amplification level of known oncogenes associated with WD/DDLPS pathogenesis

genes, was more often detected in tumors with increased genomic complexity ($p = 0.019$; Mann – Whitney test). In addition, a homozygous deletion of 155 kbp at 8p11.23p11.22, encompassing *ADAM3a* and *ADAM5* genes, was found in 10 of 23 (44%) WDLPS tumors. Quantitative PCR analysis of matched tumor and normal tissue samples revealed constitutional and not somatic character of this aberration. The overall frequency of this CNV in in-house population-matched database has been estimated at 6.5%.

DDLPS were characterized by more numerous aberrations than WDLPS, the most common being losses of chromosomes 13 and 15 (Fig. 3b). The deletions of the long arms of chromosome 15 were found exclusively in the local recurrences (6/23; 26%), while aberrations of chromosome 13, identified in 30% of DDLPS (7/23),

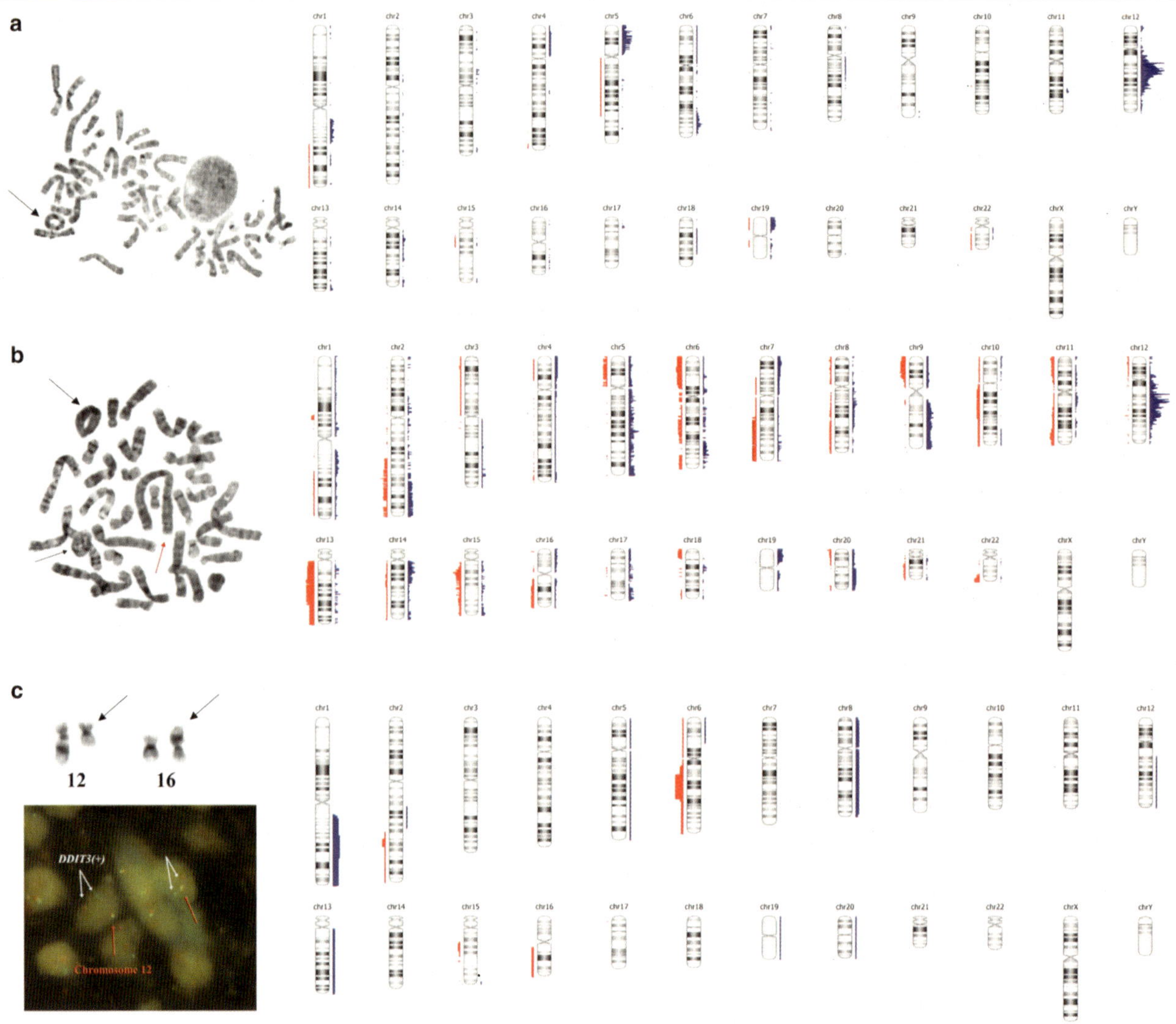


**Fig. 3** Comparison of the standard diagnostic approach and array-CGH in WDLPS, DDLPS and MLPS tumors. On the left the conventional karyotyping and/or FISH results are shown. *Black arrows* depict the supernumerary ring chromosomes in WDLPS and DDLPS tumors (**a**–**b**) and the balanced translocation t(12;16) in MLPS sample (**c**). *DDIT3* break apart probe was used in FISH analysis (one *orange* and one *green* signal pattern indicate a rearrangement of the *DDIT3* gene region). On the right the overview of all copy number aberrations (CNAs) detected by array-CGH is presented. *Red* and *blue* colors represent losses and gains, respectively

were characteristic for tumors located in the abdomen ($p = 0.058$ and $p = 0.002$, respectively). The minimal overlapping region of 65 Mb at 13q11q31.1 covered a total number of 382 genes, among which nine genes are known to be associated with cancer pathogenesis (*ZMYM2, CDX2, FLT3, BRCA2, LHFP, TTL, FOXO1, LCP1, RB1*). In addition, the losses of chromosome 11 and 13, found exclusively in DDLPS, were more frequently observed in the DDLPS tumors with increased genomic complexity ($p = 0.027$ and $p = 0.049$, respectively; Mann – Whitney test).

Genomic aberrations present considerably more (i.e. by at least 30%) often in DDLPS than in WDLPS have been classified as DDLPS-associated (Table 1). These included: losses of chromosome 6, 11 and 13q and gains of chromosome 14q. At least one of the DDLPS-associated CNA was identified in 74% of DDLPS tumors (17/23); while two such CNAs were present in 39% (9/23) and three or more in 13% (3/23) of DDPLS.

### MLPS

The presence of the specific genomic translocation t(12;16) was identified in 18 of 20 MLPS tumors (90%) by standard diagnostic testing, including karyotype and/or FISH for *DDIT3 locus*. The CNAs detected most often in MLPS were losses of 6q (8/20; 40%) and gains of 1q (6/20; 30%) (Fig. 3c). The minimal overlapping region of 36 Mbp at 6q14.1q22.31 covered a total of 175 genes, including four genes from the *Cancer Gene*

**Table 1** Copy number aberrations associated with DDLPS subtype

| Copy number aberration | WDLPS *n* (%) | DDLPS *n* (%) | *P* value (2-tailed Fisher's exact test) |
|---|---|---|---|
| **Losses of chromosome 6** | **0** | **9 (39)** | **0.002** |
| 6p23p22.2 | 0 | 6 (26) | **0.022** |
| 6q11.1q12 | 0 | 3 (13) | 0.233 |
| 6q15q22.33 | 0 | 3 (13) | 0.233 |
| **Losses of chromosome 11**[a] | **0** | **6 (26)** | **0.022** |
| 11p15.5p13 | 0 | 3 (13) | 0.233 |
| 11q23.2q24.2 | 0 | 4 (17) | 0.109 |
| **Losses of chromosome 13q**[a] | **0** | **7 (30)** | **0.009** |
| 13q11q31.1 | 0 | 7 (30) | **0.009** |
| **Gains of chromosome 14q** | **3 (13)** | **10 (43)** | **0.047**<br>OR = 0.2 95% CI [0.05 0.85] |
| 14q21.2q21.3 | 2 (9) | 9 (39) | **0.035**<br>OR = 0.2 95% CI [0.03–0.79] |
| 14q32.2q32.31 | 2 (9) | 2 (9) | 1 |

[a]CNAs associated with increased genomic complexity of DDLPS tumors

*Census* database (*PRDM1, FOX03, ROS1, GOPC*), while gains of 1q25.1q32.2 of 34 Mbp encompassed a total of 269 genes, among which six genes are known to be involved in cancer pathogenesis (*ABL2, TPR, CDC73, MDM4, ELK4, SLC45A3*). Among other CNAs present in MLPS, trisomy of chromosome 8 (3/20; 15%), 13 (2/20; 10%) and a loss of chromosome 16q (2/20; 10%) were present in more than one case each. No statistically significant correlations with the type and the location of tumors were found, but additional copies of chromosome 1 were more frequently observed in tumors with increased genomic complexity ($p = 0.035$; Mann-Whitney test).

## Discussion

In the present study, we have performed the comparison of the genomic profiles established by means of simultaneous classical and molecular cytogenetics analyses in a large series of three LPS subtypes (WDLPS, DDLPS and MLPS). In addition, we estimated the efficacy of implementation the array-CGH analyses into the panel of routine diagnostic procedures in LPS. On the other hand, evaluation of the prognostic significance of particular chromosomal abnormalities on clinical outcome of the patients is beyond the scope of current research.

The significantly higher resolution of array-CGH over conventional karyotyping allowed to detect CNAs in tumors with greater sensitivity and precision. In the current study, six tumors with apparently normal genomic profiles established by conventional technique were found to harbor unbalanced chromosomal aberrations. Certain marker and/or ring chromosomes were large enough to be identified through light microscope, however in most cases application of the molecular method allowed for identification of a number of additional events. Array-CGH screening test facilitated identification of the possible origin of the marker/ring chromosomes in 67% (31/46) of WDLPS and DDLPS cases.

Not only small genomic imbalances were identified, but this technique also allowed for estimation of the amplification frequency of specific genes (Fig. 2). Amplification of 12q, commonly observed in WDLPS and DDLPS tumors, covers *loci* of several oncogenes, including *MDM2, CDK4* and *HMGA2* that are proposed to play the role in the molecular pathogenesis of both subtypes [16]. In the current study, *MDM2, CDK4* and *HMGA2* amplifications were found in ~92% of samples what is in line with previously reported incidence [1, 4, 9, 10, 17]. Moreover, recently published data have demonstrated that the 12q14.1q21.1 amplicon may contain the other genes, presumably involved in LPS pathogenesis, such as *FRS2* (12q15) or *CPM* (12q15) [11, 17–19]. In our series, the frequency of high – level amplifications of the *FRS2* and *CPM* genes was somehow lower than previously reported (88% and 85% vs. 97% and 89%, respectively).

According to the guidelines of the *European Sarcoma Network Working Group* the genetic testing should be the mandatory part of the pathological diagnosis of soft tissue sarcomas (2014) [20]. As pointed out by Italiano et al. (2016), molecular genetic screening facilitated establishing accurate diagnosis in 14% (53/384) sarcoma cases. The highest rate of misdiagnoses prior to molecular testing was observed in the DDLPS cohort (23%, 7/30) [21]. In the current study, initially four WDLPS tumors (6%) were wrongly classified, but in light of the array-CGH profiling they were eventually diagnosed as DDLPS (Fig. 1b and Additional file 2: Table S2). The distinction between WDLPS and DDLPS is challenging, because both are characterized by the presence of ring and marker chromosomes and 12q14q15 amplification, established routinely by conventional karyotyping and FISH, respectively (Fig. 3). The application of array-CGH allowed to identify the specific set of genomic imbalances in DDLPS (Table 1; Fig. 3b) that could be used as specific marker in differential diagnosis with WDLPS. Losses of chromosomes 11 and 13, associated with increased genomic complexity of tumors, were observed exclusively in DDLPS. These CNAs encompass a number of cancer-associated genes, among which a few have already been proposed as candidate genes in the pathogenesis of soft tissue sarcomas, i.e. *RB1* [22]. It has been demonstrated that 16% of lipomas, benign fatty tumors, have harbored 13q14 losses, while in spindle cell lipomas the frequency of this aberration is almost 100% [23, 24]. Moreover, the coexistence of retinoblastoma and lipoma/liposarcoma was observed in sporadic cases, even though the role of the *RB1* gene in their pathogenesis and differentiation process remains still unknown [25, 26]. The other CNAs that are nearly specific to DDLPS included gains of chromosome 14q and losses of chromosome 6.

Overall, genomic imbalances were far more numerous in the DDLPS tumors than in WDLPS (5x) and MLPS (2.5x). Previously, Crago et al. (2012) have shown that WDLPS and DDLPS had more CNAs, affecting 5.7% and 21% of the genome, respectively [10]. The difference in the reported genomic complexity between theirs and the current study may be explained by the localization of tumors. Most of the neoplasms (89%) presented in their study were located in the retroperitoneum that is associated with poorer prognosis, compared with only 39% of such tumor location in our study.

So far, trisomy of chromosome 8 [22, 27–29] and 13q gains [30] have been reported as the CNAs with the highest prevalence in MLPS. The additional copies of chromosome 13 have been suggested to correlate with poorer prognosis of MLPS patients [30]. However, these observations were not in line with our results; gains of chromosome 8 and 13 were identified only in three and two tumors, respectively. The most frequently involved chromosomal regions in MLPS were losses of chromosome 6 and gains of chromosome 1 (Fig. 3c).

Most neoplasm disorders are characterized by chromosomal instability (CIN) that is defined as a genomic instability with observed high rate of chromosomal losses and/or gains. Even though CIN is typical for the vast majority of human cancers, its exact contribution to tumor progression is still deliberated [31]. An increasing number and size of genomic alterations from a primary tumor to its metastasis was confirmed by our studies. Nearly twofold increase in genomic complexity in recurrences and metastases was observed, compared with the primary tumors. Moreover, array-CGH analysis revealed that losses of chromosome 6 and gains of chromosome 5 were observed more frequently in the recurrences and metastases than in the primary LPS tumors regardless of their histological subtype.

The number of technical difficulties faced during cytogenetic chromosome preparations, such as high incidence of cell culture failures, contamination or normal cell growth may be overcome by using array-CGH. Array-CGH appears as a less time-consuming (analysis can be performed within 72 h) and a cost-effective genome-wide screening tool. Notwithstanding the aforesaid, array-CGH has several limitations. First of all, it does not detect balanced translocations, inversions or point mutations. In order to assess the presence of the specific balanced translocations t(12;16) or t(12;22) in MLPS tumors, classical karyotyping and/or targeted FISH has to be nonetheless performed. Furthermore, fresh frozen material is the preferred source of DNA for array-CGH analyses, because paraffin- embedded tissue (FFPE) specimens often increase experimental noise [32] leading to an elevated rate of false positive CNAs calls. That is contrary to the standard pathological procedures that prefer FFPE over fresh-frozen samples. Moreover, tumor DNA may be contaminated with DNA from non-neoplastic cells, and even the tumor cells are histologically and genetically heterogeneous. To avoid masking of acquired aberrations by normal tissue DNA it has been strongly suggested to ensure at least 25% of tumor cells in sample [33]. Constitutional normal DNA from the patient with tumor sample has been recommended as reference in array-CGH analysis, however in clinical practice it is difficult to achieve. Accordingly, to distinguish clonal from constitutional aberrations each abnormality should be verified in the databases of polymorphic, benign copy number variations (CNVs). In this study, the homozygous deletion at 8p11.23p11.22, encompassed *ADAM3a* and *ADAM5* genes, was observed in 42% cases of WDLPS tumors. Losses of 8p11.23p11.22 have been also identified in 16% of pediatric high-grade gliomas [34] and 7% of the non-small cell lung cancer samples that have been suggested to be correlated with poorer prognosis of these patients [35]. However, we demonstrated that this aberration was observed in both normal tissue and the tumor sample, implying the possibility of occurrence of nonpathogenic copy number variation (CNV) what is consistent with the findings of Li et al. [36]. Hence, it is essential to accurately identify somatic aberrations in cancer profile genome to exclude the critical errors that may cause data to be misleadingly interpreted.

## Conclusion

In conclusion, the application of array-CGH allowed to delineate clearly the genomic profiles of WDLPS,

DDLPS and MLPS that reflect biological differences between these tumors. We demonstrate that knowledge of the genome profile along with the detailed histological examination may help to reduce misdiagnoses of LPS subtypes. Specific set of genomic changes, established by array-CGH in DDLPS may facilitate diagnostic dilemma. In order to assess the significance of these alterations in LPS patients, further extensive studies on well-defined larger cohorts and correlations with clinical data should be conducted. In addition, we provide the evidence that array-CGH is an appropriate complementary method to standard diagnostic approach of conventional karyotyping and FISH, however the implementation of high-resolution profiling in routine diagnostic practice should be under taken selectively.

**Acknowledgements**

Dr Koczkowska is also affiliated with the Medical Genomics Laboratory, Department of Genetics, University of Alabama at Birmingham, AL, USA.

**Funding**

This work was supported by statutory research and young investigator research program financed by the Polish Ministry of Science and Higher Education (no. 02-0002/07 and 01-0005/08, respectively) and by a National Science Center project – 2014/13/N/NZ2/03872. MK received scholarship from the Polpharma Scientific Foundation (award 19/03/2013).

**Author's contributions**

*Study concepts*: MK, JL; *Study design*: MK, BSL-Z, JL; *Array-CGH analysis*: MK; *Karyotyping*: MI; *FISH analysis*: MI, AK; *Pathologic evaluation*: JR, MM, JL, WB, AHL; *Data analysis and interpretation*: MK, BSL-Z, JL; *Statistical analysis*: MK, BSL-Z; *Manuscript preparation*: MK, BSL-Z, JL. All authors read and approved the final manuscript.

**Competing interests**

The authors declare that they have no competing interest.

**Author details**

[1]Department of Biology and Genetics, Medical University of Gdansk, 1 Debinki Street, 80-211 Gdansk, Poland. [2]Department of Tumor Pathology, M. Sklodowska-Curie Memorial Institute of Oncology, 11 Garncarska Street, 31-115 Krakow, Poland. [3]Laboratory of Pathology, National Cancer Institute, Building 10, Room B1B47, 10 Center Drive, Bethesda 20892, MD, USA. [4]Department of Pathology, Medical University of Gdansk, 17 Smoluchowskiego Street, 80-214 Gdansk, Poland.

**References**

1. Coindre JM, Pedeutour F, Aurias A. Well-differentiated and dedifferentiated liposarcomas. Virchows Arch. 2010;456:167–79.
2. Miettinen M. Atypical lipomatous tumor and liposarcomas. In: Miettinen M, editor. Modern soft tissue pathology. New York: Cambridge University Press; 2010. p. 432–59.
3. Bridge JA. The role of cytogenetics and molecular diagnostics in the diagnosis of soft-tissue tumors. Mod Pathol. 2014;27:80–97.
4. Conyers R, Young S, Thomas DM. Liposarcoma: molecular diagnostics and therapeutics. Sarcoma. 2011;483154.
5. Dei Tos AP. Liposarcomas: diagnostic pitfalls and new insights. Histopathology. 2014;64:38–52.
6. Mastrangelo G, Coindre JM, Ducimetiere F, Dei Tos AP, Fadda E, Blay JY, Buja A, Fedeli U, Cegelon L, Frasson A, Ranchere-Vince D, Montesco C, Ray-Coquard I, Rossi CR. Incidence of soft-tissue sarcoma and beyond: a population-based prospective study in 3 European regions. Cancer. 2012; 118:5339–48.
7. Limon J, Turc-Carel C, Dal Cin P, Sandberg AA. Recurrent chromosome translocations in liposarcoma. Cancer Genet Cytogenet. 1986;22:93–4.
8. Bode-Lesniewska B, Brigerio S, Exner U, Abdou MT, Moch Z, Zimmermann DR. Relevance of translocation type in myxoid liposarcoma and identification of a novel EWSR1-DDIT3 fusion. Genes Chromosomes Cancer. 2007;46:961–71.
9. Tap WD, Eilber FC, Ginther C, Dry SM, Reese N, Barzan-Smith K, Chen HW, Wu H, Eilber FR, Slamon DJ, Anderson L. Evaluation of well-differentiated/de-differentiated liposarcomas by high-resolution oligonulceotide array-based comparative genomic hybrydization. Genes Chromosomes Cancer. 2011;50:95–112.
10. Crago AM, Socci ND, DeCarolis P, O'Connor R, Taylor BS, Qin LX, Antonescu CR, Singer S. Copy numer losses define subgroups of dedifferentiated liposarcomas with poor prognosis and genomic instability. Clin Cancer Res. 2012;18:1334–40.
11. Kanojia D, Nagata Y, Garg M, Lee DH, Sato A, Yoshida K, Sato Y, Sanada M, Mayakonda A, Bartenhagen C, Klein HU, Doan NB, Said JW, Mohith S, Gunasekar S, Shiraishi Y, Chiba K, Tanaka H, Miyano S, Myklebost O, Yang H, Dugas M, Meza-Zepeda LA, Silberman AW, Forscher C, Tyner JW, Ogawa S, Koeffler HP. Genomic landscape of liposarcoma. Oncotarget. 2015;6:42429–44.
12. Miller SA, Dykes DD, Polesky HF. A simple salting out procedure for extracting DNA from human nucleated cells. Nucleic Acids Res. 1988;16:1215.
13. Ronowicz A, Brzeskwiniewicz M, Madanecki P, Buckley PG, Orlowska E, Ochocka R, Limon J, Piotrowski A. Regeneration of comparative genomic hybridization oligonucleotide microarrays with dimethylurea. Anal Biochem. 2012;426:91–3.
14. Database of Genomic Variants. http://dgv.tcag.ca/dgv/app/home. Accessed May 2015.
15. Limon J, Dal Cin P, Sandberg AA. Application of long-term collagenase dissaggregation for the cytogenetic analysis of human solid tumors. Cancer Genet Cytogenet. 1986;23:305–13.
16. Pedeutour F, Forus A, Coindre JM, Berner JM, Nicolo G, Michniels JF, Terrier P, Ranchere-Vince D, Collin F, Myklebost O, Turc-Carcel C. Structure of the supernumerary ring and giant rod chromosomes in adipose tissue tumors. Genes Chromosomes Cancer. 1999;24:30–1.
17. Wang X, Asmann YW, Erickson-Johnson MR, Oliveira JL, Zhang H, Moura RD, Lazar AJ, Lev D, Bill K, Lloyd RV, Yaszemski MJ, Maran A, Oliveira AM. High-resolution genomic mapping reveals consistent amplification of the fibroblast growth factor receptor substrate 2 gene in well-differentiated and dedifferentiated liposarcoma. Genes Chromosomes Cancer. 2011;50:849–58.
18. Erickson-Johnson MR, Seys AR, Roth CW, King AA, Hulshizer RL, Wang X, Asmann YW, Lloyd RV, Jacob EK, Oliveira AM. Carboxypeptidase M: a biomarker for the discrimination of well differentiated liposarcoma from lipoma. Mod Pathol. 2009;22:1541–7.
19. Zhang K, Chu K, Wu X, Gao H, Wang J, Yuan YC, Loera S, Ho K, Wang Y, Chow W, Un F, Chu P, Yen Y. Amplification of FRS2 and activation of FGFR/FRS2 signaling pathway in high-grade liposarcoma. Cancer Res. 2013;73:1298–307.
20. ESMO/European Sarcoma Network Working Group. Soft tissue and visceral sarcomas: ESMO Clinical Practice Guidelines for diagnosis, treatment and follow-up. Ann Oncol. 2014;25:102–12.
21. Italiano A, Di Mauro I, Rapp J, Pierron G, Auger N, Alberti L, Chibon F, Escande F, Voegeli AC, Ghnassia JP, Keslair F, Lae M, Ranchere-Vince D, Terrier P, Baffert S, Coindre JM, Pedeutour F. Clinical effect of molecular methods in sarcoma diagnosis (GENSARC): a prospective, multicentre, observational study. Lancet Oncol. 2016;2045:1–7.
22. Mandahl N and Mertens F. Soft tissue tumors. In: Heim S and Mitelman F, editors. Cancer cytogenetics: Chromosomal and molecular genetic aberrations of tumor cells. Chichester: John Wiley & Sons, Ltd; 2015. p. 583–589.
23. Dahlen A, Debiec-Rychter M, Pedeutour F, Domanski HA, Hoglund M, Bauer HC, Rydholm A, Sciot R, Mandahl N, Mertens F. Clustering of deletions on chromosome 13 in benign and low-malignant lipomatous tumors. Int J Cancer. 2003;103:616–23.
24. Bartuma H, Nord KH, Macchia G, Isaksson M, Nilsson J, Domanski HA, Mandahl N, Mertens F. Gene expression and single nucleotide polymorphism array analyses of spindle cell lipomas and conventional lipomas with 13q14 deletion. Genes Chromosomes Cancer. 2011;50:619–32.
25. Li FP, Abramson DH, Tarone RE, Kleinerman RA, Fraumeni Jr JF, Boice Jr JD. Hereditary retinoblastoma, lipoma and second primary cases. J Natl Cancer Inst. 1997;89:83–4.
26. Genuardi M, Klutz M, Devriendt K, Caruso D, Stirpe M, Lohmann DR. Multiple lipomas linked to an RB1 gene mutation in a large pedigree with low penetrance retinoblastoma. Eur J Hum Genet. 2001;9:690–4.
27. Szymanska J, Tarkkanen M, Wiklund T, Blomgvist C, Asko-Seljavaara S, Tukiainen E, Elomaa I, Knuutila S. Gains and losses of DNA sequences in

liposarcomas evaluated by comparative genomic hybridization. Genes Chromosomes Cancer. 1996;15:89–94.

28. Parente F, Grosgeorge J, Coindre JM, Terrier P, Vilain O, Turc-Carel C. Comparative genomic hybridization reveals novel chromosome deletions in 90 primary soft tissue tumors. Cancer Genet Cytogenet. 1999;115:89–95.
29. Ohguri T, Hisaoka M, Kawauchi S, Sasaki K, Aoki T, Kanemitsu S, Matsuyam A, Korogi Y, Hashimoto H. Cytogenetic analysis of myxoid liposarcoma and myxofibrosarcoma by array-based comparative genomic hybridization. J Clin Pathol. 2006;59:978–83.
30. Schmidt H, Bartel F, Kappler M, Wurl P, Lange H, Bache M, Holzhausen HJ, Tauber H. Gains of 13q are correlated with a poor prognosis in liposarcoma. Mod Pathol. 2005;18:638–44.
31. Heng HH, Bremer SW, Stevens JB, Horne SD, Liu G, Abdallah BY, Ye KJ, Ye CJ. Chromosomal instability (CIN): what it is and why it is crucial to cancer evolution. Cancer Metastasis Rev. 2013;32:325–40.
32. Nakao K, Oikawa M, Arai J, Mussazhanova Z, Kondo H, Schichijo K, Nakashima M, Hayashi Y, Yoshiura K, Hatachi T, Nagayasu T. A predictive factor of the quality of microarray comparative genomic hybridization analysis for formalin-fixed paraffin-embedded archival tissue. Diagn Mol Pathol. 2013;22:174–80.
33. Cooley LD, Lebo M, Li MM, Slovak ML, Wolff DJ. American College of Medical Genetics and Genomics technical standards and guidelines: microarray analysis for chromosome abnormalities in neoplastic disorders. Genet Med. 2013;15:484–94.
34. Barrow J, Adamowicz-Brice M, Cartmill M, MacArthur D, Lowe J, Robson K, Brundler MA, Walker DA, Coyle B, Grundy R. Homozygous loss of ADAM3A revealed by genome - wide analysis of pediatric high - grade glioma and diffuse intrinsic pontine gliomas. Neuro Oncol. 2011;13:212–22.
35. Wang Y, Zhang Y, Wu L. Homozygous deletion of ADAM3A revealed by genome - wide analysis early - stage NSCLS in China showed to be correlated with poor prognosis. J Clin Oncol. 2011;29 Suppl:abstr e21177.
36. Li A, Liu Y, Zhao Q, Feng H, Harris L, Wang M. Genome-wide identification of somatic aberrations from paired normal-tumor samples. Plos One. 2014; 9, e87212.

# Combination of t(4;14), del(17p13), del(1p32) and 1q21 gain FISH probes identifies clonal heterogeneity and enhances the detection of adverse cytogenetic profiles in 233 newly diagnosed multiple myeloma

Thomas Smol[1,2,8*], Annika Dufour[3], Sabine Tricot[4], Mathieu Wemeau[5], Laure Stalnikiewicz[6], Franck Bernardi[7], Christine Terré[3], Benoît Ducourneau[1], Hervé Bisiau[1] and Agnès Daudignon[1]

**Abstract**

**Background:** Our aim was to set the FISH combination of del(17p13), t(4;14), 1q21 gain and del(1p32), four adverse cytogenetic factors rarely evaluated together, and compare our technical thresholds with those defined in the literature.

**Methods:** Two hundred thirty-three patients with MM at diagnosis were studied using FISH to target 4 unfavorable cytogenetic abnormalities: 17p13 deletion, t(4;14) translocation, 1p32 deletion and 1q21 gain. Technical thresholds were determined for each probe using isolated CD138-expressing PC from patients without MM.

**Results:** The FISH analysis identified abnormalities in 79.0% of patients. Del(17p13) was detected in 15.0% of cases, t(4;14) in 11.5%, 1q21 gain in 37.8% and del(1p32) in 8.7%. Adding 1p32/1q21 FISH probes has enabled us to identify adverse cytogenetic profiles in 39.0% of patients without del(17p13) or t(4;14). Clonal heterogeneity was observed in 51.1% of patients as well as an increase in the number of adverse abnormalities when related clones were greater than or equal to 2 (85.1% against 45.6%).

**Conclusion:** FISH allowed detecting accumulation of adverse abnormalities and clonal heterogeneity in MM with a combination of 4 probes. The impacts of these two parameters need to be evaluated, and could be included in future cytogenetic classifications.

**Keywords:** Multiple Myeloma, Interphase FISH, 1q21 gain, 1p32 deletion, Thresholds

## Background

Multiple Myeloma (MM) is a heterogeneous disease characterized by the clonal proliferation of abnormal plasma cells (PC), invading mainly the bone marrow (BM). MM accounts for approximately 1% of all cancers, and 10% of all hematopoietic neoplasms with a median age of 70 years at diagnosis [1]. The diagnosis of MM is based on BM infiltration by 10% or more clonal PC or dystrophic PC together with evidence of end organ damage [1].

Cytogenetic analysis plays a major role in the risk stratification of MM [2–4]. However, with a metaphase cytogenetic approach, only 35% of patients present abnormal karyotypes, often associated with an advanced stage of the disease [5]. Thus, practice guidelines now recommend interphase fluorescence in-situ hybridization (FISH) as the initial cytogenetic analysis for MM [6]. FISH is performed on isolated CD138-expressing plasma cells [7]. PC enrichment provides a pure tumour population that enables

* Correspondence: thomas.smol@chru-lille.fr
[1]Service d'Hématologie-Immunologie-Cytogénétique, CH Valenciennes, Valenciennes, France
[2]Université de Lille Nord de France, Lille, France
Full list of author information is available at the end of the article

abnormalities to be detected, irrespective of proliferation and infiltration index.

The efficiency of the cell enrichment method limits the number of targets investigated by FISH and a selection of relevant probes is required to provide information on the diagnosis and prognosis. Many combinations of cytogenetic markers have been evaluated. Routine panels mainly evaluate the deletion of 17p13 (*TP53* deletion) and the t(4;14)(p16;q32) *FGFR3-IGH* translocation but do not cover the heterogeneity of MM. The del(17p13) remains the most powerful cytogenetic factor regardless of the therapeutic choice, while t(4;14) loses its negative impact with proteasome inhibitors regimens [8]. Other rearrangements involving *IGH* genes have been reported, such as t(14;16)(q32;q23) and t(14;20)(q32;q12). The prognostic values of the latter vary depending on working groups or methods used [9–11]. In contrast, partial aneuploidies of chromosome 1 (1q21 gain and 1p32 deletion) are retained as more relevant additional markers [10, 12], even with the emerging therapeutic approaches [13, 14]. The addition of 1q21 gain probe is beginning to be integrated into the FISH panel, whereas the identification of 1p32 deletion is not widely used. Moreover, studies are focused on the presence or the absence of FISH markers without considering the clone size or the number of clones.

Our aim was to set the FISH combination of del(17p13), t(4;14), 1q21 gain and del(1p32), four adverse cytogenetic factors rarely evaluated together. In a prospective study of 233 newly diagnosed MM, we observed that the proportion of patients with unfavourable cytogenetic markers could be extended, and that a high level of clonal heterogeneity could be identified by a sufficient number of FISH probes.

## Methods

### Patient samples

Between January 2013 and August 2015, BM samples were collected from 233 patients during diagnosis at the Cytogenetic Laboratories in Valenciennes General Hospital, and Versailles General Hospital. Patients were involved on the basis of WHO 2008 diagnostic criteria for MM. The institutional ethics committee approved the study.

### Plasma cell enrichment

PC were enriched from BM mononuclear cells, using a magnetic cell-sorting CD138 MicroBeads kit (Miltenyi Biotec; BergischGlabach, Germany) according to the manufacturer's protocol. BM samples were filtered with a 70 μm filter (Miltenyi Biotec), and suspended in RPMI solution (Dutscher; Brumath, France). After centrifugation (160 G), and removal of the supernatant, mononuclear cells were marked with CD138 microbeads at 4 ° C for 15 min. The cells were then separated on a column kit separator (Miltenyi Biotec). PC enrichment was controlled on a cytospin slide by a cytologist. The median efficiency of CD138 selection was 97.5%.

### Interphase fluorescent in situ hybridization

FISH was performed on samples enriched in accordance with the manufacturer's instructions. The FISH panel included a *TP53/CEP17* probe (Amplitech, Compiègne, France), a *1p32/CDKN2C-FAF1 – 1q21/CKS1B* probe (Amplitech), a t(4;14)(p16;q32) probe (MetaSystems, Altlussheim, Germany), and an *IGH* break-apart probe (MetaSystems).

An automated reading with images captured was performed on GSL-10 Leica (Leica Biosystems; Wetzlar, Germany) and analysed with CytoVision software (Leica Biosystems). The number of PC with abnormal signal patterns was calculated as the average of data from two cytogeneticists who analysed 200 cells. The quality of hybridization was controlled for each FISH technique on metaphases from negative samples.

Technical thresholds were determined for each probe, using isolated CD138-expressing PC from patients without MM, on the basis of the same method as used with patients with MM. Between five and ten PC controls were used for each probe. Thresholds were assessed after counting 200 cells for each negative sample, and established by a "mean + 3 DS" calculation. The technical thresholds for adverse cytogenetic abnormalities were 6.5% for del(1p32), 4.5% for 1q21 gain, 4% for t(4;14) translocation, 4% for *IGH* rearrangement, and 5% for del(17p13).

Compared technical thresholds from the literature were defined as 10% for fusions and 20% for numerical abnormalities [15].

### Statistical analysis

A comparison of numerical variables between two groups was performed using the nonparametric Mann-Whitney *U* test. A comparison of qualitative variables was performed using the Fisher *F*-test. Statistical significance was defined as $p < 0.05$.

## Results

Among the 233 patients, there were 52.3% males ($n$ = 122) and 47.7% females ($n$ = 111), with a median age of 67 years (41 to 89 years-old). The repartition of ISS score was respectively 37.6%, 33.6% and 28.8% for stage I, stage II, and stage III.

Cytogenetic abnormalities were identified in 79.0% of cases (184/233) by FISH analysis (Table 1), with one or more adverse abnormalities in 51.9% (121/233). We observed a del(17p13) in 15.0%, a t(4;14) translocation in 11.5%, a 1q21 gain in 37.8%, and a del(1p32) in 8.7% of patients (Fig. 1). By adding the 1p32/1q21 FISH probe, we were able to identify one or more adverse

**Table 1** Distribution of FISH abnormalities

| Cytogenetic abnormalities [number of patients with available data] | n [%] |
|---|---|
| *1p32/CDKN2C-FAF1 – 1q21/CKS1B* probe [*n* = 230] | |
| 1q21 gain = 3 copies | 87 [37.8] |
| 1q21 gain >3 copies | 42 [18.3] |
| 1p32 monoallelic deletion | 19 [8.3] |
| 1p32 biallelic deletion | 1 [0.4] |
| monosomy 1 | 4 [1.7] |
| trisomy 1 | 7 [3.0] |
| *TP53/CEP17* probe [*n* = 233] | |
| 17p13 monoallelic deletion | 35 [15.0] |
| monosomy 17 | 11 [4.7] |
| trisomy 17 | 32 [13.7] |
| trisomy 17 with one *TP53* loss | 6 [2.6] |
| *IGH* break-apart and t(4;14)(p16;q32) - *IGH/FGFR3* probes [*n* = 217] | |
| total *IGH* rearrangements | 75 [34.6] |
| t(4;14)(p16;q32) | 25 [11.5] |
| monosomy 4 or 4p16 deletion | 4 [1.9] |
| monosomy 14 or 14q32 deletion | 12 [5.2] |
| *IGHv* loss | 17 [12.0] |
| 4p16 gain | 23 [10.9] |
| 14q32 gain | 8 [3.4] |

*Abbreviations*: *CDKN2C* Cyclin-Dependent Kinase Inhibitor 2C, *CEP17* Chromosome 17 centromere, *CKS1B* Cyclin-Dependent Kinases Regulatory Subunit 1, *FAF1* FAS-associated Factor 1, *FGFR3* Fibroblast Growth Factor Receptor 3, *FISH* fluorescence in-situ hybridization, *IGH* Immunoglobulin Heavy Locus, *IGHv* Immunoglobulin Heavy Locus variable region, *TP53* Tumour Protein P53

abnormalities in 39.0% (64/164) of patients with an absence of *TP53* deletion or t(4;14). For these patients, a 1q21 gain and a monoallelic del(1p32) were found respectively in 90.6% and 18.7% of cases. Both markers were associated in 6 cases.

When adverse cytogenetic abnormalities were present, they were isolated in 70.2% (85/121) and associated in 29.8% (36/121) of cases. In our cohort, statistically significant associations were observed between the presence of 1q21 gain and t(4;14), and between the presence of del(1p32) and del(17p13) (Fig. 1). The 1q21 gain was present in 68.0% (17/25) of patients with t(4;14) translocation versus 35.1% (67/191) of patients without t(4;14) ($p$ = *0.001*). The del(1p32) was found in 36.8% (7/19) of patients with del(17p13) versus 12.8% (27/211) of patients without del(17p13) ($p$ = *0.01*). A subgroup of 1q21 gain was identified with a number of 1q21 signals greater than 3. Between 4 and 9 signals were observed in 18.3% of cases that could be considered as 1q21 amplifications. In our cohort, this subgroup was always found as a 1q21 gain side-line, emerging in 48.3% of cases. Derivative FISH abnormalities targeting 1p32, 1q21, 4p16, 14q32, 17p13 and D17Z1 *loci* were frequently identified and are listed in Table 1 for information.

The median sizes of identified adverse clones were 50% for del(17p13), 80% for t(4;14), 52% for 1q21 gain and 77.5% for del(1p32). By applying frequently used technical thresholds to our population (10% for fusions and 20% for numerical abnormalities), 40% of del(17p13) detected would have been considered as negative, as well as 24% of 1q21 gain, 16.5% of del(1p32) and only 4% of t(4;14). These under-detected clones were mainly represented by numerical abnormalities. The difference of FISH sensibilities may be explained by the probes' design with or without internal control.

Clonal heterogeneity with at least 2 related clones was observed in 51.1% (94/184) of cases. The cases with 3 or more related clones represented 13.6% (25/184) of the population. Adverse abnormalities were significantly

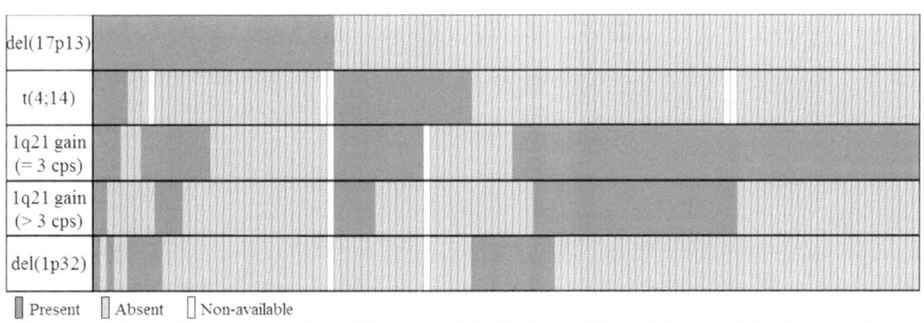


**Fig. 1** Landscape of the association of adverse abnormalities at diagnosis ($n$ = 121). Preferential associations were found between t(4;14) and 1q21 gain (68.0% of cases in t(4;14) subgroup), and between del(17p13) and del(1p32) (36.8% of cases in del(17p13)$^{+}$ subgroup). 1q21 amplification in more than 3 copies was found in 48.3% as 1q21 gain side-line. (cps = copies)

more frequent when the number of clones was greater than or equal to 2, with a frequency of 85.1% (80/94) against 45.6% (41/90) when 1 single clone was identified ($p < 0.0001$).

The distribution of adverse abnormality profiles varies with the number of identified clones (Fig. 2). When clonal heterogeneity was present (≥2 clones), a greater number of MM with 1q21 gain were found: 81.6% (71/94) compared with 18.4% (16/88) when 1 single clone was identified ($p < 0.0001$). In the case of marked clonal heterogeneity (≥3 clones), a higher involvement of del(1p32) was found with a frequency of 28.0% (7/25) against 5.8% (4/69) when only 2 related clones were present ($p = 0.002$). Del(17p13) and t(4;14) were uniformly represented, regardless of the number of clones detected. A higher number of related clones tended to be observed when the ISS stage was III, with a median of 2 clones compared with a median of 1 clone when the ISS stages were I or II ($p = 0.054$).

## Discussion

MM is characterized by the heterogeneity of cytogenetic changes, reflecting the heterogeneity of patients. Cytogenetic analyses have always played a key role in the prognostic evaluation in MM. However, low in-vitro PC proliferation index and low PC infiltration limited the conventional cytogenetic interpretation [5]. Culture failures or misinterpretations of normal karyotypes have been avoided with FISH on CD138-expressing PC [16]. In this study, we investigated 233 MM during diagnosis with a combination of four probes targeting 17p13/*TP53* deletion, t(4;14)(p16;q32) translocation, 1p32/*CDKN2C-FAF1* deletion, and 1q21/*CKS1B* gain.

The prevalence of adverse abnormalities (51.9%) in this cohort of MM at diagnosis is similar to that in previously published data [2, 3, 12, 16–18]. The combination of unfavourable conventionally used cytogenetic markers, del(17p13) and t(4;14) [19], with two more recent markers, del(1p32) and 1q21 gain, has enabled us to identify 39.0% more patients carrying chromosome 1 abnormalities. Indeed, a predominance of 1q21 gain has been observed in 37.8% of cases, as well as a significant number of del(1p32) (8.3%). The need to use a complete panel targeting these four markers in FISH can thus be confirmed.

Preferential associations between adverse abnormalities suggest a successive hits mechanism by analogy with the oncogene involvement in high-grade lymphomas. Several studies assess or stratify clinical risk by combining cytogenetic abnormalities with biomarkers. Two studies mention the accumulation of anomalies in MM with a score test based on the number of anomalies detected, combined with ISS stage [20, 21]. We observed that the accumulation of abnormalities is associated with clonal heterogeneity, considered as unfavourable in most hematologic malignancies. This parameter has not yet been integrated into prognostic models of various studies, even if a recent study indicates that the clone size affects patient outcomes [22]. As noted in previously published data, no association was observed between the number of adverse abnormalities and the ISS stage [11, 13]. Nevertheless, it seems that the clonal heterogeneity increases with the ISS stage III. This would support the idea of including clonal heterogeneity in a revised score.

The preceding remark raises the issue of how the thresholds of FISH defects are determined and used. The guidelines defined thresholds depending on the type of probe or thresholds based on prognostic switches. Such thresholds are either technical with 10% for fusions and 20% for numerical abnormalities [15], or prognostic from 60% up to 70% for del(17p13), or from 10% up to 30% for 1q21 gain and t(4;14) [12, 23–26]. In this study, we used our in-house establishment "mean + 3 standard deviation" from normal isolated PC from BM. Our technical thresholds have enabled us to compare MM data from FISH with the same matrix as that used for the negative control. Thus, we were able to report all anomalies above these thresholds and identify all determinable

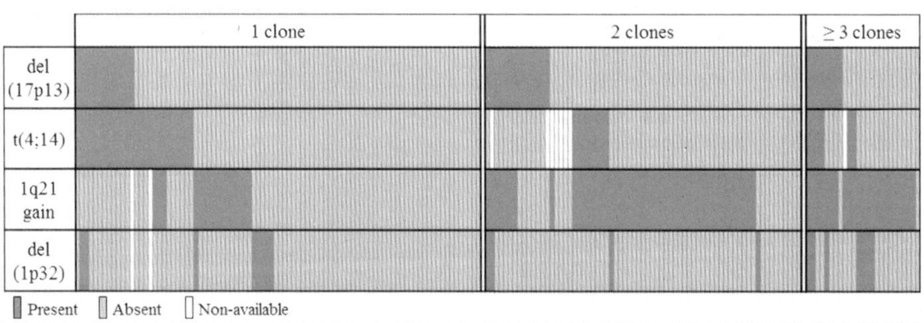


**Fig. 2** Distribution of abnormalities according to the number of clones at diagnosis ($n = 184$). 1q21 gain was more frequent in the subgroup of 2 clones or more (81.6%) compared to the subgroup of 1 clone (18.4%) ($p < 0.0001$), del(1p32) was more frequent in the subgroup of 3 clones or more (28.0%) compared to the subgroup of 1 or 2 clones (5.8%) ($p = 0.002$). No preferential distribution was observed with del(17p13) and t(4;14) translocation

clones with our four probes. Clonal heterogeneity would either have been less marked with previously published technical thresholds, or smoothed if prognostic thresholds were applied.

Detection of chromosome 1 abnormalities becomes relevant with the emergence of new therapies and therapeutic strategies. Indeed, it could identify 39.0% more patients with valuable prognostic information. Unlike t(4;14) whom negative impact can be erased by proteasome inhibitors [8], the 1q21 gain maintains a lower overall survival rate irrespective of treatment modality [13, 14]. We observed that 1q21 gain was associated with a higher clonal heterogeneity at diagnosis. Moreover, the acquisition of this anomaly is often secondary, especially with t(4;14) translocation. Studies show the lack of 1q21 gain in monoclonal gammapathy of undetermined significance compared to MM, suggesting a significant role of the 1q21 gain in MM progression [27, 28]. These data support the notion of 1q21 gain integration in the current cytogenetic classification in order to define therapeutic cytogenetic profiles, pending the establishment of consensual prognostic profiles.

The deletion of 1p32 *locus* is considered as a strong independent negative prognostic factor [12], and is associated with other adverse abnormalities in 2/3 of cases in our series. Del(1p32) potentiates the unfavourable characters of del(17p13) or t(4;14) translocation [12]. This deletion was identified in the presence of strong clonal heterogeneity (>3 related clones) reflecting a major chromosomal instability. It should therefore be a cytogenetic target in any FISH panel at MM diagnosis.

Cases with 2 or more trisomies are poorly represented in our series (7.8%) (Table 1), while hyperdiploid MM represent approximately 50–55% of cytogenetic anomalies in MM [29, 30]. This discordance arises because chromosomes 1, 4, 14 and 17 are poor indicators of hyperdiploidy in MM. Chromosomal gains affect preferentially the odd chromosomes 3, 5, 7, 9, 11, 15, 19 and 21 [31]. As a result, no conclusions about MM ploidy can be reached with our probes, unless we add a chromosomal centromeric marker among the most common trisomies, such as chromosomes 5, 9 or 15 in the set of FISH probes sorting [3, 29]. Cases with monosomies were rare, but consistent with published data, considering the non-use, in our cohort, of chromosome 13 probe known as the most frequent monosomy in MM [30].

## Conclusion

The use of FISH on sorted PC has revolutionized the genetic analysis of MM. The absence of chromosomal banding analysis complicates the process of obtaining complete data concerning the combination of cytogenetic markers. However, in this study, we were able to identify adverse abnormalities or derivative anomalies, as well as related clones or clonal evolution by FISH analysis. We also confirm the presence of clonal heterogeneity and accumulation of adverse abnormalities in the first diagnostic analysis. The prognostic impact of these parameters should be evaluated, and could be included in future cytogenetic classifications.

**Acknowledgments**
Not applicable.

**Funding**
Not applicable.

**Authors' contributions**
TS and ADu performed the research. TS wrote the paper. ADa and CT supervised molecular cytogenetic analysis. TS, ADu, ADa and CT analysed the data. ST, MW, LS, CT provided patient data. ADa supervised the project and revised the manuscript. All authors read and approved the final manuscript.

**Competing interests**
The authors declare that they have no competing interests.

**Author details**
[1]Service d'Hématologie-Immunologie-Cytogénétique, CH Valenciennes, Valenciennes, France. [2]Université de Lille Nord de France, Lille, France. [3]Laboratoire de Cytogénétique Hématologique, CH Versailles, Le Chesnay, France. [4]Service d'Hématologie Clinique, CH Valenciennes, Valenciennes, France. [5]Service d'Hématologie Clinique, CH Arras, Arras, France. [6]Service d'Hématologie Clinique, CH Lens, Lens, France. [7]Laboratoire de Biologie, CH Douai, Douai, France. [8]Institut de génétique médicale, Hôpital Jeanne de Flandre, CHRU Lille, Lille, France.

**References**
1. Vincent Rajkumar S. Multiple myeloma: 2014 Update on diagnosis, risk-stratification, and management. Am J Hematol. 2014;89:999–1009.
2. Moreau P, Cavo M, Sonneveld P, Rosinol L, Attal M, Pezzi A, et al. Combination of international scoring system 3, high lactate dehydrogenase, and t(4;14) and/or del(17p) identifies patients with multiple myeloma (MM) treated with front-line autologous stem-cell transplantation at high risk of early MM progression-related death. J Clin Oncol Off J Am Soc Clin Oncol. 2014;32:2173–80.
3. Hebraud B, Magrangeas F, Cleynen A, Lauwers-Cances V, Chretien M-L, Hulin C, et al. Role of additional chromosomal changes in the prognostic value of t(4;14) and del(17p) in multiple myeloma: the IFM experience. Blood. 2015;125:2095–100.
4. Leleu X, Karlin L, Macro M, Hulin C, Garderet L, Roussel M, et al. Pomalidomide plus low-dose dexamethasone in multiple myeloma with deletion 17p and/or translocation (4;14): IFM 2010-02 trial results. Blood. 2015;125:1411–7.
5. Liebisch P, Döhner H. Cytogenetics and molecular cytogenetics in multiple myeloma. Eur J Cancer Oxf Engl 1990. 2006;42:1520–9.
6. Hastings R, Howell R, Betts D, Porter S, Haferlach C, Dastugue N, et al. A common European framework for quality assessment for banded chromosome studies and molecular cytogenetic investigations of acquired abnormalities. Eur Cytogenet Assoc Newsl. 2013;31:7–21.
7. Kobayashi S, Hyo R, Amitani Y, Tanaka M, Hashimoto C, Sakai R, et al. Four-color flow cytometric analysis of myeloma plasma cells. Am J Clin Pathol. 2006;126:908–15.
8. Avet-Loiseau H, Leleu X, Roussel M, Moreau P, Guerin-Charbonnel C, Caillot D, et al. Bortezomib plus dexamethasone induction improves outcome of patients with t(4;14) myeloma but not outcome of patients with del(17p). J Clin Oncol Off J Am Soc Clin Oncol. 2010;28:4630–4.
9. Avet-Loiseau H, Malard F, Campion L, Magrangeas F, Sebban C, Lioure B, et al. Translocation t(14;16) and multiple myeloma: is it really an independent prognostic factor? Blood. 2011;117:2009–11.

10. Kuiper R, van Duin M, van Vliet MH, Broijl A, van der Holt B, El Jarari L, et al. Prediction of high- and low-risk multiple myeloma based on gene expression and the International Staging System. Blood. 2015; 126:1996–2004.
11. Palumbo A, Avet-Loiseau H, Oliva S, Lokhorst HM, Goldschmidt H, Rosinol L, et al. Revised International Staging System for Multiple Myeloma: A Report From International Myeloma Working Group. J Clin Oncol Off J Am Soc Clin Oncol. 2015;33:2863–9.
12. Hebraud B, Leleu X, Lauwers-Cances V, Roussel M, Caillot D, Marit G, et al. Deletion of the 1p32 region is a major independent prognostic factor in young patients with myeloma: the IFM experience on 1195 patients. Leukemia. 2014;28:675–9.
13. Nahi H, Våtsveen TK, Lund J, Heeg BMS, Preiss B, Alici E, et al. Proteasome inhibitors and IMiDs can overcome some high-risk cytogenetics in multiple myeloma but not gain 1q21. Eur J Haematol. 2015;96:46-54
14. An G, Xu Y, Shi L, Shizhen Z, Deng S, Xie Z, et al. Chromosome 1q21 gains confer inferior outcomes in multiple myeloma treated with bortezomib but copy number variation and percentage of plasma cells involved have no additional prognostic value. Haematologica. 2014;99:353–9.
15. Ross FM, Avet-Loiseau H, Ameye G, Gutiérrez NC, Liebisch P, O'Connor S, et al. Report from the European Myeloma Network on interphase FISH in multiple myeloma and related disorders. Haematologica. 2012;97:1272–7.
16. Bacher U, Haferlach T, Kern W, Alpermann T, Schnittger S, Haferlach C. Correlation of cytomorphology, immunophenotyping, and interphase fluorescence in situ hybridization in 381 patients with monoclonal gammopathy of undetermined significance and 301 patients with plasma cell myeloma. Cancer Genet Cytogenet. 2010;203:169–75.
17. Hillengass J, Zechmann CM, Nadler A, Hose D, Cremer FW, Jauch A, et al. Gain of 1q21 and distinct adverse cytogenetic abnormalities correlate with increased microcirculation in multiple myeloma. Int J Cancer. 2008;122:2871–5.
18. Nemec P, Zemanova Z, Kuglik P, Michalova K, Tajtlova J, Kaisarova P, et al. Complex karyotype and translocation t(4;14) define patients with high-risk newly diagnosed multiple myeloma: results of CMG2002 trial. Leuk Lymphoma. 2012;53:920–7.
19. Dimopoulos M, Kyle R, Fermand J-P, Rajkumar SV, San Miguel J, Chanan-Khan A, et al. Consensus recommendations for standard investigative workup: report of the International Myeloma Workshop Consensus Panel 3. Blood. 2011;117:4701–5.
20. Avet-Loiseau H, Durie BGM, Cavo M, Attal M, Gutierrez N, Haessler J, et al. Combining fluorescent in situ hybridization data with ISS staging improves risk assessment in myeloma: an International Myeloma Working Group collaborative project. Leukemia. 2013;27:711–7.
21. Boyd KD, Ross FM, Chiecchio L, Dagrada GP, Konn ZJ, Tapper WJ, et al. A novel prognostic model in myeloma based on co-segregating adverse FISH lesions and the ISS: analysis of patients treated in the MRC Myeloma IX trial. Leukemia. 2012;26:349–55.
22. An G, Li Z, Tai Y-T, Acharya C, Li Q, Qin X, et al. The Impact of Clone Size on the Prognostic Value of Chromosome Aberrations by Fluorescence In Situ Hybridization in Multiple Myeloma. Clin Cancer Res. 2015;21:2148–56.
23. Avet-Loiseau H, Attal M, Moreau P, Charbonnel C, Garban F, Hulin C, et al. Genetic abnormalities and survival in multiple myeloma: the experience of the Intergroupe Francophone du Myélome. Blood. 2007;109:3489–95.
24. Neben K, Jauch A, Bertsch U, Heiss C, Hielscher T, Seckinger A, et al. Combining information regarding chromosomal aberrations t(4;14) and del(17p13) with the International Staging System classification allows stratification of myeloma patients undergoing autologous stem cell transplantation. Haematologica. 2010;95:1150–7.
25. Neben K, Lokhorst HM, Jauch A, Bertsch U, Hielscher T, van der Holt B, et al. Administration of bortezomib before and after autologous stem cell transplantation improves outcome in multiple myeloma patients with deletion 17p. Blood. 2012;119:940–8.
26. Chang H, Jiang N, Jiang H, Saha MN, Qi C, Xu W, et al. CKS1B nuclear expression is inversely correlated with p27Kip1 expression and is predictive of an adverse survival in patients with multiple myeloma. Haematologica. 2010;95:1542–7.
27. Hanamura I, Stewart JP, Huang Y, Zhan F, Santra M, Sawyer JR, et al. Frequent gain of chromosome band 1q21 in plasma-cell dyscrasias detected by fluorescence in situ hybridization: incidence increases from MGUS to relapsed myeloma and is related to prognosis and disease progression following tandem stem-cell transplantation. Blood. 2006;108:1724–32.
28. Sawyer JR, Tian E, Heuck CJ, Johann DJ, Epstein J, Swanson CM, et al. Evidence of an epigenetic origin for high-risk 1q21 copy number aberrations in multiple myeloma. Blood. 2015;125:3756–9.
29. Wuilleme S, Robillard N, Lodé L, Magrangeas F, Beris H, Harousseau J-L, et al. Ploidy, as detected by fluorescence in situ hybridization, defines different subgroups in multiple myeloma. Leukemia. 2005;19:275–8.
30. Van Wier S, Braggio E, Baker A, Ahmann G, Levy J, Carpten JD, et al. Hypodiploid multiple myeloma is characterized by more aggressive molecular markers than non-hyperdiploid multiple myeloma. Haematologica. 2013;98:1586–92.
31. Smadja NV. Bastard C, Brigaudeau C, Leroux D, Fruchart C, Groupe Français de Cytogénétique Hématologique. Hypodiploidy is a major prognostic factor in multiple myeloma. Blood. 2001;98:2229–38.

# 14

# Inherent variability of cancer-specific aneuploidy generates metastases

Mathew Bloomfield[1,2] and Peter Duesberg[1*]

**Abstract**

**Background:** The genetic basis of metastasis is still unclear because metastases carry individual karyotypes and phenotypes, rather than consistent mutations, and are rare compared to conventional mutation. There is however correlative evidence that metastasis depends on cancer-specific aneuploidy, and that metastases are karyotypically related to parental cancers. Accordingly we propose that metastasis is a speciation event. This theory holds that cancer-specific aneuploidy varies the clonal karyotypes of cancers automatically by unbalancing thousands of genes, and that rare variants form new autonomous subspecies with metastatic or other non-parental phenotypes like drug-resistance – similar to conventional subspeciation.

**Results:** To test this theory, we analyzed the karyotypic and morphological relationships between seven cancers and corresponding metastases. We found (1) that the cellular phenotypes of metastases were closely related to those of parental cancers, (2) that metastases shared 29 to 96% of their clonal karyotypic elements or aneusomies with the clonal karyotypes of parental cancers and (3) that, unexpectedly, the karyotypic complexity of metastases was very similar to that of the parental cancer. This suggests that metastases derive cancer-specific autonomy by conserving the overall complexity of the parental karyotype. We deduced from these results that cancers cause metastases by karyotypic variations and selection for rare metastatic subspecies. Further we asked whether metastases with multiple metastasis-specific aneusomies are assembled in one or multiple, sequential steps. Since (1) no stable karyotypic intermediates of metastases were observed in cancers here and previously by others, and (2) the karyotypic complexities of cancers are conserved in metastases, we concluded that metastases are generated from cancers in one step – like subspecies in conventional speciation.

**Conclusions:** We conclude that the risk of cancers to metastasize is proportional to the degree of cancer-specific aneuploidy, because aneuploidy catalyzes the generation of subspecies, including metastases, at aneuploidy-dependent rates. Since speciation by random chromosomal rearrangements and selection is unpredictable, the theory that metastases are karyotypic subspecies of cancers also explains Foulds' rules, which hold that the origins of metastases are "abrupt" and that their phenotypes are "unpredictable."

## Background

Metastasis is defined as the development of secondary malignant growths at a distance from a primary site of cancer [1]. The relation of a metastasis to its primary cancer was described by Foulds in 1965 as a "progression" which, "is not a mere extension of a pre-existing lesion in space and time but a revolutionary change in a portion of the old lesion establishing a tumor with new properties not formerly present" [2]. Current textbooks point out that metastasis accounts for about 90% of the mortality from cancers and that, despite enormous efforts, its origins are still unclear [3, 4]. For example, *The Molecular Biology of the Cell* states that metastasis "is the most deadly – and least understood – aspect of cancer" [4].

* Correspondence: duesberg@berkeley.edu
[1]Department of Molecular and Cell Biology; Donner Laboratory, University of California at Berkeley, Berkeley, CA 94720, USA
Full list of author information is available at the end of the article

### No evidence for consistent metastasis-specific mutations

In 1954 Foulds showed that cancers progress to metastases stochastically or "abruptly" and with diverse "unpredictable" phenotypes and concluded that "it is inadvisable to attribute to mutation" the great diversity of the individual phenotypes of metastases [5]. In apparent agreement with Foulds, no consistent metastasis-specific gene mutations [6–19], aneuploidies (abnormal chromosomes) [20–48] and transcriptomes [47, 49–64] have since been found. Based on a survey of influential studies on metastasis Michaelson et al. also concluded in 2005, "There has been much uncertainty as to whether metastasis requires mutation at the time of spread" [6, 65–73]. In view of this Michaelson et al. studied the probability of metastatic spread of clinical cancers and arrived at the conclusion that metastasis follows a "nongenetic mechanism", typically at rates below 10^-8 per cancer cell [9, 10]. And *The Biology of Cancer* states in 2014–60 years after Foulds first questioned mutations - that "it is clear that the identities of many of the genes that are specifically involved in programming metastasis have been elusive." [3]. In searching for these elusive metastasis-genes, it was also observed that the proclivity of cancers to metastasize is determined prior to metastasis, is "preordained" [69] or "predetermined" [74]. Considering the elusive search for metastasis-genes and our prior work on the karyotypic basis of cancer and metastasis [43, 75–77] we have asked here, whether the proclivity of cancers to metastasize might be determined by cancer-specific aneuploidy.

**Two links between aneuploidy and metastasis**

In an effort to find a mutation-independent mechanism of metastasis, we reviewed previously unexplained findings for clues. As a result we found two conspicuous links: (1) the risk of metastasis correlates with the degrees of cancer-specific aneuploidy, and (2) the aneuploid karyotypes of metastases are related to those of primary cancers. In the following we first summarize the evidence for these two links between aneuploidy and metastasis, and then show that a karyotypic, rather than a mutational theory can explain the origins of metastasis.

***Correlations between degrees of cancer-specific aneuploidy and proclivity for metastasis***

Studying cancer cytogenetics Atkin found in 1972 that "Carcinomas of the breast fell into two discrete groups. The lower near-diploid group showed a significantly better eight year survival rate than the higher triploid-tetraploid group." [78]. Likewise, Frankfurt et al. observed in 1985, "Only 7.1% of diploid tumors with a Gleason score of 5 to 6 formed metastases, but 80% of aneuploid tumors with a higher Gleason score (7 to 10) formed metastases", and concluded, "DNA ploidy may be an important prognostic factor for human prostate cancer." [79]. In a review on "tumor progression" Wolman wrote in 1986, "There was a significantly higher survival rate and lower metastasis frequency associated with diploid tumors. A large majority (81%) of the tumors which metastasized were hyperploid." [80]. The same conclusion was reached in 1986 by Ljungberg et al., who found that "deoxyribonucleic acid content might be a useful prognostic discriminator with implications for the clinical management of patients with metastatic renal cell carcinoma" [81]. Fallenius et al. made the same observation with breast cancers in 1988, "The diploid carcinomas represent slowly growing tumors with low risk of producing metastases and consequently, a highly favorable prognosis. In contrast, aneuploid tumors are potentially highly malignant variants, mostly rapidly progressing tumors with poor prognoses" [82]. Further, Saito et al. reported in 1994, "the incidence of the cervical lymph node metastasis was significantly ($P < 0.02$) higher in the aneuploid cases (8/15) than in the diploid cases (3/21)" [83]. In 1997 Hemmer et al. reached the same conclusion based on DNA content in a study entitled, "The value of DNA flow cytometry in predicting the development of lymph node metastasis and survival in patients with locally recurrent oral squamous cell carcinoma" [84]. And Torres et al. observed in 2007 that, "the number of genomic imbalances in primary (breast) tumors was significantly higher in patients presenting lymph node metastases (median = 15.5) than in the group with no evidence" for metastasis [85]. Concurrently Jonkers et al. reached the conclusion in 2007 that "DNA copy number status is the most sensitive and efficient marker of adverse clinical outcome (of pancreatic cancers); particularly of metastatic disease" [41], which was confirmed by an independent study from Norway in 2014 [44].

Despite these consistent correlations between degrees of aneuploidy and metastasis, the functional role of aneuploidy in metastasis remained unexplained [3, 4, 86, 87].

***Karyotypic relationships between the aneuploidies of cancers and their metastases***

Numerous independent studies found that the individual aneuploid karyotypes of metastases are related to those of individual primary cancers, but not to those of metastases of other cancers [20–46, 75, 88]. Metastases also have individual transcriptomes and gene mutations that are exclusively related to those of parental cancers [3, 11–18, 49–64, 89]. The 1-to-1 correlations between the individual karyotypes and individual transcriptomes of metastases indicate that these individual transcriptomes encode the individual phenotypes of metastases.

But in view of the individuality of the karyotypes and transcriptomes of metastases, compared to the expected common metastasis-specific mutations, a coherent theory of the role of the individual karyotypes and transcriptomes of metastases has not emerged. Therefore, we test here the theory that metastasis is a form of speciation, which predicts individual metastasis-specific karyotypes and phenotypes, rather than common mutations. This theory extends and confirms preliminary karyotypic evidence for metastasis from two labs including ours [43, 75, 88].

**Karyotypic origins of metastasis**

The theory that metastases are karyotypic subspecies of cancers is a logical extension of the theory that cancers are karyotypic species of their own [75, 90, 91]. According to this theory metastasis is the end product of a sequence of karyotypic variations (Fig. 1). This sequence of variations starts with the induction of random aneuploidy in normal cells (squares in Fig. 1) by carcinogens. Aneuploidy then catalyzes further random karyotypic variation of aneuploid cells (half-squares in Fig. 1) automatically, because aneuploidy unbalances thousands of genes including mitosis-genes, at aneuploidy-dependent rates (r2, Fig. 1). Most such random variants perish. Stochastically, very rare karyotypic variants of aneuploid cells form new autonomous cancer cells (circles in Fig. 1) at very low, aneuploidy-dependent rates (r3, Fig. 1). Owing to the inherent instability of cancer-specific aneuploidy cancer karyotypes vary within margins defined by selection for cancer-specific autonomy, again at aneuploidy-dependent rates (r2, Fig. 1). Eventually, very rare new autonomous variants or new subspecies arise from cancers with metastatic or other new phenotypes, like drug-resistance at low aneuploidy-dependent rates (r4, Fig. 1).

One may argue, however, that cancers are not species, because they lack a natural habitat beyond their original host. The American evolutionary biologist Lee Van Valen acknowledged this reservation, because "cancer cells depend for their existence on the continuation of the practice of tissue culture". But Van Valen maintained that this "wholely artificial" habitat is not an argument against the species definition of cancers, "the expected persistence of its habitat is never used as a criterion for judging the reality of a species, but rather for judging its susceptibility to extinction" [92]. Moreover, unbeknown to Van Valen several cancers have found niches for infinite natural transmissions without natural graft resistance in dogs [93], Tasmanian devils [88, 93] and clams [94]. Thus cancers are species, although their natural habitats are restricted.

In the following we have tested the theory that metastases are subspecies of cancers by comparing the karyotypes of seven independent cancers with corresponding metastases.

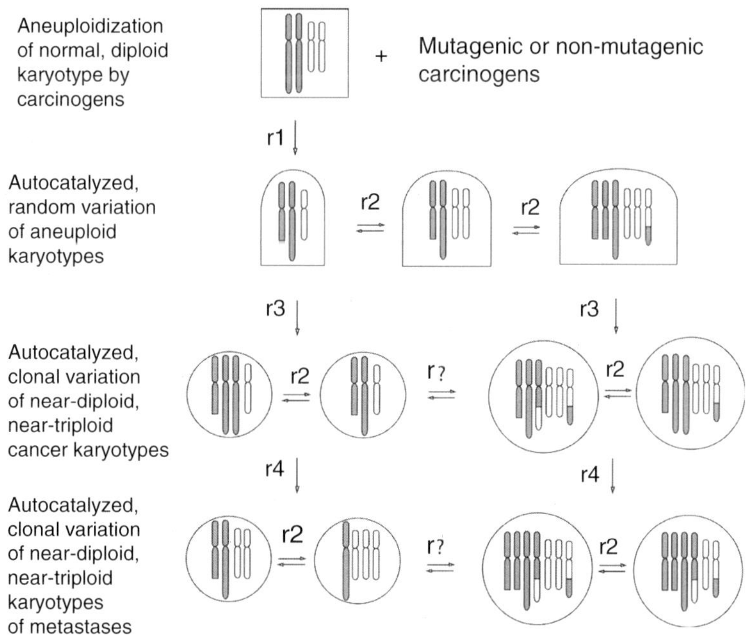


**Fig. 1** Karyotypic theory of metastasis. According to the karyotypic theory mutagenic and non-mutagenic carcinogens induce random aneuploidy in normal cells at carcinogen-dependent rates, r1. Aneuploidy then auto-catalyzes further random karyotypic variation, because it unbalances thousands of genes including mitosis-genes at aneuploidy-dependent rates, r2. Most such random variants perish. Rare karyotypic variants, however, form new autonomous cancer species with near-diploid, hypo-diploid or hyper-diploid karyotypes at very low rates, r3, because the probability to form a new autonomous cell is very low [75–77, 104, 105, 109, 135]. Owing to the inherent instability of aneuploidy, the karyotypes of new cancer species vary at aneuploidy-dependent rates, r2, within margins that are defined by selection for cancer-specific autonomy. As a result of this inherent variability of cancer karyotypes, new autonomous karyotypic subspecies with metastatic phenotypes arise stochastically. Since the probability of forming new autonomous subspecies by random variation of cancer karyotypes is very low – as in conventional subspeciation – metastases would occur typically at low rates, r4, such as the 10^-8 per-cell rate described in the Background in reference [9]. These rates are still higher than those of carcinogenesis from normal cells, r3 [136]. The Figure also records graphically our results that the karyotypic complexity of cancers is highly conserved in metastases. Thus hyper-triploid cancers formed hyper-triploid metastases and near-diploid cancers formed near-diploid metastases. There was no evidence of spontaneous alterations of the clonal karyotypic complexity of cancers or metastases; hence 'r?' in Fig. 1

## Results and discussion

### Karyotypic and phenotypic relationships between metastases and parental cancers

As a first test of our theory that metastases are subspecies of cancers, we analyzed the karyotypic and cellular phenotypic relationships between seven published pairs of cancers and metastases:

(1) The breast cancer, HIM-2 and a brain metastasis, HIM-5 [16].
(2) The melanoma, WM-115 and a metastasis of undefined origin, WM-266-4 [21–23]. It is demonstrated in Fig. 3 that both cancers analyzed here derived from an unknown common precursor.
(3) The liver cancer, H2P and a metastasis in the portal vein to the liver, H2M [35].
(4) The medulloblastoma, M-458 and a metastasis from a cerebrospinal fluid relapse, M-425 [95, 96]. A comparison between the M-458 and M-425 received in 2014 for this study with those published previously by Bigner et al. in 1991 revealed a discrepancy in chromosome copy numbers, although marker chromosomes were conserved. As a result Dr. Bigner left it up to us to decide, which variant was the original cancer or metastasis. Based on our results, e.g. the higher growth rate, growth in suspension and higher clonality of M-425 compared to M-458 described below, we named M-425 the metastasis.
(5) The colon cancer, SW-480 and a lymph node metastasis, SW-620 [97–101] with evidence, shown below, that both are derivatives of an unknown common precursor.
(6) The melanoma, IGR-39 from a leg and a metastasis from the groin, IGR-37 [102].
(7) The pancreatic cancer, A13-B and two independent metastases, a pancreatic metastasis A13-A and a liver metastasis A13-D [43].

The provenance of these cancers and corresponding metastases, and the conditions under which they were propagated are described in Methods.

The theory that metastases are subspecies of cancers makes two testable predictions: (1) Each pair of a cancer and corresponding metastasis is karyotypically related. (2) Each pair is also distinct in cancer- and metastasis-specific karyotypic and phenotypic markers. To test these predictions we compared the karyotypes and

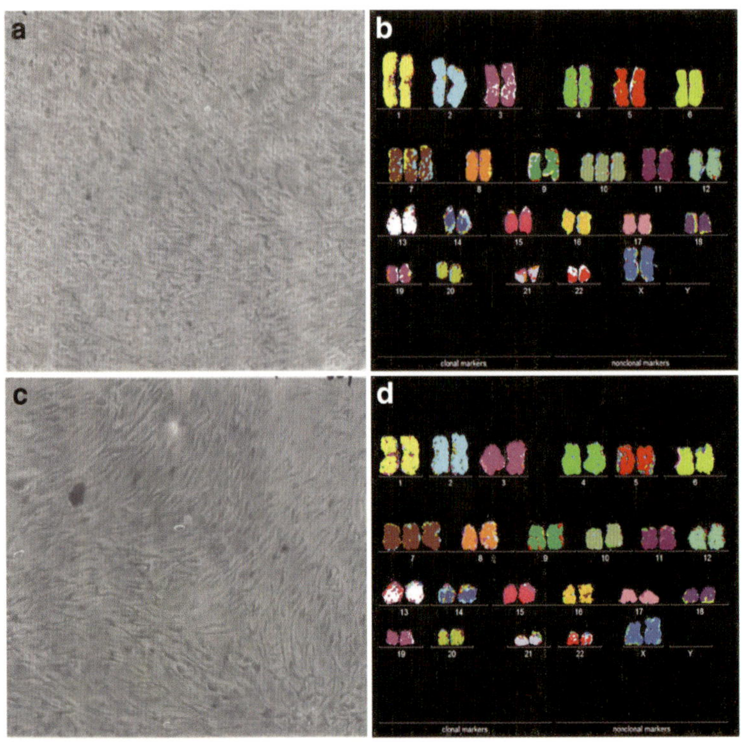


**Fig. 2** Cellular morphologies and karyotypes of breast cancer HIM-2 (**a**, **b**) and of a corresponding brain metastasis HIM-5 (**c**, **d**). The comparisons show that the primary cancer HIM-2 and corresponding metastasis HIM-5 have very similar but distinct cell morphologies (**a**, **c**) and karyotypes (**b**, **d**). Both primary cancer and metastasis have near diploid karyotypes with the same numbers and structures of chromosomes, except for a trisomy 10 that is missing in the metastasis HIM-5 (**d**). The cells were photographed at 120X in cell culture dishes (Methods). The cells of the primary cancer were found to be more refractive and growing at modestly higher rates than the metastasis. The chromosomes were prepared from metaphase-cells and color-coded as described in Methods

morphological cellular phenotypes of each of these seven cancer-metastasis pairs.

As can be seen in Figs. 2, 3, 4, 5, 6, 7, 8, the results of these tests revealed the following similarities and dissimilarities between cancers and corresponding metastases:

1) The microscopic cellular phenotypes of all seven cancers were similar to, but also distinct from those of the corresponding metastases. In addition we found non-microscopic distinctions that set apart cancers from metastases. For example, the cellular growth rate of the primary melanoma WM-115, shown in Fig. 3, was about five-fold lower than that of the metastasis WM-266-4. Likewise the growth rate of the primary melanoma IGR-37 was lower than that of the corresponding metastasis IGR-39 (Fig. 7). The primary medulloblastoma M-458 also differed from the corresponding metastasis M-425 in two physiological characteristics: The M-458 cancer cells grew slower than those of the metastasis M-425; and the M-458 cells were mostly attached to the culture dish, whereas the cells of the metastasis grew mostly in suspension, hence out of focus in Fig. 5.
2) The numbers of chromosomes of all seven cancers were very similar to, but not identical to those of the corresponding metastases.
3) The karyotypes of all seven cancers shared a majority of structurally and numerically-defined aneusomies with corresponding metastases. But they also all differed from each other in distinct cancer- and metastasis-specific aneusomies.
4) The phenotypic and karyotypic differences between cancers and metastases were roughly proportional to the degrees of cancer specific of aneuploidy: The more aneuploid the cancer, the more different are the karyotypes of cancers from those of corresponding metastases. For example, it is shown Fig. 2 that the near-diploid breast cancer HIM-2 differed from the brain metastasis HIM-5 only in the loss of one of two trisomies, namely trisomy 10. By contrast the six near-triploid cancers shown in Figs. 3, 4, 5, 6, 7, 8, differed

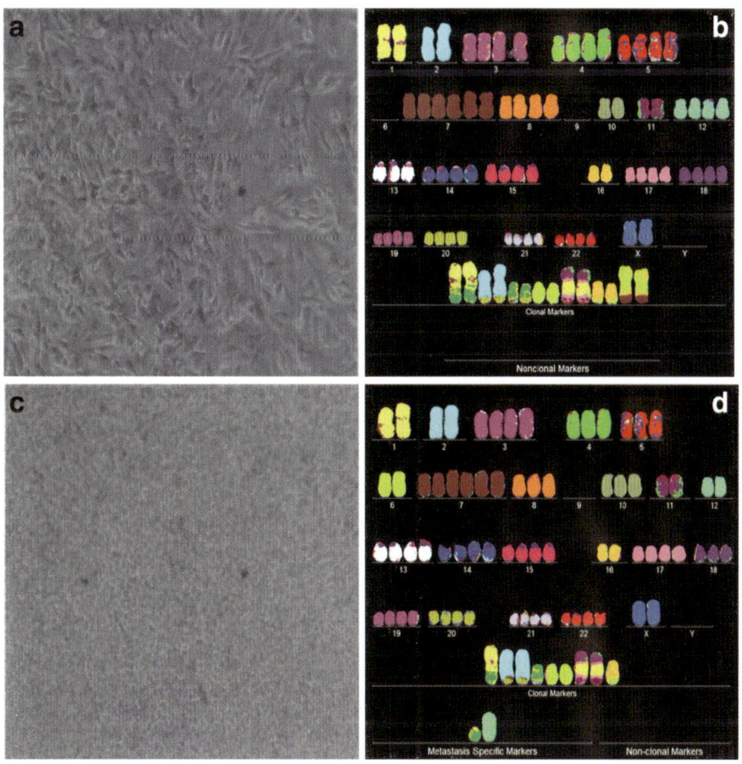


**Fig. 3** Cellular morphologies and karyotypes of melanoma WM-115 (**a**, **b**) and a corresponding metastasis WM-266-4 (**c**, **d**). The comparisons show that the primary cancer WM-115 and the corresponding metastasis WM-266-4 have similar, but distinct cell morphologies (**a**, **c**) and karyotypes (**b**, **d**). Both primary cancer and metastasis have hyper-triploid karyotypes with similar numbers of chromosomes and aneusomies and both lack intact chromosome 9. They also differ from each other in the total numbers of chromosomes and in the structures of some marker chromosomes (see Tables 1 and 2). The absence of normal chromosomes 6 from the presumed primary and the presence of "primary specific" marker chromosomes 6 indicate that both the presumed primary and the metastasis derived from an unknown primary with normal chromosomes 6. The cells were propagated and karyotyped as described for Fig. 2

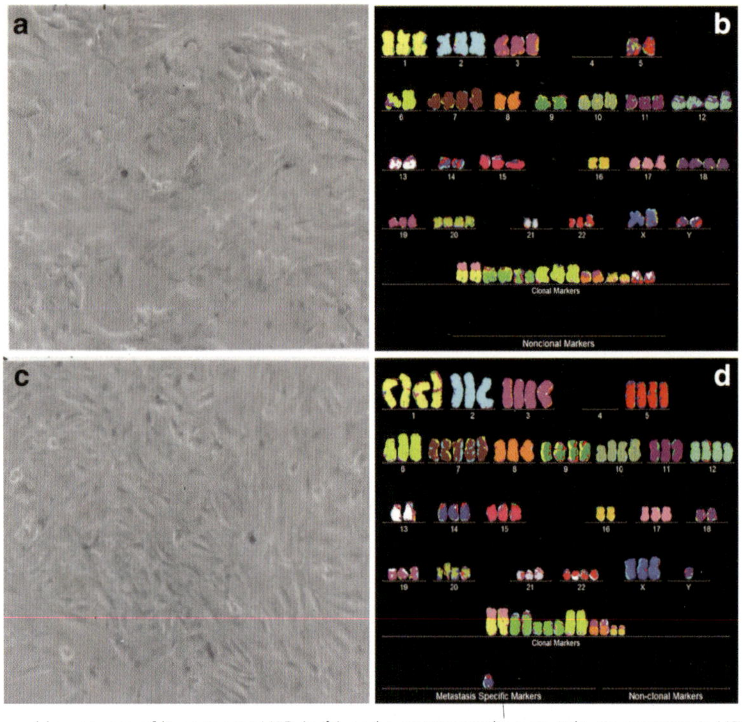


**Fig. 4** Cellular morphologies and karyotypes of liver cancer H2P (**a**, **b**) and a corresponding portal vein metastasis H2M (**c**, **d**). The comparisons show that the primary cancer H2P and the corresponding metastasis H2M have similar, but distinct cell morphologies (**a**, **c**) and karyotypes (**b**, **d**). Both primary cancer and metastasis have hyper-triploid karyotypes with similar numbers of chromosomes and aneusomies, and both lack intact chromosome 4. They differ from each other in the total numbers of chromosomes and in the structures of some marker chromosomes (see Tables 1 and 2). The cells were propagated and karyotyped as described for Fig. 2

from the corresponding metastases in high percentages of their constituent aneusomies (see also below).

We deduce from these comparative analyses that the karyotypes and phenotypes of metastases are exclusively related to, but also distinct from parental cancers – exactly as predicted by the theory that metastases are subspecies of cancers. Our observations that metastases appear to conserve the average numbers of parental chromosomes and conserve many parental aneusomies further supports the subspeciation theory – as conventional species typically conserve the genetic complexities and most of the karyotypes of their precursors [103].

It could be argued, however, that the differences setting apart the karyotypes of metastasis from parental cancers shown in Figs. 2, 3, 4, 5, 6, 7, 8 are random karyotypic variants generated by the inherent instability of cancer-specific aneuploidy, and that as yet un-identified gene mutations generate metastases from cancers. If that were correct, the karyotypes of metastases would not be stabilized by selection for autonomy and thus would not be clonal, and the numbers of their chromosomes would not, or not consistently be close to those of parental cancers.

By contrast, if metastases were karyotypic subspecies of cancers, their karyotypes would be clonally related to parental cancers and would be stabilized by selection for autonomy - like those of parental cancers and of conventional species.

To distinguish between these possibilities we next have investigated, whether the karyotypes of metastases are clonal and are clonally related to parental cancers.

### Metastases are karyotypic subspecies of cancers

To prove that cancers cause metastases by karyotypic variation rather than by gene mutation, we need evidence that the karyotypes of metastases are clonal and clonally related to parental karyotypes.

To determine karyotypic clonality, the karyotypes of multiple cells of a metastasis and of a primary cancer must be compared and shown to be identical. But, owing to the inherent variability or flexibility of cancer karyotypes and the resulting clonal heterogeneity of cancers [75, 88, 104, 105] (Background), the determination of clonality of karyotypes is often obscured in conventional karyotypic analyses of cancers by clonal heterogeneity [7, 106, 107].

Therefore, we have recently developed a technique, which determines karyotypic clonality based on the clonality of its constituent chromosomes, rather than on the karyotypes as a whole. This technique is able to detect karyotypic

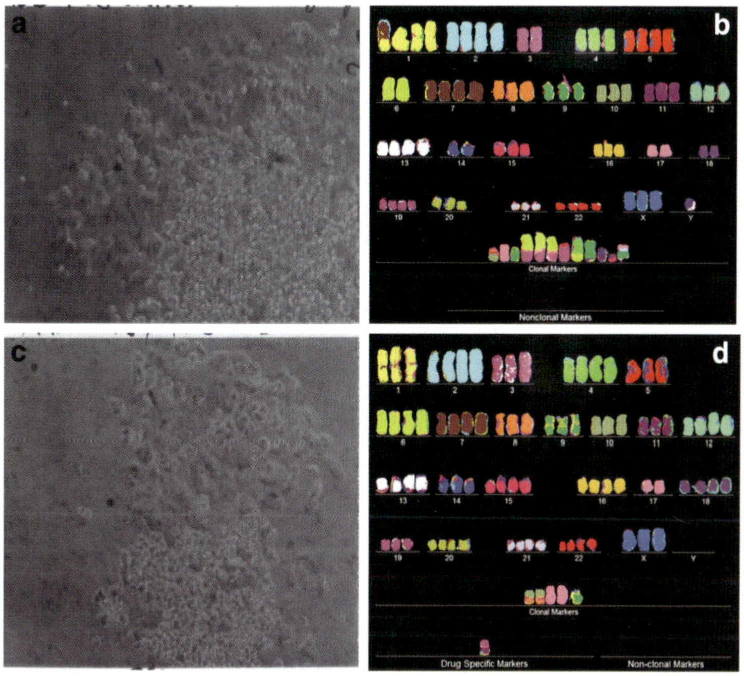


**Fig. 5** Cellular morphologies and karyotypes of medulloblastoma M-458 (**a**, **b**) and a corresponding metastasis M-425 (**c**, **d**). The comparisons show again that the primary cancer M-458 and the corresponding metastasis M-425 have similar, but distinct cell morphologies (**a**, **c**) and karyotypes (**b**, **d**). Some of the metastatic M-425 cells grew in suspension (One reason, why M-425 was named the metastasis. See note above in this section.), while the rest was attached to the culture dish. The karyotypes of both the primary cancer and the metastasis are hyper-triploid and have similar numbers of chromosomes and of aneusomies. But they also differ in the total numbers of chromosomes and in the structures of some individual marker chromosomes (see Tables 1 and 2). The cells were propagated and karyotyped as described for Fig. 2

clonality, even if a minority of the chromosomes of a given karyotype is non clonal [76, 108, 109] (Background). The technique arrays the copy numbers of individual chromosomes of 20 cancer karyotypes in 3-dimensional tables. These tables list the numbers of individual chromosomes and of individual marker chromosomes on the x-axis, the copy numbers of the chromosomes and marker chromosomes on the y-axis, and the numbers of karyotypes/metaphases analyzed on the z-axis. The resulting pattern is therefore called a karyotype array. In such arrays, karyotypes with clonal chromosome copy numbers form easily recognizable parallel lines. The arrays shown here also include tables that list the percentages of clonality of each chromosome. The percentages of chromosomal clonality have been calculated from primary data of all chromosomes of all karyotypes analyzed here (Figs. 9c, d; 10c; 11c; 12c, d; 13d,e; 14c and 15d).

As shown in the karyotype arrays of all seven cancers and of the corresponding metastases, the karyotypes of all seven cancers and corresponding metastases were mostly 70–100% clonal (Figs. 9, 10, 11, 12, 13, 14, 15). The 0–30% of non-clonal sets of chromosomes or aneusomies reflects the inherent instability of aneuploidy (Background).

We note that we have counted here all sets of identical chromosomes as aneusomies, including even diploid normal chromosomes of aneuploid cancers. This was justified by the facts that even diploid sets of normal chromosomes are less than 100% diploid in cancers owing to the inherent instability of aneuploid karyotypes (see Figs. 9, 10, 11, 12, 13, 14, 15 and [110]) and that the functions of diploid sets of normal chromosomes are altered in aneuploid karyotypes [111]. In a previous study of metastasis we have termed such aneusomies "chromosomal units" for the same reasons [43].

Table 1 presents a summary of the karyotypic relationships between the seven cancers and corresponding metastases based on shared and individual aneusomies, which is shown below on page 18. The data for this table were derived from Figs. 9, 10, 11, 12, 13, 14, 15.

As can be seen in this table, the clonal diversities between cancers and metastases increased with increasing degrees of cancer-specific aneuploidies as follows:

(1) The near-diploid breast cancer HIM-2 shared 96% and its clonal aneusomies with the near-diploid metastasis HIM-5.

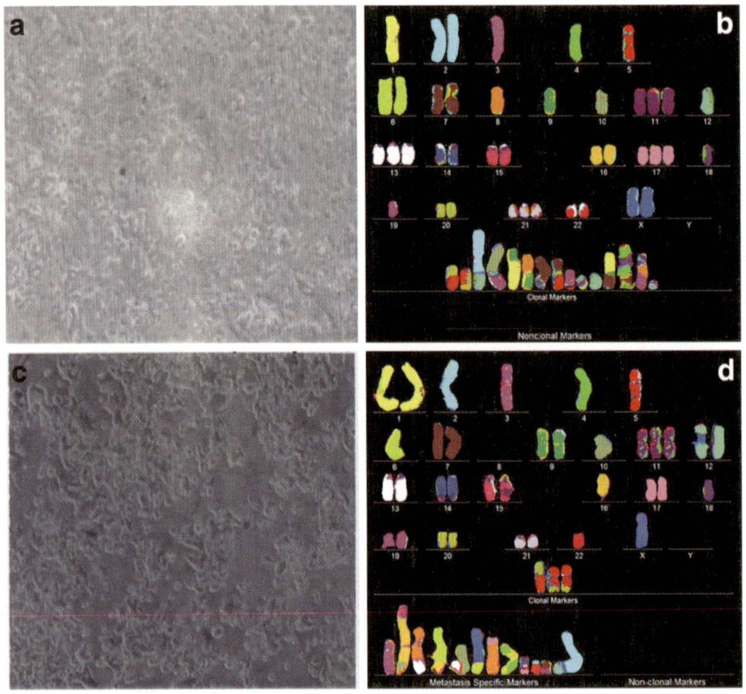


**Fig. 6** Cellular morphologies and karyotypes of colon cancer SW-480 (**a**, **b**) and of a corresponding metastasis SW-620 (**c**, **d**). The comparisons show once more that the primary cancer SW-480 and the corresponding metastasis SW-620 have similar, but distinct cell morphologies (**a**, **c**) and karyotypes (**b**, **d**). Both primary cancer and metastasis have hyper-diploid karyotypes with similar numbers of chromosomes and of aneusomies. They also differ from each other in the total numbers of chromosomes and in the structures of some marker chromosomes (see Tables 1 and 2). We adduce evidence in the text that both SW-480 and SW-620 are probably both metastases of an unknown primary. The cells were propagated and karyotyped as described for Fig. 2

(2) The hyper-diploid melanoma WM-115 shared 60% of its clonal aneusomies with the hyper-diploid metastasis WM-266-4.
(3) The hyper-triploid liver cancer H2P shared 52% of its clonal aneusomies with the hyper-triploid metastasis H2M.
(4) The hyper-triploid medulloblastoma M-458 shared 32% of its clonal aneusomies with the hyper-triploid metastasis M-425.
(5) The hyper-triploid colon cancer SW-480 Clone-1 shared 34% of its clonal aneusomies with the hyper-triploid metastasis or presumed metastasis SW-620 [97–99]. And SW-480 Clone-2 shared 29% of its clonal aneusomies with SW-620.
(6) The hyper-tetraploid melanoma IGR-39 shared 13% of its clonal aneusomies with the hyper-triploid metastasis IGR-37. But the size of this numerical discrepancy reflects in part the ploidy-shift of IGR-39 from hyper-tetraploid in the cancer to hyper-triploid in the metastasis.
(7) The hypo-triploid pancreatic cancer A13-B shared 44% of its clonal aneusomies with the hypo-triploid metastasis A13-A and 60% of its clonal aneusomies with the hypo-triploid metastasis A13-D, which confirmed and extended a previous study of ours [43].

Regarding the evaluations of the relationships between cancers and metastases based on aneusomies we point out that non-identical numerical aneusomies are typically still related, as for example the trisomy 1 of the cancer H2P versus the tetrasomy 1 in the corresponding metastasis (Fig. 11a). Likewise even structurally distinct aneusomies tend to contain common chromosomal elements. Thus the comparisons based on distinct aneusomies minimize the relationships. This effect is, however, compensated by the juxtaposition of their karyotype arrays, which favor relationships by comparing patterns of all aneusomies as a whole.

In sum all metastases analyzed here confirm the theory that metastases are individual subclones or subspecies of parental cancers, differing from parental cancers in metastasis-specific clonal aneusomies rather than in "elusive" gene mutations [3]. If gene mutations would generate metastases, metastases would have the same karyotypes as parental cancers, but this was not observed. Moreover, if gene mutations were sufficient

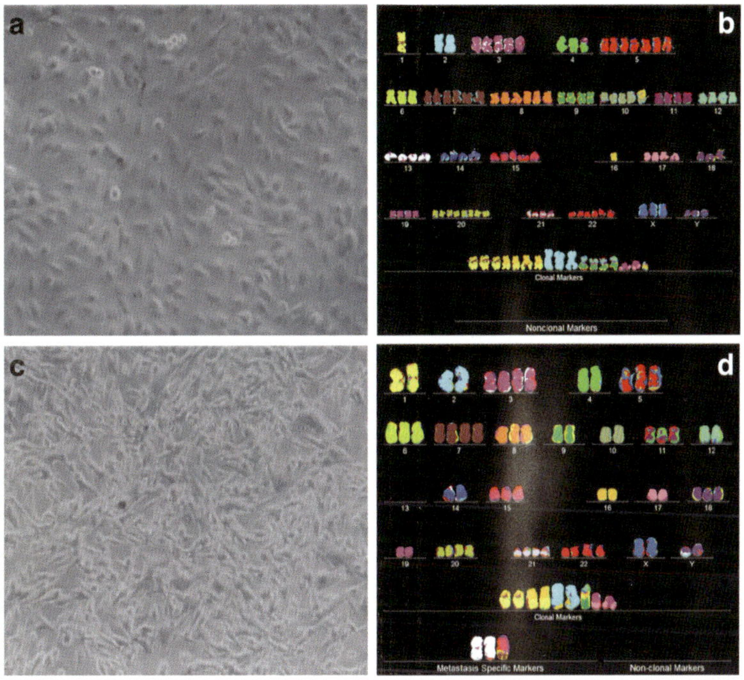

**Fig. 7** Cellular morphologies and karyotypes of melanoma IGR-39 (**a**, **b**) and of a corresponding metastasis IGR-37 (**c**, **d**). The comparisons show once more that the primary melanoma IGR-39 and the corresponding metastasis IGR-37 have similar, but distinct cell morphologies (**a**, **c**) and that their karyotypes are closely related but differ in ploidy number (**b**, **d**). The primary cancer has a hyper-tetraploid karyotype and the metastasis a closely related, but hyper-triploid karyotype. The relationship is based on chromosome copy numbers that differ from each other by the ploidy factor that sets apart the two karyotypes. The karyotypes also differ from each other in several individual chromosome numbers and in several individual marker chromosomes (see Tables 1 and 2). The cells were propagated and karyotyped as described for Fig. 2 and in the text

to confer metastatic phenotypes to cancer, the risk of metastases would be independent of the cancer karyotype. But this was also not observed here as in numerous studies in the past (see Background).

The karyotypic analyses summarized in Table 1 also show the divergence of the karyotypes of metastases from cancers was proportional to degrees of aneuploidy of the parental cancer: The more aneuploid the cancer the more it differs karyotypically from corresponding metastases. This supports the prediction of our theory that cancer-specific aneuploidy catalyzes metastasis by karyotypic variation (Background).

Unexpectedly our comparisons also showed that the total numbers of aneusomies of cancers and of corresponding metastases were consistently very close in all seven pairs of cancers and metastases compared – irrespective of the percentages of aneusomies exchanged in metastasis (Table 1). In view of this conservation of aneusomic complexity between metastases and corresponding cancers, we asked next whether this conservation of aneusomic complexity also applied to the numbers of all constituent chromosomes shared by cancers and metastases and thus to the karyotype as a whole.

### Conservation of the complexity of cancer karyotypes in metastasis

In view of the conservation of cancer-specific aneusomic complexity in metastases (Table 1) we hypothesized that the autonomy of cancers is encoded in the karyotype as a whole and that metastases conserve the specific parental autonomy via the complexity of the parental karyotype. According to this hypothesis cancers acquire new, metastasis-specific host ranges from lateral karyotypic variations between cancers and metastases that do not affect the complexity of the karyotype.

To test the conservation of the complexity of cancer karyotypes in metastases, we compared the average numbers of the chromosomes and the aneusomies of each of the seven cancers to those of the corresponding metastases based on the karyotypic data listed in Figs. 8, 9, 10, 11, 12, 13, 14, 15. The results of these comparisons are summarized in Table 2, which is shown below on page 18. As can be seen in Table 2 the average numbers of all chromosomes, like those of the aneusomies of all seven metastases were almost identical to those of the parental cancers. Even the clonal variabilities of these numbers based on standard deviations were the same. Accordingly each cancer-metastasis pair shared

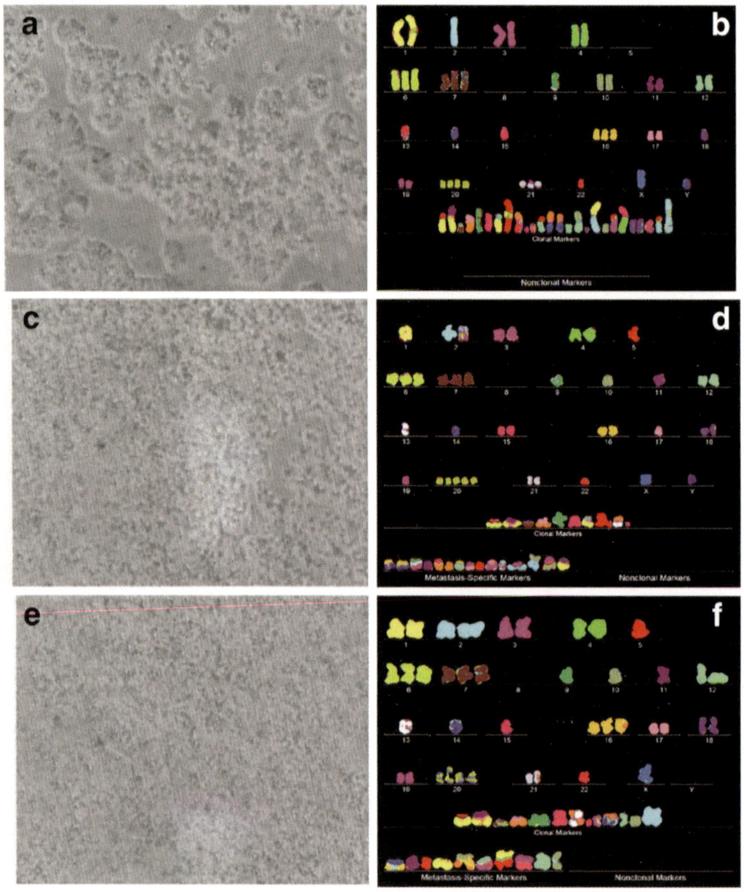


**Fig. 8** Cellular morphologies and karyotypes of pancreatic cancer A13-B (**a**, **b**) and of two corresponding metastases, a pancreatic metastasis A13-A (**c**, **d**) and a liver metastasis A13-D (**e**, **f**). The comparisons show once more that the primary cancer A13-B and the corresponding metastases A13-A and A13-D have similar, but distinct cell morphologies (**a**, **c**, **e**) and karyotypes (**b**, **d**, **f**). The primary cancer and both metastases have hyper-diploid karyotypes with similar numbers of chromosomes and of aneusomies. The primary and the two metastases differ from each other in the total numbers of chromosomes and in the structures of some individual marker chromosomes see Tables 1 and 2). The cells were propagated and karyotyped as described for Fig. 2 [103]

individual ratios of the numbers chromosomes to the numbers of aneusomies.

There was but one partial exception to this rule that cancer-specific complexity is conserved in metastasis, namely the transformation of melanoma IGR-39 to the metastasis IGR-37, which underwent an apparent ploidy reduction during transformation to metastasis (Table 2). This ploidy shift is indicated here in Table 2 by a decrease in the ratio of chromosome numbers per aneusomies from 3.5 to 2.2. The apparent ploidy shift in metastasis M-425 reflects a loss of parental marker chromosomes and a gain of copy numbers of corresponding intact chromosomes (Fig. 12), thereby maintaining the overall complexity of the cancer in the metastasis.

In view of this we note that karyotypic polyploidization or de-polyploidization does not change the relative proportions of genes within a karyotype and thus not change phenotypes directly. But ploidy variation in cancer cells is typically not exactly even, and is another independent characteristic of cancer cells that may increase or decrease oncogenicity by changing the dosage of genes evenly and non-evenly [76, 77, 112–114]. Its occurrence also seems to be proportional to the degree of cancer-specific aneuploidy [76, 115]. Balanced ploidy changes also occur in the development of some normal animal [116] and plant cells [117] and thus enhance the general output of cells.

In sum our data support the hypothesis that the autonomy of individual cancers is maintained by the karyotype as a whole and is therefore conserved in cancers and corresponding metastases within narrow limits of variation (see Fig. 1, Background). This hypothesis explains prior observations of the conservation of karyotypic complexity in metastasis described by Pearse et al. [88] and us [43, 75].

Conservation of karyotypic and genetic complexity is also observed in conventional Darwinian speciation of mammals, in which new species share with predecessors the same genetic complexity and similar karyotypes [103, 118].

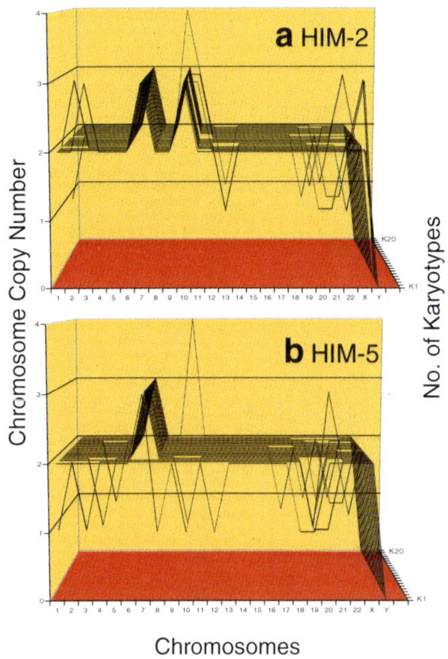


Primary Breast Cancer HIM-2 and Metastatis HIM-5

| | HIM-2 | HIM-5 |
|---|---|---|
| Avg # of chromosomes ± SD | 48±1 | 47±1.6 |
| chromosome # | copy no (% clonal) | |
| 1 | 2 (95) | 2 (95) |
| 2 | 2 (95) | 2 (100) |
| 3 | 2 (95) | 2 (95) |
| 4 | 2 (100) | 2 (90) |
| 5 | 2 (100) | 2 (100) |
| 6 | 2 (100) | 2 (100) |
| 7 | 3 (100) | 3 (90) |
| 8 | 2 (100) | 2 (95) |
| 9 | 2 (100) | 2 (100) |
| 10 | 3 (95) | 2 (85) |
| 11 | 2 (80) | 2 (100) |
| 12 | 2 (100) | 2 (95) |
| 13 | 2 (85) | 2 (100) |
| 14 | 2 (100) | 2 (100) |
| 15 | 2 (100) | 2 (100) |
| 16 | 2 (100) | 2 (100) |
| 17 | 2 (100) | 2 (95) |
| 18 | 2 (100) | 2 (95) |
| 19 | 2 (95) | 2 (75) |
| 20 | 2 (90) | 2 (85) |
| 21 | 2 (85) | 2 (90) |
| 22 | 2 (85) | 2 (90) |
| X | 2 (90) | 2 (100) |
| Y | - | - |
| Total Clonal Aneusomies | 23 | 23 |

**c** Complete karyotypes of 20 HIM-2 cells

| Total # of Chromosomes | 73 | 73 | 73 | 75 | 71 | 71 | 71 | 71 | 71 | 75 | 73 | 75 | 71 | 71 | 71 | 71 | 71 | 71 | 71 | 71 | |
|---|---|---|---|---|---|---|---|---|---|---|---|---|---|---|---|---|---|---|---|---|---|
| Chromosome # | K1 | K2 | K3 | K4 | K5 | K6 | K7 | K8 | K9 | K10 | K11 | K12 | K13 | K14 | K15 | K16 | K17 | K18 | K19 | K20 | |
| 1 | 2 | 2 | 2 | 2 | 2 | 2 | 2 | 2 | 2 | 2 | 1 | 2 | 2 | 2 | 2 | 2 | 2 | 2 | 2 | 2 | |
| 2 | 2 | 2 | 2 | 3 | 2 | 2 | 2 | 2 | 2 | 2 | 2 | 2 | 2 | 2 | 2 | 2 | 2 | 2 | 2 | 2 | |
| 3 | 3 | 2 | 2 | 2 | 2 | 2 | 2 | 2 | 2 | 2 | 2 | 2 | 2 | 2 | 2 | 2 | 2 | 2 | 2 | 2 | |
| 4 | 2 | 2 | 2 | 2 | 2 | 2 | 2 | 2 | 2 | 2 | 2 | 2 | 2 | 2 | 2 | 2 | 2 | 2 | 2 | 2 | |
| 5 | 2 | 2 | 2 | 2 | 2 | 2 | 2 | 2 | 2 | 2 | 2 | 2 | 2 | 2 | 2 | 2 | 2 | 2 | 2 | 2 | |
| 6 | 2 | 2 | 2 | 2 | 2 | 2 | 2 | 2 | 2 | 2 | 2 | 2 | 2 | 2 | 2 | 2 | 2 | 2 | 2 | 2 | |
| 7 | 3 | 3 | 3 | 3 | 3 | 3 | 3 | 3 | 3 | 3 | 3 | 3 | 3 | 3 | 3 | 3 | 3 | 3 | 3 | 3 | |
| 8 | 2 | 2 | 2 | 2 | 2 | 2 | 2 | 2 | 2 | 2 | 2 | 2 | 2 | 2 | 2 | 2 | 2 | 2 | 2 | 2 | |
| 9 | 2 | 2 | 2 | 2 | 2 | 2 | 2 | 2 | 2 | 2 | 2 | 2 | 2 | 2 | 2 | 2 | 2 | 2 | 2 | 2 | |
| 10 | 3 | 3 | 3 | 3 | 3 | 3 | 3 | 3 | 3 | 3 | 3 | 4 | 3 | 3 | 3 | 3 | 3 | 3 | 3 | 3 | |
| 11 | 2 | 3 | 2 | 2 | 2 | 2 | 2 | 2 | 2 | 3 | 3 | 3 | 2 | 2 | 2 | 2 | 2 | 2 | 2 | 2 | |
| 12 | 2 | 2 | 2 | 2 | 2 | 2 | 2 | 2 | 2 | 2 | 2 | 2 | 2 | 2 | 2 | 2 | 2 | 2 | 2 | 2 | |
| 13 | 2 | 2 | 2 | 2 | 1 | 1 | 2 | 2 | 2 | 2 | 2 | 2 | 2 | 2 | 2 | 2 | 2 | 2 | 1 | 2 | |
| 14 | 2 | 2 | 2 | 2 | 2 | 2 | 2 | 2 | 2 | 2 | 2 | 2 | 2 | 2 | 2 | 2 | 2 | 2 | 2 | 2 | |
| 15 | 2 | 2 | 2 | 2 | 2 | 2 | 2 | 2 | 2 | 2 | 2 | 2 | 2 | 2 | 2 | 2 | 2 | 2 | 2 | 2 | |
| 16 | 2 | 2 | 2 | 2 | 2 | 2 | 2 | 2 | 2 | 2 | 2 | 2 | 2 | 2 | 2 | 2 | 2 | 2 | 2 | 2 | |
| 17 | 2 | 2 | 2 | 2 | 2 | 2 | 2 | 2 | 2 | 2 | 2 | 2 | 2 | 2 | 2 | 2 | 2 | 2 | 2 | 2 | |
| 18 | 2 | 2 | 2 | 2 | 2 | 2 | 2 | 2 | 2 | 2 | 2 | 2 | 2 | 2 | 2 | 2 | 2 | 2 | 2 | 2 | |
| 19 | 2 | 2 | 2 | 2 | 2 | 2 | 2 | 2 | 2 | 2 | 2 | 1 | 2 | 2 | 2 | 2 | 2 | 2 | 2 | 2 | |
| 20 | 2 | 2 | 2 | 2 | 2 | 1 | 2 | 2 | 2 | 2 | 2 | 2 | 2 | 2 | 2 | 2 | 2 | 1 | 2 | 2 | |
| 21 | 2 | 2 | 2 | 2 | 2 | 1 | 2 | 2 | 2 | 2 | 2 | 1 | 2 | 2 | 2 | 2 | 2 | 2 | 2 | 1 | |
| 22 | 2 | 2 | 2 | 2 | 1 | 2 | 2 | 2 | 2 | 3 | 2 | 1 | 2 | 2 | 2 | 2 | 2 | 2 | 2 | 2 | |
| X | 2 | 2 | 3 | 3 | 2 | 2 | 2 | 2 | 2 | 2 | 2 | 2 | 2 | 2 | 2 | 2 | 2 | 2 | 2 | 2 | |
| Y | 0 | 0 | 0 | 0 | 0 | 0 | 0 | 0 | 0 | 0 | 0 | 0 | 0 | 0 | 0 | 0 | 0 | 0 | 0 | 0 | **Average±SD** |
| **Non-Clonal Aneusomies** | **1** | **1** | **1** | **2** | **2** | **3** | **0** | **0** | **0** | **2** | **2** | **5** | **0** | **0** | **0** | **0** | **0** | **1** | **1** | **1** | **1±1** |
| **Aneusomies per Karyotype** | **23** | **23** | **23** | **23** | **23** | **23** | **23** | **23** | **23** | **23** | **23** | **23** | **23** | **23** | **23** | **23** | **23** | **23** | **23** | **23** | **23±0** |

**d** Complete karyotypes of 20 HIM-5 cells

| Total No of Chromosomes | 42 | 42 | 46 | 45 | 46 | 47 | 47 | 47 | 46 | 47 | 47 | 46 | 47 | 47 | 45 | 45 | 47 | 45 | 47 | 49 | |
|---|---|---|---|---|---|---|---|---|---|---|---|---|---|---|---|---|---|---|---|---|---|
| Chromosome # | K1 | K2 | K3 | K4 | K5 | K6 | K7 | K8 | K9 | K10 | K11 | K12 | K13 | K14 | K15 | K16 | K17 | K18 | K19 | K20 | |
| 1 | 2 | 1 | 2 | 2 | 2 | 2 | 2 | 2 | 2 | 2 | 2 | 2 | 2 | 2 | 2 | 2 | 2 | 2 | 2 | 2 | |
| 2 | 2 | 2 | 2 | 2 | 2 | 2 | 2 | 2 | 2 | 2 | 2 | 2 | 2 | 2 | 2 | 2 | 2 | 2 | 2 | 2 | |
| 3 | 2 | 1 | 2 | 2 | 2 | 2 | 2 | 2 | 2 | 2 | 2 | 2 | 2 | 2 | 2 | 2 | 2 | 2 | 2 | 2 | |
| 4 | 2 | 2 | 2 | 1 | 2 | 2 | 2 | 2 | 2 | 2 | 2 | 2 | 2 | 2 | 2 | 1 | 2 | 2 | 2 | 2 | |
| 5 | 2 | 2 | 2 | 2 | 2 | 2 | 2 | 2 | 2 | 2 | 2 | 2 | 2 | 2 | 2 | 2 | 2 | 2 | 2 | 2 | |
| 6 | 2 | 2 | 2 | 2 | 2 | 2 | 2 | 2 | 2 | 2 | 2 | 2 | 2 | 2 | 2 | 2 | 2 | 2 | 2 | 2 | |
| 7 | 3 | 2 | 2 | 3 | 3 | 3 | 3 | 3 | 3 | 3 | 3 | 3 | 3 | 3 | 3 | 3 | 3 | 3 | 3 | 3 | |
| 8 | 1 | 2 | 2 | 2 | 2 | 2 | 2 | 2 | 2 | 2 | 2 | 2 | 2 | 2 | 2 | 2 | 2 | 2 | 2 | 2 | |
| 9 | 2 | 2 | 2 | 2 | 2 | 2 | 2 | 2 | 2 | 2 | 2 | 2 | 2 | 2 | 2 | 2 | 2 | 2 | 2 | 2 | |
| 10 | 1 | 2 | 2 | 2 | 1 | 2 | 2 | 2 | 2 | 2 | 2 | 2 | 2 | 2 | 2 | 2 | 2 | 2 | 2 | 4 | |
| 11 | 2 | 2 | 2 | 2 | 2 | 2 | 2 | 2 | 2 | 2 | 2 | 2 | 2 | 2 | 2 | 2 | 2 | 2 | 2 | 2 | |
| 12 | 1 | 2 | 2 | 2 | 2 | 2 | 2 | 2 | 2 | 2 | 2 | 2 | 2 | 2 | 2 | 2 | 2 | 2 | 2 | 2 | |
| 13 | 2 | 2 | 2 | 2 | 2 | 2 | 2 | 2 | 2 | 2 | 2 | 2 | 2 | 2 | 2 | 2 | 2 | 2 | 2 | 2 | |
| 14 | 2 | 2 | 2 | 2 | 2 | 2 | 2 | 2 | 2 | 2 | 2 | 2 | 2 | 2 | 2 | 2 | 2 | 2 | 2 | 2 | |
| 15 | 2 | 2 | 2 | 2 | 2 | 2 | 2 | 2 | 2 | 2 | 2 | 2 | 2 | 2 | 2 | 2 | 2 | 2 | 2 | 2 | |
| 16 | 2 | 2 | 2 | 2 | 2 | 2 | 2 | 2 | 2 | 2 | 2 | 2 | 2 | 2 | 2 | 2 | 2 | 2 | 2 | 2 | |
| 17 | 2 | 2 | 2 | 2 | 2 | 2 | 2 | 2 | 2 | 2 | 2 | 1 | 2 | 2 | 2 | 2 | 2 | 2 | 2 | 2 | |
| 18 | 1 | 2 | 2 | 2 | 2 | 2 | 2 | 2 | 2 | 2 | 2 | 2 | 2 | 2 | 2 | 2 | 2 | 2 | 2 | 2 | |
| 19 | 1 | 1 | 1 | 1 | 2 | 2 | 2 | 2 | 2 | 2 | 2 | 2 | 2 | 2 | 2 | 2 | 2 | 1 | 2 | 2 | |
| 20 | 2 | 1 | 3 | 2 | 2 | 2 | 2 | 2 | 2 | 2 | 2 | 2 | 2 | 2 | 2 | 1 | 2 | 2 | 2 | 2 | |
| 21 | 2 | 2 | 2 | 2 | 2 | 2 | 2 | 2 | 2 | 2 | 2 | 2 | 2 | 2 | 1 | 2 | 2 | 1 | 2 | 2 | |
| 22 | 2 | 2 | 2 | 2 | 2 | 2 | 2 | 2 | 1 | 2 | 2 | 2 | 2 | 2 | 1 | 2 | 2 | 2 | 2 | 2 | |
| X | 2 | 2 | 2 | 2 | 2 | 2 | 2 | 2 | 2 | 2 | 2 | 2 | 2 | 2 | 2 | 2 | 2 | 2 | 2 | 2 | |
| Y | 0 | 0 | 0 | 0 | 0 | 0 | 0 | 0 | 0 | 0 | 0 | 0 | 0 | 0 | 0 | 0 | 0 | 0 | 0 | 0 | **Average±SD** |
| **Non-Clonal Aneusomies** | **5** | **5** | **3** | **2** | **1** | **0** | **0** | **0** | **1** | **0** | **0** | **1** | **0** | **0** | **2** | **2** | **0** | **2** | **0** | **1** | **1.3±1.6** |
| **Aneusomies per Karyotype** | **23** | **23** | **23** | **23** | **23** | **23** | **23** | **23** | **23** | **20** | **22** | **21** | **23** | **23** | **23** | **23** | **23** | **23** | **23** | **23** | **23±0** |

**Fig. 9 a**, **b**, **c**, **d** Karyotypic evidence that the brain metastasis HIM-5 is an individual subspecies of the breast cancer HIM-2. The karyotypic theory of metastasis predicts that metastases have individual clonal karyotypes that differ from those of parental cancers in individual metastasis-specific aneusomies. To test this theory we have compared karyotype-arrays of the brain metastasis HIM-5 to that of the primary cancer HIM-2. Karyotype arrays are three-dimensional tables of 20 karyotypes, which list the chromosome numbers of arrayed karyotypes on the x-axis, the copy numbers of each chromosome on the y-axis, and the number of karyotypes arrayed on the z-axis, as detailed in Results (Section, Metastases are karyotypic subspecies of cancers). Figure 9 **a**, **b** and the attached table show that 85 to 100% of the chromosomes of the cancer HIM-2 and the metastasis HIM-5 were clonal, and that cancer and metastasis formed very similar clonal patterns. The karyotype of the metastasis differed from that of the primary only in the loss of trisomy 10. The copy numbers of the non-clonal chromosomes differed from the clonal averages typically ±1 (see Fig. 9 **a**,**b** and specifically Fig. 9 **c**,**d**). These non-clonal copy numbers represent the ongoing karyotypic variation predicted by the inherent variability of cancer-specific aneuploidy (Background). We conclude that the brain metastasis HIM-5 is a subspecies of the parental breast cancer HIM-2

In the following we ask, whether the qualitative karyotypic replacements of multiple cancer-specific aneusomies by metastatic counterparts, shown in Tables 1 and 2, occur simultaneously, in single steps or sequentially in multiple independent steps.

### Are metastases with multiple new aneusomies generated in single or in multiple sequential steps?

The currently prevailing model of carcinogenesis and progressions of cancers holds that normal karyotypes are gradually converted to those of cancer cells - and from cancer cells to variant cancer cells, such as metastases by sequential gene mutations or karyotypic alterations that alter the dosage or structures of certain genes [3, 4, 13, 69, 119–124]. According to this model the numbers of precursors with cancer-specific aneusomies would decrease with increasing numbers of linearly acquired metastasis-specific aneusomies and thus form the pyramids of intermediates predicted by the step-wise or linear model [3, 4, 69]. To generate from cancers the metastases with multiple metastasis-specific aneusomies described in Table 1, 13 to 27 such steps would be needed, because these metastases differ from parental cancers in 13 to 27 metastasis-specific aneusomies. If so many precursors do indeed exist, they should show up among the many variants of parental cancer karyotypes before or at metastasis. But no such hypothetical karyotypic precursors were found in our karyotype arrays of the six cancers that spawned metastases with multiple aneusomies (Table 1). This conclusion is based on complete analyses of all aneusomies of 20 karyotypes of the six cancers from which metastases with multiple new aneusomies arose (and even of corresponding metastases) that are shown in Figs. 10c, 11c, 12c, 13d and e, 14c and 15d.

This result can, however, be explained by an alternative model, which holds that all chromosomal alterations setting apart cancers from normal cells, and likewise all chromosome alterations setting apart metastases from cancers occur simultaneously in a single step. This proposal is based on the absence of the many intermediates

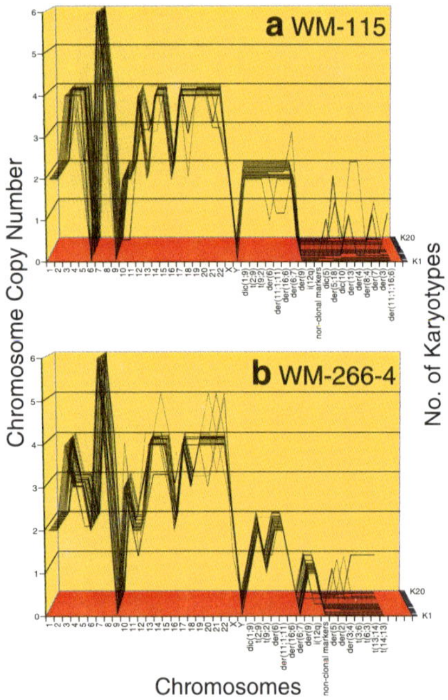


Primary Melanoma WM-115 and Metastatic WM-266-4

| | WM-115 | WM-266-4 |
|---|---|---|
| Avg # of chromosomes ± SD | 86±1 | 82±2 |
| chromosome # | copy no (% clonal) | |
| 1 | 2 (100) | 2 (100) |
| 2 | 2 (100) | 2 (100) |
| 3 | 4 (95) | 4 (90) |
| 4 | 4 (95) | 3 (100) |
| 5 | 4 (85) | 3 (90) |
| 6 | 0 | 2 (100) |
| 7 | 6 (95) | 6 (90) |
| 8 | 4 (90) | 3 (85) |
| 9 | 0 | 0 |
| 10 | 2 (95) | 3 (85) |
| 11 | 2 (100) | 2 (90) |
| 12 | 4 (90) | 2 (75) |
| 13 | 3 (45)/2 (40) | 4 (95) |
| 14 | 4 (95) | 4 (90) |
| 15 | 4 (95) | 4 (75) |
| 16 | 2 (100) | 2 (95) |
| 17 | 4 (100) | 4 (100) |
| 18 | 4 (80) | 3 (75) |
| 19 | 4 (100) | 4 (95) |
| 20 | 4 (100) | 4 (85) |
| 21 | 4 (90) | 4 (90) |
| 22 | 4 (90) | 4 (85) |
| X | 2 (100) | 2 (95) |
| Y | 0 | 0 |
| clonal markers | - | - |
| dic(1;9) | 2 (100) | 1 (100) |
| t(2;9) | 2 (100) | 2 (100) |
| t(9;2) | 2 (100) | 1 (95) |
| der(6) | 2 (95) | 2 (95) |
| der(11;1;11) | 2 (95) | 2 (100) |
| der(16;6) | 2 (95) | 1 (100) |
| der(6;7) | 2 (95) | - |
| der(9) | - | 1 (95) |
| i(12q) | - | 1 (75) |
| Total Clonal Aneusomies | 30 | 31 |

**c** Complete karyotypes of melanoma WM-115

| Total # of Chromosomes | 84 | 85 | 86 | 84 | 87 | 86 | 85 | 87 | 85 | 87 | 86 | 85 | 84 | 86 | 87 | 87 | 87 | 87 | 87 | 87 | |
|---|---|---|---|---|---|---|---|---|---|---|---|---|---|---|---|---|---|---|---|---|---|
| Chromosome # | K1 | K2 | K3 | K4 | K5 | K6 | K7 | K8 | K9 | K10 | K11 | K12 | K13 | K14 | K15 | K16 | K17 | K18 | K19 | K20 | |
| 1 | 2 | 2 | 2 | 2 | 2 | 2 | 2 | 2 | 2 | 2 | 2 | 2 | 2 | 2 | 2 | 2 | 2 | 2 | 2 | 2 | |
| 2 | 2 | 2 | 2 | 2 | 2 | 2 | 2 | 2 | 2 | 2 | 2 | 2 | 2 | 2 | 2 | 2 | 2 | 2 | 2 | 2 | |
| 3 | 4 | 4 | 4 | 4 | 4 | 4 | 4 | 4 | 4 | 4 | 4 | 4 | 4 | 4 | 4 | 4 | 3 | 4 | 4 | 4 | |
| 4 | 4 | 4 | 4 | 4 | 4 | 4 | 4 | 4 | 4 | 4 | 4 | 4 | 4 | 4 | 4 | 4 | 4 | 4 | 2 | 4 | |
| 5 | 4 | 2 | 4 | 2 | 4 | 4 | 4 | 4 | 4 | 4 | 4 | 4 | 4 | 4 | 4 | 4 | 4 | 4 | 3 | 4 | |
| 6 | 0 | 0 | 0 | 0 | 0 | 0 | 0 | 0 | 0 | 0 | 0 | 0 | 0 | 0 | 0 | 0 | 0 | 0 | 0 | 0 | |
| 7 | 6 | 6 | 6 | 6 | 6 | 6 | 6 | 6 | 5 | 6 | 6 | 6 | 6 | 6 | 6 | 6 | 6 | 6 | 6 | 6 | |
| 8 | 3 | 4 | 4 | 4 | 4 | 4 | 4 | 4 | 4 | 4 | 4 | 4 | 4 | 4 | 4 | 4 | 4 | 4 | 2 | 4 | |
| 9 | 0 | 0 | 0 | 0 | 0 | 0 | 0 | 0 | 0 | 0 | 0 | 0 | 0 | 0 | 0 | 0 | 0 | 0 | 0 | 0 | |
| 10 | 2 | 2 | 2 | 2 | 2 | 2 | 2 | 2 | 2 | 2 | 2 | 2 | 2 | 2 | 2 | 2 | 2 | 0 | 2 | 2 | |
| 11 | 2 | 2 | 2 | 2 | 2 | 2 | 2 | 2 | 2 | 2 | 2 | 2 | 2 | 2 | 2 | 2 | 2 | 2 | 2 | 2 | |
| 12 | 4 | 4 | 4 | 4 | 4 | 4 | 4 | 4 | 4 | 4 | 3 | 3 | 4 | 4 | 4 | 4 | 4 | 4 | 4 | 4 | |
| 13 | 2 | 2 | 2 | 2 | 2 | 2 | 2 | 2 | 3 | 3 | 3 | 3 | 3 | 3 | 3 | 3 | 3 | 4 | 4 | 4 | |
| 14 | 4 | 4 | 4 | 4 | 4 | 4 | 4 | 4 | 3 | 4 | 4 | 4 | 4 | 4 | 4 | 4 | 4 | 4 | 4 | 4 | |
| 15 | 4 | 4 | 4 | 4 | 4 | 4 | 4 | 4 | 4 | 4 | 4 | 3 | 4 | 4 | 4 | 4 | 4 | 4 | 4 | 4 | |
| 16 | 2 | 2 | 2 | 2 | 2 | 2 | 2 | 2 | 2 | 2 | 2 | 2 | 2 | 2 | 2 | 2 | 2 | 2 | 2 | 2 | |
| 17 | 4 | 4 | 4 | 4 | 4 | 4 | 4 | 4 | 4 | 4 | 4 | 4 | 4 | 4 | 4 | 4 | 4 | 4 | 4 | 4 | |
| 18 | 4 | 4 | 4 | 2 | 4 | 3 | 4 | 4 | 4 | 4 | 4 | 4 | 3 | 3 | 4 | 4 | 4 | 4 | 4 | 4 | |
| 19 | 4 | 4 | 4 | 4 | 4 | 4 | 4 | 4 | 4 | 4 | 4 | 4 | 4 | 4 | 4 | 4 | 4 | 4 | 4 | 4 | |
| 20 | 4 | 4 | 4 | 4 | 4 | 4 | 4 | 4 | 4 | 4 | 4 | 4 | 4 | 4 | 4 | 4 | 4 | 4 | 4 | 4 | |
| 21 | 4 | 4 | 4 | 4 | 4 | 4 | 4 | 4 | 4 | 4 | 4 | 4 | 3 | 4 | 4 | 4 | 4 | 4 | 4 | 3 | |
| 22 | 4 | 4 | 4 | 4 | 4 | 3 | 4 | 4 | 4 | 4 | 4 | 4 | 3 | 4 | 4 | 4 | 4 | 4 | 4 | 4 | |
| X | 2 | 2 | 2 | 2 | 2 | 2 | 2 | 2 | 2 | 2 | 2 | 2 | 2 | 2 | 2 | 2 | 2 | 2 | 2 | 2 | |
| Y | 0 | 0 | 0 | 0 | 0 | 0 | 0 | 0 | 0 | 0 | 0 | 0 | 0 | 0 | 0 | 0 | 0 | 0 | 0 | 0 | |
| dic(1;9) | 2 | 2 | 2 | 2 | 2 | 2 | 2 | 2 | 2 | 2 | 2 | 2 | 2 | 2 | 2 | 2 | 2 | 2 | 2 | 2 | |
| t(2;9) | 2 | 2 | 2 | 2 | 2 | 2 | 2 | 2 | 2 | 2 | 2 | 2 | 2 | 2 | 2 | 2 | 2 | 2 | 2 | 2 | |
| t(9;2) | 2 | 2 | 2 | 2 | 2 | 2 | 2 | 2 | 2 | 2 | 2 | 2 | 2 | 2 | 2 | 2 | 2 | 2 | 2 | 2 | |
| der(6) | 1 | 2 | 2 | 2 | 2 | 2 | 2 | 2 | 2 | 2 | 2 | 2 | 2 | 2 | 2 | 2 | 2 | 2 | 2 | 2 | |
| der(11;1;11) | 2 | 2 | 2 | 2 | 2 | 2 | 1 | 2 | 2 | 2 | 2 | 2 | 2 | 2 | 2 | 2 | 2 | 2 | 2 | 2 | |
| der(16;6) | 2 | 2 | 2 | 2 | 2 | 2 | 1 | 2 | 2 | 2 | 2 | 2 | 2 | 2 | 2 | 2 | 2 | 2 | 2 | 2 | |
| der(6;7) | 2 | 2 | 2 | 2 | 2 | 2 | 2 | 3 | 2 | 2 | 2 | 2 | 2 | 2 | 2 | 2 | 2 | 2 | 2 | 2 | |
| dic(5) | | 1 | | | | | | | | | | | | | | | | | | | |
| der(5;18) | | | | 2 | | | | | | | | | | | | | | | | | |
| dic(10) | | | | | | | | | | | | | | | | | | 1 | | | |
| der(13) | | | | | 1 | 1 | | | | | | | | | | | | | | | |
| der(4) | | | | | | | | | | | | | | | | | | | 2 | | |
| der(8;4) | | | | | | | | | | | | | | | | | | | 2 | | |
| der(7) | | | | | | 1 | | | | | | | | | | | | | | | |
| der(3) | | | | | | | | | | | | | | | | | 1 | | | | |
| der(11;1;16;6) | | | | | | | 1 | | | | | | | | | | | | | | Average±SD |
| **Non-Clonal Aneusomies** | **2** | **2** | **0** | **3** | **1** | **4** | **3** | **0** | **2** | **0** | **1** | **2** | **3** | **1** | **0** | **0** | **2** | **3** | **6** | **2** | **2±2** |
| **Aneusomies per Karyotype** | **30** | **31** | **30** | **31** | **31** | **32** | **31** | **30** | **30** | **30** | **30** | **30** | **30** | **30** | **30** | **30** | **31** | **31** | **32** | **30** | **30±1** |

**Fig. 10 a, b, c** Karyotypic evidence that the metastasis WM-266-4 is an individual subspecies of melanoma WM-115. The karyotypic theory of metastasis predicts that metastases have individual clonal karyotypes that differ from those of parental cancers in individual metastasis-specific aneusomies. To test this theory we have compared karyotype-arrays of the melanoma metastasis WM-266-4 to that of the primary cancer WM-115 prepared as described for Fig. 9. Figure 10 **a**, **b** and the attached table show that 80 to 100% of the chromosomes of the metastasis WM-266-4 and of the cancer WM-115 were clonal, and that cancer and metastasis both formed very similar clonal patterns. The karyotype of the metastasis differed from that of the primary cancer in about 13 of an average of 31 aneusomies (Fig. 10 **a**, **b**, **c** and Table 1). The copy numbers of the non-clonal chromosomes differed from clonal averages ± 1; there were also several non-clonal marker chromosomes (Fig. 10 **a**, **b**, **c**). These non-clonal chromosomes represent the ongoing karyotypic variation predicted by the inherent variability of cancer-specific aneuploidy (see Fig. 10 **a**, **b** and specifically Fig. 10**c**, and Background). We conclude that the melanoma metastasis WM-266-4 is a subspecies of the parental melanoma WM-115

or precursors predicted by the linear model, which are probably absent, because they are not viable [43, 76, 77, 125–127] and the finding of others that all aneusomies of the cancers analyzed carried genetic markers only from one, instead of both sets of normal parental chromosomes of an organism [128, 129].

This single-step model predicts that (1) there would be no stable precursors of metastases with less than the full set of authentic metastasis-specific aneusomies, and that (2) all metastases retain the karyotypic complexity of parental cancer as a whole, despite metastasis-specific aneusomic variations (see previous section). At the same time the single-step model also predicts there would be no precursors of the many non-clonal, non-metastatic variants of cancer-karyotypes with multiple non-parental aneusomies (See Figs. 8, 9, 10, 11, 12, 13, 14, 15).

As pointed out above and summarized in Table 2 our karyotypic analyses shown in Figs. 10, 11, 12, 13, 14, 15 exactly confirm these predictions of the single-step model: (1) There were no intermediates of metastases with subsets of the aneusomies of authentic metastases in Figs. 10, 11, 12, 13, 14, 15; and (2) The karyotypic complexity of metastases with multiple non-parental aneusomies was practically the same as that of parental cancers (Table 2).

This absence of precursors of metastases confirms previous results from others including us [43, 76, 77, 126, 127]. In addition our results confirm the predicted absence of precursors of the many non-metastatic variants with multiple aneusomies and with the same complexities as their metastatic counterparts (Figs. 10, 11, 12, 13, 14, 15). In view of this we conclude that our data support the single-step model of metastasis.

In agreement with the single-step model we found, unexpectedly, one specific cell, in which the whole karyotype of the metastatic medulloblastoma M-425 with all of its 24 individual aneusomies was already or was still present in the primary cancer, M-458 (marked yellow in Fig. 12c). This result argues against the sequential theory, because predictably more precursors with less than the 24 new metastasis-specific aneusomies of M-425 should have been present in this cancer than the 1 in 20 with all 24 M-425-specific aneusomies we found. But this was not the case.

The simplest explanation for this result suggests that metastasis is a stochastic single-step variation of the

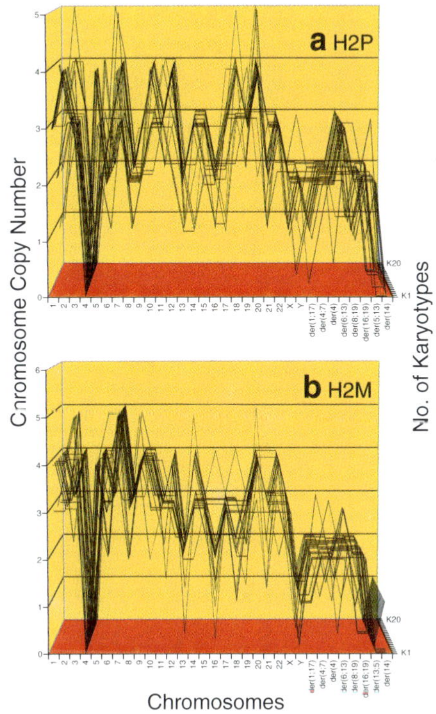


Primary Liver Cancer H2P and Metastatis H2M

| | H2P | H2M |
|---|---|---|
| Avg # of chromosomes ± SD | 78±7 | 86±4 |
| chromosome # | copy no (% clonal) | |
| 1 | 3 (45) | 4 (75) |
| 2 | 3 (50) | 3 (70) |
| 3 | 3 (70) | 4 (60) |
| 4 | 0 | 0 (95) |
| 5 | 2 (40)/4 (35) | 4 (80) |
| 6 | 2 (70) | 3 (55) |
| 7 | 4 (50) | 5 (85) |
| 8 | 2 (80) | 3 (85) |
| 9 | 2 (65) | 4 (85) |
| 10 | 3 (50) | 4 (65) |
| 11 | 3 (70) | 3 (80) |
| 12 | 4 (60) | 4 (55) |
| 13 | 2 (70) | 2 (90) |
| 14 | 3 (75) | 3 (50) |
| 15 | 3 (70) | 3 (90) |
| 16 | 2 (80) | 2 (50) |
| 17 | 3 (60) | 3 (95) |
| 18 | 4 (60) | 2 (45)/3 (35) |
| 19 | 3 (75) | 3 (70) |
| 20 | 4 (70) | 4 (80) |
| 21 | 2 (40)/3 (40) | 3 (70) |
| 22 | 3 (90) | 4 (50) |
| X | 2 (75) | 3 (65) |
| Y | 2 (75) | 1 (75) |
| clonal markers | - | - |
| der(1;17) | 2 (50) | 2 (80) |
| der(4;7) | 2 (95) | 2 (90) |
| der(4) | 2 (100) | 2 (80) |
| der(6;13) | 3 (70) | 2 (65) |
| der(8;19) | 2 (55) | 2 (95) |
| der(16;19) | 2 (90) | 2 (70) |
| der(13;5) | 2 (55) | - |
| der(14) | - | 1 (85) |
| Total Clonal Aneusomies | 31 | 31 |

**c** Complete karyotypes of liver cancer H2P

| Total # of Chromosomes | 80 | 83 | 86 | 86 | 85 | 81 | 68 | 73 | 64 | 86 | 74 | 64 | 74 | 81 | 80 | 74 | 70 | 78 | 83 | 87 | |
|---|---|---|---|---|---|---|---|---|---|---|---|---|---|---|---|---|---|---|---|---|---|
| Chromosome # | K1 | K2 | K3 | K4 | K5 | K6 | K7 | K8 | K9 | K10 | K11 | K12 | K13 | K14 | K15 | K16 | K17 | K18 | K19 | K20 | |
| 1 | 3 | 3 | 3 | 3 | 3 | 2 | 2 | 2 | 1 | 4 | 4 | 2 | 1 | 2 | 3 | 1 | 3 | 3 | 3 | 4 | |
| 2 | 4 | 4 | 3 | 4 | 4 | 3 | 3 | 4 | 2 | 3 | 3 | 3 | 3 | 3 | 4 | 3 | 3 | 5 | 4 | 4 | |
| 3 | 3 | 3 | 4 | 3 | 3 | 3 | 3 | 3 | 3 | 3 | 2 | 2 | 3 | 2 | 4 | 3 | 2 | 3 | 3 | 3 | |
| 4 | 0 | 0 | 0 | 0 | 0 | 0 | 0 | 0 | 0 | 0 | 0 | 0 | 0 | 0 | 0 | 0 | 0 | 0 | 0 | 0 | |
| 5 | 4 | 4 | 4 | 3 | 4 | 4 | 3 | 2 | 2 | 2 | 3 | 3 | 2 | 2 | 2 | 2 | 4 | 3 | 4 | 2 | |
| 6 | 2 | 2 | 2 | 2 | 2 | 2 | 2 | 2 | 1 | 2 | 3 | 2 | 3 | 3 | 2 | 3 | 2 | 2 | 2 | 5 | |
| 7 | 4 | 3 | 4 | 3 | 5 | 4 | 3 | 3 | 3 | 4 | 3 | 3 | 4 | 4 | 4 | 4 | 3 | 3 | 4 | 4 | |
| 8 | 2 | 3 | 2 | 2 | 2 | 2 | 2 | 2 | 1 | 2 | 1 | 1 | 2 | 2 | 2 | 2 | 2 | 2 | 2 | 2 | |
| 9 | 3 | 2 | 2 | 2 | 2 | 2 | 2 | 2 | 2 | 2 | 2 | 2 | 3 | 3 | 2 | 3 | 3 | 2 | 3 | 3 | |
| 10 | 3 | 3 | 4 | 4 | 3 | 3 | 3 | 4 | 2 | 3 | 3 | 2 | 4 | 4 | 4 | 4 | 3 | 3 | 3 | 4 | |
| 11 | 3 | 3 | 3 | 3 | 3 | 3 | 3 | 3 | 3 | 4 | 3 | 3 | 3 | 3 | 2 | 3 | 2 | 2 | 4 | 4 | |
| 12 | 4 | 3 | 4 | 4 | 4 | 4 | 2 | 4 | 2 | 3 | 4 | 3 | 4 | 4 | 4 | 4 | 3 | 2 | 4 | 3 | |
| 13 | 2 | 2 | 2 | 2 | 2 | 2 | 1 | 2 | 1 | 2 | 1 | 2 | 1 | 2 | 2 | 1 | 2 | 2 | 2 | 3 | |
| 14 | 3 | 3 | 3 | 3 | 3 | 3 | 1 | 1 | 2 | 3 | 3 | 1 | 3 | 3 | 3 | 3 | 2 | 3 | 3 | 3 | |
| 15 | 2 | 3 | 3 | 3 | 3 | 3 | 3 | 2 | 3 | 3 | 2 | 2 | 2 | 3 | 3 | 2 | 3 | 3 | 3 | 3 | |
| 16 | 2 | 2 | 3 | 2 | 2 | 2 | 2 | 2 | 1 | 2 | 1 | 1 | 2 | 2 | 2 | 2 | 2 | 2 | 2 | 2 | |
| 17 | 3 | 3 | 3 | 4 | 2 | 3 | 1 | 3 | 3 | 3 | 3 | 1 | 2 | 3 | 3 | 2 | 1 | 2 | 3 | 3 | |
| 18 | 4 | 4 | 4 | 4 | 4 | 4 | 3 | 4 | 4 | 5 | 3 | 3 | 3 | 4 | 3 | 3 | 4 | 2 | 4 | 4 | |
| 19 | 3 | 3 | 3 | 3 | 3 | 3 | 4 | 3 | 3 | 3 | 3 | 3 | 3 | 2 | 2 | 3 | 2 | 3 | 2 | 3 | |
| 20 | 4 | 4 | 4 | 4 | 4 | 4 | 2 | 4 | 4 | 5 | 3 | 4 | 4 | 5 | 4 | 4 | 4 | 3 | 4 | 5 | |
| 21 | 2 | 3 | 3 | 3 | 3 | 2 | 3 | 2 | 1 | 2 | 1 | 1 | 2 | 2 | 3 | 2 | 2 | 3 | 3 | 1 | |
| 22 | 3 | 3 | 3 | 3 | 3 | 3 | 3 | 3 | 3 | 3 | 2 | 3 | 3 | 3 | 3 | 3 | 3 | 3 | 2 | 3 | |
| X | 2 | 2 | 2 | 1 | 2 | 2 | 2 | 1 | 1 | 2 | 2 | 1 | 2 | 2 | 2 | 2 | 2 | 1 | 2 | 2 | |
| Y | 1 | 2 | 2 | 2 | 2 | 2 | 2 | 2 | 2 | 2 | 2 | 2 | 0 | 1 | 3 | 0 | 2 | 2 | 2 | 2 | |
| der(1;17) | 2 | 1 | 2 | 2 | 2 | 2 | 1 | 0 | 1 | 1 | 2 | 1 | 1 | 2 | 2 | 1 | 1 | 2 | 2 | 1 | |
| der(4;7) | 2 | 2 | 2 | 2 | 2 | 2 | 2 | 1 | 2 | 2 | 2 | 2 | 2 | 2 | 2 | 2 | 2 | 2 | 2 | 2 | |
| der(4) | 2 | 2 | 2 | 2 | 2 | 2 | 2 | 2 | 2 | 2 | 2 | 2 | 2 | 2 | 2 | 2 | 2 | 2 | 2 | 2 | |
| der(6;13) | 3 | 3 | 3 | 2 | 3 | 3 | 3 | 3 | 2 | 3 | 2 | 3 | 3 | 3 | 2 | 3 | 1 | 3 | 3 | 0 | |
| der(8;19) | 1 | 2 | 2 | 1 | 2 | 3 | 1 | 1 | 2 | 2 | 2 | 2 | 1 | 2 | 2 | 1 | 1 | 1 | 2 | 2 | |
| der(16;19) | 2 | 1 | 2 | 2 | 2 | 2 | 2 | 2 | 2 | 2 | 2 | 2 | 2 | 2 | 2 | 2 | 1 | 2 | 2 | 2 | |
| der(13;5) | 0 | 2 | 2 | 2 | 2 | 0 | 2 | 2 | 1 | 3 | 2 | 1 | 0 | 1 | 0 | 0 | 2 | 2 | 2 | 2 | |
| i(5q) | | | | | | | | | 1 | | | | 1 | 1 | 1 | 1 | | | | | |
| der(10;15) | 2 | | | | | | | | | | | | | | | | | | | | |
| dic(16;9;17) | | 1 | | | | | | | | | | | | | | | | | | | |
| dic(7;9) | | 1 | | | | | | | | | | | | | | | | | | | |
| der(5) | | 1 | | | | | | | | | | | | | | | | | | | |
| del(9q) | | | 1 | 1 | | | | | | | | | | | | | | | | | |
| dic(7;8) | | | | 1 | | | | | | | | | | | | | | | | | |
| der(6;5) | | | | 1 | | | | | | | | | | | | | | | | | |
| der(5;?) | | | | 1 | | | | | | | | | | | | | | | | | |
| del(Xq) | | | | 1 | | | | | | | | | | | | | | | | | |
| del(8q) | | | | 1 | | | | | | | | | | | | | | | | | |
| der(9;17) | | | | | 1 | | | | | | | | | | | | | | | | |
| del(10p) | | | | | 1 | | | | | | | | | | | | | | | | |
| dic(1;9) | | | | | | 1 | | | | | | | | | | | | | | | |
| der(17;21) | | | | | | 1 | | | | | | | | | | | | | | | |
| dic(9;1;17) | | | | | | | | 1 | | | | | | | | | | | | | |
| der(14;1;12) | | | | | | | | 1 | | | | | | | | | | | | | |
| der(X;9) | | | | | | | | | 1 | | | | | | | | | | | | |
| dic(2;9) | | | | | | | | | | 1 | | | | | | | | | | | |
| der(5;17)long | | | | | | | | | | 1 | | | | | | | | | | | |
| der(5;17)short | | | | | | | | | | 2 | | | | | | | | | | | |
| der(8;18) | | | | | | | | | | | 1 | | | | | | | | | | |
| der(7;20) | | | | | | | | | | | 1 | | | | | | | | | | |
| der(9;21) | | | | | | | | | | | 1 | | | | | | | | | | |
| der(1;17)small | | | | | | | | | | | | 1 | | | | | | | | | |
| del(1p) | | | | | | | | | | | | | 1 | | | 1 | | | | | |
| del(1q) | | | | | | | | | | | | | 1 | | | 1 | | | | | |
| der(2;17) | | | | | | | | | | | | | 1 | | | | | | | | |
| der(1) | | | | | | | | | | | | | | 1 | | | | | | | |
| der(19;17) | | | | | | | | | | | | | | 1 | | | | | | | |
| der(9;11) | | | | | | | | | | | | | | | 1 | 1 | | | | | |
| der(2;17) | | | | | | | | | | | | | | | | 1 | | | | | |
| del(17q) | | | | | | | | | | | | | | | | | 1 | | | | |
| del(7p) | | | | | | | | | | | | | | | | | | 1 | | | |
| der(10;7) | | | | | | | | | | | | | | | | | | 1 | | | |
| mar(X?) | | | | | | | | | | | | | | | | | | 3 | | | |
| der(5;17) | | | | | | | | | | | | | | | | | | | | 1 | |
| der(17;5) | | | | | | | | | | | | | | | | | | | | 2 | |
| der(18;21) | | | | | | | | | | | | | | | | | | | | 1 | Average±SD |
| **Non-clonal Aneusomies** | 6 | 8 | 4 | 14 | 5 | 5 | 11 | 12 | 16 | 9 | 17 | 16 | 15 | 12 | 11 | 15 | 12 | 13 | 5 | 14 | 12±4 |
| **Aneusomies per Karyotype** | 32 | 34 | 32 | 37 | 33 | 33 | 31 | 33 | 32 | 34 | 34 | 32 | 34 | 33 | 32 | 34 | 32 | 34 | 31 | 34 | 33±1 |

**Fig. 11 a, b, c** Karyotypic evidence that the metastasis H2M is an individual subspecies of liver cancer H2P. The karyotypic theory of metastasis predicts that metastases have individual clonal karyotypes that differ from those of parental cancers in individual metastasis-specific aneusomies. To test this theory we have compared karyotype-arrays of the metastasis H2M to that of the primary cancer H2P prepared as described for Fig. 9. Figure 11 **a**, **b** and the attached table show that 45–80% of the chromosomes of cancer H2P and 50–90% of the chromosomes of metastasis H2M were clonal, and that cancer and metastasis formed similar clonal patterns. The karyotype of the metastasis differed from that of the primary cancer in about 15 of an average of 31 H2M aneusomies (Fig. 11 **a**, **b**, **c** and Table 1). The copy numbers of non-clonal chromosomes including marker chromosomes differed from clonal averages ± 1 (see Fig. 11 **a**, **b** and specifically Fig. 11**c**). The chromosomes with non-clonal copy numbers represent the ongoing karyotypic variation predicted by the inherent variability of cancer-specific aneuploidy (See Fig. 11**c** and Background). We conclude that the metastasis H2M is a subspecies of the parental liver cancer H2P

parental cancer karyotype, which expands the host-range of the parental clone to non-native tissues and thus favors metastasis while retaining its native host range. So this M-425 'metastasis' would have continued to replicate in the primary cancer after a sibling had metastasized to a new site. Thus, this observation lends further support to our theory that metastases are single-step karyotypic variants of clonal cancer karyotypes.

By contrast generation of metastases by independent sequential karyotypic variations of precursors, would predict metastases with unpredictable complexities that would not necessarily match those of parental cancers. In addition the sequential model would predict intermediates with aneusomies shared with authentic metastases in M-458, which we did not observe, as shown by the complete karyotypic analyses of M-458 in Fig. 12c.

### Is metastasis a model for Darwinian speciation?

Our results on the karyotypic evolution of metastatic subspecies from cancers may also serve as an experimental model for theories that karyotypic alterations, rather than gene mutations [130], have generated new conventional species such as those proposed by Goldschmidt (1940) [131], White (1978) [118], King (1993) [132], Vincent (2011) [90] and Heng (2015) [133].

In contrast to these karyotypic theories of speciation, the evolution of Darwinian species is widely presented as a stepwise accumulations of genetic mutations [130], much like the currently established models of carcinogenesis [3, 4]. But testable mutations of this "Neo-Darwinian theory" have not been described [103, 130]. Moreover, the Neo-Darwinian theory does not explain the karyotypic individuality of all species [103] and of all cancers [75]. Instead, mutations predict common targets on common karyotypes rather than karyotypic individuality [90, 134].

Thus our results on the origins of metastases from cancers offer a testable karyotypic model for the origins of conventional species, especially the mammals, from their immediate precursors [103, 118].

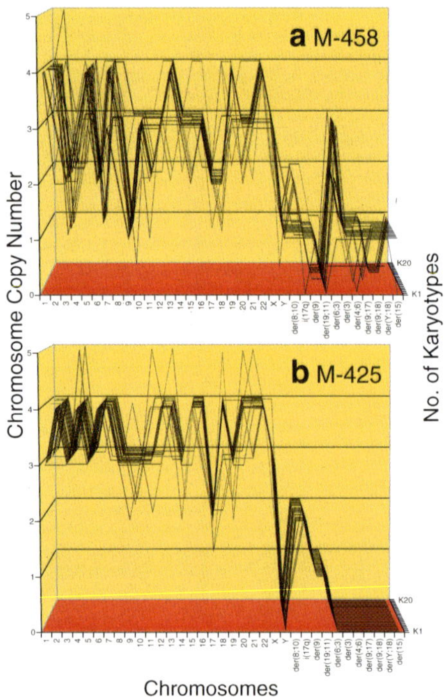


| Primary Medulloblastoma M-458 and Metastasis M-425 | M-458 | M-425 |
|---|---|---|
| Avg # of chromosomes ± SD | 81±2.5 | 85±2 |
| chromosome # | copy no (% clonal) | |
| 1 | 4 (80) | 3 (85) |
| 2 | 4 (55) | 4 (85) |
| 3 | 2 (70) | 3 (100) |
| 4 | 3 (60) | 4 (80) |
| 5 | 4 (70) | 3 (100) |
| 6 | 2 (60) | 4 (95) |
| 7 | 4 (65) | 4 (85) |
| 8 | 3 (65) | 3 (100) |
| 9 | 1 (65) | 3 (80) |
| 10 | 3 (95) | 3 (100) |
| 11 | 3 (50) | 3 (70) |
| 12 | 3 (90) | 4 (70) |
| 13 | 4 (75) | 4 (75) |
| 14 | 3 (95) | 3 (90) |
| 15 | 3 (75) | 4 (90) |
| 16 | 3 (90) | 4 (85) |
| 17 | 2 (95) | 2 (90) |
| 18 | 2 (60) | 4 (70) |
| 19 | 4 (55) | 3 (85) |
| 20 | 3 (70) | 4 (80) |
| 21 | 3 (90) | 4 (80) |
| 22 | 4 (80) | 4 (100) |
| X | 3 (85) | 3 (90) |
| Y | 1 (75) | 0 |
| clonal markers | - | - |
| der(8;10) | 1 (60) | 2 (85) |
| i(17q) | 1 (90) | 2 (100) |
| del(9p) | 1 (70) | 1 (100) |
| der(6;3) | 3 (50) | - |
| der(3) | 1 (95) | - |
| der(4;6) | 1 (80) | - |
| der(9;18) | 1 (70) | - |
| der(Y;18) | 1 (70) | - |
| der(15) | 1 (90) | |
| der(9;17) | 1 (85) | - |
| Total Clonal Aneusomies | 34 | 28 |

**c** Complete karyotypes of 20 M-458 cells

| Total # of Chromosomes | 79 | 77 | 79 | 81 | 84 | 83 | 83 | 78 | 78 | 82 | 77 | 80 | 81 | 81 | 78 | 83 | 82 | 86 | 79 | 79 | |
|---|---|---|---|---|---|---|---|---|---|---|---|---|---|---|---|---|---|---|---|---|---|
| Chromosome # | K1 | K2 | K3 | K4 | K5 | K6 | K7 | K8 | K9 | K10 | K11 | K12 | K13 | K14 | K15 | K16 | K17 | K18 | K19 | K20 | |
| 1 | 4 | 4 | 4 | 3 | 4 | 4 | 4 | 4 | 4 | 4 | 4 | 3 | 4 | 2 | 4 | 4 | 4 | 3 | 4 | 4 | |
| 2 | 2 | 3 | 3 | 4 | 4 | 4 | 4 | 3 | 4 | 4 | 4 | 4 | 4 | 3 | 2 | 5 | 3 | 4 | 3 | 4 | |
| 3 | 2 | 2 | 2 | 1 | 2 | 2 | 2 | 1 | 1 | 2 | 2 | 1 | 1 | 2 | 2 | 2 | 2 | 3 | 2 | 2 | |
| 4 | 3 | 3 | 2 | 2 | 3 | 3 | 3 | 3 | 2 | 3 | 3 | 3 | 2 | 2 | 2 | 3 | 3 | 4 | 2 | 3 | |
| 5 | 4 | 4 | 4 | 3 | 4 | 4 | 4 | 4 | 4 | 4 | 3 | 4 | 4 | 3 | 4 | 3 | 3 | 3 | 4 | 4 | |
| 6 | 2 | 2 | 2 | 2 | 2 | 2 | 2 | 2 | 2 | 2 | 2 | 1 | 1 | 1 | 1 | 1 | 1 | 4 | 1 | 2 | |
| 7 | 3 | 3 | 4 | 3 | 4 | 4 | 4 | 4 | 4 | 3 | 4 | 3 | 3 | 3 | 4 | 4 | 4 | 4 | 4 | 4 | |
| 8 | 2 | 2 | 3 | 3 | 3 | 3 | 3 | 2 | 3 | 3 | 3 | 3 | 3 | 3 | 3 | 4 | 4 | 3 | 2 | 2 | |
| 9 | 1 | 1 | 1 | 1 | 1 | 1 | 1 | 1 | 1 | 1 | 1 | 1 | 1 | 3 | 3 | 3 | 3 | 3 | 3 | 0 | |
| 10 | 3 | 3 | 3 | 3 | 3 | 2 | 3 | 3 | 3 | 3 | 3 | 3 | 3 | 3 | 3 | 3 | 3 | 3 | 3 | 3 | |
| 11 | 3 | 1 | 2 | 3 | 3 | 2 | 2 | 2 | 2 | 2 | 2 | 3 | 3 | 3 | 2 | 3 | 3 | 3 | 3 | 2 | |
| 12 | 3 | 3 | 3 | 3 | 3 | 3 | 3 | 3 | 3 | 3 | 2 | 3 | 3 | 3 | 3 | 3 | 3 | 4 | 3 | 3 | |
| 13 | 4 | 4 | 4 | 2 | 3 | 4 | 4 | 4 | 3 | 4 | 4 | 2 | 3 | 4 | 4 | 4 | 4 | 4 | 4 | 4 | |
| 14 | 3 | 3 | 3 | 3 | 3 | 3 | 3 | 3 | 3 | 3 | 2 | 3 | 3 | 3 | 3 | 3 | 3 | 3 | 3 | 3 | |
| 15 | 2 | 3 | 2 | 3 | 3 | 3 | 3 | 2 | 3 | 3 | 3 | 2 | 3 | 3 | 3 | 3 | 3 | 4 | 3 | 3 | |
| 16 | 3 | 3 | 3 | 3 | 3 | 3 | 3 | 3 | 3 | 3 | 3 | 3 | 3 | 3 | 2 | 3 | 3 | 4 | 3 | 3 | |
| 17 | 2 | 2 | 2 | 2 | 2 | 2 | 2 | 2 | 1 | 2 | 2 | 2 | 2 | 2 | 2 | 2 | 2 | 2 | 2 | 2 | |
| 18 | 2 | 2 | 2 | 2 | 2 | 1 | 2 | 2 | 2 | 2 | 1 | 2 | 2 | 3 | 3 | 4 | 4 | 4 | 1 | 2 | |
| 19 | 4 | 3 | 4 | 4 | 4 | 4 | 4 | 3 | 4 | 3 | 3 | 4 | 4 | 3 | 3 | 2 | 4 | 3 | 4 | 3 | |
| 20 | 2 | 3 | 3 | 2 | 3 | 3 | 3 | 3 | 3 | 3 | 3 | 3 | 3 | 2 | 3 | 3 | 2 | 4 | 2 | 3 | |
| 21 | 3 | 3 | 3 | 3 | 2 | 3 | 3 | 3 | 3 | 3 | 3 | 3 | 3 | 3 | 3 | 3 | 3 | 4 | 3 | 3 | |
| 22 | 3 | 4 | 4 | 4 | 4 | 4 | 3 | 3 | 4 | 4 | 3 | 4 | 4 | 4 | 4 | 4 | 4 | 4 | 4 | 4 | |
| X | 3 | 2 | 3 | 3 | 3 | 3 | 3 | 3 | 2 | 3 | 3 | 3 | 3 | 2 | 3 | 3 | 3 | 3 | 3 | 3 | |
| Y | 1 | 1 | 1 | 2 | 1 | 1 | 1 | 1 | 1 | 1 | 1 | 1 | 2 | 1 | 2 | 1 | 1 | 0 | 2 | 1 | |
| der(8;10) | 2 | 1 | 2 | 1 | 2 | 1 | 1 | 1 | 1 | 1 | 1 | 2 | 1 | 1 | 2 | 2 | 2 | 2 | 1 | 1 | |
| i(17q) | 0 | 1 | 1 | 1 | 1 | 1 | 1 | 1 | 1 | 1 | 1 | 1 | 1 | 1 | 1 | 1 | 1 | 2 | 1 | 1 | |
| del(9p) | 1 | 1 | 1 | 1 | 1 | 1 | 1 | 1 | 1 | 0 | 1 | 1 | 1 | 0 | 0 | 0 | 0 | 1 | 0 | 1 | |
| der(6;3) | 1 | 3 | 2 | 3 | 2 | 2 | 3 | 3 | 3 | 3 | 3 | 3 | 3 | 2 | 2 | 2 | 2 | 0 | 2 | 3 | |
| der(3) | 1 | 1 | 1 | 1 | 1 | 1 | 1 | 1 | 1 | 1 | 1 | 1 | 1 | 1 | 1 | 1 | 1 | 0 | 1 | 1 | |
| der(4;6) | 1 | 0 | 1 | 1 | 1 | 1 | 1 | 0 | 1 | 1 | 1 | 1 | 1 | 1 | 1 | 1 | 1 | 0 | 1 | 0 | |
| der(9;18) | 1 | 1 | 1 | 1 | 1 | 1 | 1 | 1 | 1 | 1 | 1 | 1 | 1 | 0 | 0 | 0 | 0 | 0 | 0 | 1 | |
| der(Y;18) | 1 | 1 | 1 | 1 | 1 | 1 | 1 | 1 | 1 | 1 | 1 | 1 | 1 | 0 | 0 | 0 | 0 | 0 | 0 | 1 | |
| der(15) | 0 | 1 | 1 | 1 | 1 | 1 | 1 | 1 | 1 | 1 | 1 | 1 | 1 | 1 | 1 | 1 | 1 | 0 | 1 | 1 | |
| der(9;17) | 1 | 1 | 1 | 1 | 1 | 1 | 1 | 1 | 0 | 1 | 0 | 1 | 1 | 1 | 1 | 1 | 1 | 0 | 1 | 1 | |
| der(19;11) | | | | | | | | | | | | | | | | | | 1 | | | |
| der(11;8) | | | | | | 1 | 1 | | 1 | 1 | 1 | | | | | | | | | | |
| der(12) | 1 | | | | 1 | 1 | 1 | | 1 | 1 | 1 | 1 | | | | | | | | | |
| der(3;9) | | | | | | | | | | 1 | | | | | | | | | | | |
| der(1) | | | | 1 | | | | | | | | 1 | | | | | | | | | |
| der(3;13) | | | | | | | | | | | | 1 | | | | | | | | | |
| der(13;3;6;16) | | | | | | | | | | | | | | | | 1 | | | | | |
| del(2p) | 1 | | | | | | | | | | | | | | | | | | | | |
| del(2q) | 1 | | | | | | | | | | | | | | | | | | | | |
| der(8;17) | 1 | | | | | | | | | | | | | | | | | | | | |
| der(17;8) | 1 | | | | | | | | | | | | | | | | | | | | |
| der(6;7) | 1 | | | | | | | | | | | | | | | | | | | | |
| der(8) | | 1 | | | | | | 1 | | | | | | | | | | | | 1 | |
| del(3q) | | | | | | | | 1 | | | | | | | | | | | | | |
| del(3p) | | | | | | | | 1 | | | | | | | | | | | | | |
| der(3)long | | | | 1 | | | | | | | | | 1 | | | | | | | | |
| der(4) | | | | | | | | | | | | | 1 | | | | | | | | |
| der(13;21) | | | | | 1 | | | | | | | | | | | | | | | | |
| der(6;14?) | | | | | 1 | | | | | | | | | | | | | | | | |
| der(18;10) | | | | | | 1 | | | | | | | | | | | | | | | |
| der(10) | | | | | | 1 | | | | | | | | | | | | | | | |
| der(11;2) | | 1 | | | | | | | | | | | | | | | | | | | |
| der(4;1) | | | | | | | | | | | | | | 1 | | | | | | | |
| der(1;7) | | | | | | | | | | | | | | 1 | | | | | | | |
| der(1;3) | | | | | | | | | | | | | | 1 | | | | | | | |
| der(20;7) | | | | | | | | | | | | | | 1 | | | | | | | |
| der(19;5) | | | | | | | | | | | | | | 1 | | | | | | | |
| der(6) | | | | | | | | | | | | | | 1 | | | | | | | |
| mar(Y?) | | | | | | | | | | | | | | 2 | | | | | | | |
| del(Xq) | | | | | | | | | | | | | | 1 | | | | | | | |
| der(4) | | | | 1 | | | | | | | | | | | | | | | | | |
| mar(5) | | | | 2 | | | | | | | | | | | | | | | | | |
| der(6;16) | | | | | | | | | | | | | | | 1 | | | | 1 | | |
| der(16;6;3;4;3;13) | | | | | | | | | | | | | | | | | 1 | | | | |
| t(18;20) | | | | | | | | | | | | | | | | | | | 1 | | |
| t(20;18) | | | | | | | | | | | | | | | | | | | 1 | | Average±SD |
| **Non-Clonal Aneusomies** | **16** | **9** | **4** | **12** | **6** | **6** | **3** | **10** | **8** | **6** | **9** | **10** | **8** | **22** | **13** | **12** | **12** | **24** | **13** | **5** | **10±5** |
| **Aneusomies per Karyotype** | **40** | **36** | **34** | **38** | **37** | **38** | **36** | **37** | **36** | **37** | **36** | **37** | **36** | **42** | **35** | **35** | **35** | **35** | **37** | **35** | **37±2** |

**d** Complete karyotypes of 20 M-425 cells

| Total # of Chromosomes | 85 | 84 | 86 | 87 | 85 | 85 | 85 | 82 | 89 | 81 | 87 | 83 | 85 | 86 | 84 | 85 | 87 | 81 | 84 | 84 | |
|---|---|---|---|---|---|---|---|---|---|---|---|---|---|---|---|---|---|---|---|---|---|
| Chromosome # | K1 | K2 | K3 | K4 | K5 | K6 | K7 | K8 | K9 | K10 | K11 | K12 | K13 | K14 | K15 | K16 | K17 | K18 | K19 | K20 | |
| 1 | 3 | 3 | 3 | 3 | 3 | 3 | 3 | 3 | 4 | 3 | 3 | 3 | 3 | 4 | 3 | 4 | 3 | 3 | 3 | 3 | |
| 2 | 3 | 4 | 4 | 4 | 4 | 4 | 4 | 4 | 4 | 3 | 4 | 4 | 4 | 4 | 4 | 4 | 4 | 4 | 4 | 3 | |
| 3 | 3 | 3 | 3 | 3 | 3 | 3 | 3 | 3 | 3 | 3 | 3 | 3 | 3 | 3 | 3 | 3 | 3 | 3 | 3 | 3 | |
| 4 | 4 | 3 | 4 | 4 | 4 | 4 | 5 | 4 | 4 | 4 | 4 | 4 | 4 | 4 | 4 | 5 | 4 | 3 | 4 | 4 | |
| 5 | 3 | 3 | 3 | 3 | 3 | 3 | 3 | 3 | 3 | 3 | 3 | 3 | 3 | 3 | 3 | 3 | 3 | 3 | 3 | 3 | |
| 6 | 4 | 4 | 4 | 4 | 4 | 4 | 4 | 4 | 4 | 4 | 4 | 4 | 4 | 4 | 3 | 4 | 4 | 4 | 4 | 4 | |
| 7 | 4 | 4 | 4 | 4 | 4 | 3 | 4 | 4 | 4 | 3 | 4 | 4 | 4 | 4 | 4 | 4 | 4 | 3 | 4 | 4 | |
| 8 | 3 | 3 | 3 | 3 | 3 | 3 | 3 | 3 | 3 | 3 | 3 | 3 | 3 | 3 | 3 | 3 | 3 | 3 | 3 | 3 | |
| 9 | 3 | 2 | 3 | 3 | 3 | 3 | 3 | 3 | 3 | 4 | 3 | 3 | 3 | 3 | 2 | 3 | 3 | 3 | 3 | 2 | |
| 10 | 3 | 3 | 3 | 3 | 3 | 3 | 3 | 3 | 3 | 3 | 3 | 3 | 3 | 3 | 3 | 3 | 3 | 3 | 3 | 3 | |
| 11 | 4 | 3 | 3 | 4 | 3 | 3 | 3 | 2 | 5 | 3 | 3 | 3 | 3 | 3 | 3 | 3 | 4 | 3 | 4 | 3 | |
| 12 | 4 | 3 | 4 | 4 | 4 | 4 | 4 | 3 | 4 | 3 | 4 | 3 | 4 | 3 | 4 | 3 | 4 | 4 | 4 | 4 | |
| 13 | 4 | 4 | 4 | 4 | 4 | 4 | 3 | 4 | 4 | 3 | 5 | 4 | 4 | 4 | 4 | 3 | 4 | 3 | 4 | 4 | |
| 14 | 3* | 2 | 3 | 3 | 3 | 3 | 3 | 3 | 3 | 3 | 3 | 3 | 3 | 3 | 3 | 3 | 3 | 3 | 3 | 2 | |
| 15 | 3 | 4 | 4 | 4 | 4 | 4 | 4 | 4 | 4 | 4 | 4 | 4 | 4 | 4 | 4 | 3 | 4 | 4 | 4 | 4 | |
| 16 | 4 | 3 | 4 | 4 | 4 | 3 | 4 | 4 | 4 | 4 | 4 | 4 | 4 | 3 | 4 | 4 | 4 | 4 | 4 | 4 | |
| 17 | 2 | 2 | 2 | 2 | 2 | 2 | 2 | 2 | 2 | 2 | 2 | 2 | 2 | 2 | 2 | 2 | 2 | 1 | 1 | 2 | |
| 18 | 4 | 5 | 4 | 4 | 4 | 4 | 3 | 4 | 4 | 2 | 4 | 3 | 4 | 4 | 4 | 4 | 4 | 3 | 2 | 4 | |
| 19 | 3 | 2 | 3 | 3 | 3 | 3 | 3 | 3 | 3 | 3 | 3 | 3 | 3 | 4 | 3 | 3 | 3 | 2 | 3 | 3 | |
| 20 | 3 | 4 | 4 | 4 | 4 | 5 | 4 | 3 | 4 | 4 | 4 | 4 | 4 | 4 | 4 | 3 | 4 | 4 | 4 | 4 | |
| 21 | 4 | 4 | 4 | 4 | 4 | 4 | 5 | 3 | 4 | 3 | 4 | 3 | 4 | 4 | 4 | 4 | 4 | 4 | 4 | 4 | |
| 22 | 4 | 4 | 4 | 4 | 4 | 4 | 4 | 4 | 4 | 4 | 4 | 4 | 4 | 4 | 4 | 4 | 4 | 4 | 4 | 4 | |
| X | 3 | 3 | 3 | 3 | 2 | 3 | 3 | 3 | 3 | 3 | 3 | 3 | 3 | 3 | 3 | 4 | 3 | 3 | 3 | 3 | |
| Y | 0 | 0 | 0 | 0 | 0 | 0 | 0 | 0 | 0 | 0 | 0 | 0 | 0 | 0 | 0 | 0 | 0 | 0 | 0 | 0 | |
| der(8;10) | 2 | 2 | 2 | 2 | 1 | 2 | 1 | 2 | 2 | 2 | 2 | 2 | 1 | 2 | 2 | 2 | 2 | 2 | 2 | 2 | |
| i(17q) | 2 | 2 | 2 | 2 | 2 | 2 | 2 | 2 | 2 | 2 | 2 | 2 | 2 | 2 | 2 | 2 | 2 | 2 | 2 | 2 | |
| del(9p) | 1 | 1 | 1 | 1 | 1 | 1 | 1 | 1 | 1 | 1 | 1 | 1 | 1 | 1 | 1 | 1 | 1 | 1 | 1 | 1 | |
| der(19;11) | 1 | 1 | 1 | 1 | 1 | 1 | 1 | 1 | 1 | 1 | 1 | 1 | 1 | 1 | 1 | 1 | 1 | 1 | 1 | 1 | |
| der(16) | 1 | | | | | | | | | | | | | | | | | | | | |
| der(12;2) | | 1 | | | | | | | | | | | | | | | | | | | |
| del(16p) | | 1 | | | | | | | | | | | | | | | | | | | |
| del(19q) | | 1 | | | | | | | | | | | | | | | | | | | |
| del(Xq) | | | | | 1 | | | | | | | | | | | | | | | | |
| der(2;17) | | | | | | | | | | 1 | | | | | | | | | | | |
| del(17q) | | | | | | | | | | | | | | | | | | 1 | | | |
| der(11;14) | | | | | | | | | | | | | | | | | | | | 1 | Average±SD |
| **Non-Clonal Aneusomies** | **5** | **10** | **0** | **1** | **3** | **3** | **5** | **4** | **2** | **8** | **1** | **3** | **1** | **4** | **2** | **7** | **1** | **7** | **3** | **4** | **3.7±2.6** |
| **Aneusomies per Karyotype** | **29** | **31** | **28** | **28** | **29** | **28** | **28** | **28** | **28** | **29** | **28** | **28** | **28** | **28** | **28** | **28** | **28** | **29** | **28** | **29** | **28±1** |

**Fig. 12 a, b, c, d** Karyotypic evidence that the metastasis M-425 is an individual subspecies of medulloblastoma M-458. The karyotypic theory of metastasis predicts that metastases have individual clonal karyotypes that differ from those of parental cancers in individual metastasis-specific aneusomies. To test this theory we have compared karyotype-arrays of the metastasis M-425 to that of the primary cancer M-458 prepared as described for Fig. 9. Figure 12 **a**, **b** and the attached table show that 55–90% of the chromosomes of the cancer M-458 and 70–100% of the chromosomes of the metastasis M-425 were clonal, and that cancer and metastasis formed similar clonal patterns. The fact that the karyotype of M-425 was more clonal than that of M-458, again supports the view that M-425 is the metastasis and M-458 the original cancer (See comment regarding this question in section "Karyotypic and phenotypic relationships between metastases and parental cancers"). The karyotype of the metastasis differed from that of the primary cancer in about 17 of an average of 28 M-425 aneusomies (Fig. 12 **a**, **b**, **c**, **d** and Table 1). The copy numbers of most non-clonal chromosomes including marker chromosomes differed from clonal averages ± 1 (see Fig. 12 **a**, **b** and specifically Fig. 12 **c**, **d**). The chromosomes with non-clonal copy numbers represent the ongoing karyotypic variation predicted by the inherent variability of cancer-specific aneuploidy (See Fig. 11**c** and Background). We conclude that the metastasis M-425 is subspecies of the parental medulloblastoma M-458

## Conclusions

The theory that cancer-specific aneuploidy catalyzes the karyotypic evolution of metastases from cancers, explains the following characteristics of metastasis, which are not predictable by the competing mutation theory:

1) The dependence of metastasis on the degree of cancer-specific aneuploidy, because aneuploidy catalyzes karyotypic variations from which metastases arise at aneuploidy-dependent rates: the more aneuploid the cancer the higher its proclivity to

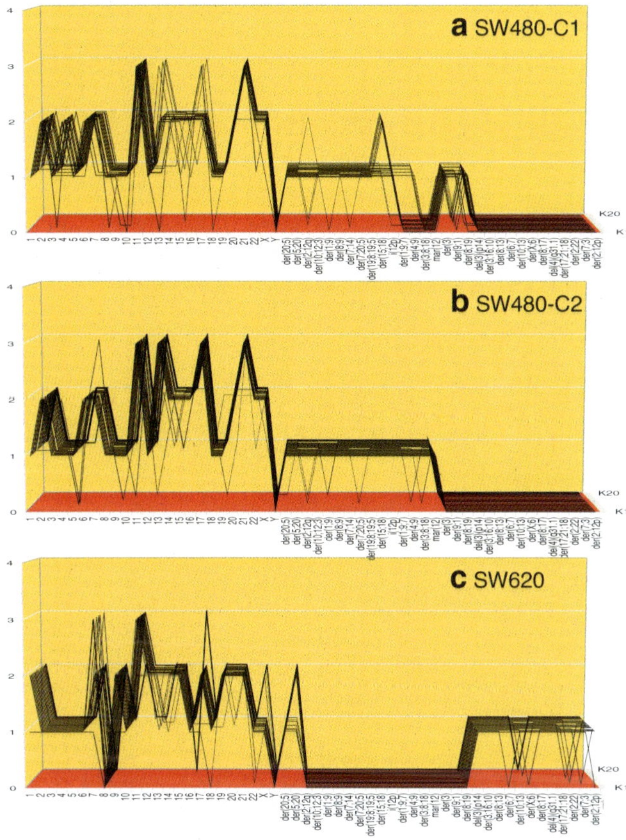


## d Complete karyotypes of 20 cells of SW-480 C1

| Total # of Chromosomes | 53 | 54 | 53 | 54 | 53 | 52 | 55 | 51 | 55 | 53 | 55 | 55 | 54 | 54 | 53 | 55 | 53 | 56 | 53 | |
|---|---|---|---|---|---|---|---|---|---|---|---|---|---|---|---|---|---|---|---|---|
| Chromosome # | K1 | K2 | K3 | K4 | K5 | K6 | K7 | K8 | K9 | K10 | K11 | K12 | K13 | K14 | K15 | K16 | K17 | K18 | K19 | |
| 1 | 1 | 1 | 1 | 1 | 1 | 1 | 1 | 1 | 1 | 1 | 1 | 1 | 1 | 1 | 1 | 1 | 1 | 1 | 1 | |
| 2 | 2 | 2 | 2 | 2 | 2 | 2 | 2 | 2 | 2 | 2 | 1 | 2 | 2 | 2 | 2 | 2 | 1 | 1 | 2 | |
| 3 | 1 | 1 | 1 | 1 | 1 | 0 | 1 | 1 | 1 | 1 | 1 | 1 | 1 | 1 | 1 | 1 | 1 | 1 | 1 | |
| 4 | 2 | 2 | 1 | 2 | 2 | 2 | 1 | 2 | 2 | 2 | 1 | 2 | 2 | 2 | 1 | 1 | 1 | 1 | 2 | |
| 5 | 1 | 1 | 1 | 1 | 1 | 1 | 1 | 1 | 1 | 1 | 1 | 1 | 1 | 1 | 1 | 1 | 1 | 1 | 1 | |
| 6 | 2 | 1 | 2 | 2 | 2 | 2 | 2 | 2 | 2 | 2 | 2 | 2 | 2 | 2 | 2 | 2 | 2 | 2 | 2 | |
| 7 | 2 | 2 | 1 | 2 | 2 | 2 | 1 | 2 | 2 | 2 | 2 | 2 | 2 | 2 | 1 | 2 | 2 | 1 | 2 | |
| 8 | 1 | 1 | 1 | 1 | 1 | 0 | 1 | 1 | 1 | 1 | 1 | 1 | 1 | 1 | 1 | 1 | 1 | 1 | 1 | |
| 9 | 1 | 1 | 1 | 1 | 1 | 1 | 1 | 0 | 1 | 1 | 1 | 1 | 1 | 1 | 1 | 1 | 1 | 1 | 1 | |
| 10 | 0 | 1 | 1 | 1 | 1 | 1 | 1 | 0 | 1 | 1 | 1 | 1 | 1 | 1 | 1 | 1 | 1 | 1 | 1 | |
| 11 | 3 | 3 | 3 | 3 | 3 | 3 | 3 | 3 | 3 | 3 | 3 | 2 | 3 | 3 | 3 | 3 | 3 | 3 | 3 | |
| 12 | 1 | 1 | 1 | 1 | 1 | 1 | 1 | 1 | 1 | 1 | 1 | 1 | 1 | 1 | 1 | 1 | 1 | 1 | 1 | |
| 13 | 2 | 0 | 3 | 2 | 2 | 1 | 1 | 2 | 2 | 2 | 3 | 1 | 2 | 2 | 1 | 3 | 2 | 3 | 2 | |
| 14 | 2 | 2 | 2 | 2 | 2 | 2 | 2 | 2 | 2 | 2 | 2 | 2 | 2 | 2 | 1 | 2 | 2 | 2 | 2 | |
| 15 | 2 | 1 | 2 | 2 | 2 | 2 | 2 | 2 | 2 | 2 | 1 | 0 | 2 | 2 | 2 | 2 | 2 | 2 | 2 | |
| 16 | 1 | 2 | 2 | 2 | 2 | 2 | 2 | 2 | 2 | 2 | 2 | 2 | 2 | 2 | 2 | 2 | 1 | 2 | 2 | |
| 17 | 2 | 3 | 3 | 2 | 2 | 2 | 3 | 2 | 2 | 2 | 2 | 2 | 2 | 2 | 2 | 2 | 2 | 3 | 2 | |
| 18 | 1 | 1 | 0 | 1 | 1 | 1 | 1 | 1 | 1 | 1 | 1 | 1 | 1 | 1 | 1 | 1 | 1 | 1 | 1 | |
| 19 | 1 | 1 | 1 | 1 | 1 | 1 | 1 | 1 | 1 | 1 | 1 | 1 | 1 | 1 | 1 | 1 | 1 | 1 | 1 | |
| 20 | 2 | 2 | 2 | 2 | 2 | 2 | 2 | 2 | 2 | 2 | 2 | 2 | 2 | 2 | 2 | 2 | 2 | 2 | 2 | |
| 21 | 3 | 3 | 3 | 3 | 2 | 3 | 3 | 3 | 3 | 3 | 3 | 3 | 3 | 3 | 3 | 3 | 3 | 3 | 3 | |
| 22 | 2 | 2 | 2 | 2 | 2 | 2 | 2 | 1 | 2 | 1 | 2 | 2 | 2 | 2 | 2 | 2 | 2 | 2 | 2 | |
| X | 2 | 1 | 2 | 2 | 2 | 2 | 2 | 2 | 2 | 2 | 2 | 2 | 2 | 2 | 2 | 2 | 2 | 2 | 2 | |
| Y | 0 | 0 | 0 | 0 | 0 | 0 | 0 | 0 | 0 | 0 | 0 | 0 | 0 | 0 | 0 | 0 | 0 | 0 | 0 | |
| der(20;5) | 1 | 1 | 1 | 1 | 1 | 1 | 1 | 1 | 1 | 1 | 1 | 1 | 1 | 1 | 1 | 1 | 1 | 1 | 1 | |
| der(5;20) | 1 | 1 | 1 | 1 | 1 | 1 | 1 | 1 | 1 | 1 | 1 | 1 | 1 | 1 | 1 | 1 | 1 | 1 | 1 | |
| der(2;12q) | 1 | 1 | 1 | 1 | 1 | 1 | 1 | 0 | 2 | 1 | 1 | 1 | 1 | 1 | 0 | 1 | 1 | 1 | 1 | |
| der(10;12;3) | 1 | 1 | 1 | 1 | 1 | 1 | 1 | 1 | 1 | 1 | 1 | 1 | 1 | 1 | 1 | 1 | 1 | 1 | 1 | |
| der(1;9) | 1 | 1 | 0 | 1 | 1 | 1 | 1 | 1 | 1 | 1 | 1 | 1 | 1 | 1 | 1 | 1 | 1 | 1 | 1 | |
| der(8;9) | 1 | 1 | 1 | 1 | 1 | 1 | 1 | 1 | 1 | 1 | 1 | 1 | 1 | 1 | 1 | 1 | 1 | 1 | 1 | |
| der(7;14) | 1 | 1 | 1 | 1 | 1 | 0 | 1 | 1 | 1 | 1 | 1 | 1 | 1 | 1 | 1 | 1 | 1 | 1 | 1 | |
| der(7;20;5) | 1 | 1 | 1 | 1 | 1 | 1 | 1 | 1 | 1 | 1 | 1 | 1 | 1 | 1 | 1 | 1 | 1 | 1 | 1 | |
| der(19;8;19;5) | 1 | 1 | 1 | 1 | 1 | 1 | 1 | 1 | 1 | 1 | 1 | 1 | 1 | 1 | 1 | 1 | 1 | 1 | 1 | |
| der(15;18) | 2 | 1 | 1 | 2 | 1 | 2 | 1 | 1 | 1 | 2 | 1 | 1 | 2 | 2 | 1 | 1 | 2 | 1 | 1 | |
| i(12p) | 1 | 1 | 1 | 1 | 1 | 1 | 1 | 0 | 1 | 1 | 1 | 1 | 1 | 1 | 1 | 1 | 1 | 1 | 0 | |
| der(1;9;7) | 0 | 0 | 1 | 0 | 0 | 0 | 1 | 0 | 0 | 0 | 1 | 0 | 0 | 0 | 1 | 1 | 0 | 1 | 0 | |
| der(4;9) | 0 | 0 | 1 | 0 | 0 | 0 | 1 | 0 | 0 | 0 | 1 | 0 | 0 | 0 | 1 | 1 | 0 | 1 | 0 | |
| mar(12) | 0 | 1 | 0 | 0 | 0 | 0 | 0 | 0 | 0 | 0 | 0 | 0 | 0 | 0 | 0 | 0 | 0 | 0 | 0 | |
| der(3) | 1 | 1 | 1 | 1 | 1 | 1 | 1 | 1 | 1 | 1 | 1 | 1 | 1 | 1 | 1 | 1 | 1 | 1 | 1 | |
| der(9;1) | 1 | 1 | 0 | 1 | 1 | 1 | 0 | 1 | 1 | 1 | 0 | 0 | 1 | 1 | 0 | 0 | 1 | 0 | 1 | |
| der(8;19) | 0 | 0 | 1 | 1 | 1 | 1 | 1 | 0 | 1 | 0 | 1 | 1 | 1 | 1 | 1 | 1 | 1 | 1 | 1 | |
| dic(8;16;10) | 1 | | | | | | | | | | | | | | | | | | | |
| del(16p) | 1 | | | | | | | | | | | | | | | | | | | |
| dic(X;6) | | 1 | | | | | | | | | | | | | | | | | | |
| der(8;13) | | 1 | | | | | | | | | | | | | | | | | | |
| der(13;9) | | 1 | | | | | | | | | | | | | | | | | | |
| der(13;18) | | 1 | | | | | | | | | | 1 | | | | | | | | |
| der(13;15) | | 1 | | | | | | | | | | 1 | | | | | | | | |
| dic(1;9;18) | | | 1 | | | | | | | | | | | | | | | | | |
| mar(18) | | | | | 1 | | | | 1 | | | 1 | | | | | | | 1 | |
| der(3;13) | | | | | | 1 | | | | | | | | | | | | | | |
| dic(8;7;14) | | | | | | 1 | | | | | | | | | | | | | | |
| der(4;13) | | | | | | | 1 | | | | | | | | | | | | | |
| der(7;13) | | | | | | | 1 | | | | | | | | 1 | | | | | |
| i(18p) | | | | | | | 1 | | | | | | | | 1 | 1 | | 1 | | |
| dic(8;2;12) | | | | | | | | 1 | | | | | | | | | | | | |
| der(9;17) | | | | | | | | 1 | | | | | | | | | | | | |
| dic(10;12;10;12) | | | | | | | | 1 | | | | | | | | | | | | |
| dic(15;18;22) | | | | | | | | 1 | | | | | | | | | | | | |
| dic(8;22) | | | | | | | | | | 1 | | | | | | | | | | |
| der(2;15) | | | | | | | | | | | 1 | | | | | | | | | |
| der(17;18) | | | | | | | | | | | 1 | | | | | | | | | |
| del(17q) | | | | | | | | | | | 1 | | | | | | | | | |
| der(1;9;18) | | | | | | | | | | | | 1 | | | | | | | | |
| der(15;17) | | | | | | | | | | | | 1 | | | | | | | | |
| der(11) | | | | | | | | | | | | 1 | | | | | | | | |
| mar(17) | | | | | | | | | | | | 1 | | | 1 | | | | | |
| der(15;2;12) | | | | | | | | | | | | | | | 1 | | | | | |
| der(2;4) | | | | | | | | | | | | | | | | | 1 | | | |
| der(16;4) | | | | | | | | | | | | | | | | | 1 | | | |
| del(7q) | | | | | | | | | | | | | | | | | | 1 | | |
| der(2) | | | | | | | | | | | | | | | | | | 1 | | Average±SD |
| **Non-Clonal Aneusomies** | **6** | **12** | **10** | **1** | **2** | **7** | **10** | **10** | **2** | **4** | **10** | **11** | **1** | **1** | **12** | **6** | **6** | **11** | **2** | **6.5±4** |
| **Aneusomies per Karyotype** | **39** | **43** | **40** | **38** | **39** | **40** | **42** | **41** | **39** | **38** | **42** | **44** | **38** | **38** | **43** | **40** | **40** | **42** | **39** | **40±2** |

| Primary Colon Cancer SW480-1, SW480-2 and Metastatis SW620 | | | | | | | |
|---|---|---|---|---|---|---|---|
| | SW480-C1 | SW480-C2 | SW620 | | SW480-C1 | SW480-C2 | SW620 |
| Avg # of chromosomes ± SD | 53±1 | 54±2 | 49±2 | clonal markers | copy no (% clonal) | | |
| chromosome # | copy no (% clonal) | | | der(20;5) | 1 (100) | 1 (95) | 1 (100) |
| 1 | 1 (100) | 1 (100) | 2 (95) | der(5;20) | 1 (100) | 1 (100) | 2 (65) |
| 2 | 2 (84) | 2 (95) | 1 (100) | der(2;12q) | 1 (84) | 1 (90) | - |
| 3 | 1 (95) | 1 (100) | 1 (100) | der(10;12;3) | 1 (100) | 1 (100) | - |
| 4 | 2 (63) | 1 (95) | 1 (100) | der(1;9) | 1 (95) | 1 (90) | - |
| 5 | 1 (100) | 1 (90) | 1 (100) | der(8;9) | 1 (100) | 1 (100) | - |
| 6 | 2 (95) | 2 (90) | 1 (100) | der(7;14) | 1 (95) | 1 (100) | - |
| 7 | 2 (79) | 2 (95) | 2 (65) | der(7;20;5) | 1 (100) | 1 (95) | - |
| 8 | 1 (95) | 1 (95) | 0 | der(19;8;19;5) | 1 (100) | 1 (100) | - |
| 9 | 1 (95) | 1 (95) | 2 (95) | der(15;18) | 1 (63) | 1 (100) | - |
| 10 | 1 (89) | 1 (95) | 1 (100) | i(12p) | 1 (89) | 1 (100) | - |
| 11 | 3 (95) | 3 (86) | 3 (85) | der(1;9;7) | 1 (32) | 1 (100) | - |
| 12 | 1 (100) | 1 (95) | 2 (90) | der(4;9) | 1 (32) | 1 (95) | - |
| 13 | 2 (53) | 3 (86) | 2 (75) | der(3;8;18) | - | 1 (95) | - |
| 14 | 2 (95) | 2 (90) | 2 (90) | mar(12) | 1 (5) | 1 (100) | - |
| 15 | 2 (84) | 2 (90) | 2 (100) | der(3) | 1 (100) | - | - |
| 16 | 2 (89) | 2 (100) | 1 (95) | der(9;1) | 1 (63) | - | - |
| 17 | 2 (79) | 3 (95) | 2 (85) | der(8;19) | 1 (79) | - | - |
| 18 | 1 (95) | 1 (100) | 1 (95) | del(3)(p14) | - | - | 1 (100) |
| 19 | 1 (100) | 1 (90) | 2 (95) | der(3;16;10) | - | - | 1 (100) |
| 20 | 2 (100) | 2 (95) | 2 (90) | der(8;13) | - | - | 1 (100) |
| 21 | 3 (95) | 3 (90) | 2 (100) | der(6;7) | - | - | 1 (95) |
| 22 | 2 (89) | 2 (95) | 1 (90) | der(10;13) | - | - | 1 (100) |
| X | 2 (95) | 2 (95) | 1 (85) | der(X;6) | - | - | 1 (85) |
| Y | 0 | 0 | 0 | der(8;17) | - | - | 1 (100) |
| | | | | del(4)(q31.1) | - | - | 1 (100) |
| | | | | der(17;21;18) | - | - | 1 (100) |
| | | | | der(2;22) | - | - | 1 (90) |
| | | | | der(7;3) | - | - | 1 (90) |
| | | | | der(2;12p) | - | - | 1 (95) |
| | | | | Total Clonal Aneusomies | 38 | 39 | 38 |

## e Complete karyotypes of 20 cells of SW-480 C2

| Total # of Chromosomes | 57 | 55 | 55 | 55 | 55 | 55 | 55 | 54 | 56 | 53 | 54 | 55 | 51 | 55 | 55 | 55 | 53 | 51 | 46 | 55 | 55 | |
|---|---|---|---|---|---|---|---|---|---|---|---|---|---|---|---|---|---|---|---|---|---|---|
| Chromosome # | K1 | K2 | K3 | K4 | K5 | K6 | K7 | K8 | K9 | K10 | K11 | K12 | K13 | K14 | K15 | K16 | K17 | K18 | K19 | K20 | K21 | |
| 1 | 1 | 1 | 1 | 1 | 1 | 1 | 1 | 1 | 1 | 1 | 1 | 1 | 1 | 1 | 1 | 1 | 1 | 1 | 1 | 1 | 1 | |
| 2 | 2 | 2 | 2 | 2 | 2 | 2 | 2 | 1 | 2 | 2 | 2 | 2 | 2 | 2 | 2 | 2 | 2 | 2 | 2 | 2 | 2 | |
| 3 | 1 | 1 | 1 | 1 | 1 | 1 | 1 | 1 | 1 | 1 | 1 | 1 | 1 | 1 | 1 | 1 | 1 | 1 | 1 | 1 | 1 | |
| 4 | 2 | 1 | 1 | 1 | 1 | 1 | 1 | 1 | 1 | 1 | 1 | 1 | 1 | 1 | 1 | 1 | 1 | 1 | 1 | 1 | 1 | |
| 5 | 1 | 1 | 1 | 1 | 1 | 1 | 1 | 0 | 1 | 0 | 1 | 1 | 1 | 1 | 1 | 1 | 1 | 1 | 1 | 1 | 1 | |
| 6 | 2 | 2 | 2 | 2 | 2 | 2 | 2 | 2 | 2 | 2 | 2 | 2 | 2 | 2 | 2 | 2 | 1 | 1 | 2 | 2 | 2 | |
| 7 | 2 | 2 | 2 | 2 | 2 | 2 | 2 | 2 | 2 | 3 | 2 | 2 | 2 | 2 | 2 | 2 | 2 | 2 | 2 | 2 | 2 | |
| 8 | 2 | 1 | 1 | 1 | 1 | 1 | 1 | 1 | 1 | 1 | 1 | 1 | 1 | 1 | 1 | 1 | 1 | 1 | 1 | 1 | 1 | |
| 9 | 1 | 1 | 1 | 1 | 1 | 1 | 1 | 1 | 1 | 1 | 1 | 1 | 0 | 1 | 1 | 1 | 1 | 1 | 1 | 1 | 1 | |
| 10 | 1 | 1 | 1 | 1 | 1 | 1 | 1 | 1 | 1 | 1 | 1 | 1 | 1 | 1 | 1 | 1 | 0 | 1 | 1 | 1 | 1 | |
| 11 | 3 | 3 | 3 | 3 | 3 | 3 | 3 | 3 | 3 | 3 | 3 | 3 | 2 | 3 | 3 | 3 | 2 | 3 | 2 | 3 | 3 | |
| 12 | 1 | 1 | 1 | 1 | 1 | 1 | 1 | 1 | 1 | 1 | 1 | 1 | 1 | 1 | 1 | 1 | 1 | 1 | 0 | 1 | 1 | |
| 13 | 3 | 3 | 3 | 3 | 3 | 3 | 3 | 3 | 3 | 3 | 3 | 3 | 2 | 3 | 3 | 3 | 3 | 2 | 1 | 3 | 3 | |
| 14 | 2 | 2 | 2 | 2 | 2 | 2 | 2 | 2 | 2 | 2 | 2 | 2 | 1 | 2 | 2 | 2 | 2 | 1 | 2 | 2 | 2 | |
| 15 | 2 | 2 | 2 | 2 | 2 | 2 | 2 | 2 | 2 | 1 | 1 | 2 | 2 | 2 | 2 | 2 | 2 | 2 | 2 | 2 | 2 | |
| 16 | 2 | 2 | 2 | 2 | 2 | 2 | 2 | 2 | 2 | 2 | 2 | 2 | 2 | 2 | 2 | 2 | 2 | 2 | 2 | 2 | 2 | |
| 17 | 3 | 3 | 3 | 3 | 3 | 3 | 3 | 3 | 3 | 3 | 3 | 3 | 3 | 3 | 3 | 3 | 3 | 3 | 2 | 3 | 3 | |
| 18 | 1 | 1 | 1 | 1 | 1 | 1 | 1 | 1 | 1 | 1 | 1 | 1 | 1 | 1 | 1 | 1 | 1 | 1 | 1 | 1 | 1 | |
| 19 | 1 | 1 | 1 | 1 | 1 | 1 | 1 | 1 | 2 | 1 | 1 | 1 | 1 | 1 | 1 | 1 | 1 | 1 | 0 | 1 | 1 | |
| 20 | 2 | 2 | 2 | 2 | 2 | 2 | 2 | 2 | 2 | 2 | 2 | 2 | 2 | 2 | 2 | 2 | 2 | 2 | 1 | 2 | 2 | |
| 21 | 3 | 3 | 3 | 3 | 3 | 3 | 3 | 2 | 3 | 3 | 3 | 3 | 3 | 3 | 3 | 3 | 3 | 2 | 3 | 3 | 3 | |
| 22 | 2 | 2 | 2 | 2 | 2 | 2 | 2 | 2 | 2 | 1 | 2 | 2 | 2 | 2 | 2 | 2 | 2 | 2 | 2 | 2 | 2 | |
| X | 2 | 2 | 2 | 2 | 2 | 2 | 2 | 2 | 2 | 2 | 2 | 2 | 2 | 2 | 2 | 2 | 1 | 2 | 2 | 2 | 2 | |
| Y | 0 | 0 | 0 | 0 | 0 | 0 | 0 | 0 | 0 | 0 | 0 | 0 | 0 | 0 | 0 | 0 | 0 | 0 | 0 | 0 | 0 | |
| der(20;5) | 1 | 1 | 1 | 1 | 1 | 1 | 1 | 1 | 1 | 1 | 1 | 1 | 1 | 1 | 1 | 1 | 1 | 1 | 0 | 1 | 1 | |
| der(5;20) | 1 | 1 | 1 | 1 | 1 | 1 | 1 | 1 | 1 | 1 | 1 | 1 | 1 | 1 | 1 | 1 | 1 | 1 | 1 | 1 | 1 | |
| der(2;12q) | 1 | 1 | 1 | 1 | 1 | 1 | 1 | 1 | 1 | 0 | 1 | 1 | 1 | 1 | 1 | 1 | 1 | 0 | 1 | 1 | 1 | |
| der(10;12;3) | 1 | 1 | 1 | 1 | 1 | 1 | 1 | 1 | 1 | 1 | 1 | 1 | 1 | 1 | 1 | 1 | 1 | 1 | 1 | 1 | 1 | |
| der(1;9) | 1 | 1 | 1 | 1 | 1 | 1 | 1 | 1 | 1 | 1 | 1 | 1 | 1 | 1 | 1 | 1 | 1 | 0 | 0 | 1 | 1 | |
| der(8;9) | 1 | 1 | 1 | 1 | 1 | 1 | 1 | 1 | 1 | 1 | 1 | 1 | 1 | 1 | 1 | 1 | 1 | 1 | 1 | 1 | 1 | |
| der(7;14) | 1 | 1 | 1 | 1 | 1 | 1 | 1 | 1 | 1 | 1 | 1 | 1 | 1 | 1 | 1 | 1 | 1 | 1 | 1 | 1 | 1 | |
| der(7;20;5) | 1 | 1 | 1 | 1 | 1 | 1 | 1 | 1 | 1 | 0 | 1 | 1 | 1 | 1 | 1 | 1 | 1 | 1 | 1 | 1 | 1 | |
| der(19;8;19;5) | 1 | 1 | 1 | 1 | 1 | 1 | 1 | 1 | 1 | 1 | 1 | 1 | 1 | 1 | 1 | 1 | 1 | 1 | 1 | 1 | 1 | |
| der(15;18) | 1 | 1 | 1 | 1 | 1 | 1 | 1 | 1 | 1 | 1 | 1 | 1 | 1 | 1 | 1 | 1 | 1 | 1 | 1 | 1 | 1 | |
| i(12p) | 1 | 1 | 1 | 1 | 1 | 1 | 1 | 1 | 1 | 1 | 1 | 1 | 1 | 1 | 1 | 1 | 1 | 1 | 1 | 1 | 1 | |
| der(1;9;7) | 1 | 1 | 1 | 1 | 1 | 1 | 1 | 1 | 1 | 1 | 1 | 1 | 1 | 1 | 1 | 1 | 1 | 1 | 1 | 1 | 1 | |
| der(4;9) | 1 | 1 | 1 | 1 | 1 | 1 | 1 | 1 | 1 | 1 | 0 | 1 | 1 | 1 | 1 | 1 | 1 | 1 | 1 | 1 | 1 | |
| der(3;8;18) | 1 | 1 | 1 | 1 | 1 | 1 | 1 | 1 | 1 | 0 | 1 | 1 | 1 | 1 | 1 | 1 | 1 | 1 | 1 | 1 | 1 | |
| mar(12) | 1 | 1 | 1 | 1 | 1 | 1 | 1 | 1 | 1 | 1 | 1 | 1 | 1 | 1 | 1 | 1 | 1 | 1 | 1 | 1 | 1 | |
| dic(15;2;12) | 0 | 0 | 0 | 0 | 0 | 0 | 0 | 0 | 0 | 1 | 0 | 0 | 0 | 0 | 0 | 0 | 0 | 0 | 0 | 0 | 0 | |
| dic(18;8;3;5;7;22) | 0 | 0 | 0 | 0 | 0 | 0 | 0 | 0 | 0 | 1 | 0 | 0 | 0 | 0 | 0 | 0 | 0 | 0 | 0 | 0 | 0 | |
| der(3;7;5) | 0 | 0 | 0 | 0 | 0 | 0 | 0 | 0 | 0 | 1 | 0 | 0 | 0 | 0 | 0 | 0 | 0 | 0 | 0 | 0 | 0 | |
| der(2;5) | 0 | 0 | 0 | 0 | 0 | 0 | 0 | 1 | 0 | 0 | 0 | 0 | 0 | 0 | 0 | 0 | 0 | 0 | 0 | 0 | 0 | |
| dup(21) | 0 | 0 | 0 | 0 | 0 | 0 | 0 | 1 | 0 | 0 | 0 | 0 | 0 | 0 | 0 | 0 | 0 | 0 | 0 | 0 | 0 | |
| dic(15;4;9) | 0 | 0 | 0 | 0 | 0 | 0 | 0 | 0 | 0 | 0 | 1 | 0 | 0 | 0 | 0 | 0 | 0 | 0 | 0 | 0 | 0 | |
| dic(X;10) | 0 | 0 | 0 | 0 | 0 | 0 | 0 | 0 | 0 | 0 | 0 | 0 | 0 | 0 | 0 | 0 | 1 | 0 | 0 | 0 | 0 | |
| der(6) | 0 | 0 | 0 | 0 | 0 | 0 | 0 | 0 | 0 | 0 | 0 | 0 | 0 | 0 | 0 | 0 | 1 | 0 | 0 | 0 | 0 | |
| der(2;15) | 0 | 0 | 0 | 0 | 0 | 0 | 0 | 0 | 0 | 0 | 0 | 0 | 0 | 0 | 0 | 0 | 0 | 1 | 0 | 0 | 0 | |
| der(2;12)short | 0 | 0 | 0 | 0 | 0 | 0 | 0 | 0 | 0 | 0 | 0 | 0 | 0 | 0 | 0 | 0 | 0 | 1 | 0 | 0 | 0 | Average±SD |
| **Non-Clonal Aneusomies** | **2** | **0** | **0** | **0** | **0** | **0** | **0** | **5** | **1** | **10** | **3** | **0** | **4** | **0** | **0** | **0** | **6** | **8** | **8** | **0** | **0** | **2±3** |
| **Aneusomies per Karyotype** | **39** | **39** | **39** | **39** | **39** | **39** | **39** | **41** | **39** | **42** | **40** | **39** | **39** | **39** | **39** | **39** | **41** | **41** | **39** | **39** | **39** | **40±1** |

**Fig. 13** (See legend on next page.)

(See figure on previous page.)
**Fig. 13** **a**, **b**, **c**, **d**, **e** Karyotypic evidence that the metastasis SW-620 is an individual subspecies of SW-480 or of an unknown common precursor. The karyotypic theory of metastasis predicts that metastases have individual clonal karyotypes that differ from those of parental cancers in individual metastasis-specific aneusomies. To test this theory we have compared karyotype-arrays of the metastasis SW-620 to that of two clones of the presumed primary SW-480, prepared as described for Fig. 9. Figure 13 **a**, **b**, **c** and the attached table show that 75 - 100% of the chromosomes of SW-620 and 53–100% of the chromosomes of SW-480 C1 and 75-100% of the chromosomes of SW-480 C2 were clonal, and that the two cancer clones and the metastasis formed similar clonal patterns. The karyotype of the metastasis differed from that of the primary cancer SW-480 C1 in 25 of 38 average SW-480 C1 aneusomies and differed from SW-480 C2 in 27 of 38 average aneusomies (Fig. 13**a**, **b**, **c**, **d**, **e** and Table 1). The copy numbers of most non-clonal chromosomes including marker chromosomes differed from clonal averages ± 1 (Fig. 13**a**, **b**, **c** and specifically Fig. 13**d**, **e**). The chromosomes with non-clonal copy numbers represent the ongoing karyotypic variation predicted by the inherent variability of cancer-specific aneuploidy (See Fig. 11**d**, **e** and Background). We conclude that the metastasis SW-620 is a subspecies of the parental colon cancer SW-480 or of a common unknown precursor

metastasize. This explains the early studies summarized in the Background that have linked the risk of metastasis to the degrees of cancer-specific aneuploidy. Catalysis by cancer-specific aneuploidy further suggests that the "mutant alleles" thought to "preordain" or "pre-determine" the proclivity of cancers to metastasize [69, 74] are instead cancer-specific aneuploidies.

2) The individuality of metastases as results of unpredictable stochastic karyotypic variations that convert cancers to metastases - much like random karyotypic variantions explain the individuality of conventional species.
3) The conservation of the complexities of cancer karyotypes in metastasis - as in conventional speciation [103].

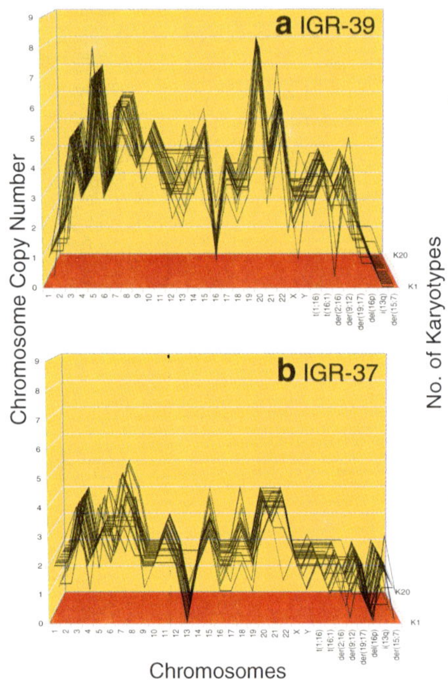


Primary Melanoma IGR-39 and Metastatis IGR-37

| | IGR-39 | IGR-37 |
|---|---|---|
| Avg # of chromosomes ± SD | 111±3 | 73±4 |
| chromosome # | copy no (% clonal) | |
| 1 | 1 (95) | 2 (75) |
| 2 | 2 (60) | 2 (90) |
| 3 | 5 (80) | 4 (85) |
| 4 | 3 (100) | 2 (90) |
| 5 | 7 (85) | 3 (70) |
| 6 | 3 (100) | 3 (60) |
| 7 | 6 (70) | 5 (35)/4 (35) |
| 8 | 6 (65) | 3 (50) |
| 9 | 4 (90) | 2 (95) |
| 10 | 5 (85) | 2 (100) |
| 11 | 4 (90) | 3 (75) |
| 12 | 3 (75) | 2 (100) |
| 13 | 4 (45)/3 (35) | 0 (85) |
| 14 | 4 (70) | 2 (100) |
| 15 | 5 (55) | 3 (75) |
| 16 | 1 (85) | 2 (75) |
| 17 | 4 (80) | 2 (90) |
| 18 | 3 (80) | 3 (45)/2 (35) |
| 19 | 4 (60) | 2 (90) |
| 20 | 8 (65) | 4 (85) |
| 21 | 4 (60) | 4 (65) |
| 22 | 6 (80) | 4 (85) |
| X | 3 (70) | 2 (100) |
| Y | 3 (75) | 2 (70) |
| clonal markers | - | - |
| t(1;16) | 3 (75) | 2 (100) |
| t(16;1) | 4 (85) | 2 (55) |
| der(2;16) | 3 (65) | 2 (80) |
| der(9;12) | 4 (50) | 1 (70) |
| der(19;17) | 2 (75) | 2 (80) |
| del(16p) | 1 (85) | 0 (95) |
| i(13q) | 1 (10) | 2 (70) |
| der(15;7) | - | 1 (60) |
| Total Clonal Aneusomies | 30 | 31 |

**C** Complete karyotypes of 20 IGR-39 cells

| Total # of Chromosomes | 115 | 115 | 111 | 107 | 111 | 114 | 109 | 113 | 110 | 107 | 111 | 108 | 108 | 116 | 115 | 111 | 111 | 104 | 111 | 114 | |
|---|---|---|---|---|---|---|---|---|---|---|---|---|---|---|---|---|---|---|---|---|---|
| Chromosome # | K1 | K2 | K3 | K4 | K5 | K6 | K7 | K8 | K9 | K10 | K11 | K12 | K13 | K14 | K15 | K16 | K17 | K18 | K19 | K20 | |
| 1 | 1 | 1 | 1 | 1 | 1 | 1 | 0 | 1 | 1 | 1 | 1 | 1 | 1 | 1 | 1 | 1 | 1 | 1 | 1 | 1 | |
| 2 | 2 | 2 | 3 | 2 | 1 | 2 | 3 | 2 | 2 | 1 | 2 | 2 | 1 | 3 | 2 | 2 | 2 | 2 | 3 | 3 | |
| 3 | 5 | 5 | 5 | 5 | 5 | 5 | 4 | 5 | 5 | 5 | 5 | 5 | 5 | 5 | 4 | 5 | 4 | 5 | 4 | 5 | |
| 4 | 3 | 3 | 3 | 3 | 3 | 3 | 3 | 3 | 3 | 3 | 3 | 3 | 3 | 3 | 3 | 3 | 3 | 3 | 3 | 3 | |
| 5 | 7 | 7 | 8 | 7 | 7 | 7 | 7 | 7 | 7 | 7 | 6 | 7 | 7 | 7 | 7 | 7 | 7 | 5 | 7 | 7 | |
| 6 | 3 | 3 | 3 | 3 | 3 | 3 | 3 | 3 | 3 | 3 | 3 | 3 | 3 | 3 | 3 | 3 | 3 | 3 | 3 | 3 | |
| 7 | 6 | 6 | 6 | 5 | 5 | 6 | 6 | 5 | 6 | 6 | 6 | 5 | 6 | 6 | 6 | 6 | 6 | 5 | 4 | 6 | |
| 8 | 5 | 6 | 6 | 5 | 6 | 6 | 5 | 6 | 6 | 5 | 5 | 4 | 6 | 6 | 6 | 6 | 6 | 6 | 5 | 6 | |
| 9 | 4 | 4 | 4 | 4 | 4 | 4 | 4 | 4 | 4 | 4 | 4 | 4 | 3 | 4 | 3 | 4 | 4 | 4 | 4 | 4 | |
| 10 | 5 | 5 | 5 | 5 | 4 | 5 | 5 | 5 | 5 | 5 | 5 | 5 | 4 | 5 | 4 | 5 | 5 | 5 | 5 | 5 | |
| 11 | 4 | 4 | 4 | 4 | 4 | 4 | 4 | 3 | 4 | 4 | 4 | 3 | 4 | 4 | 4 | 4 | 4 | 4 | 4 | 4 | |
| 12 | 3 | 3 | 3 | 3 | 3 | 3 | 2 | 3 | 3 | 4 | 3 | 3 | 3 | 4 | 3 | 3 | 4 | 4 | 3 | 3 | |
| 13 | 4 | 2 | 4 | 3 | 4 | 3 | 3 | 3 | 2 | 3 | 3 | 4 | 3 | 4 | 5 | 2 | 4 | 4 | 4 | 4 | |
| 14 | 5 | 4 | 3 | 3 | 4 | 4 | 4 | 4 | 3 | 4 | 4 | 4 | 5 | 4 | 3 | 4 | 4 | 4 | 4 | 4 | |
| 15 | 6 | 5 | 4 | 4 | 5 | 5 | 4 | 5 | 5 | 4 | 5 | 4 | 4 | 5 | 5 | 5 | 5 | 2 | 4 | 5 | |
| 16 | 1 | 1 | 1 | 1 | 1 | 1 | 1 | 1 | 1 | 1 | 1 | 1 | 1 | 1 | 2 | 1 | 0 | 1 | 1 | 2 | |
| 17 | 4 | 4 | 4 | 3 | 4 | 4 | 4 | 4 | 4 | 4 | 3 | 4 | 4 | 4 | 3 | 3 | 4 | 4 | 4 | 4 | |
| 18 | 3 | 3 | 3 | 2 | 4 | 3 | 3 | 3 | 3 | 3 | 3 | 2 | 3 | 3 | 3 | 3 | 3 | 2 | 3 | 3 | |
| 19 | 4 | 4 | 4 | 3 | 5 | 4 | 3 | 4 | 3 | 3 | 4 | 4 | 4 | 4 | 3 | 3 | 4 | 4 | 5 | 4 | |
| 20 | 8 | 7 | 8 | 8 | 7 | 8 | 7 | 7 | 6 | 4 | 8 | 7 | 8 | 8 | 8 | 8 | 8 | 8 | 8 | 8 | |
| 21 | 4 | 4 | 3 | 4 | 5 | 4 | 4 | 4 | 4 | 4 | 4 | 3 | 4 | 4 | 5 | 4 | 3 | 2 | 3 | 3 | |
| 22 | 6 | 6 | 5 | 6 | 6 | 6 | 6 | 6 | 6 | 6 | 6 | 5 | 6 | 6 | 6 | 6 | 5 | 6 | 7 | 6 | |
| X | 2 | 3 | 3 | 2 | 2 | 3 | 3 | 3 | 3 | 3 | 2 | 3 | 2 | 3 | 3 | 3 | 1 | 3 | 3 | 3 | |
| Y | 3 | 3 | 3 | 3 | 3 | 3 | 3 | 3 | 3 | 3 | 3 | 2 | 3 | 3 | 3 | 3 | 4 | 0 | 2 | 2 | |
| t(1;16) | 3 | 3 | 3 | 4 | 3 | 3 | 4 | 4 | 2 | 3 | 3 | 3 | 3 | 4 | 3 | 3 | 3 | 3 | 3 | 3 | |
| t(16;1) | 4 | 4 | 4 | 4 | 4 | 4 | 4 | 4 | 4 | 3 | 4 | 4 | 4 | 4 | 4 | 4 | 4 | 3 | 4 | 3 | |
| der(2;16) | 3 | 3 | 1 | 3 | 3 | 3 | 0 | 3 | 3 | 3 | 3 | 2 | 3 | 2 | 3 | 3 | 2 | 3 | 2 | 2 | |
| der(9;12) | 4 | 5 | 4 | 4 | 2 | 4 | 4 | 3 | 4 | 3 | 3 | 4 | 2 | 3 | 4 | 4 | 2 | 4 | 3 | 3 | |
| der(19;17) | 2 | 2 | 2 | 2 | 2 | 2 | 1 | 2 | 2 | 2 | 2 | 1 | 1 | 2 | 3 | 1 | 2 | 2 | 2 | 2 | |
| del(16p) | 1 | 2 | 1 | 1 | 1 | 1 | 1 | 1 | 1 | 1 | 1 | 1 | 1 | 1 | 0 | 1 | 1 | 1 | 0 | 1 | |
| i(13q) | | 1 | | | | | | | | | 1 | | | | | | | | | | |
| der(2;1) | | | | | | | 1 | | | | | | | | | | | | | | |
| der(2;13) | | | | | | | 1 | | | | | | | | | | | | | | |
| der(3;15) | | | | | | | 1 | | | | | | | | | | | | 1 | | |
| der(12) | | | | | | | 1 | | | | | 1 | | | | | | | | 1 | |
| der(11;7) | | | | | | | | 1 | | | | | | | | | | | | | |
| der(7) | | | | | | | | 1 | | | | | | | | | | | | | |
| der(1;14) | | | | | | | | | 1 | | | | | | | | | | | | |
| der(13;20) | | | | | | | | | 1 | | | | | | | | | | | | |
| der(1;16;18) | | | | | | | | | | 1 | | | | | | | | | | | |
| dic(9;15) | | | | | | | | | | 1 | | | | | | | | | | | |
| der(12;17) | | | | | | | | | | | 1 | | | | | | | | | | |
| der(2;21) | | | | | | | | | | | | 1 | | | | | | | | | |
| der(20;11) | | | | | | | | | | | | 1 | | | | | | | | | |
| der(18;8) | | | | | | | | | | | | 1 | | | | | | | | | |
| der(15;22) | | | | | | | | | | | | 1 | | | | | | | | | |
| der(9;13) | | | | | | | | | | | | | 1 | | | | | | | | |
| der(3;17) | | | | | | | | | | | | | | | 1 | | | | | | |
| der(5) | | | | | | | | | | | | | | | 1 | | | | | | |
| del(9p) | | | | | | | | | | | | | | | 1 | | | | | | |
| der(13;19;17) | | | | | | | | | | | | | | | | 1 | | | | | |
| del(Xq) | | | | | | | | | | | | | | | | | 1 | | | | |
| der(3p) | | | | | | | | | | | | | | | | | 1 | | | | |
| del(3q) | | | | | | | | | | | | | | | | | 1 | | | | |
| dic(16;15) | | | | | | | | | | | | | | | | | | 1 | | | |
| der(16;21) | | | | | | | | | | | | | | | | | | | 1 | | |
| der(Y;12) | | | | | | | | | | | | | | | | | | | 1 | | |
| der(9;17) | | | | | | | | | | | | | | | | | | | | 1 | **Average±SD** |
| **Non-Clonal Aneusomies** | **4** | **5** | **7** | **9** | **9** | **0** | **15** | **7** | **7** | **10** | **7** | **16** | **9** | **5** | **14** | **5** | **12** | **9** | **15** | **9** | **11±4** |
| **Aneusomies per Karyotype** | **30** | **31** | **30** | **30** | **30** | **30** | **34** | **32** | **32** | **32** | **32** | **35** | **31** | **30** | **33** | **31** | **33** | **31** | **33** | **32** | **32±1** |

**Fig. 14** **a**, **b**, **c** Karyotypic evidence that the metastasis IGR-37 is an individual subspecies of melanoma IGR-39. The karyotypic theory of metastasis predicts that metastases have individual clonal karyotypes that differ from those of parental cancers in individual metastasis-specific aneusomies. To test this theory we have compared karyotype-arrays of the metastasis IGR-37 to that of the primary cancer IGR-39 prepared as described for Fig. 9. Figure 14 **a**, **b**, **c** and the attached table show that 55–100% of the chromosomes of the parental cancer IGR-39 and 50–100% of the chromosomes of the metastasis IGR-37 were clonal, and that cancer and metastasis formed similar clonal patterns. These patterns show, however, that metastasis coincided with a reduction in the ploidy of the parental cancer from hyper-tetraploid to hyper-triploid. Moreover, the karyotype of the metastasis differed from that of the primary cancer in about 27 of an average of 31 metastasis-specific aneusomies (Fig. 14 **a**, **b**, **c** and Table 1). Since the ploidy-shift changed the relative chromosome copy numbers of many aneusomies, the percentage of metastasis-specific aneusomies is, however, larger than if it were based on qualitative differences only (see Table 1). As in all other hyper-diploid cancers, the copy numbers of most non-clonal chromosomes including marker chromosomes differed from clonal averages ± 1 (Fig. 14 **a**, **b** and specifically Fig. 14**c**). Again, the chromosomes with non-clonal copy numbers represent the ongoing karyotypic variation predicted by the inherent variability of cancer-specific aneuploidy (See Background). We conclude that the metastasis IGR-37 is a subspecies of the parental melanoma IGR-39

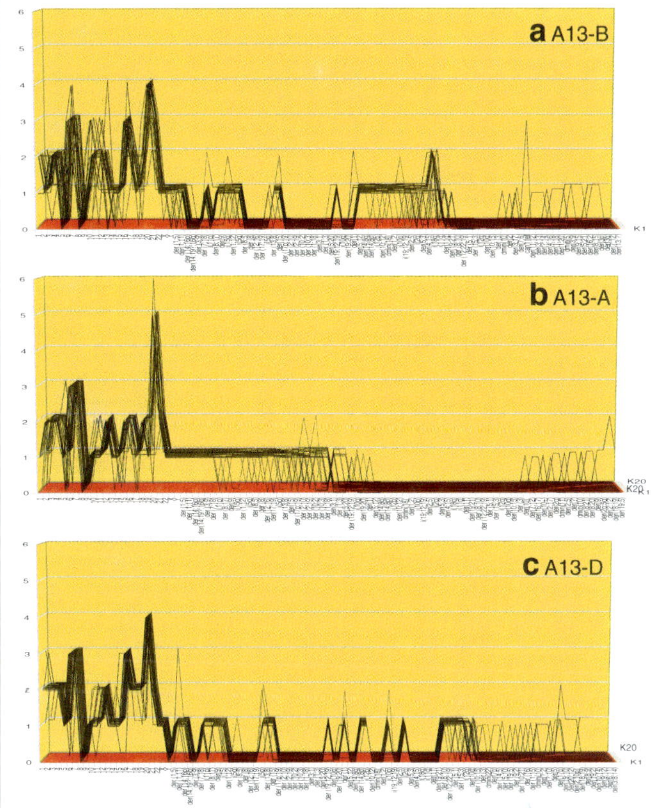


**d.** Complete karyotypes of 20 A13-B cells

| Total # of Chromosomes | 67 | 65 | 63 | 63 | 67 | 67 | 67 | 65 | 51 | 67 | 68 | 70 | 66 | 68 | 68 | 48 | 67 | 54 | 69 | 68 | |
|---|---|---|---|---|---|---|---|---|---|---|---|---|---|---|---|---|---|---|---|---|---|
| Chromosome # | K1 | K2 | K3 | K4 | K5 | K6 | K7 | K8 | K9 | K10 | K11 | K12 | K13 | K14 | K15 | K16 | K17 | K18 | K19 | K20 | |
| 1 | 1 | 1 | 2 | 2 | 2 | 2 | 2 | 2 | 2 | 1 | 2 | 1 | 1 | 1 | 2 | 1 | 1 | 1 | 2 | 2 | |
| 2 | 1 | 1 | 1 | 1 | 2 | 2 | 1 | 1 | 1 | 1 | 1 | 1 | 1 | 2 | 1 | 0 | 1 | 1 | 1 | 1 | |
| 3 | 2 | 2 | 1 | 2 | 2 | 2 | 2 | 2 | 2 | 2 | 2 | 2 | 2 | 2 | 2 | 1 | 2 | 1 | 2 | 1 | |
| 4 | 2 | 2 | 2 | 2 | 2 | 2 | 2 | 2 | 2 | 2 | 2 | 2 | 2 | 2 | 2 | 1 | 2 | 1 | 2 | 2 | |
| 5 | 0 | 0 | 0 | 0 | 0 | 1 | 0 | 0 | 1 | 0 | 0 | 0 | 0 | 0 | 0 | 0 | 0 | 0 | 1 | 0 | |
| 6 | 3 | 3 | 3 | 2 | 3 | 3 | 3 | 3 | 2 | 3 | 3 | 3 | 3 | 3 | 3 | 2 | 3 | 2 | 3 | 3 | |
| 7 | 4 | 2 | 3 | 4 | 2 | 3 | 3 | 3 | 1 | 3 | 3 | 3 | 2 | 2 | 3 | 2 | 3 | 3 | 3 | 2 | |
| 8 | 0 | 0 | 0 | 0 | 0 | 0 | 0 | 0 | 0 | 0 | 0 | 0 | 0 | 0 | 0 | 0 | 0 | 0 | 0 | 0 | |
| 9 | 1 | 1 | 1 | 2 | 1 | 2 | 1 | 1 | 1 | 1 | 1 | 1 | 1 | 1 | 1 | 1 | 1 | 0 | 0 | 1 | |
| 10 | 2 | 1 | 2 | 3 | 3 | 3 | 2 | 2 | 2 | 2 | 2 | 3 | 2 | 2 | 2 | 1 | 2 | 1 | 2 | 2 | |
| 11 | 2 | 2 | 2 | 2 | 3 | 2 | 2 | 0 | 1 | 2 | 2 | 2 | 3 | 1 | 2 | 2 | 2 | 2 | 2 | 2 | |
| 12 | 2 | 2 | 1 | 2 | 2 | 3 | 2 | 2 | 1 | 2 | 2 | 2 | 2 | 2 | 2 | 1 | 2 | 1 | 2 | 4 | |
| 13 | 0 | 0 | 1 | 0 | 1 | 1 | 1 | 1 | 1 | 1 | 1 | 1 | 1 | 1 | 1 | 0 | 1 | 0 | 1 | 0 | |
| 14 | 1 | 1 | 1 | 1 | 1 | 0 | 1 | 1 | 1 | 1 | 1 | 1 | 1 | 1 | 1 | 1 | 1 | 0 | 1 | 1 | |
| 15 | 1 | 1 | 1 | 1 | 1 | 1 | 1 | 1 | 1 | 0 | 1 | 1 | 1 | 1 | 1 | 1 | 1 | 0 | 1 | 1 | |
| 16 | 3 | 3 | 3 | 2 | 3 | 2 | 3 | 3 | 3 | 3 | 3 | 4 | 3 | 3 | 3 | 3 | 3 | 1 | 3 | 3 | |
| 17 | 2 | 2 | 2 | 2 | 2 | 2 | 2 | 2 | 1 | 2 | 2 | 2 | 1 | 2 | 2 | 1 | 2 | 2 | 2 | 2 | |
| 18 | 1 | 1 | 1 | 2 | 1 | 1 | 2 | 0 | 1 | 1 | 1 | 1 | 1 | 1 | 1 | 1 | 1 | 0 | 1 | 1 | |
| 19 | 2 | 3 | 2 | 2 | 1 | 2 | 2 | 2 | 1 | 2 | 2 | 2 | 2 | 2 | 2 | 1 | 2 | 2 | 2 | 2 | |
| 20 | 3 | 4 | 4 | 4 | 3 | 4 | 4 | 4 | 4 | 3 | 4 | 4 | 4 | 4 | 4 | 2 | 4 | 3 | 4 | 4 | |
| 21 | 3 | 2 | 3 | 2 | 3 | 3 | 3 | 3 | 1 | 3 | 3 | 3 | 3 | 3 | 3 | 2 | 3 | 2 | 2 | 3 | |
| 22 | 1 | 1 | 1 | 1 | 1 | 1 | 1 | 1 | 1 | 1 | 1 | 1 | 1 | 1 | 1 | 0 | 1 | 1 | 1 | 1 | |
| X | 1 | 1 | 1 | 1 | 1 | 1 | 1 | 1 | 1 | 1 | 1 | 1 | 1 | 1 | 1 | 1 | 1 | 1 | 1 | 0 | |
| Y | 1 | 1 | 0 | 1 | 0 | 1 | 1 | 1 | 1 | 1 | 1 | 1 | 1 | 1 | 1 | 1 | 1 | 1 | 1 | 1 | |
| der (1;5) | 1 | 0 | 1 | 1 | 1 | 0 | 1 | 1 | 1 | 1 | 1 | 1 | 1 | 1 | 1 | 1 | 1 | 1 | 1 | 1 | |
| der(1;11) | 0 | 1 | 1 | 1 | 1 | 1 | 1 | 1 | 0 | 1 | 1 | 1 | 1 | 1 | 1 | 1 | 1 | 1 | 1 | 1 | |
| der (7;18) | 1 | 1 | 1 | 0 | 1 | 0 | 1 | 1 | 1 | 1 | 1 | 1 | 1 | 2 | 1 | 0 | 1 | 1 | 1 | 1 | |
| der(8;17) | 1 | 1 | 1 | 1 | 1 | 1 | 1 | 1 | 0 | 1 | 1 | 1 | 1 | 1 | 1 | 1 | 1 | 0 | 1 | 0 | |
| der(9) | 1 | 1 | 1 | 1 | 1 | 1 | 1 | 1 | 0 | 1 | 1 | 1 | 1 | 1 | 1 | 0 | 1 | 1 | 1 | 1 | |
| i(15q) | 1 | 1 | 1 | 1 | 2 | 1 | 1 | 1 | 1 | 1 | 1 | 0 | 1 | 1 | 1 | 1 | 1 | 1 | 1 | 1 | |
| der(1;12) | 1 | 1 | 1 | 1 | 1 | 1 | 1 | 1 | 1 | 0 | 1 | 1 | 1 | 1 | 1 | 0 | 1 | 1 | 1 | 1 | |
| i(5q) | 1 | 1 | 1 | 1 | 1 | 0 | 1 | 1 | 0 | 1 | 1 | 1 | 1 | 1 | 1 | 1 | 1 | 1 | 1 | 1 | |
| der (13;8) | 1 | 0 | 1 | 0 | 1 | 1 | 1 | 1 | 1 | 1 | 1 | 1 | 1 | 1 | 1 | 1 | 1 | 0 | 1 | 1 | |
| der(15) | 1 | 1 | 1 | 1 | 2 | 1 | 1 | 1 | 1 | 1 | 1 | 1 | 1 | 1 | 1 | 0 | 1 | 1 | 1 | 1 | |
| der(19;12;19) | 1 | 1 | 1 | 0 | 1 | 0 | 1 | 1 | 0 | 1 | 1 | 1 | 1 | 1 | 1 | 0 | 1 | 1 | 1 | 1 | |
| der(5;12) | 1 | 1 | 1 | 1 | 1 | 1 | 1 | 1 | 1 | 1 | 1 | 1 | 1 | 1 | 1 | 1 | 1 | 1 | 1 | 1 | |
| der(14;8q) | 1 | 1 | 1 | 1 | 1 | 1 | 1 | 1 | 1 | 1 | 1 | 1 | 1 | 1 | 1 | 1 | 1 | 1 | 1 | 1 | |
| der(14;8p) | 1 | 1 | 1 | 1 | 1 | 1 | 1 | 1 | 1 | 1 | 1 | 1 | 1 | 1 | 1 | 0 | 1 | 1 | 1 | 1 | |
| i(12p) | 1 | 1 | 0 | 1 | 1 | 1 | 1 | 1 | 1 | 1 | 1 | 1 | 1 | 1 | 1 | 1 | 1 | 1 | 1 | 1 | |
| der(10;12) | 1 | 1 | 1 | 1 | 1 | 1 | 1 | 1 | 0 | 1 | 1 | 1 | 1 | 1 | 1 | 1 | 1 | 1 | 1 | 1 | |
| dmin(18) | 1 | 1 | 1 | 1 | 1 | 1 | 1 | 1 | 1 | 1 | 1 | 1 | 1 | 1 | 1 | 1 | 1 | 1 | 1 | 0 | |
| der(1;2) | 1 | 1 | 1 | 0 | 1 | 1 | 1 | 1 | 1 | 1 | 1 | 1 | 1 | 1 | 1 | 1 | 1 | 1 | 1 | 1 | |
| i(10p) | 1 | 2 | 1 | 0 | 1 | 1 | 1 | 1 | 0 | 1 | 1 | 1 | 1 | 1 | 1 | 1 | 1 | 1 | 1 | 1 | |
| i(19;12;19) | 1 | 1 | 1 | 0 | 1 | 1 | 0 | 1 | 1 | 1 | 1 | 1 | 1 | 1 | 1 | 1 | 0 | 1 | 1 | 1 | |
| der(2;5) | 1 | 1 | 1 | 0 | 1 | 1 | 1 | 1 | 1 | 1 | 1 | 1 | 0 | 1 | 1 | 1 | 1 | 1 | 0 | 1 | |
| i(2q) | 1 | 1 | 0 | 1 | 0 | 0 | 1 | 1 | 1 | 1 | 1 | 1 | 1 | 0 | 1 | 1 | 1 | 1 | 1 | 1 | |
| der(5;3) | 1 | 0 | 1 | 1 | 1 | 1 | 1 | 1 | 0 | 1 | 1 | 1 | 1 | 1 | 1 | 1 | 1 | 0 | 0 | 1 | |
| der(4;15) | 1 | 1 | 0 | 1 | 0 | 1 | 1 | 1 | 0 | 1 | 1 | 2 | 1 | 1 | 1 | 1 | 1 | 0 | 1 | 1 | |
| i(18q) | 2 | 2 | 1 | 0 | 2 | 1 | 1 | 2 | 1 | 2 | 2 | 2 | 2 | 2 | 2 | 2 | 2 | 1 | 1 | 2 | |
| i(11q) | 1 | 1 | 0 | 1 | 1 | 1 | 1 | 0 | 1 | 1 | 0 | 1 | 0 | 2 | 1 | 0 | 1 | 0 | 2 | 1 | |
| der(11q) | 1 | | | | | 1 | | 1 | | | 1 | | | | | | | | | | |
| der(1) | | | | | | | | | | | | 1 | 1 | | | 2 | 1 | | | | |
| i(5p) | | 1 | | | | | | | | | | | | | | | | 1 | | | |
| der(19;21) | | 1 | | 1 | | | | | | | | | | | | | | | | | |
| der (14;16p) | | | | | | | | | | | | | | | | | | 1 | | | |
| i(11p) | | | | | | | | | | | | | | 1 | | | | | | | |
| der(5;20) | | | | | | | | | | | | | | | | | | 1 | | | |
| dmin(10) | | | | | | 1 | | | | | | | | | | | | | | | |
| der(2) | 1 | | | | | | | | | | | | | | | | | | | | |
| der(3;17) | | 1 | | | | | | | | | | | | | | | | | | | |
| der(7;6) | | | | | | | | | | | | | 1 | | | | | | | | |
| can't tell | | | | 3 | | | | | | | | | | | | | | | | | |
| der(11;12) | | | 1 | | | | | | | | | | | | | | | | | | |
| der(3;13) | | | 1 | | | | | | | | | | | | | | | | | | |
| der(?;14) | | | 1 | | | | | | | | | | | | | | | | | | |
| der(4;16) | | | | | | | | | 1 | | | | | | | | | | | | |
| der(1;18) | | | | | | | | | | 1 | | | | | | | | | | | |
| der(1;20) | | | | | | | | | | 1 | | | | | | | | | | | |
| dmin(5) | | | | | | | | | | 1 | | | | | | | | | | | |
| der(3;9) | | | | | | | | | | | | | | | | | | | 1 | | |
| der(9;15) | | | | | | | | | | | | | | | | | | 1 | 1 | | |
| der(5;21) | | | | | | | | | | | | | | | | | | | 1 | | |
| der(16;2) | | | | | | | | | | | | | | | | | | | 1 | | |
| der(8;15) | | | | | | | | | | | | | | | | | | 1 | | | |
| der(3p) | | | | | | | | | | | | | | | | | | 1 | | 1 | |
| der(3q) | | | | | | | | | | | | | | | | | | 1 | | 1 | |
| der(7;12) | | | | | | | | | | | | | | | | | | | | 1 | |
| der(13;?) | | | | | | | | | | | | | | | | | | | | 1 | Average±SD |
| **Non-Clonal Aneusomies** | 7 | 13 | 11 | 18 | 11 | 15 | 3 | 4 | 18 | 7 | 2 | 6 | 8 | 8 | 0 | 20 | 3 | 26 | 11 | 11 | 10±7 |
| **Aneusomies per Karyotype** | 52 | 53 | 53 | 52 | 50 | 52 | 50 | 51 | 51 | 53 | 51 | 51 | 52 | 51 | 50 | 51 | 51 | 57 | 54 | 54 | 52±2 |

Primary Pancreatic Cancer A13-B and Metastases A13-A and A13-D

| | A13-B | A13-A | A13-D | | A13-B | A13-A | A13-D |
|---|---|---|---|---|---|---|---|
| Avg # of chromosomes ± SD | 64±6.0 | 62±3.6 | 62±1.8 | | Copy No (% clonal) | | |
| chromosome # | Copy No (% clonal) | | | der (8;5) | 0 | 1(95) | 0 |
| 1 | 2(55) | 1(75) | 2(80) | der (8) | 0 | 1(95) | 0 |
| 2 | 1(80) | 2(85) | 2(90) | der (12;16) | 0 | 1(95) | 0 |
| 3 | 2(80) | 2(100) | 2(100) | der(17;19) | 0 | 1(95) | 0 |
| 4 | 2(90) | 2(90) | 2(100) | i(5p) | 0(90) | 1(85) | 1(80) |
| 5 | 0(85) | 1(75) | 1(90) | der (13;8) | 1(85) | 1(85) | 1(95) |
| 6 | 3(80) | 3(95) | 3(95) | der(15) | 1(90) | 1(85) | 1(85) |
| 7 | 3(55) | 3(85) | 3(95) | der (17p;19) | 0 | 1(85) | 0 |
| 8 | 0 | 0(95) | 0 | der (2;10) | 0 | 1(80) | 0 |
| 9 | 1(80) | 1(95) | 1(95) | der (2;19) | 0 | 1(80) | 0 |
| 10 | 2(65) | 1(80) | 1(80) | der (10;2) | 0 | 1(75) | 0 |
| 11 | 2(75) | 1(95) | 1(80) | der (10;3) | 0 | 1(70) | 0 |
| 12 | 2(70) | 2(95) | 2(95) | der (1;18) | 0 | 1(50) | 0 |
| 13 | 1(70) | 1(90) | 1(95) | der (19;12;19) | 1(80) | 1(10) | 1(80) |
| 14 | 1(90) | 1(90) | 1(90) | der(1) | 0(80) | 1(5) | 1(85) |
| 15 | 1(90) | 2(90) | 1(90) | der(5;12) | 1(100) | 0 | 0 |
| 16 | 3(80) | 2(85) | 3(100) | der(14;8q) | 1(100) | 0 | 0 |
| 17 | 2(85) | 1(90) | 2(95) | der(14;8p) | 1(95) | 0 | 1(95) |
| 18 | 1(80) | 2(85) | 2(95) | i(12p) | 1(95) | 0 | 1(100) |
| 19 | 2(80) | 1(50) | 2(80) | der(10;12) | 1(95) | 0 | 0 |
| 20 | 4(75) | 5(45) | 4(100) | dmin(18) | 1(95) | 0 | 0 |
| 21 | 3(70) | 2(95) | 2(90) | der(1;2) | 1(95) | 0 | 0 |
| 22 | 1(95) | 1(100) | 1(100) | i(10p) | 1(85) | 0 | 1(70) |
| X | 1(95) | 1(100) | 1(100) | i(19;12;19) | 1(85) | 0 | 0 |
| Y | 1(90) | 1(100) | 0 | der(2;5) | 1(85) | 0 | 0 |
| der (1;5) | 1(90) | 1(100) | 1(90) | i(2q) | 1(80) | 0 | 1(95) |
| der (1;11) | 1(90) | 1(100) | 1(100) | der(5;3) | 1(80) | 0 | 0 |
| der (14;16p) | 0(95) | 1(100) | 1(90) | der(4;15) | 1(75) | 0 | 0 |
| der(14;19?;16q) | 0 | 1(100) | 0 | i(18q) | 2(65) | 0 | 0 |
| der (3;9) | 0 | 1(100) | 0 | i(11q) | 1(60) | 0 | 0 |
| der (7;18) | 1(80) | 1(95) | 1(100) | der (8;10) | 0 | 0 | 1(100) |
| i(11p) | 0(95) | 1(95) | 1(75) | der (12;22;19) | 0 | 0 | 1(95) |
| der (8;17) | 1(85) | 1(95) | 1(95) | der (5;1) | 0 | 0 | 1(90) |
| der(9) | 1(90) | 1(95) | 1(95) | der (15;3) | 0 | 0 | 1(90) |
| i(15q) | 1(90) | 1(95) | 1(80) | i(12q) | 0 | 0 | 1(90) |
| der (1;12) | 1(90) | 1(95) | 0 | Total Clonal Aneusomies | 50 | 49 | 46 |
| i(5q) | 1(90) | 1(95) | 0(95) | | | | |

**Fig. 15** (See legend on next page.)

(See figure on previous page.)
**Fig. 15 a, b, c, d** Karyotypic evidence that the metastases A13-A and A13-D are individual subspecies of the pancreatic cancer A-13B. The karyotypic theory of metastasis predicts that metastases have individual clonal karyotypes that differ from those of parental cancers in individual metastasis-specific aneusomies. To test this theory we have compared the karyotype-arrays of the metastases A13-A and A13-D to that of the primary cancer A-3B. The karyotype arrays were again prepared as described for Fig. 9. Figure 15 **a**, **b**, **c** and the attached table show that the chromosomes of the cancer were 55–95% clonal and that of the chromosomes of metastasis A13-A were 75–100% and those of metastasis A13-D were 75–100% clonal, and that all three cancers formed related clonal patterns. As shown in Table 1, the karyotype of the metastasis A13-A differed from that of the primary cancer A13-B in 27 of 49 aneusomies and metastasis A13-D differed from that of the primary in 16 of 49 aneusomies (Fig. 15 **a**, **b**, **c**, **d**). The copy numbers of most non-clonal chromosomes including marker chromosomes differed from clonal averages ± 1 (Fig. 15 **a**, **b**, **c** and specifically Fig. 15**d**). The chromosomes with non-clonal copy numbers represent the ongoing karyotypic variation predicted by the inherent variability of cancer-specific aneuploidy (See Background). We conclude that the metastases A13-A and D are subspecies of the parental pancreatic cancer A13-B

4) The "abrupt" origins and the "unpredictable" and "independent" phenotypes of cancers in metastasis, known as Foulds rules of progression [5], by the low probability and phenotypic unpredictability of new subspecies generated by random chromosomal rearrangements - much like the abrupt origins of new species in conventional speciation.

## Methods

### Origins of seven cancer cells and corresponding metastases

(1) A near-diploid breast cancer, termed HIM-2 and a brain metastasis, termed HIM-5 were a generous gift of Elaine Mardis. They were isolated and sequenced as described by her and her collaborators in 2010 [16]. (2) A hyper-triploid primary melanoma WM-115 and a metastasis of undefined origin, termed WM-266-4 [21–23] were obtained from American Type Culture Collection. (3) A liver cancer termed H2P and a metastasis in the portal vein to the liver termed H2M was isolated and provided by Xin-Yuan Guan [35]. (4) A hyper-triploid medulloblastoma termed Med-458 and a metastasis from a cerebrospinal fluid relapse termed Med-425 [95, 96] were kindly transferred to us by the senior author of this study, Darell D. Bigner (personal communication, 2014). (5) A hyper-diploid colon cancer SW-480 and a lymph node metastasis SW-620 [97–101] with evidence shown above that both are metastases from an unknown common precursor were obtained from two sources, SW-480 was a purchase from American Type Culture Collection and SW-620 was a kind gift from Josh Nicholson (Virginia Polytechnic Institute and State University, Blacksburg, Virginia). (6) A hyper-tetraploid melanoma from the leg, termed IGR-39 and a hyper-triploid metastasis from the groin of young male patient, termed IGR-37 [102] were purchased from DSMZ-Deutsche Sammlung von Mikroorganismen und Zellkulturen GmbH, Braunschweig,

**Table 1** Individual and shared clonal aneusomies of metastases and parental cancers

| Primary/Metastasis | Total clonal aneusomies | Aneusomies shared with cancer | Metastasis-specific, clonal aneusomies (% of total) |
|---|---|---|---|
| 1)Breast, HIM-2 | 23 | - | - |
| Metastasis, HIM-5 | 23 | 22 | 1 (4%) |
| 2)Melanoma, WM-115 | 30 | - | - |
| Metastasis, WM-266-4 | 31 | 18 | 13 (42%) |
| 3)Liver, H2P | 31 | - | - |
| Metastasis, H2M | 31 | 16 | 15 (48%) |
| 4)Medulloblastoma M-458 | 34 | | |
| Metastasis, M-425 | 28 | 11 | 17 (61%) |
| 5)Colon, SW480-C1 | 38 | - | - |
| Colon SW480-C2 | 39 | - | - |
| Metastasis, SW620 vs C1 | 38 | 13 | 25 (66%) |
| SW620 vs C2 | 38 | 11 | 27 (71%) |
| 6)Melanoma, IGR-39 | 30 | - | - |
| Metastasis, IGR-37 | 31 | 4 | 27 (87%)[a] |
| 7)Pancreas, A13-B | 50 | | |
| Metastases, A13-A | 49 | 22 | 27 (55%) |
| and A13-D | 46 | 30 | 16 (35%) |

[a]High percentage of individuality reflects ploidy shift (see below, Table 2)

**Table 2** Conservation of karyotypic complexity of cancers in metastasis based on their numbers of clonal chromosomes and aneusomies

| Cancer-Metastasis pair | Average numbers of chromosomes ± SE | Average numbers of aneusomies ± SE | Ratio chromosomes per aneusomy[a] |
|---|---|---|---|
| 1)BrCa HIM-2 | 48 ± 1 | 23 ± 0 | 2.1 |
| Metas HIM-5 | 47 ± 1.6 | 23 ± 0 | 2 |
| 2)Mela WM-115 | 86 ± 1 | 30 ± 1 | 2.9 |
| Metas WM-266-4 | 82 ± 2 | 31 ± 1 | 2.7 |
| 3)Liver H2P | 78 ± 7 | 33 ± 1 | 2.4 |
| Meta H2M | 86 ± 4 | 34 ± 2 | 2.5 |
| 4)Medullob - 458 | 81 ± 2.5 | 37 ± 2 | 2.2 |
| Metas- 425 | 85 ± 2 | 28 ± 1 | 3.0 |
| 5)Colon SW480-C1 | 53 ± 1 | 40 ± 2 | 1.3 |
| SW480-C2 | 54 ± 2 | 40 ± 1 | 1.4 |
| Metas SW-620 | 49 ± 2 | 39 ± 1 | 1.3 |
| 6)Mela IGR-39 | 111 ± 3 | 32 ± 1 | 3.5 |
| Metas IGR-37 | 73 ± 4[b] | 33 ± 1 | 2.2 |
| 7)Panc A-13B | 64 ± 6 | 52 ± 2 | 1.2 |
| Metas A-13-A | 62 ± 2.6 | 51 ± 1 | 1.2 |
| Metas A-13-D | 62 ± 1.8 | 48 ± 2 | 1.3 |

[a]Numbers of chromosomes divided by numbers of aneusomies generates a form of ploidy; [b]ploidy shift

Germany. (7) A hypo-triploid pancreatic cancer termed A13-B and two independent hypo-triploid metastases, a pancreatic metastasis A13-A and a liver metastasis A13-D, were obtained as described previously [43]. All cultures were grown in RPMI 1640 medium (Sigma Co.) supplemented with 3 to 5% fetal calf serum and antibiotics as described previously [101, 102].

## Karyotype analyses

One to two days before karyotyping, cells were seeded at about 50% confluence in a 5-cm culture dish with 3 ml of the medium described above. After reaching ~75% confluence, 250–300 ng colcemid in 25–30 μl solution (KaryoMax, Gibco) was added to 3 ml medium. The culture was then incubated at 37 °C for 4–8 h. Subsequently cells were washed once with 3 ml of physiological saline, dissociated with trypsin, pelleted and then incubated in 0.075 molar KCl at 37 °C for 15 min. The cell suspension was then cooled in ice-water, mixed ('prefixed') with 0.1 volume of the freshly mixed glacial acetic acid-methanol (1:3, vol. per vol.) and centrifuged at 800 g for 6 min at room temperature. The cell pellet was then suspended in about 100 μl supernatant and mixed drop-wise with 5 ml of the ice-cold acetic acid-methanol solution and then incubated at room temperature for 15–30 min or overnight at -20C. This cell suspension was then pelleted and was then either once more re-suspended in fixative and pelleted, or was directly re-suspended in a small volume of the acetic acid-methanol solution for microscopic examination. For this purpose an aliquot of a visually turbid suspension was transferred with a micropipette tip to a glass microscope slide, allowed to evaporate at room temperature and inspected under the microscope at x 200 for an adequate, non-overlapping density of metaphase chromosomes. Metaphase chromosomes attached to glass slides were then hybridized to color-coded, chromosome-specific DNA probes as described by the manufacturer, MetaSystems (Newton, MA 02458). Karyotypes were analyzed under a fluorescence microscope, as described by us previously [17, 49].


#### Acknowledgments

We thank Thomas Liehr and his laboratory (Universitaetsklinikum-Jena and Institut fuer Humangenetik, Kollegiengasse, Jena, Germany) for discussions and review of early drafts of this manuscript, and Peter Walian (Lawrence Berkeley National Laboratory, Donner Lab, Berkeley CA) for critical reviews of this manuscript and for stimulating discussions and ideas. We thank Elaine R Mardis (Washington University School of Medicine, St Louis, Missouri, USA) and Xin-Yuan Guan (Department of Clinical Oncology, The University of Hong Kong, School of Chinese Medicine,Hong Kong, China) for the cancer-metastasis pairs HIM-2 and HIM-5 and H2P and H2M respectively. We gratefully acknowledge Henry Heng (Center for Molecular Medicine and Genetics Wayne State University School of Medicine, Detroit), David Rasnick (Oakland CA, former visiting scholar at UC Berkeley), Mark Vincent (Department of Medical Oncology, London Regional Cancer Center, London, Ontario, Canada) for valuable information, inspiring questions and critical comments on the experiments and theories in this manuscript. Bong-Gyoon Han (Lawrence Berkeley National Laboratory, Donner Lab at UC Berkeley) is specifically thanked for drafting and designing Fig. 1. Our study would not have been possible without the generous support of the philanthropists Robert Leppo (San Francisco CA, USA), Christian Fiala (Gynmed Ambulatorium, Mariahilferguertel 37, Vienna, Austria), Peter Rozsa (Taubert Memorial Foundation, Los Angeles CA, USA) and several anonymous private sources.

#### Funding

Private sources (see Acknowledgements).


#### Authors' contribution

MB and PD equally participated in planning and conducting experiments and writing of the manuscript. Both authors read and approved the final manuscript.

#### Competing interests

The authors declare that they have no competing interests.


#### Author details

[1]Department of Molecular and Cell Biology; Donner Laboratory, University of California at Berkeley, Berkeley, CA 94720, USA. [2]Present address: Department of Natural Sciences and Mathematics, Dominican University of California, San Rafael, CA, USA.


#### References


1. New Oxford American Dictionary: 2010, 2013 by Oxford University Press, Inc
2. Foulds L. Multiple etiologic factors in neoplastic development. Cancer Res. 1965;25(8):1339–47.
3. Weinberg RA. The biology of cancer, Second edition. New York; London: Garland Science; 2014.
4. Alberts B, Johnson A, Lewis J, Raff M, Roberts K, Walter P. Molecular Biology of the Cell. New York: Garland; 2014.
5. Foulds L. Tumor progression: a review. Cancer Res. 1954;14:327–39.
6. Fidler IJ. The Ernst W. Bertner Memorial Award lecture: the evolution of biological heterogeneity in metastatic neoplasms. Symp Fundam Cancer Res. 1983;36:5–26.
7. Heppner GH. Tumor heterogeneity. Cancer Res. 1984;44(6):2259–65.
8. Fidler IJ, Kripke ML. Genomic analysis of primary tumors does not address the prevalence of metastatic cells in the population. Nat Genet. 2003;34(1):23. author reply 25.
9. Michaelson JS, Cheongsiatmoy JA, Dewey F, Silverstein MJ, Sgroi D, Smith B, Tanabe KK. Spread of human cancer cells occurs with probabilities indicative of a nongenetic mechanism. Br J Cancer. 2005;93(11):1244–9.
10. Michaelson JS, Chen LL, Silverstein MJ, Cheongsiatmoy JA, Mihm Jr MC, Sober AJ, Tanabe KK, Smith BL, Younger J. Why cancer at the primary site and in the lymph nodes contributes to the risk of cancer death. Cancer. 2009;115(21):5084–94.
11. Jones S, Chen WD, Parmigiani G, Diehl F, Beerenwinkel N, Antal T, Traulsen A, Nowak MA, Siegel C, Velculescu VE, et al. Comparative lesion sequencing provides insights into tumor evolution. Proc Natl Acad Sci U S A. 2008;105(11):4283–8.
12. Yachida S, Jones S, Bozic I, Antal T, Leary R, Fu B, Kamiyama M, Hruban RH, Eshleman JR, Nowak MA, et al. Distant metastasis occurs late during the genetic evolution of pancreatic cancer. Nature. 2010;467(7319):1114–7.
13. Bozic I, Antal T, Ohtsuki H, Carter H, Kim D, Chen S, Karchin R, Kinzler KW, Vogelstein B, Nowak MA. Accumulation of driver and passenger mutations during tumor progression. Proc Natl Acad Sci U S A. 2010;107(43):18545–50.
14. Campbell PJ, Yachida S, Mudie LJ, Stephens PJ, Pleasance ED, Stebbings LA, Morsberger LA, Latimer C, McLaren S, Lin ML, et al. The patterns and

dynamics of genomic instability in metastatic pancreatic cancer. Nature. 2010;467(7319):1109–13.
15. Ostrovnaya I, Olshen AB, Seshan VE, Orlow I, Albertson DG, Begg CB. A metastasis or a second independent cancer? Evaluating the clonal origin of tumors using array copy number data. Stat Med. 2010;29(15):1608–21.
16. Ding L, Ellis MJ, Li S, Larson DE, Chen K, Wallis JW, Harris CC, McLellan MD, Fulton RS, Fulton LL, et al. Genome remodelling in a basal-like breast cancer metastasis and xenograft. Nature. 2010;464(7291):999–1005.
17. Gerlinger M, Rowan AJ, Horswell S, Larkin J, Endesfelder D, Gronroos E, Martinez P, Matthews N, Stewart A, Tarpey P, et al. Intratumor heterogeneity and branched evolution revealed by multiregion sequencing. N Engl J Med. 2012;366(10):883–92.
18. Jacob LS, Vanharanta S, Obenauf AC, Pirun M, Viale A, Socci ND, Massague J. Metastatic Competence Can Emerge with Selection of Preexisting Oncogenic Alleles without a Need of New Mutations. Cancer Res. 2015;75(18):3713–9.
19. Klein CA. Cancer. The metastasis cascade. Science. 2008;321(5897):1785–7.
20. Hagemeijer A, Hoehn W, Smit EM. Cytogenetic analysis of human renal carcinoma cell lines of common origin (NC 65). Cancer Res. 1979;39(11): 4662–7.
21. Balaban G, Herlyn M, Guerry D, Bartolo R, Koprowski H, Clark WH, Nowell PC. Cytogenetics of human malignant melanoma and premalignant lesions. Cancer Genet Cytogenet. 1984;11(4):429–39.
22. Herlyn M, Balaban G, Bennicelli J, Guerry D, Halaban R, Herlyn D, Elder DE, Maul GG, Steplewski Z, Nowell PC, et al. Primary melanoma cells of the vertical growth phase: similarities to metastatic cells. J Natl Cancer Inst. 1985;74(2):283–9.
23. Balaban GB, Herlyn M, Clark Jr WH, Nowell PC. Karyotypic evolution in human malignant melanoma. Cancer Genet Cytogenet. 1986;19(1–2):113–22.
24. Frankfurt OS, Slocum HK, Rustum YM, Arbuck SG, Pavelic ZP, Petrelli N, Huben RP, Pontes EJ, Greco WR. Flow cytometric analysis of DNA aneuploidy in primary and metastatic human solid tumors. Cytometry. 1984;5(1):71–80.
25. Minke JM, Cornelisse CJ, Stolwijk JA, Kuipers-Dijkshoorn NJ, Rutteman GR, Misdorp W. Flow cytometric DNA ploidy analysis of feline mammary tumors. Cancer Res. 1990;50(13):4003–7.
26. Gronwald J, Storkel S, Holtgreve-Grez H, Hadaczek P, Brinkschmidt C, Jauch A, Lubinski J, Cremer T. Comparison of DNA gains and losses in primary renal clear cell carcinomas and metastatic sites: importance of 1q and 3p copy number changes in metastatic events. Cancer Res. 1997;57(3):481–7.
27. Kuukasjarvi T, Karhu R, Tanner M, Kahkonen M, Schaffer A, Nupponen N, Pennanen S, Kallioniemi A, Kallioniemi OP, Isola J. Genetic heterogeneity and clonal evolution underlying development of asynchronous metastasis in human breast cancer. Cancer Res. 1997;57(8):1597–604.
28. Mahlamaki EH, Hoglund M, Gorunova L, Karhu R, Dawiskiba S, Andren-Sandberg A, Kallioniemi OP, Johansson B. Comparative genomic hybridization reveals frequent gains of 20q, 8q, 11q, 12p, and 17q, and losses of 18q, 9p, and 15q in pancreatic cancer. Genes Chromosomes Cancer. 1997;20(4):383–91.
29. Pandis N, Teixeira MR, Adeyinka A, Rizou H, Bardi G, Mertens F, Andersen JA, Bondeson L, Sfikas K, Qvist H, et al. Cytogenetic comparison of primary tumors and lymph node metastases in breast cancer patients. Genes Chromosomes Cancer. 1998;22(2):122–9.
30. Al-Mulla F, Keith WN, Pickford IR, Going JJ, Birnie GD. Comparative genomic hybridization analysis of primary colorectal carcinomas and their synchronous metastases. Gen Chrom Canc. 1999;24(4):306–14.
31. Fadl-Elmula I, Gorunova L, Mandahl N, Elfving P, Lundgren R, Mitelman F, Heim S. Cytogenetic monoclonality in multifocal uroepithelial carcinomas: evidence of intraluminal tumour seeding. Br J Cancer. 1999;81(1):6–12.
32. Adeyinka A, Kytola S, Mertens F, Pandis N, Larsson C. Spectral karyotyping and chromosome banding studies of primary breast carcinomas and their lymph node metastases. Int J Mol Med. 2000;5(3):235–40.
33. Petersen S, Aninat-Meyer M, Schluns K, Gellert K, Dietel M, Petersen I. Chromosomal alterations in the clonal evolution to the metastatic stage of squamous cell carcinomas of the lung. Br J Cancer. 2000;82(1):65–73.
34. Alcock HE, Stephenson TJ, Royds JA, Hammond DW. Analysis of colorectal tumor progression by microdissection and comparative genomic hybridization. Genes Chromosomes Cancer. 2003;37(4):369–80.
35. Hu L, Wen JM, Sham JS, Wang W, Xie D, Tjia WM, Huang JF, Zhang M, Zeng WF, Guan XY. Establishment of cell lines from a primary hepatocellular carcinoma and its metastatis. Cancer Genet Cytogenet. 2004;148(1):80–4.
36. Knosel T, Schluns K, Stein U, Schwabe H, Schlag PM, Dietel M, Petersen I. Chromosomal alterations during lymphatic and liver metastasis formation of colorectal cancer. Neoplasia. 2004;6(1):23–8.
37. Knosel T, Schluns K, Dietel M, Petersen I. Chromosomal alterations in lung metastases of colorectal carcinomas: associations with tissue specific tumor dissemination. Clin Exp Metastasis. 2005;22(7):533–8.
38. Jiang JK, Chen YJ, Lin CH, Yu IT, Lin JK. Genetic changes and clonality relationship between primary colorectal cancers and their pulmonary metastases–an analysis by comparative genomic hybridization. Genes Chromosomes Cancer. 2005;43(1):25–36.
39. Jin Y, Jin C, Lv M, Tsao SW, Zhu J, Wennerberg J, Mertens F, Kwong YL. Karyotypic evolution and tumor progression in head and neck squamous cell carcinomas. Cancer Genet Cytogenet. 2005;156(1):1–7.
40. Jonkers YM, Claessen SM, Perren A, Schmid S, Komminoth P, Verhofstad AA, Hofland LJ, de Krijger RR, Slootweg PJ, Ramaekers FC, et al. Chromosomal instability predicts metastatic disease in patients with insulinomas. Endocr Relat Cancer. 2005;12(2):435–47.
41. Jonkers YM, Claessen SM, Perren A, Schmitt AM, Hofland LJ, de Herder W, de Krijger RR, Verhofstad AA, Hermus AR, Kummer JA, et al. DNA copy number status is a powerful predictor of poor survival in endocrine pancreatic tumor patients. Endocr Relat Cancer. 2007;14(3):769–79.
42. Liu W, Laitinen S, Khan S, Vihinen M, Kowalski J, Yu G, Chen L, Ewing CM, Eisenberger MA, Carducci MA, et al. Copy number analysis indicates monoclonal origin of lethal metastatic prostate cancer. Nat Med. 2009;15(5):559–65.
43. Duesberg P, Iacobuzio-Donahue C, Brosnan JA, McCormack A, Mandrioli D, Chen L. Origin of metastases: Subspecies of cancers generated by intrinsic karyotypic variations. Cell Cycle. 2012;11(6):1151–66.
44. Haugvik SP, Gorunova I , Haugom L, Eibak AM, Gladhaug IP, Heim S, Micci F. Loss of 11p11 is a frequent and early event in sporadic nonfunctioning pancreatic neuroendocrine neoplasms. Oncol Rep. 2014;32(3):906–12.
45. Backdahl M, Cohn K, Auer G, Forsslund G, Granberg PO, Lundell G, Lowhagen T, Willems JS, Zetterberg A. Comparison of nuclear DNA content in primary and metastatic papillary thyroid carcinoma. Cancer Res. 1985; 45(6):2890–4.
46. Bissig H, Richter J, Desper R, Meier V, Schraml P, Schaffer AA, Sauter G, Mihatsch MJ, Moch H. Evaluation of the clonal relationship between primary and metastatic renal cell carcinoma by comparative genomic hybridization. Am J Pathol. 1999;155(1):267–74.
47. Marusyk A, Polyak K. Tumor heterogeneity: causes and consequences. Biochim Biophys Acta. 2010;1805(1):105–17.
48. Almendro V, Kim HJ, Cheng YK, Gonen M, Itzkovitz S, Argani P, van Oudenaarden A, Sukumar S, Michor F, Polyak K. Genetic and phenotypic diversity in breast tumor metastases. Cancer Res. 2014;74(5):1338–48.
49. Clarke PA, te Poele R, Wooster R, Workman P. Gene expression microarray analysis in cancer biology, pharmacology, and drug development: progress and potential. Biochem Pharmacol. 2001;62(10):1311–36.
50. Chen X, Cheung ST, So S, Fan ST, Barry C, Higgins J, Lai KM, Ji J, Dudoit S, Ng IO, et al. Gene expression patterns in human liver cancers. Mol Biol Cell. 2002;13(6):1929–39.
51. Chung CH, Bernard PS, Perou CM. Molecular portraits and the family tree of cancer. Nat Genet. 2002;32(Suppl):533–40.
52. Perou CM, Sorlie T, Eisen MB, van de Rijn M, Jeffrey SS, Rees CA, Pollack JR, Ross DT, Johnsen H, Akslen LA, et al. Molecular portraits of human breast tumours. Nature. 2000;406(6797):747–52.
53. van't Veer LJ, Dai H, van de Vijver MJ, He YD, Hart AA, Mao M, Peterse HL, van der Kooy K, Marton MJ, Witteveen AT, et al. Gene expression profiling predicts clinical outcome of breast cancer. Nature. 2002;415:530–6.
54. Ramaswamy S, Ross KN, Lander ES, Golub TR. A molecular signature of metastasis in primary solid tumors. Nat Genet. 2003;33(1):49–54.
55. Weigelt B, Glas AM, Wessels LF, Witteveen AT, Peterse JL, van't Veer LJ. Gene expression profiles of primary breast tumors maintained in distant metastases. Proc Natl Acad Sci U S A. 2003;100(26):15901–5.
56. Weigelt B, Hu Z, He X, Livasy C, Carey LA, Ewend MG, Glas AM, Perou CM, Van't Veer LJ. Molecular portraits and 70-gene prognosis signature are preserved throughout the metastatic process of breast cancer. Cancer Res. 2005;65(20):9155–8.
57. Weigelt B, Wessels LF, Bosma AJ, Glas AM, Nuyten DS, He YD, Dai H, Peterse JL, van't Veer LJ. No common denominator for breast cancer lymph node metastasis. Br J Cancer. 2005;93(8):924–32.
58. Grade M, Hormann P, Becker S, Hummon AB, Wangsa D, Varma S, Simon R, Liersch T, Becker H, Difilippantonio MJ, et al. Gene expression profiling reveals a massive, aneuploidy-dependent transcriptional deregulation and distinct differences between lymph node-negative and lymph node-positive colon carcinomas. Cancer Res. 2007;67(1):41–56.

59. Suzuki M, Tarin D. Gene expression profiling of human lymph node metastases and matched primary breast carcinomas: clinical implications. Mol Oncol. 2007;1(2):172–80.
60. Thomassen M, Tan Q, Kruse TA. Gene expression meta-analysis identifies chromosomal regions and candidate genes involved in breast cancer metastasis. Breast Cancer Res Treat. 2009;113(2):239–49.
61. Chen GK, Lacayo NJ, Duran GE, Wang Y, Bangs CD, Rea S, Kovacs M, Cherry AM, Brown JM, Sikic BI. Preferential expression of a mutant allele of the amplified MDR1 (ABCB1) gene in drug-resistant variants of a human sarcoma. Genes Chromosomes Cancer. 2002;34(4):372–83.
62. Hao X, Sun B, Hu L, Lahdesmaki H, Dunmire V, Feng Y, Zhang SW, Wang H, Wu C, Wang H, et al. Differential gene and protein expression in primary breast malignancies and their lymph node metastases as revealed by combined cDNA microarray and tissue microarray analysis. Cancer. 2004;100(6):1110–22.
63. Wang Y, Klijn JG, Zhang Y, Sieuwerts AM, Look MP, Yang F, Talantov D, Timmermans M, Meijer-van Gelder ME, Yu J, et al. Gene-expression profiles to predict distant metastasis of lymph node negative primary breast cancer. Lancet. 2005;365(9460):671–9.
64. Fridlyand J, Snijders AM, Ylstra B, Li H, Olshen A, Segraves R, Dairkee S, Tokuyasu T, Ljung BM, Jain AN, et al. Breast tumor copy number aberration phenotypes and genomic instability. BMC Cancer. 2006;6:96.
65. Cifone MA, Fidler IJ. Increasing metastatic potential is associated with increasing genetic instability of clones isolated from murine neoplasms. Proc Natl Acad Sci U S A. 1981;78(11):6949–52.
66. Sobel ME. Metastasis suppressor genes. J Natl Cancer Inst. 1990;82(4):267–76.
67. Welch DR, Steeg PS, Rinker-Schaeffer CW. Molecular biology of breast cancer metastasis. Genetic regulation of human breast carcinoma metastasis. Breast Cancer Res. 2000;2(6):408–16.
68. Yokota J. Tumor progression and metastasis. Carcinogenesis. 2000;21(3):497–503.
69. Bernards R, Weinberg RA. A progression puzzle. Nature. 2002;418(6900):823.
70. Couzin J. Medicine. A clash over genes that foretell metastasis. Science. 2003;299(5609):1005.
71. Bernards R. Cancer: cues for migration. Nature. 2003;425(6955):247–8.
72. Van't Veer LJ, Weigelt B. Road map to metastasis. Nat Med. 2003;9(8):999–1000.
73. Yang J, Mani SA, Donaher JL, Ramaswamy S, Itzykson RA, Come C, Savagner P, Gitelman I, Richardson A, Weinberg RA. Twist, a master regulator of morphogenesis, plays an essential role in tumor metastasis. Cell. 2004;117(7):927–39.
74. Weinberg RA. Is metastasis predetermined? Mol Oncol. 2007;1(3):263–4. author reply 265–266.
75. Duesberg P, Mandrioli D, McCormack A, Nicholson JM. Is carcinogenesis a form of speciation? Cell Cycle. 2011;10(13):2100–14.
76. Bloomfield M, Duesberg P. Karyotype alteration generates the neoplastic phenotypes of SV40-infected human and rodent cells. Mol Cytogenet. 2015;8:79.
77. Bloomfield M, McCormack A, Mandrioli D, Fiala C, Aldaz CM, Duesberg P. Karyotypic evolutions of cancer species in rats during the long latent periods after injection of nitrosourea. Mol Cytogenet. 2014;7(1):71.
78. Atkin NB. Modal deoxyribonucleic acid value and survival in carcinoma of the breast. Br Med J. 1972;1(5795):271–2.
79. Frankfurt OS, Chin JL, Englander LS, Greco WR, Pontes JE, Rustum YM. Relationship between DNA ploidy, glandular differentiation, and tumor spread in human prostate cancer. Cancer Res. 1985;45(3):1418–23.
80. Wolman SR. Cytogenetic heterogeneity: its role in tumor evolution. Cancer Genet Cytogenet. 1986;19(1–2):129–40.
81. Ljungberg B, Stenling R, Roos G. Prognostic value of deoxyribonucleic acid content in metastatic renal cell carcinoma. J Urol. 1986;136(4):801–4.
82. Fallenius AG, Franzen SA, Auer GU. Predictive value of nuclear DNA content in breast cancer in relation to clinical and morphologic factors. A retrospective study of 227 consecutive cases. Cancer. 1988;62(3):521–30.
83. Saito T, Sato J, Satoh A, Notani K, Fukuda H, Mizuno S, Shindoh M, Amemiya A. Flow cytometric analysis of nuclear DNA content in tongue squamous cell carcinoma: relation to cervical lymph node metastasis. Int J Oral Maxillofac Surg. 1994;23(1):28–31.
84. Hemmer J, Thein T, Van Heerden WF. The value of DNA flow cytometry in predicting the development of lymph node metastasis and survival in patients with locally recurrent oral squamous cell carcinoma. Cancer. 1997;79(12):2309–13.
85. Torres L, Ribeiro FR, Pandis N, Andersen JA, Heim S, Teixeira MR. Intratumor genomic heterogeneity in breast cancer with clonal divergence between primary carcinomas and lymph node metastases. Breast Cancer Res Treat. 2007;102(2):143–55.
86. Tarin D, Price JE, Kettlewell MG, Souter RG, Vass AC, Crossley B. Mechanisms of human tumor metastasis studied in patients with peritoneovenous shunts. Cancer Res. 1984;44(8):3584–92.
87. Weinberg RA. Coming full circle-from endless complexity to simplicity and back again. Cell. 2014;157(1):267–71.
88. Pearse AM, Swift K, Hodson P, Hua B, McCallum H, Pyecroft S, Taylor R, Eldridge MD, Belov K. Evolution in a transmissible cancer: a study of the chromosomal changes in devil facial tumor (DFT) as it spreads through the wild Tasmanian devil population. Cancer Genet. 2012;205(3):101–12.
89. Bayani J, Brenton JD, Macgregor PF, Beheshti B, Albert M, Nallainathan D, Karaskova J, Rosen B, Murphy J, Laframboise S, et al. Parallel analysis of sporadic primary ovarian carcinomas by spectral karyotyping, comparative genomic hybridization, and expression microarrays. Cancer Res. 2002;62(12): 3466–76.
90. Vincent MD. Cancer: beyond speciation. Adv Cancer Res. 2011;112:283–350.
91. Heng HH, Stevens JB, Bremer SW, Liu G, Abdallah BY, Ye CJ. Evolutionary mechanisms and diversity in cancer. Adv Cancer Res. 2011;112:217–53.
92. Van Valen L, Maiorana V. HeLa, a new microbial species. Evolutionary Theory. 1991;10:71–4.
93. Makino S. Cytogenetics of canine venereal tumors: Worldwide distribution and a common karyotype. In: German J, editor. Chromosomes and Cancer. New Yor: Wiley; 1974. p. 336–72.
94. Weiss RA, Fassati A. The clammy grip of parasitic tumors. Cell. 2015;161(2):191–2.
95. Friedman HS, Oakes WJ, Bigner SH, Wikstrand CJ, Bigner DD. Medulloblastoma: tumor biological and clinical perspectives. J Neurooncol. 1991;11(1):1–15.
96. He XM, Wikstrand CJ, Friedman HS, Bigner SH, Pleasure S, Trojanowski JQ, Bigner DD. Differentiation characteristics of newly established medulloblastoma cell lines (D384 Med, D425 Med, and D458 Med) and their transplantable xenografts. Lab Invest. 1991;64(6):833–43.
97. Leibovitz A, Stinson JC, McCombs 3rd WB, McCoy CE, Mazur KC, Mabry ND. Classification of human colorectal adenocarcinoma cell lines. Cancer Res. 1976;36(12):4562–9.
98. Gagos S, Hopwood VL, Iliopoulos D, Kostakis A, Karayannakos P, Yatzides H, Skalkeas GD, Pathak S. Chromosomal markers associated with metastasis in two colon cancer cell lines established from the same patient. Anticancer Res. 1995;15(2):369–78.
99. Gagos S, Iliopoulos D, Tseleni-Balafouta S, Agapitos M, Antachopoulos C, Kostakis A, Karayannakos P, Skalkeas G. Cell senescence and a mechanism of clonal evolution leading to continuous cell proliferation, loss of heterozygosity, and tumor heterogeneity: studies on two immortal colon cancer cell lines. Cancer Genet Cytogenet. 1996;90(2):157–65.
100. Melcher R, Steinlein C, Feichtinger W, Muller CR, Menzel T, Luhrs H, Scheppach W, Schmid M. Spectral karyotyping of the human colon cancer cell lines SW480 and SW620. Cytogenet Cell Genet. 2000;88(1–2):145–52.
101. Knutsen T, Padilla-Nash HM, Wangsa D, Barenboim-Stapleton L, Camps J, McNeil N, Difilippantonio MJ, Ried T. Definitive molecular cytogenetic characterization of 15 colorectal cancer cell lines. Genes Chromosomes Cancer. 2010;49(3):204–23.
102. Aubert C, Rouge F, Galindo JR. Tumorigenicity of human malignant melanocytes in nude mice in relation to their differentiation in vitro. J Natl Cancer Inst. 1980;64(5):1029–40.
103. O'Brien S, Menotti-Raymond M, Murphy W, Nash W, Wirnberg J, Stanyon R, Copeland N, Jenkins N, Womack J, Marshall Graves J. The promise of comparative genomics in mammals. Science. 1999;286:458–81.
104. Duesberg P, Rausch C, Rasnick D, Hehlmann R. Genetic instability of cancer cells is proportional to their degree of aneuploidy. Proc Natl Acad Sci U S A. 1998;95(23):13692–7.
105. Duesberg PH. Does aneuploidy destabilize karyotypes automatically? Proc Natl Acad Sci U S A. 2014;111:E974.
106. Heim S, Mitelman F. Cancer Cytogenetics. 2nd ed. New York: Wiley-Liss; 1995.
107. Mitelman F (ed.): ISCN (1991) - An International System for Human Cytogenetic Nomenclature. Basel: S. Karger; 1995.
108. Nicholson JM, Duesberg P. On the karyotypic origin and evolution of cancer cells. Cancer Genet Cytogenet. 2009;194(2):96–110.
109. McCormack A, Fan JL, Duesberg M, Bloomfield M, Fiala C, Duesberg P. Individual karyotypes at the origins of cervical carcinomas. Mol Cytogenet. 2013;6(1):44.
110. Sneige N, Liu B, Yin G, Gong Y, Arun BK. Correlation of cytologic findings and chromosomal instability detected by fluorescence in situ hybridization in breast fine-needle aspiration specimens from women at high risk for breast cancer. Mod Pathol. 2006;19(5):622–9.

111. Lockstone HE, Harris LW, Swatton JE, Wayland MT, Holland AJ, Bahn S. Gene expression profiling in the adult Down syndrome brain. Genomics. 2007;90(6):647–60.
112. Levan A, Hauschka TS. Endomitotic reduplication mechanisms in ascites tumors of the mouse. J Natl Cancer Inst. 1953;14(1):1–43.
113. Li R, Hehlman R, Sachs R, Duesberg P. Chromosomal alterations cause the high rates and wide ranges of drug resistance in cancer cells. Cancer Genet Cytogenet. 2005;163(1):44–56.
114. Seltenhammer MH, Sundstrom E, Meisslitzer-Ruppitsch C, Cejka P, Kosiuk J, Neumuller J, Almeder M, Majdic O, Steinberger P, Losert UM, et al. Establishment and characterization of a primary and a metastatic melanoma cell line from Grey horses. In Vitro Cell Dev Biol Anim. 2014;50(1):56–65.
115. Li L, McCormack AA, Nicholson JM, Fabarius A, Hehlmann R, Sachs RK, Duesberg PH. Cancer-causing karyotypes: chromosomal equilibria between destabilizing aneuploidy and stabilizing selection for oncogenic function. Cancer Genet Cytogenet. 2009;188(1):1–25.
116. Pandit SK, Westendorp B, de Bruin A. Physiological significance of polyploidization in mammalian cells. Trends Cell Biol. 2013;23(11):556–66.
117. Nei M, Nozawa M. Roles of mutation and selection in speciation: from Hugo de Vries to the modern genomic era. Genome Biol Evol. 2011;3:812–29.
118. White MJD. Modes of speciation. San Francisco: W H Freeman and Co.; 1978.
119. Nowell PC. The clonal evolution of tumor cell populations. Science. 1976; 194(4260):23–8.
120. Fearon ER, Vogelstein B. A genetic model for colorectal tumorigenesis. Cell. 1990;61:759–67.
121. Vogelstein B, Kinzler KW. The multistep nature of cancer. Trends Genet. 1993;9(4):138–41.
122. Hanahan D, Weinberg RA. The hallmarks of cancer. Cell. 2000;100(1):57–70.
123. Hoglund M, Gisselsson D, Mandahl N, Johansson B, Mertens F, Mitelman F, Sall T. Multivariate analyses of genomic imbalances in solid tumors reveal distinct and converging pathways of karyotypic evolution. Gen Chrom Canc. 2001;31(2):156–71.
124. Hoglund M, Gisselsson D, Hansen GB, Sall T, Mitelman F. Multivariate analysis of chromosomal imbalances in breast cancer delineates cytogenetic pathways and reveals complex relationships among imbalances. Cancer Res. 2002;62(9):2675–80.
125. Wollweber L, Munster H, Hoffmann S, Siller K, Greulich KO. Early phase karyotype analysis of chromosome segregation after formation of mouse-mouse hybridomas with chromosome painting probes. Chromosome Res. 2000;8(1):37–44.
126. Paulsson K, Morse H, Fioretos T, Behrendtz M, Strombeck B, Johansson B. Evidence for a single-step mechanism in the origin of hyperdiploid childhood acute lymphoblastic leukemia. Genes Chromosomes Cancer. 2005;44(2):113–22.
127. Gao R, Davis A, McDonald TO, Sei E, Shi X, Wang Y, Tsai PC, Casasent A, Waters J, Zhang H, et al. Punctuated copy number evolution and clonal stasis in triple-negative breast cancer. Nat Genet. 2016;48:1119–30.
128. Onodera N, McCabe NR, Nachman JB, Johnson FL, Le Beau MM, Rowley JD, Rubin CM. Hyperdiploidy arising from near-haploidy in childhood acute lymphoblastic leukemia. Genes Chromosomes Cancer. 1992;4(4):331–6.
129. Onodera N, McCabe NR, Rubin CM. Formation of a hyperdiploid karyotype in childhood acute lymphoblastic leukemia. Blood. 1992;80(1):203–8.
130. Charlesworth B, Lande R, Slatkin M. A neo-darwinian commentary on macroevolution. Evolution. 1982;36:474–98.
131. Goldschmidt RB. The material basis of evolution. New Haven: Yale University Press; 1940.
132. King M. Species evolution: the role of chromosome change. Cambridge: Cambridge University Press; 1993.
133. Heng HH. Debating cancer: the paradox in cancer research. Hackensack: World Scientific; 2015.
134. Goymer P. Natural selection: The evolution of cancer. Nature. 2008; 454(7208):1046–8.
135. Duesberg P, McCormack A. Immortality of cancers: A consequence of inherent karyotypic variations and selections for autonomy. Cell Cycle. 2013;12(5):783–802.
136. Cairns J. Cancer: Science and Society. San Francisco: W. H. Freeman; 1978.

# 15

# Comparative cytogenetics in three Sciaenid species (Teleostei, Perciformes): evidence of interspecific chromosomal diversification

Dongdong Xu[1*], Wagner Franco Molina[2], Cassia Fernanda Yano[3], Yurong Zhang[1], Ezequiel Aguiar de Oliveira[3,4], Bao Lou[1] and Marcelo de Bello Cioffi[3]

## Abstract

**Background:** Species belonging to the Sciaenidae family present a karyotype composed by 48 acrocentric chromosomes and are thus considered a striking example of chromosomal conservation. In this family, three species are extensively studied including *Larimichthys crocea*, *Larimichthys polyactis* and *Nibea albiflora* due to their importance in fishery and aquaculture in East Asia. Despite abundant data of population genetics available for some of them, cytogenetic information on these species is still scarce and obtained by conventional cytogenetic protocols. Therefore, a more detailed cytogenomic investigation was performed in these species to analyze their karyotype differentiation using conventional staining techniques and fluorescence in situ hybridization to map several repetitive DNAs.

**Results:** The three species showed a slight karyotype differentiation with 4sm + 2st + 42a in *L. polyactis*, 20st + 28a in *L. crocea* and 48a in *N. albiflora*. Additionally, the mapping of repetitive sequences further revealed a number of interspecific differences among them. Particularly, 18S and 5S rDNA sites showed syntenic arrangements in *N. albiflora* and non-syntenic arrangements in both *Larimichthys* species. The microsatellites $(CA)_{15}$ and $(GA)_{15}$ showed conspicuous terminal clusters in some chromosomes of all species. On the other hand, $(CGG)_{10}$ repeats, *Rex6* elements and U2 snRNA displayed a scattered distribution on the chromosomes.

**Conclusions:** Although the three Sciaenid species examined displayed a general pattern of karyotypic conservatism, we explored chromosomal diversification among them. The diversificated karyotypic macrostructure is followed by intergeneric evolutionary diversification of the repetitive sequences. The data indicate some degree of intergeneric evolutionary diversification at chromosomal level, and suggest the evolutionary dynamics among Sciaenid species, higher than previously thought. The present cytogenetic data provide new insight into the chromosomal diversification in Sciaenidae, and contribute to inferring the chromosomal rearrangements and trends of karyotype evolution in this fish group.

**Keywords:** Sciaenidae, Chromosome evolution, Repetitive sequences, Pericentric inversions, U2 snRNA

## Background

Sciaenidae form one of the largest Perciformes' families, comprising 66 genera and approximately 291 species [1]. They are commonly called croakers or drums because of their propensity to produce sounds using sonic muscles and swim bladder. Sciaenid fishes are among the top priced seafood species in Asian cuisine due to their delicate flavor and rich nutritional value. The genera *Larimichthys* and *Nibea* include three of the most popular species in this family, which are the large yellow croaker (*Larimichthys crocea*), the small yellow croaker (*Larimichthys polyactis*) and the yellow drum (*Nibea albiflora*) [2]. They are commercially important species distributed along the coasts of East Asia (Fig. 1). In fact, *L. crocea* is one of the most highlighted aquaculture species in China, with the annual yield exceeding any other net-cage-farmed marine fish species [3], while *L. polyactis* is one of the principal marine fishery species in China and

* Correspondence: xudong0580@163.com
[1]Marine Fishery Institute of Zhejiang Province, Key Lab of Mariculture and Enhancement of Zhejiang Province, 316100 Zhoushan, Zhejiang Province, People's Republic of China
Full list of author information is available at the end of the article

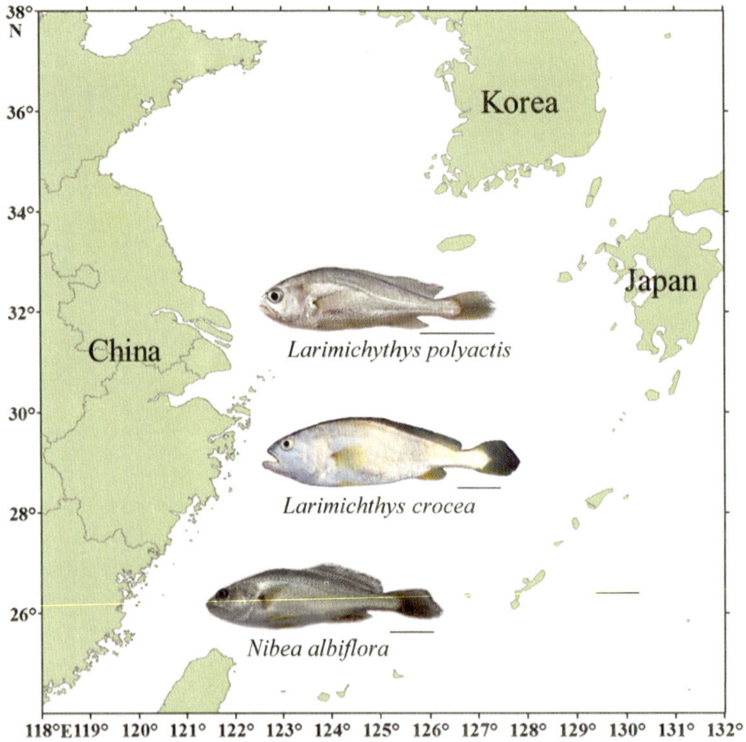


**Fig. 1** Sciaenidae species analyzed in this study and distribution regions in the China Sea. Scale bars = 5 cm

East Asian countries [4]. Phylogenetically related to *Larimichthys*, *Nibea albiflora* has great importance for commercial fisheries and is a promising candidate for aquaculture in China [5]. Together, these species have been significantly overfished, putting them at risk, therefore, over the last years initiatives have been made to preserve the wild stocks. Due to its importance, deep efforts have been applied in understanding their genetic aspects, including the analysis of population genetic structure, genetic map, and genomic prospections [3, 6–9].

In spite of the cumulative genetic information in others areas, the chromosomal data for Sciaenids are restricted to few conventional cytogenetic analyses, in which karyotypes are reported for 38 (14%) species [10]. Most of the Sciaenids examined have a diploid number (2n) of 48 chromosomes (95% of species), nearly all acrocentric (85% of species) [10, 11], revealing a remarkable example of chromosomal stability and conservation among Perciform fishes. Previous conventional cytogenetic data also showed 48 chromosomes in *L. polyactis*, *L. crocea* and *N. albiflora* [12–14]. However, the karyotype formulas of these species revealed discrepant differences, especially for *L. crocea* [14–16]. Moreover, very little is known about other important cytogenetic features, such as the incidence of chromosomal repetitive DNA elements and their evolutionary role in this fish group. Therefore, processes involved in macro-structural karyotype changes, chromosomal diversification, and genomic restructuring can be overlooked.

Molecular cytogenetics provides valuable tools and insights for comparative genomic research and has emerged as promising for understanding genome evolution and organization. In particular, the molecular organization and cytogenetic mapping of repetitive DNA elements, including satellites, multigene families and microsatellite repeats, have been analyzed in a large number of species [17]. These studies have demonstrated the enormous potential that the investigation of repetitive DNAs offers toward extending our knowledge of karyotype differentiation.

In this sense, we performed conventional (Giemsa staining and C-banding) and molecular (in situ mapping of 7 different repetitive DNAs) cytogenetic approaches in three Sciaenid species. Besides providing new cytogenetic data to this family, the present study is useful to infer the chromosomal rearrangements and trends of karyotype evolution in this fish group.

## Methods

### Materials

Fishes were sampled from the research station of Marine Fishery Institute of Zhejiang Province (Xishan Island, City of Zhoushan, China). Three species were analyzed: *Larimichthys crocea* (six males an seven females),

*Larimichthys polyactis* (seven males and eight females), and *Nibea albiflora* (six males and six females).

#### Mitotic chromosome preparation and chromosome banding

Mitotic chromosome preparations were obtained by the air-drying method, following Bertollo et al. (2015) [18]. The specimens were injected with 0.05% colchicine for 3 h. The kidney tissue was collected and placed in hypotonic 0.075 mol/l KCl solution for 30 min, to obtaining a cell suspension. The cells were fixed in Carnoy's solution (methanol: acetic acid, 3: 1). Afterwards, the cells were dropped on cooled clean glass slides, air-dried and stained with 15% Giemsa solution diluted with phosphate buffer (pH 6.8). C-bands were obtained according to the method described by Sumner (1972) [19].

#### Probes preparation

Two tandemly-arrayed DNA sequences isolated from the genome of an Erythrinidae fish species, *Hoplias malabaricus*, were used as probes. The first probe contained a 5S rDNA repeat copy and included 120 base pairs (bp) of the 5S rRNA transcribed gene and 200 bp of the non-transcribed spacer (NTS) sequence [20]. The second probe contained a 1400 bp segment of the 18S rRNA gene obtained via PCR from the nuclear DNA [21]. The 5S rDNA partial sequence were cloned into plasmid vectors and propagated in DH5α *E. coli* competent cells (Invitrogen, San Diego, CA, USA). The 18S and 5S rDNA probe were labeled with DIG-11-dUTP and biotin-14-dATP, respectively, by nick translation according to manufacturer's recommendations (Invitrogen, San Diego, CA, USA).

The microsatellites $d(CA)_{15}$, $d(GA)_{15}$, and $d(CGG)_{10}$ were synthesized according to Kubat et al. (2008) [22]. These sequences were directly labeled with Cy3 at 5′ terminal during synthesis by Sigma (St. Louis, MO, USA). The probes for retrotransposable element *Rex6* and the multigene family U2 snDNA were produced by PCR using primers described in Volff et al. (2001) [23] and Úbeda-Manzanaro et al. (2010) [24], respectively. Both U2 snDNA and *Rex6* probes were directly labeled with Spectrum Orange-dUTP by nick translation, according to the manufacturer's recommendations (Roche, Mannheim, Germany).

#### Fluorescence in situ hybridization and signal detection

Fluorescence in situ hybridization (FISH) experiments were performed as described in Yano et al. (2017) [25], with slight modifications. The experiment was performed under high stringency conditions on mitotic chromosome spreads. Metaphase chromosome slides were incubated with RNase (40 μg/ml) for 1.5 h at 37 ° C. After denaturation of the chromosomal DNA in 70% formamide/2× SSC at 72 °C for 3 min, the hybridization mixture (2.5 ng/μl probes, 2 μg/μl salmon sperm DNA, 50% deionized formamide, 10% dextran sulphate) was dropped on the slides, and the hybridization was performed overnight at 37 °C in a moist chamber containing 2× SSC. The first post-hybridization wash was performed with 2× SSC for 5 min at 42 °C, and a final wash was performed at room temperature in 1× SSC for 5 min. The signal detection was performed using anti-digoxigenin rhodamine (Roche) for the 18S rDNA probe and with avidin-FITC (Sigma) for 5S rDNA. Subsequently, the slides were dehydrated again in an ethanol series (70%, 85% and 100%), 2 min each. Finally, the slides were counterstained with DAPI and mounted in an antifading solution (Vectashield from Vector Laboratories).

#### Microscopy analyses and image processing

The chromosomes were analyzed in an epifluorescence microscope Olympus BX50 (Olympus Corporation, Ishikawa, Japan). Approximately 30 metaphase spreads were analyzed per specimen to determine the diploid chromosome number and karyotype structure. The chromosomes were classified as metacentric (m), submetacentric (sm), subtelocentric (st) or acrocentric (a) according to arm ratios (Levan et al. 1964) [26]. The count of fundamental arm number (NF) considered m, sm, and st as bi-brachial chromosomes, while terminal, as mono-brachial.

## Results

All the species presented the same diploid number (2n = 48), with karyotypes composed by 4sm + 2st +42a in *L. polyactis*, 20st + 28a in *L. crocea* and 48a in *N. albiflora* (Fig. 2). No differences between male and female karyotypes were observed in all the species. The C-positive heterochromatic blocks preferentially located in the centromeric regions, with some pairs exhibiting additional blocks in the telomeric region (Fig. 2).

Mapping of 5S rDNA and 18 rDNA showed single sites for all the species analyzed, but exhibited different distribution patterns. In *L. polyactis* and *L. crocea*, both genes were located in the terminal position of short arms of two distinct sm chromosomal pairs (Figs. 3 and 4). On the other hand, in *N. albiflora* the 18S rDNA and 5S rDNA sites have a syntenic organization, with the 18S rDNA sequences located in the terminal region of the short arms and the 5S rDNA cluster in the proximal region of the long arms of an acrocentric chromosome pair (Fig. 5).

The chromosomal mapping of microsatellites $(CA)_{15}$ and $(GA)_{15}$ showed similar patterns for all species, with a remarkable accumulation in the subtelomeric regions of some chromosomes. However, different patterns were observed among species with $(CGG)_{10}$, since, in addition to the presence of scattered signals, a considerable

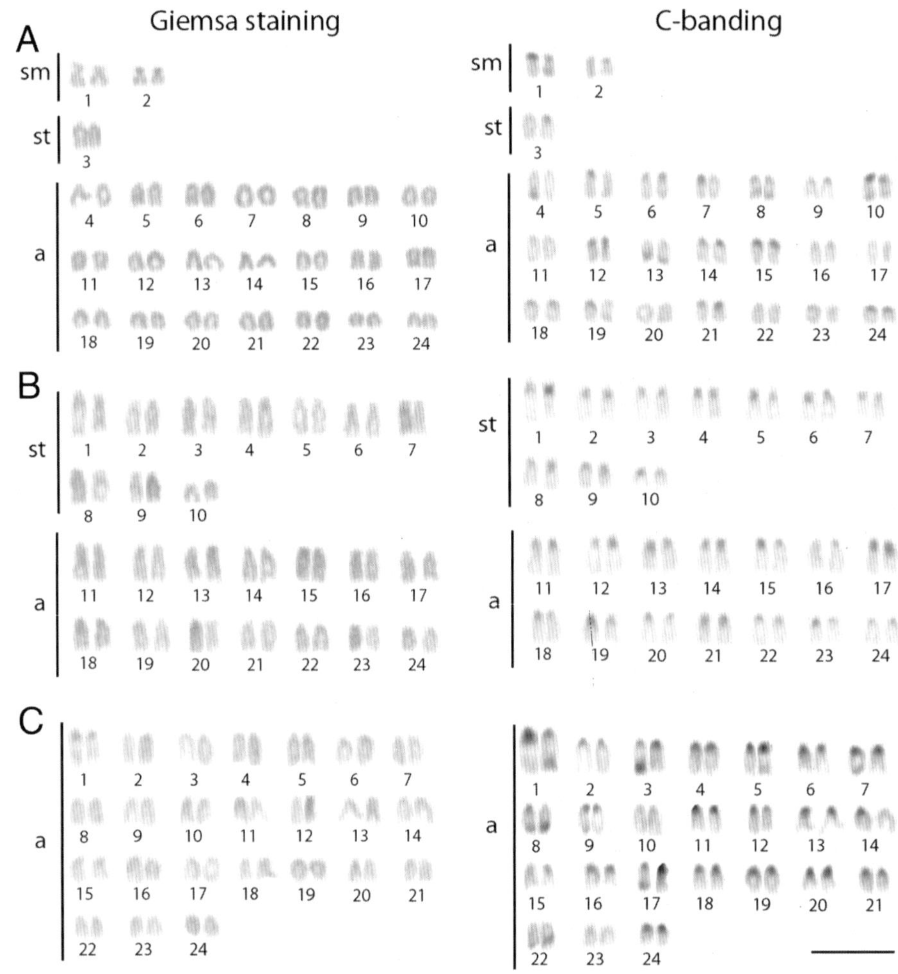


**Fig. 2** Karyotypes of *Larimichthys polyactis*, *Larimichthys crocea* and *Nibea albiflora* after Giemsa and C-banding staining. Scale bar = 5 μm

accumulation of this sequence was detected in both *Larimichthys* species (Figs. 3 and 4); while very weak and disperse signals were observed in the chromosomes of *N. albiflora* (Fig. 5). FISH using the PCR fragments of *Rex6* and U2 snDNA, presented a similar dispersion pattern in which the signals were abundantly distributed in the chromosomes of all the species (Figs. 3, 4, 5).

## Discussion

### Karyotype differentiation

In the present study, we characterized the karyotypes and chromosomal features of three croaker fishes using conventional and molecular cytogenetic approaches. To our knowledge, these are the first molecular cytogenetic data for any Sciaenid species.

The karyotypes for the three fish species exhibited basal chromosome number (2n = 48) and predominance of acrocentric chromosomes. The results are basically consistent with that reported in previous Giemsa staining analyses. However, different chromosomal formulas were reported for *L. crocea* and *L. polyactis* in previous studies. In *L. crocea*, the cryptic classification among the subtelocentric and acrocentric chromosomes has caused divergences in the chromosomal formulas reported by different authors [15, 16]. However, the cytogenetic analysis in *L. polyactis* reveals a yelling karyotype discrepancy with previous studies in this species. In fact, our study showed the presence of three bi-brachial chromosome pairs not identified in previous reports [12]. The detection of discrete chromosome differences in *L. crocea* and more conspicuous in *L. polyactis* may show evidence of polymorphism in these species. Nevertheless, the small chromosomal size and the lack of notable technical improvement in fish chromosome obtainment and analysis not rule out the possibility of chromosomal artifacts. Our study is a step forward to clarifying these issues and understanding the biodiversity of marine Sciaenidae.

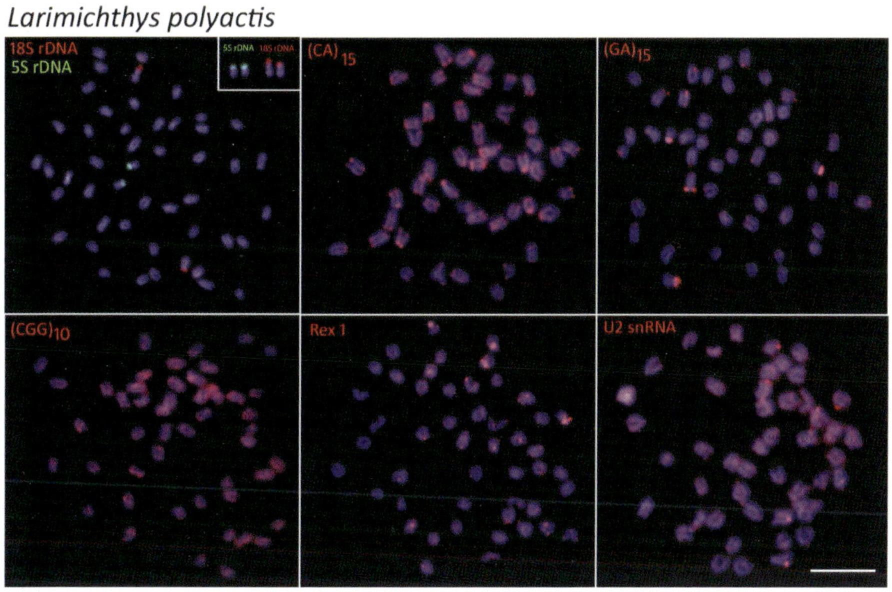


**Fig. 3** Metaphase plates of *Larimichthys polyactis* mapped with different repeated DNAs. 5S rDNA (green), 18S rDNA, di-and trinucleotide microsatellites, *Rex*1 and U2 snRNA (red) as probes. The chromosomes bearing 18S rDNA sites are shown in enlarged forms boxes. Scale bar = 5 μm

Sciaenidae is characterized by a symmetrical and conservative karyotypic pattern, with most of them displaying 2n = 48 and karyotypes with a high number of acrocentric chromosomes [10]. This conservative pattern is recurrent in Atlantic species analyzed [11]. Similarly, the three species analyzed also displayed the conserved karyotype observed for most marine fishes, especially in *N. albiflora* which is a remarkable example with a chromosome set made up of 48 acrocentric chromosomes. Nevertheless, significant karyotypic differentiations were observed in genus *Larimichthys*. Indeed, *L. polyactis* shows two sm chromosomes pairs and one pair of st chromosomes (NF = 54), while *L. crocea* possesses 10 pairs of st (NF = 68). Such variations in chromosomal morphology indicate that pericentric inversions, like in other Perciformes [27], are the primary mechanisms for karyotype diversification among them

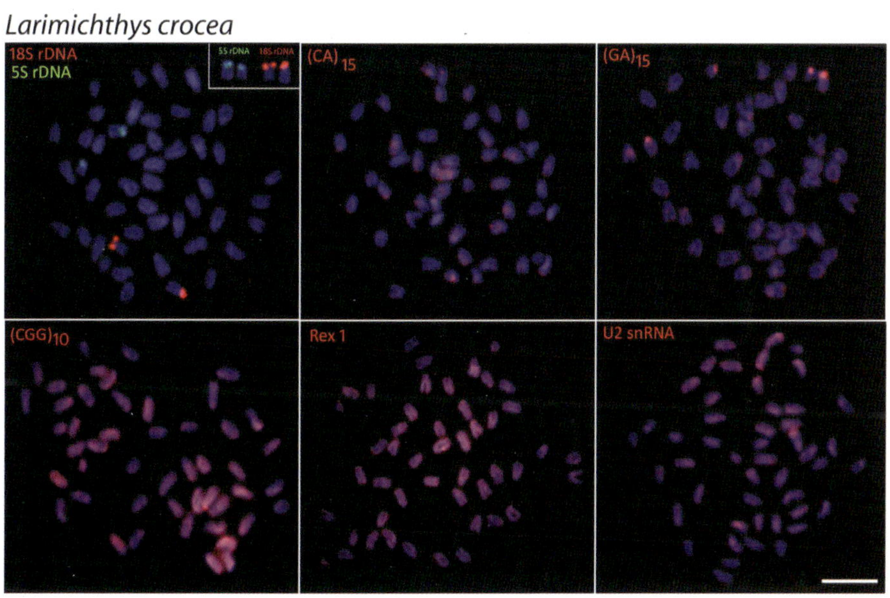


**Fig. 4** Metaphase plates of *Larimichthys crocea* mapped with different repeated DNAs. 5S rDNA (green), 18S rDNA, di-and trinucleotide microsatellites, *Rex*1 and U2 snRNA (red) as probes. The chromosomes bearing 18S rDNA sites are shown in enlarged forms boxes. Scale bar = 5 μm

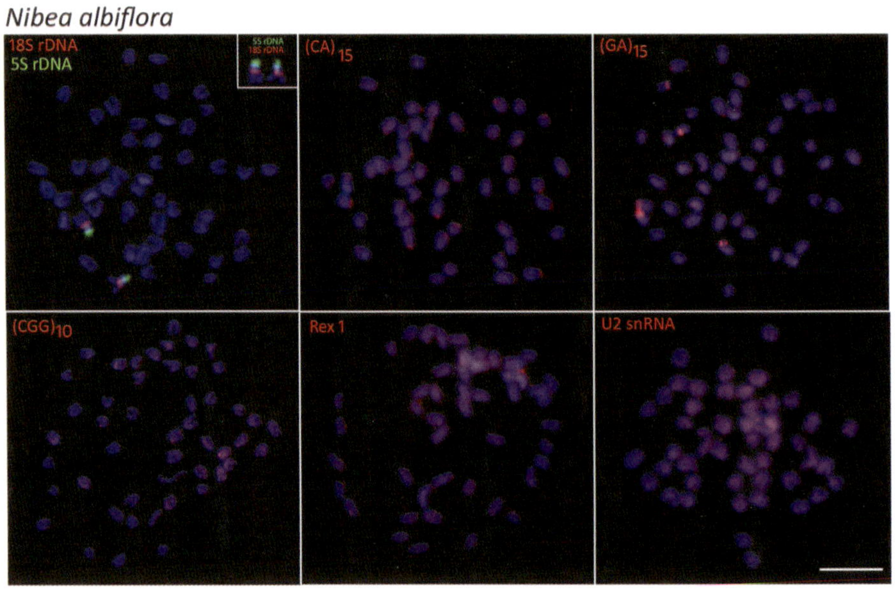


**Fig. 5** Metaphase plates of *Nibea albiflora* mapped with different repeated DNAs. 5S rDNA (green), 18S rDNA, di-and trinucleotide microsatellites, *Rex*1 and U2 snRNA (red) as probes. The chromosomes bearing 18S rDNA sites are shown in enlarged forms boxes. Scale bar = 5 μm

**Chromosomal distribution of repetitive sequences**

The in situ localization and chromosome mapping of seven classes of repetitive DNA sequences resulted in useful characteristics for comparative genomics at chromosomal level. Among these DNA classes, the ribosomal RNA genes are the most mapped sequences for purposes of chromosomal evolution analysis in fishes. Accordingly, chromosomal distribution of rDNA clusters can be informative for comparative analysis of closely related species or even to the characterization of population variations.

The 18S rDNA sites were located on the terminal position in a sm chromosome pair of *L. polyactis* and in a st chromosome pair of *L. crocea*, suggesting that rearrangements involving 18S rDNA loci in the homologous chromosome occurred during the divergence of these congeneric species of *Larimichthys*. The 5S and 18S rDNA sites display non-syntenic arrangements in the genus *Larimichthys*, while notably, these genes occur in a syntenic array in *N. albiflora*. The non-syntenic arrangements of 5S and 18S rDNA loci are the most common features in chromosomes of fishes, indicating independent evolution of these loci [28, 29]. On the contrary, the syntenic association of 5S and 18S rDNA sites evidenced in *N. albiflora* is infrequent in fishes, despite these gene arrays have been reported to several species among them [30, 31]. Taken together, the different syntenic patterns of 5S and 18S rDNA sites found here suggest that these regions may represent an important feature for karyotype diversification in the three Sciaenides.

Some repetitive sequences, especially the microsatellites, are particularly variable in fish chromosomes and linked to karyotype diversification. In the analyzed species, microsatellites $(CGG)_{10}$ were strongly distributed in the chromosomes of *Larimichthys*, but with a distinct and more discrete distribution pattern in *N. albiflora*. The organization of $(CGG)_{10}$ in fish chromosomes have demonstrated that these repeat motifs can show particular arrangements among different species [17]. Since these sequences are subjected to high rates of changes, their distribution indicate distinct evolutionary pathways concerning the genome organization among genus *Larimichthys* and *Nibea*.

*Rex* is comprised of various families of transposable elements that are abundant in teleosts, and their distribution varies from a scattered pattern to preferential accumulation in certain regions of the chromosomes [32]. Our data show that *Rex*1 elements display a diffuse and sparse distribution, as similarly described for some fishes, as in naked catfish *Mystus bocourti* [33], cichlids [34] and several Atlantic snappers [35]. Generally this distribution pattern is nonrandom and seems to have some relation to specific characteristics of sub-regions of the host genomes, indicating that TEs are important structural components of the heterochromatic regions and have played an important role in dynamic processes of fish karyotype evolution.

The multi-gene family U2 snRNA, which is one of the components of the small nuclear ribonucleoprotein particles (snDNA) and responsible for mRNA splicing, exhibited a very widely scattered pattern in the three analyzed species, with intense hybridization signals in some specific regions. This genomic organization of the three species is quite similar to the one found for the fishes *Amphichthys cryptocentrus*, *Porichthys plectrodon* and *Abudefduf* species [24, 36]. Contrasted with the aforementioned results, most of the data available for different groups showed that these conserved genes are organized in a single or a small number of chromosomal clusters [33]. It has been proposed a trend for the U2 snRNA genes to accumulate in a specific chromosome pair over the course of the evolutionary history in the Batrachoididae family [24]. It would be interesting to study this gene in more members of Sciaenid family to deduce its distribution trend in the chromosomes.

### Chromosomal differentiation and speciation

Sciaenid fishes displayed extensive phenotypic diversity, especially for the species distributed in Eastern Pacific. However, the speciation process is not considered to be followed by significant karyotype differentiation [11, 15]. In the present study, significant karyotype and macro-karyotype differentiation were explored among the three Schianid species, allowing a connection between the chromosomal data and the biogeographic events related to this group of fish. It is hypothesized that historical environmental variations caused by glacial events gave rise to the initial diversification in this family [37], leading to population restrictions and the fixation of genetic divergences, such as the chromosomal arrangements. The role of glacial events in fractioning and restricting population is considered relevant for the chromosomal diversification and transitory polymorphisms present in marine species of the genus *Chromis* [38].

It is noteworthy that *L. polyactis* and *L. crocea* share morphological characteristics [2] and have similar mtDNA barcodes [4]. Molecular analyses show that these two congeneric species are closely related, with divergence estimated at around 4.62 Mya [37], suggesting a recent sympatric speciation. The cytogenetic divergences promoted by pericentric inversions could lead to the effective postzygotic reproductive isolation between both species during that time. However, wild stocks of genus *Larimichthys* were severely depleted, since they have been extensively explored in the past decades, especially *L. crocea* [16]. These anthropogenic factors lead to the changes in life history and expansion of the distribution area, and thereby promoting hybridization events as demonstrated in various marine species [39]. These conditions are particularly worrisome in *Larimichthys* because interspecific breeding between *L. polyactis* and *L. crocea* were found to produce viable hybrid offspring (data unpublished). The potential fragility of the reproductive isolation mechanisms among *Larimichthys* species and their considerable degree of chromosomal similarity promote low protection to ensure the preservation of the genetic cohesion of the species. Ineffective reproductive blocking may cause reverse speciation, a condition that enables the mixture or the genetic submersion of the gene pool of a species into another [40]. In this sense, extending analyses are required to clarify the hybrid events between *L. polyactis* and *L. crocea*.

## Conclusions

Sciaenid fishes are valuable in Asian fishery and aquaculture, especially the species analyzed in the present study. Our results showed significant interspecific chromosomal diversification among the three Sciaenid fishes examined, incorporated a general pattern of karyotypic conservatism. *N. albiflora* is characterized by a basal karyotype, while *Larimichthys* shows karyotype diversifications promoted by pericentric inversions. Moreover, such variability is also reinforced by the dynamism of repetitive elements in the genome, especially by the differential distribution and accumulation of rDNA sequences among chromosomes.

The karyotype divergences between *L. polyactis* and *L. crocea* could act as post-zygotic chromosomal barriers. On the other hand, these species showed a remarkable similarity of chromosomal organization of repetitive sequences and functional genes. Thus, the anthropological activities such as overfishing, stock enhancement, and changes in marine environment could breakdown the "calm sea of speciation". In this aspect, extending cytogenetic and molecular studies are relevant to provide informative data for diagnosing possible interspecific hybridization and introgression between them.

**Acknowledgements**
Not applicable

**Funding**
This work was supported by grants from the National Natural Science Foundation of China (41106114), the Project of Zhejiang Province of China (2017C04003, 2017C02013) and by the Brazilian agency Fundação de Amparo à Pesquisa do Estado de São Paulo - FAPESP (2016/22196–2).

**Authors' contributions**
XD carried out the conventional cytogenetic analysis, coordinated the study and drafted and revised the manuscript. ZY and LB helped in the conventional cytogenetic analysis and drafted the manuscript. MWF drafted and revised the manuscript. YCF, OEA and MBC carried out the molecular cytogenetic analysis, drafted and revised the manuscript. All authors read and approved the final version of the manuscript.

### Competing interests
The authors declare that they have no competing interests.

### Author details
[1]Marine Fishery Institute of Zhejiang Province, Key Lab of Mariculture and Enhancement of Zhejiang Province, 316100 Zhoushan, Zhejiang Province, People's Republic of China. [2]Departamento de Biologia Celular e Genética, Centro de Biociências, Universidade Federal do Rio Grande do Norte, Campus Universitário, Lagoa Nova, 3000, Natal, RN 59078-970, Brazil. [3]Departamento de Genética e Evolução, Universidade Federal de São Carlos, Rodovia Washington Luís, km 235, São Carlos, SP 13565-905, Brazil. [4]Secretaria de Estado de Educação de Mato Grosso – SEDUÇ-MT, Cuiabá, MT, Brazil.

### References
1. Eschmeyer WN, Fricke R, Van der Laan R. Catalog of fishes: genera, species, references. http://researcharchive.calacademy.org/research/ichthyology/catalog/fishcatmain.asp. Accessed 24 Apr 2017.
2. Zhu YD, Luo YL, Wu HL. A study on the classification of the Sciaenoid fishes of China, with description of new genera and species. China: Shanghai Scientific and Technical Press; 1963.
3. Wu C, Zhang D, Kan M, Lv Z, Zhu A, Su Y, et al. The draft genome of the large yellow croaker reveals well-developed innate immunity. Nat Commun. 2014;5:5227.
4. Zhang YR, Yang F, Wang Z, You Q, Lou B, Xu D, et al. Mitochondrial DNA variation and population genetic structure in the small yellow croaker at the coast of Yellow Sea and East China Sea. Biochem Syst Ecol. 2017;71:236–43.
5. Hong W, Zhang Q. Review of captive bred species and fry production of marine fish in China. Aquaculture. 2003;227:305–18.
6. Xu ZL, Chen JJ. Population division of *Larimichthys polyactis* in China Sea. Chinese J Appl Ecol. 2010;21:2856–64. (In Chinese with English abstract)
7. Xu D, Lou B, Shi H, Geng Z, Li S, Zhang Y. Genetic diversity and population structure of *Nibea albiflora* in the China Sea revealed by mitochondrial COI sequences. Biochem Syst Ecol. 2012;45:158–65.
8. Xiao S, Wang P, Zhang Y, Fang L, Liu Y, Li JT, et al. Gene map of large yellow croaker (*Larimichthys crocea*) provides insights into teleost genome evolution and conserved regions associated with growth. Sci Rep. 2015;5:18661.
9. Ao JQ, Mu Y, Xiang LX, Fan DD, Feng MJ, Zhang SC, et al. Genome sequencing of the Perciform fish *Larimichthys crocea* provides insights into molecular and genetic mechanisms of stress adaptation. PLoS Genet. 2015; 11(4):e1005118.
10. Arai R. Fish Karyotypes: A Check List. Tokyo: Springer; 2011.
11. Accioly IV, Molina WF. Cytogenetic studies in Brazilian marine Sciaenidae and Sparidae fishes (Perciformes). Genet Mol Res. 2008;7:358–70.
12. Wang JX, Zhao XF, Wang XM, Tian MC. Karyotype analysis for seven species of clupeiform and perciform fishes. Zool Res. 1994;15:76–9. (In Chinese with English abstract)
13. Yu ZI, Kong XY, Xie ZY, Dai JX. Studies on the chromosomes of five species of marine fish. J Ocean Univ Qingdao. 1996;26:44–8. (In Chinese with English abstract)
14. Zou SM, Li SF, Zhao JL, Cai WQ, Liu JF. Karyotype of *Pseudosciaena crocea* in Guanjingyang of Fujian. J Shanghai Fisheries Univ. 2003;12:179–81. (In Chinese with English abstract)
15. Niu WT, Cai ZP. Review on karyotype study marine fishes in China. J Xiamen Univ (Natural Science). 2006;45:125–31. (In Chinese with English abstract)
16. Lou J, Lei S, Zhu J, Wu X. Chromosome karyotype of *Pseudosciaena crocea* Daiqu population. Chin J Zool. 2015;50:148–52. (In Chinese with English abstract)
17. Cioffi MB, Bertollo LAC. Chromosomal distribution and evolution of repetitive DNAs in fish. In Repetitive DNA (Vol. 7). Basel: Karger Publishers; 2012. p. 197-221.
18. Bertollo LAC, Cioffi MB, Moreira O. Filho. Direct chromosome preparations from Freshwater teleost fishes. In: Catherine Ozouf-Costaz, Eva Pisano, Fausto Foresti, Lurdes Foresti de Almeida Toledo, editors. Fish cytogenetic techniques (Chondrichthyans and Teleosts). Enfield: CRC Press; 2015. p. 21–6.
19. Sumner AT. A simple technique for demonstrating centromeric heterochromatin. Expl Cell Res. 1972;75:304–6.
20. Martins C, Ferreira IA, Oliveira C, Foresti F, Galetti PM Jr. A tandemly repetitive centromeric DNA sequence of the fish *Hoplias malabaricus* (Characiformes: Erythrinidae) is derived from 5S rDNA. Genetica. 2006;127:133–41.
21. Cioffi MB, Martins C, Centofante L, Jacobina U, Bertollo LAC. Chromosomal variability among allopatric populations of Erythrinidae fish *Hoplias malabaricus*: mapping of three classes of repetitive DNAs. Cytogenet Genome Res. 2009;125:132–41.
22. Kubat Z, Hobza R, Vyskot B, Kejnovsky E. Microsatellite accumulation in the Y chromosome of *Silene latifolia*. Genome. 2008;51:350–6.
23. Volff JN, Körting C, Froschauer A, Sweeney K, Schartl M. Non-LTR retrotransposons encoding a restriction enzyme-like endonuclease in vertebrates. J Mol Evol. 2001;52:351–60.
24. Úbeda-Manzanaro M, Merlo MA, Palazón JLI, Cross I, Sarasquete C, Rebordinos L. Chromosomal mapping of the major and minor ribosomal genes, (GATA)n and U2 snRNA gene by double-colour FISH in species of the Batrachoididae Family. Genetica. 2010;138:787–94.
25. Yano CF, Bertollo LAC, Cioffi MB. FISH-FISH: molecular Cytogenetics in fish species. In: Liehr T, editor. Fluorescence in situ Hybridization (FISH)-Application Guide. 2ed ed. Berlin: Springer; 2017. p. 429–44.
26. Levan A, Fredga K, Sandberg AA. Nomenclature for centromeric position on chromosomes. Hereditas. 1964;52:201–20.
27. Galetti PM Jr, Aguilar CT, Molina WF. An overview of marine fish cytogenetics. Hydrobiologia. 2000;420:55–62.
28. Motta-Neto CC, Cioffi MB, Bertollo LAC, Molina WF. Molecular cytogenetic analysis of Haemulidae fish (Perciformes): evidence of evolutionary conservation. J Exp Mar Biol Ecol. 2011;407:97–100.
29. Costa GWWF, Cioffi MB, Bertollo LAC, Molina WF. Transposable elements in fish chromosomes: a study in the marine cobia species. Cytogenet Genome Res. 2013;141:126–32.
30. Fujiwara A, Fujiwara M, Nishida-Umehara C, Abe S, Masaoka T. Characterization of Japanese flounder karyotype by chromosome bandings and fluorescence in situ hybridization with DNA markers. Genetica. 2007; 131:267–74.
31. Amorim KDJ, Cioffi MB, Bertollo LAC, Soares RX, Souza AS, Costa GWWF, Molina WF. Co-located 18S/5S rDNA arrays: an ancient and unusual chromosomal trait in Julidini species (Labridae, Perciformes). Comp Cytogenet. 2016;10:555–70.
32. Ferreira DC, Oliveira C, Foresti F. Chromosome mapping of retrotransposable elements Rex1 and Rex3 in three fish species in the subfamily Hypoptopomatinae (Teleostei, Siluriformes, Loricariidae). Cytogenet Genome Res. 2011;132:64–70.
33. Supiwong W, Liehr T, Cioffi MB, Chaveerach A, Kosyakova N, Pinthong K, Tanee T, Tanomtong A. Karyotype and cytogenetic mapping of 9 classes of repetitive DNAs in the genome of the naked catfish *Mystus bocourti* (Siluriformes, Bagridae). Mol Cytogenet. 2013;6:51.
34. Schneider CH, Gross MC, Terencio ML, Do Carmo EJ, Martins C, Feldberg E. Evolutionary dynamics of retrotransposable elements Rex 1, Rex 3 and Rex 6 in neotropical cichlid genomes. BMC Evol Biol. 2013;13:152.
35. Costa GWWF, Cioffi MB, Bertollo LAC, Molina WF. The evolutionary dynamics of ribosomal genes, histone H3, and transposable Rex elements in the genome of Atlantic snappers. J Hered. 2016;107:173–80.
36. Getlekha NMB, Cioffi YCF, Maneechot N, Bertollo LAC, Supiwong W, Tanomtong A, Molina WF. Chromosome mapping of repetitive DNAs in sergeant major fishes (Abudefdufinae, Pomacentridae): a general view on the chromosomal conservatism of genus. Genetica. 2016a;144:567–76.
37. Lo PC, Liu SH, Chao NL, Nunoo FK, Mok HK. Chen WJ.A multi-gene dataset reveals a tropical new world origin and early Miocene diversification of croakers (Perciformes: Sciaenidae). Mol Phylogenet Evol. 2015;88:132–43.
38. Molina WF, Galetti PM Jr. Robertsonian rearrangements in the reef fish *Chromis* (Perciformes, Pomacentridae) involving chromosomes bearing 5S rRNA genes. Genet Mol Biol. 2002;25:373–7.
39. Coleman RR, Gaither MR, Kimokeo B, Stanton FG, Bowen BW, Toonen RJ. Large-scale introduction of the Indo-Pacific damselfish *Abudefduf vaigiensis* into Hawai'i promotes genetic swamping of the endemic congener *A. abdominalis*. Mol Ecol. 2014;23:5552–65.
40. Getlekha N, Molina WF, Cioffi MB, Yano CF, Maneechot N, Bertollo LAC, Supiwong W, Tanomtong A. Repetitive DNAs highlight the role of chromosomal fusions in the karyotype evolution of *Dascyllus* species (Pomacentridae, Perciformes). Genetica. 2016b;144:203–11.

# 16

# A *Gossypium* BAC clone contains key repeat components distinguishing sub-genome of allotetraploidy cottons

Yuling Liu[1,2], Renhai Peng[1,3], Fang Liu[1], Xingxing Wang[1], Xinglei Cui[1], Zhongli Zhou[1], Chunying Wang[1], Xiaoyan Cai[1], Yuhong Wang[1], Zhongxu Lin[2*] and Kunbo Wang[1*]

**Abstract**

**Background:** Dissecting genome organization is indispensable for further functional and applied studies. As genome sequences data shown, cotton genomes contain more than 60 % repetitive sequences, so study on repetitive sequences composition, structure, and distribution is the key step to dissect cotton genome.

**Results:** In this study, a bacterial artificial chromosome (BAC) clone enriched in repetitive sequences, was discovered initiatively by fluorescence in situ hybridization (FISH). FISHing with allotetraploidy cotton as target DNA, dispersed signals on most regions of all A sub-genome chromosomes, and only middle regions of all D sub-genome chromosomes were detected. Further FISHing with other cotton species bearing A or D genome as target DNA, specific signals were viewed. After BAC sequencing and bioinformational analysis, 129 repeat elements, size about 57,172 bp were found, accounting for more than 62 % of the BAC sequence (91,238 bp). Among them, a type of long terminal repeat-retrotransposon (LTR-RT), LTR/Gypsy was the key element causing the specific FISH results. Using the fragments of BAC matching with the identified Gypsy-like LTR as probes, the BAC-57I23-like FISH signals were reappeared. Running BLASTN, the fragments had good match with all chromosomes of *G. arboreum* ($A_2$) genome and A sub-genome of *G. hirsutum* ($AD_1$), and had relatively inferior match with all chromosomes of D sub-genome of $AD_1$, but had little match with the chromosomes of *G. raimondii* ($D_5$) genome, which was consistent with the FISH results.

**Conclusion:** A repeats-enriched cytogenetic marker to identify A and D sub genomes of *Gossypium* was discovered by FISH. Combined sequences analysis with FISH verification, the assembly quality of repetitive sequences in the allotetraploidy cotton draft genome was assessed, and better chromosome belonging was verified. We also found the genomic distribution of the identified Gypsy-LTR-RT was similar to the distribution of heterochromatin. The expansion of this type of Gypsy-LTR-RT in heterochromatic regions may be one of the major reasons for the size gap between A and D genome. The findings showed here will help to understand the composition, structure, and evolution of cotton genome, and contribute to the further perfection of the draft genomes of cotton.

**Keywords:** *Gossypium*, BAC, Repetitive sequences, LTR-RT, FISH

## Background

*Gossypium*, as one of the best-characterized allopolyploid species, is divided into eight diploid genome groups (2n = 2× = 26), namely A-G and K, and one allotetraploidy genome group (2n = 4× = 52), which is allotetraploid bearing A and D genomes [1, 2]. So far, approximately 45 diploid and 6 tetrapolyploid *Gossypium* species are recognized [3, 4]. Among them, four cultivated species, the New World allopolyploids *G. hirsutum* and *G. barbadense* (2n = 4× = 52), and the Old World diploids *G. arboreum* and *G. herbaceum* (2n = 2× = 26), especially *G. hirsutum*, dominate worldwide cotton production. For a long time, cotton has been firmly established as the world's most important fiber crop and an important source of seed oil and protein meal [5].

* Correspondence: linzhongxu@mail.hzau.edu.cn; wkbcri@163.com
[2]National Key Laboratory of Crop Genetic Improvement, Huazhong Agricultural University, Wuhan 430070, China
[1]State Key Laboratory of Cotton Biology, Institute of Cotton Research of Chinese Academy of Agricultural Science, Anyang, Henan 455000, China
Full list of author information is available at the end of the article

The two progenitors of allotetraploidy cotton diverged 4–8 million years ago, and re-hybridized about 1–2 million years ago [6, 7]. There is enough time for sequence divergence, as well as subsequent genome stability. What's more, there is a wide range in genome size across closely related diploid species (from 880 Mb to 2572 Mb per haploid nucleus) and well-established phylogeny in *Gossypium* [8]. So, cotton is also an excellent model system for studying polyploidization, genomic organization, and genome-size variation. To dissect the genomic complexity in allotetraploidy cotton, extensive efforts have been performed. The ployploid parentage had been explained with the help of series of cytogenetic data combined with the observation derived from different studies. In early years, based on some classic cytogenetic and cytological studies, genome composition of the polyploids was investigated, which confirmed that the American allotetraploidy species are allopolyploids containing two resident genomes, an A-genome from Africa or Asia, and a D-genome similar to those found in the American diploids [9–11]. With the extensive application of FISH, more evidences that allotetraploidy cottons may be polyphyly have been obtained [12, 13].

It is believed that the proportion of protein-coding sequences is generally similar in different plant species [14], and repetitive DNA sequences are important factors in genome size variation [15–17]. Repetitive sequences can be classified into two categories: tandem repeats and transposable elements [18]. The former, which is usually found in specific genomic regions, such as centromeres or telomeres, has been extensively studied in different plant species [19–24]. Among the latter, retrotransposons replicating through a 'copy and paste' mechanism can result in the increase of the genome size to a great extent. Different methods had been used for analysis of repetitive DNA sequences, such as the low $C_0t$ analysis [25, 26], bacterial artificial chromosome (BAC) end sequences analysis [27], full-length BAC sequences analysis [28, 29]. To date, the most powerful method to characterize the high copy fraction of a genome is next generation sequencing and subsequent bioinformatic analysis [30, 31]. Recently, the draft assemblies of cotton genomes have been reported. More than 60 % of repetitive DNA sequences in genomes were revealed [32–36]. So dissecting the repetitive DNA sequences of genome is helpful to further understand the composition, evolution, and function of the cotton genome.

Fluorescence in situ hybridization (FISH), which allows direct mapping of DNA sequences on chromosomes, has become the most important technique in plant molecular cytogenetics [37]. Unique distribution patterns of repetitive DNA sequences on chromosomes has been revealed by FISH [38, 39], which provided a wealth of information regarding the chromosomal location of repetitive DNA sequences and their evolution in polyploidy genomes.

Here we analyzed a repeats-rich BAC clone combining FISH verification with sequence analysis, and identified the key elements resulting in specific FISH signal patterns, that is, a type of long terminal repeat-retrotransposon (LTR-RT). Simultaneous FISH with different cotton species as target chromosomes provided visual cytogenetic evidences of the colonization and size variation of the genomes. Moreover, by integrating FISH results with the cotton draft genomes, we preliminarily assessed the assembly quality of the draft genome assemblies.

## Methods

### Plant materials and BAC library

The cultivated *Gossypium* species, *G. hirsutum* ($AD_1$) (accession TM-1), *G. barbadense* ($AD_2$) (cultivar Hai-7124), and *G. arboreum* ($A_2$) (cultivar Shixiya-1) were planted at Institute of Cotton Research of Chinese Academy of Agricultural Sciences (CRI-CAAS) in Anyang City, Henan Province, China. The wild species *G. tomentosum* ($AD_3$) (accession P0601211), *G. mustelinum* ($AD_4$) (accession P0811704), *G. darwinii* ($AD_5$) (accession $AD_5$-7), *G. raimondii* ($D_5$) (accession $D_5$-2), and the artificial hexaploid cotton (*G. hirsutum* ($AD_1$) x *G. stocksii* ($E_1$)) are perennially growing in National Wild Cotton Nursery in Sanya city, Hainan Island, China. The BAC library of *G. herbaceum* var. *africanum* was constructed by Gao et al. [40].

### BAC clone screening

During the screening of the $1^{th}$ chromosome-specific BACs from the BAC library of *G. herbaceum* var. *africanum*, with SSR markers derived from a whole-genome marker map [41], the BAC clone 57I23 enriched in repeats was found. The corresponding SSR marker Gh216, with primers (F/R): TCCACATTCCCATGCACTACTC/ CTAAAACCTTATACATACAAAATGCAGC was used to screen the BAC library according to Cheng et al. [42] with a few modifications.

### BAC sequencing and repeats identification

The screened BAC clone 57I23 was sequenced and assembled by Shanghai Invitrogen Inc. Then BLASTN searches were performed using the BAC sequence as query, the draft genomes of cotton [33, 34, 36] as subjects respectively to detect the high copy repeats consisted in the BAC sequence. To further identify repeats types, online programs CENSOR (http://www.girinst.org/) [43], LTR-FINDER (http://tlife.fudan.edu.cn/ltr_finder/) [44] were used with the default parameters.

### Isolation of repeats

The primers of the selected repeats, with better match to genome or higher score in CENSOR results, were designed using NCBI primer-BLAST (http://www.ncbi.nlm.nih.gov/tools/primer-blast/). Touchdown PCR was performed to obtain amplification products with the BAC-57I23 bacterium as template. The amplification procedure was as follows: firstly, 98 °C 5 min for pre-degeneration; then 98 °C for 11 s, 52 + 1 °C for 18 s, 68 °C for 2.5 min for 10 cycles; 98 °C for 11 s, 57 °C for 18 s, 68 °C for 2.5 min for 30 cycles with a final extension at 68 °C for 6 min.

### DNA probes preparation

To visualize the distribution of the BAC-57I23 and its repeat elements, FISH was performed using BAC-DNA and repeat elements as probes respectively. BAC-DNA was isolated using Plasmid Miniprep Kit (Biomiga) according to the handbook. The PCR products were purified using Wizard SV Gel and PCR Clean-up System (Promega). They were labeled with DIG-nick translation Mix, according to the instructions of the manufacturer (Roche, USA).

### Chromosome preparation and FISH

Chromosome Preparation and the FISH procedure were conducted according to the previous protocols [45, 46]. The probes were detected with anti-digoxigenin-rhodamine (red) (Roche, USA). Images were captured using a CCD camera attached to a Zeiss Imager M1 microscope. Images were processed using Photoshop CS3.

## Results

### Discovery of the repeat-rich BAC clone 57I23

During the screening of the 1$^{th}$ chromosome-specific BACs from the BAC library of *G. herbaceum* var. *africanum*, a genome-specific BAC clone 57I23 was obtained using SSR marker Gh216, which was genetically mapped to AD_chr.01 ($A_t$01) [47, 48]. FISHing with AD genome species as target DNA, the signals dispersed on the all chromosomes except the terminal areas of A sub-genome, and only middle areas of all D sub-genome chromosomes (Fig. 1a-e). So the FISH with BAC-57I23 can distinguish A sub-genome from D sub-genome simultaneously. Further FISHing with diploid A and D species, high coverage signals on all chromosomes of A genome were found (Fig. 1g), but hardly any signal on chromosomes of D genome (Fig. 1h). When using the artificial hexaploid hybrid (*G. hirsutum* x *G. stocksii*) preparation as target chromosomes, the similar A and D sub-genome signal patterns were observed, and none signal on E sub-genome (Fig. 1f). More than 15 metaphase cells with clear chromosome spreads were chosen to analyze the distribution of the FISH signals along the chromosomes. Based on the signal pattern, we deduced that the BAC clone 57I23 enriched in some types of repetitive elements.

### BAC sequencing and BLASTN analysis

To further understand the composition of BAC-57I23, BAC sequencing was performed by Shanghai Invitrogen Inc. Due to the existence of enriched repetitive sequences, three scaffolds with size of scaffold1-42,338 bp, scaffold2-26,803 bp, scaffold3-22,097 bp were obtained, respectively.

By BLASTN using the BAC sequence as query and $A_2$ draft genome (*G. arboretum*) [34] as subject sequence, we obtained ten DNA fragments (named after its sequence location in corresponding scaffold) from the BAC sequence, based on the more-than-80 % similarity and zero or approximate zero e-value. With the ten selected DNA fragments as query sequences, BLASTN

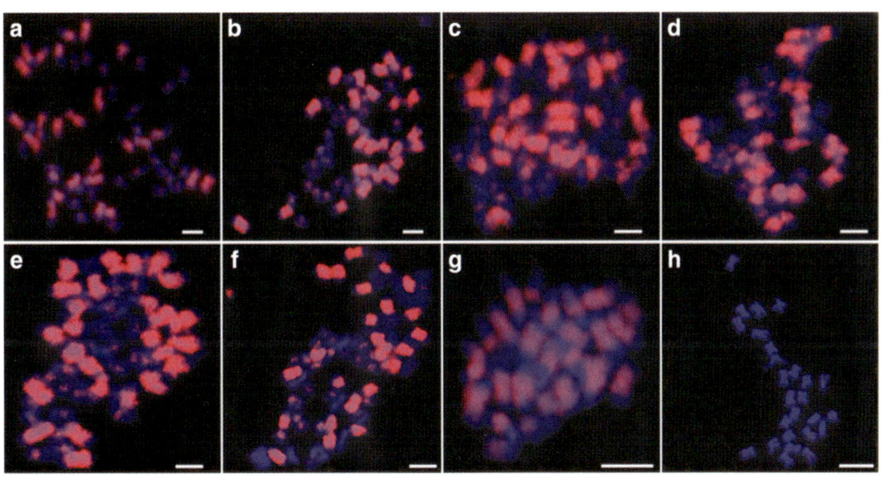


**Fig. 1** FISH mapping of BAC clone 57I23 on metaphase chromosomes of different *Gossypium* species. **a**-**h**: *G. hirsutum* ($AD_1$, 2n = 4x = 52), *G. barbadense* ($AD_2$, 2n = 4x = 52), *G. tomentosum* ($AD_3$, 2n = 4x = 52), *G. mustelinum* ($AD_4$, 2n = 4x = 52), *G. darwinii* ($AD_5$, 2n = 4x = 52), hexaploid hybrid (*G. hirsutum* x *G. stocksii*) (AADDEE, 3n = 6x = 78), *G. arboreum* ($A_2$, 2n = 2x = 26), *G. raimondii* ($D_5$, 2n = 2x = 26). *Red*: the signal of BAC-57I23. Bar = 5 μm

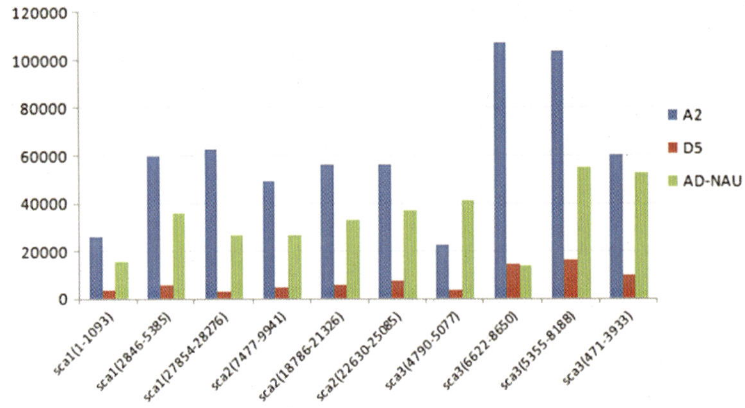


**Fig. 2** Copy number of the ten selected DNA fragments in $A_2$, $D_5$, and $AD_1$ (Zhang et al. 2015 [36]) (hereafter we named it as $AD_1$-NAU) genomes by BLASTN

were performed against $D_5$ (*G. raimondii*) and $AD_1$ (*G. hirsutum*) draft genomes [33, 36] respectively. After comparing the distribution of the ten fragments in different cotton genomes, it was found that the copy number was the highest in $A_2$ genome, but 10–25 times lower in $D_5$ genome (Fig. 2), and with very bad match hits (data not shown), which maybe partially explain the FISH results in D genome species. We extracted the sequences of the ten fragments from the BAC sequence for the following analysis.

At the same time, taking into account the FISH results of BAC-57I23 in AD genome species, we compared the total repeated numbers of ten fragments in every chromosome of AD genome (Fig. 3). Result showed that the A sub-genome chromosomes had more than 10 times of repeats copy numbers than D sub-genome, and better consistency with the FISH results was viewed.

### Identification of repetitive sequences

Based on CENSOR results, DNA transposon, LTR-RT, Non-LTR-RT, and other repetitive elements were identified from the BAC sequences, which account for more than 62 % of the assembled BAC sequence. Among them, LTR-RT was predominant, accounting for 88.11 % of total identified repetitive elements (55.21 to 62.66 %) (Fig. 4 and Table 1). The identified LTR-RTs were classified into LTR/Gypsy, LTR/Copia, LTR/BEL families. Especially, LTR/Gypsy accounted for more than 91 % of the total identified LTR-RTs. By combining the CENSOR with BLASTN analysis results, we selected 12 LTR-RTs with higher score value (Table 2), and extracted the corresponding sequences from the BAC sequences for FISH verification.

When running LTR-FINDER (version 1.05) using BAC sequence as query sequence, a 4118 bp full-length LTR-RT was identified in sequence region of scaffold1 (13558-17675). It belonged to the LTR/Copia family, and overlapped with Copia-80_ST-I identified by CENSOR.

By RepeatMasker (RepeatMasker vesion open-4.0.5) analysis, a 659 bp (sca2 (20662-21331)) Gypsy/DIRSI LTR element was identified, which had overlap region with sca2 (18785-21330) from the CENSOR results.

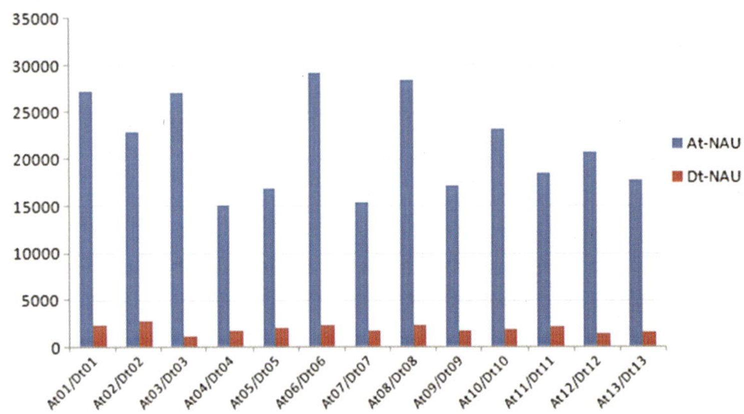


**Fig. 3** Total copy number of the ten fragments in every chromosome of $AD_1$-NAU genome (At/Dt)

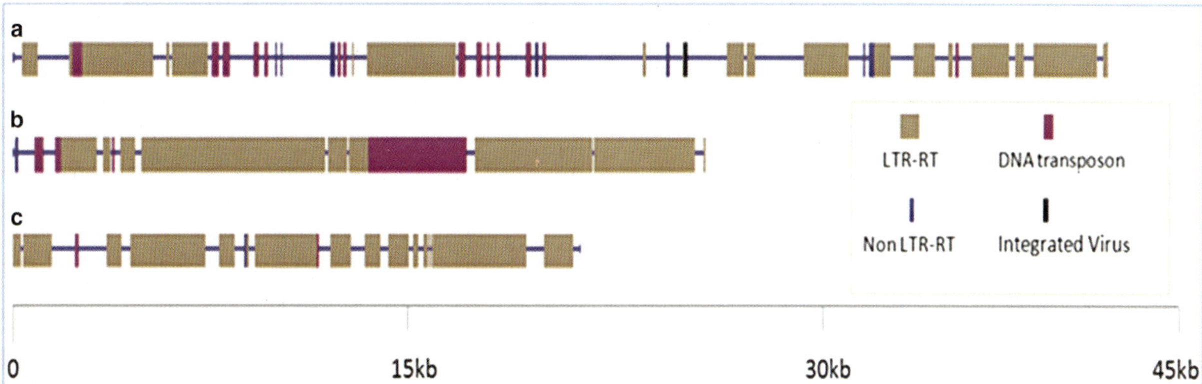


**Fig. 4** Sequence analysis graphical map of the repeat-rich bacterial artificial chromosome (BAC) clone 57123. *Horizontal blue bars* represent the BAC sequence, *vertical bars* represent different repeat elements. *a*, scaffold1-42338 bp; *b*, scaffold2-26803 bp; *c*, scaffold3-22097 bp

For further FISH verification, the partial above-mentioned fragments and LTR-RTs were PCR amplified and purified. Each purified DNA fragment had single band and expected size, which suited for the following work.

### Distribution of LTR-RTs in the cotton genomes

The FISH analysis of somatic metaphase chromosomes showed differential distribution patterns for each LTR-RT subfamily. When using Gypsy-48_GR-I-like LTR-RTs as probes, BAC-57123-like signals were reappeared (Fig. 5a, d-i). Using sca3 (5355-8188) as probes, the FISH signals only were observed on chromosomes of A sub-genome with lower coverage relative to BAC 57123 (Fig. 5b), and no signal on *G. raimondii* chromosomes (Fig. 5c). Using sca1 (13558-17675), a 4118 bp-LTR/Copia element as probe, only a few dotty signals appeared (Fig. 5j). But using sca2 (23904-25399), a Non-Gypsy-48_GR-I-like LTR-RT as probe, no signal appeared (Fig. 5k).

Pachytene chromosomes can display a differentiated pattern of heterochromatic and euchromatic regions [46, 49]. The pachytene-FISH results of *G. hirsutum* using fragment sca2 (18785-21330) as probe, which belonging to Gypsy-48_GR-I-like LTR-RT, showed high signal density throughout the partial pachytene chromosomes mainly following the distribution of heterochromatin, as white arrow shown (Fig. 5l).

**Table 1** Summary of identified repeats in BAC sequence by CENSOR

| Repeat class | Fragments | Length (bp) | Percentage accounting for BAC sequence |
|---|---|---|---|
| Integrated Virus | 1 | 86 | 0.09 % |
| DNA transposon | 25 | 6086 | 6.67 % |
| LTR Retrotransposon | 94 | 50373 | 55.21 % |
| BEL | 1 | 65 | 0.07 % |
| Copia | 4 | 4251 | 4.66 % |
| Gypsy | 89 | 46057 | 50.48 % |
| Non-LTR Retrotransposon | 9 | 627 | 0.69 % |
| Total | 129 | 57172 | 62.66 % |

## Discussion

### Sub-genome-specific cytogenetic marker

In early times, cotton chromosome identification was mainly based on the analysis of cytological characters, such as chromosomal relative lengths, arm ratios, and nuclear organization regions (NORs) in the mitotic or meiotic metaphase [50]. Because of the big number and small size of the chromosomes in cotton, the cytological identification of the chromosome has been hitherto limited. With the development of FISH, chromosome-specific FISH markers are effective tools for chromosome identification, analysis of genetic stocks, and physical mapping [13, 51–53]. BAC-57123 displayed here can be used as a sub-genome specific FISH marker to identify A and D sub-genomes simultaneously in AD genome cotton species or allohexaploids containing A and D sub-genomes, due to the different FISH signal patterns on A and D sub-genome chromosomes. The discovery of BAC-57123 provided a new FISH marker for identification of two or three sub-genomes at the same time, so the one-BAC FISH with 57123 can take the place of GISH (genomic in situ hybridization) with two or three genomes DNA to achieve the identification of the sub-genomes.

### Assembly quality of repetitive sequences in allotetraploidy cotton draft genome

Decoding cotton genomes is a foundation for understanding the functional and agronomic significance of polyploidy and genome size variation within the *Gossypium* genus. But high-quality assembly of allopolyploid plant genomes is a formidable task because of the large genomes and the existence of highly homeologous sub-

**Table 2** Selected LTR-RTs from CENSOR results

| Name | From | To | Name | From | To | Class | Name |
|---|---|---|---|---|---|---|---|
| scaffold1\|size42338 | 4200 | 5326 | Gypsy-48_GR-I | 1376 | 2498 | LTR/Gypsy | sca1 (4200-5326) |
| scaffold1\|size42338 | 13782 | 17200 | Copia-80_ST-I | 194 | 3604 | LTR/Copia | sca1 (13782-17200) |
| scaffold1\|size42338 | 31153 | 32254 | Gypsy-48_GR-I | 3205 | 4308 | LTR/Gypsy | sca1 (31153-32254) |
| scaffold2\|size26803 | 7498 | 8637 | Gypsy-48_GR-I | 76 | 1221 | LTR/Gypsy | sca2 (7498-8637) |
| scaffold2\|size26803 | 23904 | 25399 | Gypsy-18_GR-I | 1326 | 2899 | LTR/Gypsy | sca2 (23904-25399) |
| scaffold3\|size22097 | 10623 | 11420 | Gypsy-18_GR-I | 2893 | 3697 | LTR/Gypsy | sca3 (10623-11420) |
| scaffold3\|size22097 | 17834 | 19556 | Gypsy-48_GR-I | 2773 | 4562 | LTR/Gypsy | sca3 (17834-19556) |
| scaffold3\|size22097 | 20731 | 21832 | Gypsy-48_GR-I | 3260 | 4363 | LTR/Gypsy | sca3 (20731-21832) |
| scaffold2\|size26803 | 13047 | 13565 | Copia-2_JC-I | 4861 | 5382 | LTR/Copia | sca2 (13047-13565) |
| scaffold2\|size26803 | 19133 | 19572 | Gypsy-1_JC-I | 276 | 715 | LTR/Gypsy | sca2 (19133-19572) |
| scaffold2\|size26803 | 18785 | 21330 | Gypsy-48_GR-I | 50 | 2596 | LTR/Gypsy | sca2 (18785-21330) |
| scaffold3\|size22907 | 5533 | 6040 | Gypsy-1_JC-I | 269 | 774 | LTR/Gypsy | sca3 (5533-6040) |

genomes [36]. Mis-assemblies are common when draft genome sequences have been generated by de novo assembly of sequences obtained with NGS technologies [54]. It's possible that regions with repeated sequences might not be assembled successfully. FISH, allowing directly mapping of DNA sequences on chromosomes, has become an important technique in plant molecular cytogenetic research and can be used to guide draft genome assembly [37, 55, 56]. In this study, when blasting against the $AD_1$-NAU draft genome using the identified repeats, the results had good consistency with the BAC-FISH results (Figs. 1 and 3). Based on this result, we can infer the assembly of the identified repetitive sequences in $AD_1$-NAU draft genome has better matchup on their chromosome belonging.

### Genome size expansion and LTR-RTs

In diploid cottons, the A genome (1697 Mb) has nearly twice the size of the D genome (885 Mb) [1, 5]. The sequences analysis of cotton draft genome indicates that

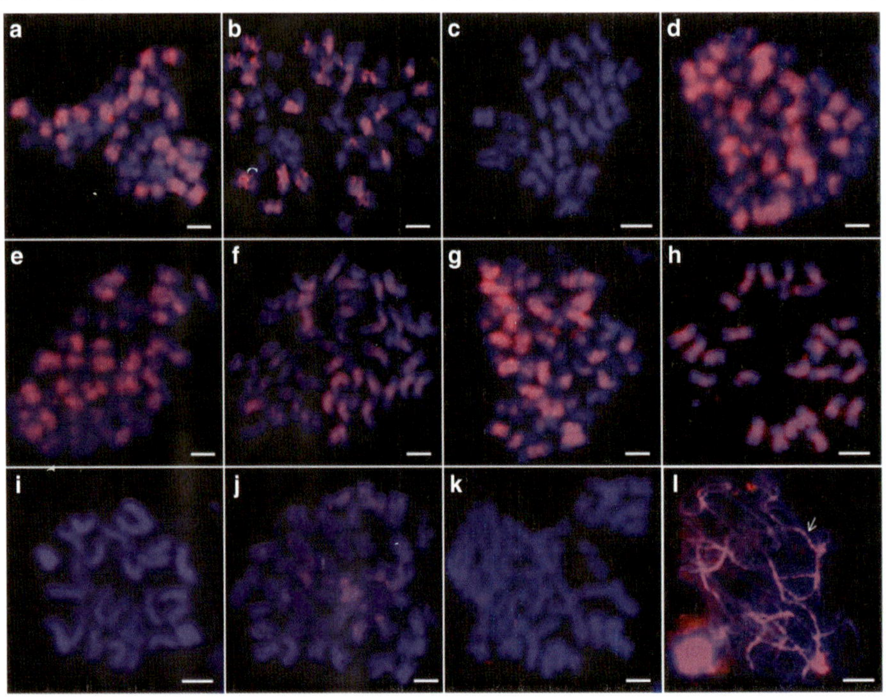


**Fig. 5** FISH analysis of distribution of identified LTR-RTs in cotton genome. **a**, sca2 (18785-21330)- *G. hirsutum*; **b**, sca3 (5355-8188)- *G. hirsutum*; **c**, sca3 (5355-8188)- *G. raimondii*.; **d**, sca1 (4200-5326)- *G. hirsutum*; **e**, sca2 (7498-8637)- *G. hirsutum*; **f**, sca3 (17834-19556)- *G. hirsutum*; **g**, sca3 (20731-21832)- *G. hirsutum*; **h**, sca1 (4200-5326)- *G. arboreum*; **i**, sca1 (4200-5326)- *G. raimondii*; **j**, scaffold1 (13558-17675)- *G. hirsutum*; **k**, sca2 (23904-25399)- *G. hirsutum*; **l**, sca2 (18785-21330)- *G. hirsutum* (pachytene). Bar = 5 μm

the amount of sequence encompassing LTR-type retrotransposons increased from 348 Mb in *G. raimondii* to 1145 Mb in *G. arboreum*, whereas the protein-coding capacities of these two species remained largely unchanged [32, 34]. In this study, the significant difference of FISH signal patterns of the BAC-57I23 between A and D genomes indicated that the BAC-57I23 should have specific composition, which can partly explain the size gap between A and D genome (Fig. 1g, h). By sequence analysis, a type of Gypsy-like LTR-RTs was identified as the key element in the BAC. The genomic distribution of the identified Gypsy-LTR-RT was similar to the distribution of heterochromatin (Fig. 5l). The expansion of this type of Gypsy-LTR-RT in heterochromatic regions may be one of the major reasons for the size gap between A and D genome. Here we provided visualized evidence by FISH that the proliferation of a type of Gypsy-like LTR-RTs is one of the major reasons for genome size diversity between A and D, which further supported the former studies results [8, 57, 58].

### The colonization of the genome

The previous studies showed that A-genome-specific dispersed repetitive sequences at the diploid level have colonized the D-genome at the polyploid level [38, 59]. Similarly, another study showed that a family of copia-like retrotransposable elements "horizontally" transferred across genomes following allopolyploid formation [60]. Page et al. discovered that approximately 900 kp of sequence in the polyploid genome have been converted from one genome to another in separate conversion events scattered across the genome by whole-genome re-sequencing [61]. Here, our results combined BAC-sequencing with FISH verification showed that a type of Gypsy-like LTR-RTs had high copies in *G. arboreum* ($A_2$) genome, but none in the *G. raimondii.* (D5) genome (Fig. 5), however at the polyploidy level, obviously sequence expansion and colonization from A to D sub-genomes occurred, which dispersed on all D sub-genome chromosomes middle areas.

## Conclusions

As an excellent system for studying genome evolution and polyploidization, cotton cytogenetic study is increasingly on the agenda. Combined sequences analysis with FISH verification, a new genome-specific cytogenetic marker for identification of sub-genome was discovered. The repetitive sequences assembly quality of the allotetraploidy cotton draft genome was verified preliminarily, that is, the chromosome belonging of the repeats in $AD_1$ draft genome has good consistency with the BAC-FISH results. A type of Gypsy-like LTR-RTs identified from the BAC-57I23 can partially explain the size gap between A and D genome. During the process of polyploidization of cotton, "horizontally" transferred from the A sub-genome to D sub-genome The findings showed here will help to understand the composition, structure, and evolution of cotton genome, and also will contribute to the further perfection of the draft genomes of cotton, as well as provided the cytogenetic evidence for polyploidy formation.

#### Competing interests

The authors declare that they have no competing interests.

#### Authors' contributions

YL: Design of the study; Performed most of the experiments, manuscript writing. KW, RP, FL, ZL: Design of the study; Manuscript corrections; Supervision. XW, XC, CW, XC, YW, ZZ: Participated in the experiments, Manuscript corrections. All authors read and approved the final version of the manuscript.

#### Funding

This study was financially supported in part by a grant from the National Natural Science Foundation of China (No. 31471548), State Key Laboratory of Cotton Biology Open Fund (No.CB2014A07), National High Technology Research and Development Program (No.2013AA102601).

#### Author details

[1]State Key Laboratory of Cotton Biology, Institute of Cotton Research of Chinese Academy of Agricultural Science, Anyang, Henan 455000, China. [2]National Key Laboratory of Crop Genetic Improvement, Huazhong Agricultural University, Wuhan 430070, China. [3]Anyang Institute of Technology, Anyang, Henan 455000, China.

#### References

1. Endrizzi JE, Turcotte EL, Kohel RJ. Genetics, cytogenetics, and evolution of *Gossypium*. Adv Genet. 1985;23:271–375.
2. Wendel JF, Schnabel A, Seelanan T. Bidirectional interlocus concerted evolution following allopolyploid speciation in cotton (*Gossypium*). Proc Natl Acad Sci U S A. 1995;92(1):280–4.
3. Fryxell PA. A revised taxonomic interpretation of *Gossypium* L. (Malvaceae). Rheedea. 1992;2:108–65.
4. Stewart JM, Craven LA, Brubaker C, Wendel JF. *Gossypium* anapoides (Malvaceae), a New Species from Western Australia. Novon. 2015;23(4):447–51.
5. Wendel JF, Cronn RC. Polyploidy and the evolutionary history of cotton. Adv Agron. 2003;78:139–86.
6. Seelanan T, Schnabel A, Wendel JF. Congruence and consensus in the cotton tribe. Syst Bot. 1997;22:259–90.
7. Wendel JF, Albert VA. Phylogenetics of the cotton genus (*Gossypium* L.): character-state weighted parsimony analysis of chloroplast DNA restriction site data and its systematic and biogeographic implications. Syst Bot. 1992;17:115–43.
8. Hawkins JS, Kim H, Nason JD, Wing RA, Wendel JF. Differential lineage-specific amplification of transposable elements is responsible for genome size variation in *Gossypium*. Genome Res. 2006;16(10):1252–61.
9. Webber JM. Interspecific hybridization in *Gossypium* and the meiotic behavior of F1 plants. J Agric Res. 1935;51:1047–70.
10. Skovsted A. Cytological studies in cotton. II. Two interspecific hybrids between Asiatic and New World cottons. J. Genet. 1934;28:407–24.
11. Beasley JO. The origin of American tetraploid *Gossypium* species. Am Nat. 1940;74:285–6.
12. Liu SH, Wang KB, Song GL, Wang CY, Liu F, Li SH, et al. Primary investigation on GISH-NOR in cotton. Chinese Sci Bull. 2005;50(5):425–9.
13. Gan YM, Chen D, Liu F, Wang CY, Li SH, Zhang XD, et al. Individual chromosome assignment and chromosomal collinearity in *Gossypium thurberi*, *G. trilobum* and D subgenome of *G. barbadense* revealed by BAC-FISH. Genes Genet Syst. 2011;86(3):165–74.
14. SanMiguel P, Tikhonov A, Jin YK, Motchoulskaia N, Zakharov D, Melake-Berhan A, et al. Nested retrotransposons in the intergenic regions of the maize genome. Science. 1996;274(5288):765–8.

15. Soltis DE, Soltis PS, Bennett MD, Leitch IJ. Evolution of genome size in the angiosperms. Am J Bot. 2003;90(11):1596–603.
16. Bennetzen JL, Ma J, Devos KM. Mechanisms of recent genome size variation in flowering plants. Ann Bot. 2005;95(1):127–32.
17. Lysak MA, Koch MA, Beaulieu JM, Meister A, Leitch IJ. The dynamic ups and downs of genome size evolution in Brassicaceae. Mol Biol Evol. 2009;26(1):85–98.
18. Kubis S, Schmidt T, Heslop-Harrison JS. Repetitive DNA elements as a major component of plant genomes. Ann Bot. 1998;82(Suppl):45–55.
19. Ananiev EV, Phillips RL, Rines HW. Chromosome-specific molecular organization of maize (*Zea mays* L.) centromeric regions. Proc Natl Acad Sci U S A. 1998;95(22):13073–8.
20. Copenhaver GP, Nickel K, Kuromori T, Benito MI, Kaul S, Lin X, et al. Genetic definition and sequence analysis of *Arabidopsis* centromeres. Science. 1999;286(5449):2468–74.
21. Kishii M, Nagaki K, Tsujimoto HA. Tandem repetitive sequence located in the centromeric region of common wheat (*Triticum aestivum*) chromosomes. Chromosome Res. 2001;9(5):417–28.
22. Cheng ZK, Dong GF, Langdon TL, Ouyang S, Buell CR, Gu MH, et al. Functional rice centromeres are marked by a satellite repeat and a centromere-specific retrotransposon. Plant Cell. 2002;14(8):1691–704.
23. Kulikova O, Geurts R, Lamine M, Kim DJ, Cook DR, Leunissen J, et al. Satellite repeats in the functional centromere and pericentromeric heterochromatin of *Medicago truncatula*. Chromosoma. 2004;113(6):276–83.
24. Fajkus J, Sykorova E, Leitch AR. Telomeres in evolution and evolution of telomeres. Chromosome Res. 2005;13(5):469–79.
25. Ho ISH, Leung FC. Isolation and characterization of repetitive DNA sequences from *Panax ginseng*. Mol Genet Genomics. 2002;266(6):951–61.
26. Liu WX, Thummasuwan S, Sehgal SK, Chouvarine P, Peterson DG. Characterization of the genome of bald cypress. BMC Genomics. 2011;12:553.
27. Hong CP, Lee SJ, Park JY, Plaha P, Park YS, Lee YK, et al. Construction of a BAC library of Korean ginseng and initial analysis of BAC-end sequences. Mol Genet Genomics. 2004;271(6):709–16.
28. Choi HI, Waminal NE, Park HM, Kim NH, Choi BS, Park M, et al. Major repeat components covering one-third of the ginseng (*Panax ginseng* C.A. Meyer) genome and evidence for allotetraploidy. Plant J. 2014;77(6):906–16.
29. Tamura M, Hisataka Y, Moritsuka E, Watanabe A, Uchiyama K, Futamura N, et al. Analyses of random BAC clone sequences of Japanese cedar, *Cryptomeria japonica*. Tree Genet Genomes. 2015;11(3):50.
30. Macas J, Neumann P, Navratilova A. Repetitive DNA in the pea (Pisum sativum L.) genome: comprehensive characterization using 454 sequencing and comparison to soybean and Medicago truncatula. BMC Genomics. 2007;8:427.
31. Novak P, Neumann P, Macas J. Graph-based clustering and characterization of repetitive sequences in next-generation sequencing data. BMC Bioinformatics. 2010;11:378. doi:10.1186/1471-2105-11-378.
32. Wang KB, Wang ZW, Li FG, Ye WW, Wang JY, Song GL, et al. The draft genome of a diploid cotton *Gossypium raimondii*. Nat Genet. 2012;44(10):1098–103.
33. Paterson AH, Wendel JF, Gundlach H, Guo H, Jenkins J, Jin DC, et al. Repeated polyploidization of *Gossypium* genomes and the evolution of spinnable cotton fibres. Nature. 2012;492(7429):423–7.
34. Li FG, Fan GY, Wang KB, Sun FM, Yuan YL, Song GL, et al. Genome sequence of the cultivated cotton *Gossypium arboreum*. Nat Genet. 2014;46(6):567–72.
35. Li FG, Fan GY, Lu CR, Xiao GH, Zou CS, Kohel RJ, et al. Genome sequence of cultivated Upland cotton (*Gossypium hirsutum* TM-1) provides insights into genome evolution. Nat Biotechnol. 2015;33(5):524–30.
36. Zhang TZ, Hu Y, Jiang WK, Fang L, Guan XY, Chen JD, et al. Sequencing of allotetraploid cotton (*Gossypium hirsutum* L. acc. TM-1) provides a resource for fiber improvement. Nat Biotechnol. 2015;33(5):531–7.
37. Jiang JM, Gill BS. Current status and the future of fluorescence in situ hybridization (FISH) in plant genome research. Genome. 2006;49(9):1057–68.
38. Hanson RE, Zhao XP, Islam-Faridi MN, Paterson AH, Zwick MS, Crane CF, et al. Evolution of interspersed repetitive elements in *Gossypium* (Malvaceae). Am J Bot. 1998;85(10):1364–8.
39. Luo S, Mach J, Abramson B, Ramirez R, Schurr R, Barone P, et al. The cotton centromere contains a Ty3-gypsy-like LTR Retroelement. PLoS ONE. 2012; 7(4): doi:10.1371/journal.pone.0035261
40. Gao HY, Wang HF, Liu F, Peng RH, Zhang Y, Cheng H, et al. Construction of the bacterial artificial chromosome library of *G. herbaceum* var. *africanum*. Chinese Sci Bull. 2013;58(26):3199–201.
41. Wang ZN, Zhang D, Wang XY, Tan X, Guo H, Paterson AH. A whole-genome DNA marker map for cotton based on the D-genome sequence of *Gossypium raimondii* L. Genes Genom Genet. 2013;3(10):1759–67.
42. Cheng H, Peng RH, Zhang XD, Liu F, Wang CY, Wang KB. A rapid method to screen BAC library in cotton. Biotechnology (In Chinese). 2012;22(3):55–7.
43. Kohany O, Gentles AJ, Hankus L, Jurka J. Annotation, submission and screening of repetitive elements in Repbase: RepbaseSubmitter and Censor. BMC Bioinformatics. 2006;7:474.
44. Xu Z, Wang H. LTR_FINDER: an efficient tool for the prediction of full-length LTR retrotransposons. Nucleic Acids Res. 2007;35(Web Server issue):W265–8. http://tlife.fudan.edu.cn/ltr_finder/.
45. Jiang JM, Gill BS, Wang GL, Ronald PC, Ward DC. Metaphase and interphase fluorescence in situ hybridization mapping of the rice genome with bacterial artificial chromosomes. Proc Natl Acad Sci U S A. 1995;92(10):4487–91.
46. Peng RH, Zhang T, Liu F, Ling J, Wang CY, Li SH, et al. Preparations of miotic pachytene chromosomes and extended DNA fibers from cotton suitable for fluorescence in situ hybridization. PLoS ONE. 2012; 7(3): doi:10.1371/journal.pone.0033847.
47. Yu Y, Yuan D, Liang S, Li X, Wang X, Lin Z, et al. Genome structure of cotton revealed by a genome-wide SSR genetic map constructed from a BC1 population between *gossypium hirsutum* and *G. barbadense*. BMC Genomics. 2011;12:15. doi:10.1186/1471-2164-12-15.
48. Yu JZ, Kohel RJ, Fang DD, Cho J, Van Deynze A, Ulloa M, et al. A high-density simple sequence repeat and single nucleotide polymorphism genetic map of the tetraploid cotton genome. Genes Genom Genet. 2012;2(1):43–58.
49. De Jong JH, Fransz P, Zabel P. High resolution FISH in plants – techniques and applications. Trends Plant Sci. 1999;4(7):258–63.
50. Wang KB, Li MX. The karyotype variation and evolution of D genome in *Gossypium*. Acta Agron Sin. 1990;16(3):200–7.
51. Kim JS, Childs KL, Islam-Faridi MN, Menz MA, Klein RR, Klein PE, et al. Integrated karyotyping of sorghum by in situ hybridization of landed BACs. Genome. 2002;45(2):402–12.
52. Wang K, Guo W, Zhang T. Development of one set of chromosome-specific microsatellite-containing BACs and their physical mapping in *Gossypium hirsutum* L. Theor Appl Genet. 2007;115(5):675–82.
53. Gan YM, Liu F, Peng RH, Wang CY, Li SH, Zhang XD, et al. Individual chromosome identification, chromosomal collinearity and genetic physical integrated map in *Gossypium darwinii* and four D genome cotton species revealed by BAC-FISH. Genes Genet Syst. 2012;87(4):233–41.
54. Alkan C, Sajjadian S, Eichler EE. Limitations of next-generation genome sequence assembly. Nat Methods. 2011;8(1):61–5.
55. Yang L, Koo DH, Li Y, Zhang X, Luan F, Havey MJ, et al. Chromosome rearrangements during domestication of cucumber as revealed by high-density genetic mapping and draft genome assembly. Plant J. 2012;71(6):895–906.
56. Sun JY, Zhang ZH, Zong X, Huang SW, Li ZY, Han YH. A high-resolution cucumber cytogenetic map integrated with the genome assembly. BMC Genomics. 2013;14:461.
57. Hawkins JS, Proulx SR, Rapp RA, Wendel JF. Rapid DNA loss as a counterbalance to genome expansion through retrotransposon proliferation in plants. Proc Natl Acad Sci U S A. 2009;106(42):17811–6.
58. Grover CE, Wendel JF. Recent insights into mechanisms of genome size change in plants. J Bot. 2010. doi:10.1155/2010/382732.
59. Zhao XP, Si Y, Hanson RE, Crane CF, Price HJ, Stelly DM, et al. Dispersed repetitive DNA has spread to new genomes since polyploid formation in cotton. Genome Res. 1998;8(5):479–92.
60. Hanson RE, Islam-Faridi MN, Crane CF, Zwick MS, Czeschin DG, Wendel JF, et al. Ty1-copia-retrotransposon behavior in a polyploid cotton. Chromosome Res. 1999;8(1):73–6.
61. Page JT, Huynh MD, Liechty ZS, Grupp K, Stelly D, Ashrafi AH, et al. Insights into the evolution of cotton diploids and polyploids from whole-genome resequencing. Genes Genom Genet. 2013;3(10):1809–18.

# 17

# High chromosomal instability in workers occupationally exposed to solvents and paint removers

Mónica Villalba-Campos[1], Lilian Chuaire-Noack[1], Magda Carolina Sánchez-Corredor[1] and Milena Rondón-Lagos[1,2*]

**Abstract**

**Background:** Painters are exposed to an extensive variety of harmful substances like aromatic hydrocarbons used as solvents and paint removers, some of which have shown clastogenic activity. These substances constitute a complex mixture of chemicals which contain well-known genotoxicants, such as Benzene, Toluene and Xylene. Thus, chronic occupational exposure to such substances may be considered to possess genotoxic risk. In Colombia the information available around the genotoxic damage (Chromosomal and DNA damage) in car paint shop workers is limited and the knowledge of this damage could contribute not only to a better understanding of the carcinogenic effect of this kind of substances but also could be used as biomarkers of occupational exposure to genotoxic agents.

**Results:** In this study, the genotoxic effect of aromatic hydrocarbons was assessed in peripheral blood lymphocytes of 24 workers occupationally exposed and 24 unexposed donors, by using Cytogenetic analysis and comet assay. A high frequency of Chromosomal alterations was found in the exposed group in comparison with those observed in the unexposed group. Among the total of CAs observed in the exposed group, fragilities were most frequently found (100 %), followed by chromosomal breaks (58 %), structural (41.2 %) and numerical chromosomal alterations (21 %). Numerical chromosomal alterations, fragilities and chromosomal breaks showed significant differences between exposed and unexposed groups. Among the fragilities, fra(9)(q12) was the most frequently observed. DNA damage Index was also significantly higher in the exposed group compared to the unexposed group ($p < 0.000$).

**Conclusions:** Our results revealed that occupational exposure to aromatic hydrocarbons is significantly associated with Chromosomal and DNA damage in car paint shops workers and are also indicative of high chromosomal instability. The high frequency of both Chromosomal Alterations and DNA Damage Index observed in this study indicates an urgent need of intervention not only to prevent the increased risk of developing cancer but also to the application of strict health control and motivation to the use of appropriate protecting devices during work.

**Keywords:** Chromosomal alterations, Chromosomal instability, Occupational exposure, Aromatic hydrocarbons, Comet assay

## Background

Occupational aromatic hydrocarbons exposure (Benzene, Toluene and Xylene - BTX), mainly via inhalation, occurs most frequently as result of various activities in which these substances are processed, generated or used [1]. These are present in both evaporative and combustive automobile emissions, in cigarette smoke and are commonly used as an industrial solvent in the workplace. Recently, the International Agency for Research on Cancer 2010 (IARC) [2], included in group 1 carcinogens, some aromatic hydrocarbons used as solvents and paint removers, like Benzene, Toluene and Xylene.

Benzene, is a chemical potentially carcinogenic (leukaemogenic) in humans due to the ultimate carcinogen hydroquinone and 1,4-benzoquinone metabolised by cytochrome P450 enzymes (CYP2E1) in the liver [3–6]. Toluene, the methyl- substituted derivative of benzene,

* Correspondence: srondonl@unito.it
[1]Facultad de Ciencias Naturales y Matemáticas, Universidad del Rosario, Bogotá, DC, Colombia
[2]Department of Medical Sciences, University of Turin, Via Santena 7, 10126 Turin, Italy

is also metabolized by CYP450 enzymes [7]. Although the main products of the benzene metabolism (acid S-phenylmercapturic and trans -trans -muconic) and toluene (hippuric acid) are eliminated through the urine, some intermediate metabolites may generate reactive oxygen species (ROS) and can cause oxidative stress and genetic damage [8]. This genetic damage is mainly represented by DNA adduct formation and impairment of DNA repair mechanisms, DNA single-strand breaks, sister-chromatid exchanges (SCE), micronuclei (MN), DNA cross-linking and Chromosomal Alterations (CAs) in peripheral blood lymphocytes (PBLs) [9–14]. In addition, have been reported that benzene can cause an increased risk of developing cancer in various organs, such as lung, bladder, pancreas and lymphatic and hematopoietic tumors, being it cataloged as clastogenic to human PBLs [10, 15–17].

CAs in PBLs reflect inter-individual sensitivity to exogenous and endogenous genotoxic substances and can be used as biomarkers of genotoxic damage and carcinogenic risk [17–20]. In fact, according to recent reports, CAs represent one of the best internationally standardized and validated biomarkers of early biological effects in human biomonitoring [18, 21, 22]. However, the type and frequency of such CAs have not been carefully characterized in a Colombian population and these could be used as markers of cytogenotoxic damage.

Additional methods are also used in human biomonitoring studies, as the comet assay (gel electrophoresis of individual cells). The comet assay, has proved its usefulness and versatility in human biomonitoring, ecogenotoxicology, genotoxicity testing and basic research into the mechanisms of DNA damage and repair [23–25]. It detects strand breaks and alkali-labile sites at frequencies from a few hundred to several thousand breaks per cell. The use of this assay have greatly increased during the past few decades [26, 27] and allowed evaluating the DNA damage index (DNA-DI) caused by occupational exposure to chemicals.

The aim of the present study was to evaluate the genotoxic effect of occupational exposure to aromatic hydrocarbons used as solvents and paint removers, on the frequency of CAs and on the DNA-DI in PBLs of workers at ten car paint shops at the "7 de agosto" neighborhood in Bogota DC, Colombia.

## Methods

### Study population

The study was carried out in a group of 24 men selected at random and routinely "exposed" to solved paints, at ten car paint shops at the "7 de agosto" neighborhood in Bogota DC, Colombia. The exposed donors consisted of men between 21 and 73 years old and a work time exposed to organic solvents of at least 1 year. Individuals who had suffered from hepatitis or cancer, or had been under chemotherapy or radiotherapy or any other recent prolonged medical treatment were excluded of this study.

The unexposed group was recruited in another area within the same neighborhood, with similar characteristics except for the presence of nearby car paint shops. This group consisted of 24 healthy men, without indication of previous occupational exposure to aromatic hydrocarbons and whose ages were similar to the exposed donors (between 20 and 72 years old) (Table 1).

Data from the 24 exposed donors were compared with those of the unexposed donors. Each donor was personally interviewed by filling in a routine questionnaire including age, smoking and drinking habits, exposure to organic solvents, diseases, occupational history including duration of exposure to chemicals and the use of protecting devices during work (Table 1).

### Blood sampling

Two peripheral blood samples were collected from exposed and unexposed donors by venipuncture. One blood sample was used for Cytogenetic analysis and the other for lymphocytes isolation and further comet assay. The samples were labeled, transported to the laboratory and processed within 3 to 4 h.

### Metaphase spreads and high-resolution GTG

Metaphases were obtained using standardized harvesting protocols for conventional cytogenetic analysis. Briefly, 0.8 ml of heparinised peripheral blood were cultured in duplicates in 10 ml RPMI-1640 medium (Sigma, St. Louis, MO, USA), supplemented with 10 % fetal bovine serum (FBS) (Sigma) and 0.5 % phytohemaglutinin-M (Gibco, Life Technologies, Nebraska, USA). The cultures were incubated at 37 °C and 5 % $CO_2$ for 72 h. After this, colcemid solution (N-Deacetyl-N-methylcolchicine, 0.0001 g/ml final conc.) (Sigma) was added to cultures 25 min before cell harvesting [28]. Cells were then

**Table 1** Characteristics of the Study population

| | Exposed | | | Unexposed | | |
|---|---|---|---|---|---|---|
| Characteristic | N | Mean ± SD/% | Range | N | Mean ± SD/% | Range |
| Age (years) | 24 | 44.25 ± 13.42 | 21–73 | 24 | 44.45 ± 12.91 | 20–72 |
| Exposure time (years) | 24 | 18.4 ± 11.1 | 1–35 | 24 | 0 | 0 |
| Smoking habits | | | | | | |
| Smokers | 3 | 12.5 | | 3 | 12.5 | |
| No smokers | 21 | 87.5 | | 21 | 87.5 | |
| Alcohol consumption | | | | | | |
| Drinkers | 21 | 87.5 | | 17 | 70.9 | |
| No drinkers | 3 | 12.5 | | 7 | 29.1 | |

*SD* Standard Deviation

treated with hypotonic solution (KCl 0.075 M), fixed three times with Carnoy's fixative (3:1 methanol to acetic acid) and spread on glass. Glass slides were baked at 80 °C for 2 h, incubated in 2xSSC buffer, placed in trypsin solution (0,25 %) (Gibco) before treatment with Giemsa stain (Sigma).

### Chromosome analysis

Characterisation of CAs was performed in a total of 1018 metaphases. Image acquisition and subsequent karyotyping of metaphases was performed using a Nikon microscope (Applied Imaging, Santa Clara, CA, USA). Numerical (NCAs) and structural chromosomal alterations (SCAs), Fragilities (FRA), chromosome breaks (chrb) and chromatid breaks (chrtb), present in at least two or three metaphases were evaluated. All CAs were described according to the International System for Human Cytogenetic Nomenclature (ISCN) 2013 [29].

### Lymphocyte separation

To perform the comet assay the lymphocytes were isolated by Ficoll-1077 (Sigma Aldrich, St. Louis, MO, USA) density gradient centrifugation and washed in phosphate buffered saline (PBS 1X) (Gibco, Life Technologies, Nebraska, USA). The viability of the cells was tested by trypan blue test (Life Technologies, Nebraska, USA) and was kept greater than 90 %. The volume of cell suspension used in the test was $4\times10^3$ lymphocytes.

### Comet assay

We used the standard procedure of alkaline comet assay described by Collins et al 2001 [30] using the Trevigen Comet Assay Kit (Trevigen, Gaithersburg, USA).

In order to calculate DNA damage, 100 cells per individual was analyzed by using fluorescence microscope (Nikon Instruments Inc, USA), with a magnification of 100X. All assays were performed in duplicate. The comets were classified through the Comet Score publisher program, in five categories according to the percentage of DNA in the tail, as follows: 0: No damage (<5 %), 1: Low damage (6–25 %), 2: moderate damage (26–50 %), 3: high damage (51–75 %) and 4: severe damage (>76 %) [30–32]. DNA-DI was then calculated according to the formula proposed by Collins et al 2004 [27]: $DI = 0(n) + 1(n) + 2(n) + 3(n) + 4(n)$, where "n" indicates number of cells in each class. Therefore, a DNA-DI could range from 0 (all cells with no tail, 100 cells × 0) to 400 (all cells with maximally long tails, 100 cells × 4).

### Data analysis

All statistical analyses were performed using IBM-SPSS Statistics Developer (Version 21.0 IBM Company, Chicago, IL). Normality of the data was evaluated by Shapiro-Wilk test. Fisher's exact test and Wilcoxon test were performed to compare the cytogenetic data with parametric a non-parametric distribution, respectively. The comet assay data, which was normally distributed, were analyzed using Student's *T*-test. *P* values less than 0.05 were considered significant ($^*p \le 0.05$ $^{**}p \le 0.01$).

## Results

### Characteristics of study groups

The effect of occupational exposure to aromatic hydrocarbons on DNA in car paint workers and unexposed donors was assessed by Conventional Cytogenetics and the comet assay.

Detailed information of researched groups is displayed in the Table 1. For the exposed group the median time of exposure to aromatic hydrocarbons was 18.4 years and their median age was 44.25 years. A low prevalence of smoking (12.5 %) and a high consumption of alcoholic beverage (87.5 %) were reported in this group. Also a low prevalence of smoking (12.5 %) and a high consumption of alcoholic beverage (70.9 %) were reported in the unexposed group. The results were expressed as mean ± standard deviation (SD).

### Cytogenetic data

In order to define CAs (Numerical and structural chromosomal alterations, Fragilities, chromosome breaks and chromatid breaks), between 14 and 26 metaphases with good chromosome dispersion and morphology were analyzed for both exposed and unexposed groups. Cytogenetic analysis for both groups demonstrated a modal number diploid (2n). As shown in Table 2 and Fig. 1a, a significant high frequency of CAs was found in the exposed group (119 CAs) in comparison with those observed in the unexposed group (33 CAs) ($p \le 5.261e\text{-}06$)

Among the total of CAs observed in the exposed group, Fragilities (FRA) were most frequently found (68/119) (Table 3, Figs. 2, 3a and b), followed by chromosome breaks (chrb) (22/119) and chromatid breaks (chtb) (5/119) (Fig. 3c), structural chromosomal alterations (SCAs) (13/119) (Fig. 3c) and numerical chromosomal alterations (NCAs) (11/119) (Fig. 2). NCAs, FRA, chrb and chtb showed significant differences when exposed and unexposed groups were compared ($p \le 0.01$, $p \le 0.000001$ and $p \le 0.017$ respectively) (Table 3). No significant differences were found in the number of CAs between smokers and nonsmokers.

#### *Structural and numerical chromosomal alterations*

A higher frequency of NCAs and SCAs was identified in the exposed group (11 and 13 respectively) compared to those observed in the unexposed group (4 and 8 respectively). However SCAs alterations were observed only in individual cases and no statistically significant differences

**Table 2** Total number of CAs (by donor) found in the exposed and unexposed groups

| No | Exposed | Unexposed | $p$ |
|---|---|---|---|
| 1 | 8 | 5 | |
| 2 | 1 | 2 | |
| 3 | 7 | 0 | |
| 4 | 6 | 0 | |
| 5 | 9 | 4 | |
| 6 | 15 | 3 | |
| 7 | 3 | 4 | |
| 8 | 4 | 1 | |
| 9 | 6 | 1 | |
| 10 | 5 | 1 | |
| 11 | 2 | 0 | |
| 12 | 6 | 2 | |
| 13 | 1 | 2 | |
| 14 | 6 | 1 | |
| 15 | 8 | 0 | |
| 16 | 6 | 1 | |
| 17 | 3 | 0 | |
| 18 | 2 | 0 | |
| 19 | 2 | 2 | |
| 20 | 4 | 0 | |
| 21 | 5 | 0 | |
| 22 | 2 | 2 | |
| 23 | 3 | 2 | |
| 24 | 5 | 0 | |
| Total | 119 | 33 | 5.261e-06** |
| Mean | 4.95 | 1.37 | |
| SD | 3.12 | 1.46 | |

**Difference significant relative to unexposed group at $p \leq 0.01$ (Wilcoxon test); *SD* Standard Deviation

were found in the number of donors affected by them (Table 3).

The NCAs identify in both groups were mainly represented by monosomies, whereas trisomies were absent. In the exposed group were found monosomies of the chromosomes 6, 8, 18, 19 and 21, while in the unexposed group were observed monosomies of chromosomes Y and 22.

In the exposed group were observed 13 SCAs in seven donors, including deletions (del), duplications (dup), translocations (t and der), additional material of unknown origin (add) and isochromosomes (i) (Table 4). Among the total of SCAs, deletions were most frequently found (38.5 %), followed by translocations (30 %) and duplications (15 %) (Fig. 3c). In the unexposed group were observed 8 SCAs (deletions and isochromosomes) in four donors (Table 4).

### *Fragilities*

A high frequency of FRA was found in the exposed group (68 fragilities) which showed a statistically significant difference ($p \leq 0.0001$) as compared to unexposed group (14 fragilities) (Table 3). In the exposed group, the chromosomes X, 1, 2, 3, 5, 6, 8, 9, 10 and 12 showed higher number of fragilities, being the fra(9)(q12) the most frequent (29/68) and present in the 75 % of the exposed ($p \leq 0.0001$) (Table 5, Fig. 3a and b), followed by fra(1p) and fra(8q) (Table 5). In the unexposed group the fra(9)(q12) was also the most frequent (5/14) in the 16.6 % of the donors.

### *Chromosome and chromatid breaks*

In addition to fragilities, a higher frequency of chrb and chtb were also observed in the exposed group (22 and 5 breaks respectively) compared to those observed in the unexposed group (6 and 1 breaks respectively). Chromosomes most affected by such changes in the exposed group were chromosomes 1, 3, 6 and 9 (Table 6, Fig. 3c). Comparison of presence of chrb and chtb between exposed and unexposed donors showed a significant difference ($p \leq 0.0023$ and $p \leq 0.0004$ respectively) (Table 3).

### Comet assay

The comet assay data for exposed and unexposed groups are presented in Table 7 and Fig. 1b. The DNA damage index (DNA-DI) observed in the exposed group was significantly higher than that observed in the unexposed group (235.7 ± 29.2 and 193.7 ± 22.2, $p < 0.000$, respectively). Smoking habits had no significant effect on DNA-DI among the exposed and unexposed groups.

## Discussion

The aim of the present study was to evaluate the genotoxic effect of occupational exposure to aromatic hydrocarbons used as solvents and paint removers, on the frequency of CAs and on the DNA-DI in PBLs of workers at ten car paint shops at the "7 de agosto" neighborhood in Bogota DC, Colombia.

Car paints shop workers are occupationally exposed to a wide range of aromatic hydrocarbons including BTX. Exposure to aromatic hydrocarbons, may take place via vapor inhalation or absorption through the intact skin. Many epidemiological studies have showed a clear relationship between the increase genotoxic damage and exposure to aromatic hydrocarbons, being neccesary to provide more relevant information regarding to the possible deleterious damage upon chromosomes. Although many studies have been conducted around of this topic, the specific type and frequency of such CAs have not been carefully characterized and these could be used as biomarkers of genotoxic damage and as predictors of future cancer risk. To the above is added that in Colombia

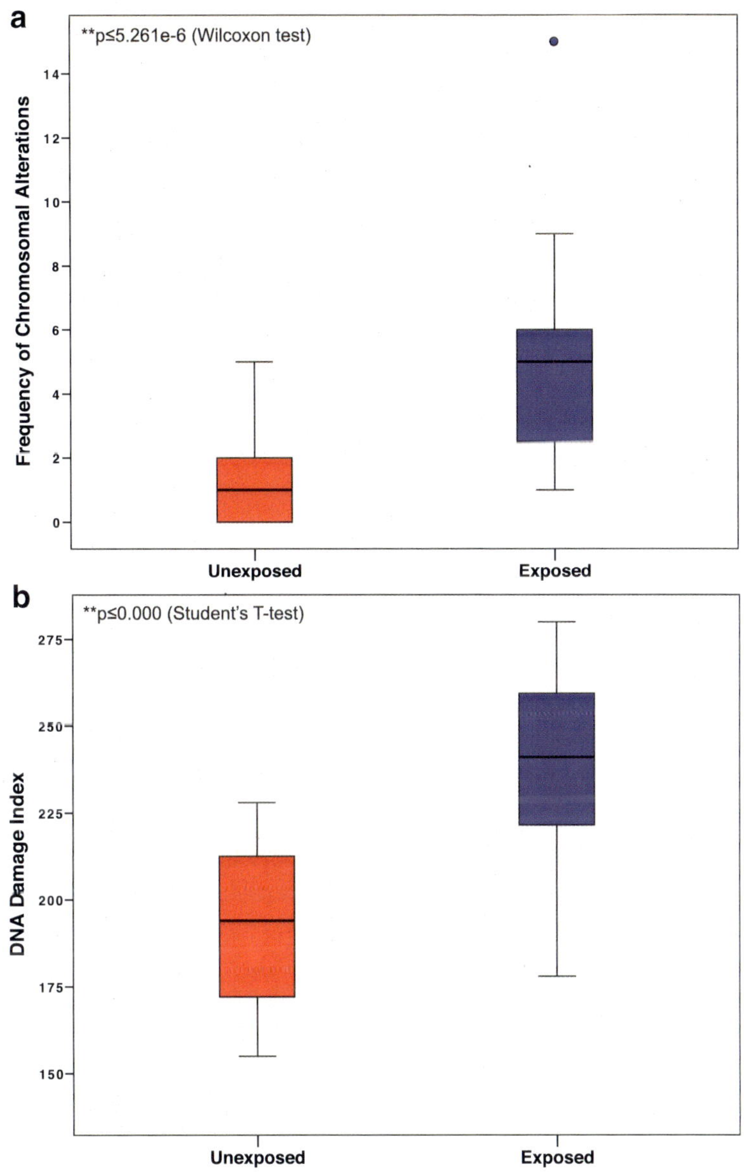


**Fig. 1** Boxplot of the genotoxic damage observed in the exposed and unexposed groups. **a** Frequency of CAs. The single point at the top of the exposed boxplot represents the maximum number of CAs within this group. **b** DNA damage index (DNA DI). The black line represents the CAs median values. The bottom and top of the boxes represent the 25th and 75th percentile respectively, whereas the box represents the interquartile range

**Table 3** Percentage of chromosomal alterations identify in the exposed and unexposed groups

| Chromosomal alterations | Exposed % | Unexposed % | *p* |
|---|---|---|---|
| NCAs | 21 | 8.3 | 0.01** |
| SCAs | 29 | 16.6 | 0.06 |
| FRA | 100 | 37.5 | 0.0001** |
| chrb | 37.5 | 16.6 | 0.0023** |
| chtb | 21 | 4.1 | 0.0004** |

*NCAs* Numerical chromosomal alterations, *SCAs* Structural chromosomal alterations, *FRA* Fragilities, *chrb* Chromosomal breaks, *chtb* Chromatid breaks
**Statistically significant difference relative to unexposed group at $p \leq 0.01$ (Fisher's exact test)

the information available around the cytogenotoxic damage in car paint shop workers is limited.

The results obtained using high-resolution G-Banding analyses of a large number of metaphases, allowed us to detect previously unreported CAs in individuals exposed to BTX. The mean of CAs found in the exposed group was 3.6 times higher than in the unexposed group, thus indicating a potential cytogenetic hazard due to exposure to aromatic hydrocarbons used as solvents and paint removers in car paint shops.

Among the chromosomal alterations observed at high frequency in the exposed group, monosomies, fragilities,

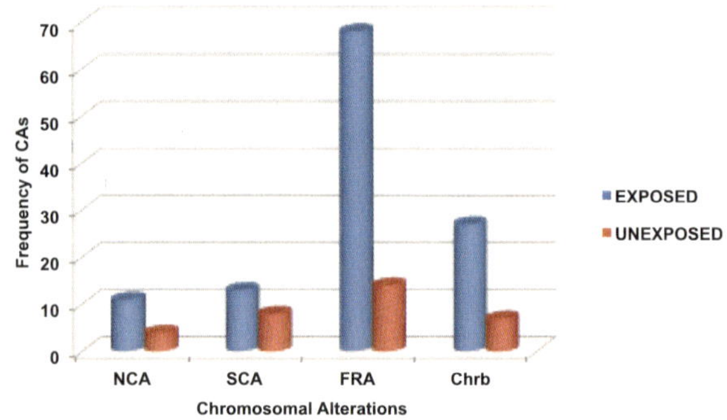


**Fig. 2** Frequencies of CAs in the PBLs of exposed and unexposed groups. NCAs: Numerical chromosomal alterations; SCAs: Structural chromosomal alterations; FRA: Fragilities: Chrb: Chromosomal breaks

**Table 4** Structural chromosomal alterations observed in the exposed and unexposed groups

| Number | Structural alterations | |
|---|---|---|
| | Exposed | Unexposed |
| 1 | del(Y)(q12) | del(2)(q16) |
| 2 | del(2)(q32) | del(6)(q22) |
| 3 | ?i(5)(q10) | add(7)(p22) |
| 4 | del(5)(q11.2) | inv(7)(p21q36) |
| 5 | dup(6)(p22p23) | del(9)(p21) |
| 6 | der(7)t(2;7)(q32;q36) | del(10)(p12) |
| 7 | der(7)t(7;14)(q32;q22) | del(10)(p13) |
| 8 | add(11)(p15) | i(11)(q10) |
| 9 | der(11)t(4;11)(q13;q23) | |
| 10 | t(13;14)(q34;q32) | |
| 11 | del(14)(q22) | |
| 12 | del(17)(q24) | |
| 13 | ?dup(17)(q22q25) | |

chbr and chrb showed statistically significant differences when were compared to those observed in the unexposed group. In several recent studies, this type of chromosomal alterations have been correlated with a heightened risk of cancer, especially hematological malignancies [33, 34]. For instance, monosomies, observed in gas station attendants and in individuals occupationally exposed to formaldehyde [35, 36], were associated with myeloid malignancies [37]. Further, monosomies of chromosomes 18 and 19, observed by us in the exposed group, were associated with risk of developing leukemia in individuals occupationally exposed to benzene [33]. Nevertheless, although the structural chromosomal alterations identify in the exposed group were not significant, some of them, including del(5)(q) and t(11)(q23), were detected in leukemia patients with likely prior exposure to benzene [12, 38].

In addition, a significant increase in the frequency of FRA, chrb and chtb in exposed compared to unexposed group was also observed. FRA, chrb and chtb are unstable CAs and regions of potential genome instability [39] that can lead to the formation of cancer-specific CAs such as translocations, deletions [39–43], duplications, amplifications [44, 45], sister chromatid exchanges [46], intrachromosomal gene amplification [47] and other chromosomal changes associated with human diseases [48, 49]. Further, many genes identified as tumor suppressors or oncogenes are located at or within fragile sites [50].

Among the FRA identified in this study, fra(9q12) was the most frequently observed in the exposed group. High frequency of this fragility was previously reported by us in a Colombian population with breast cancer [51]. On chromosome 9 are located the tumor suppressor genes *CDKN2A*, *PIPSK1B*, *BTEB1*, *RECK* and *BAG1*, the latter associated with antiapoptotic functions and overexpressed in invasive breast carcinomas.

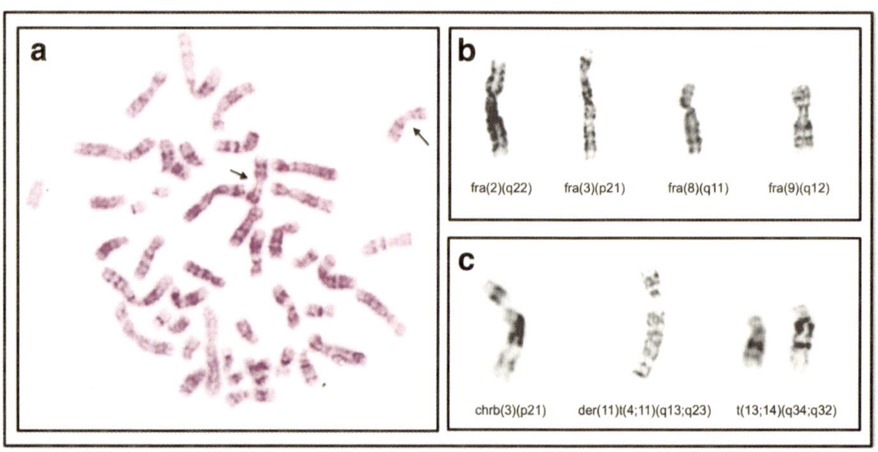


**Fig. 3** Representative images of CAs observed in the exposed group. **a** G-banding metaphase showing fragility of both chromosomes 9 (fra(9)(q12) (*indicated by arrows*). **b** Chromosomes showing fragilities found in higher frequency. **c** Chromosomes showing chrb and chtb and SCAs

**Table 5** Fragilities more frequently observed in the exposed and unexposed groups

| Fragilities | Exposed % | Unexposed % | p |
|---|---|---|---|
| fra(1)(p) | 21 | 4 | 0.0004** |
| fra(2)(q) | 16.6 | 8 | 0.08 |
| fra(3)(p) | 21 | 12.5 | 0.18 |
| fra(8)(q) | 21 | 0 | 0.0001** |
| fra(9)(q12) | 75 | 16.6 | 0.0001** |

**Statistically significant difference relative to unexposed group at $p \leq 0.01$ (Fisher's exact test)

Given the significantly high frequency of **fra(9)(q12)** in the exposed group, as well as its previous observation in patients with breast cancer, we considered that this fragility could be postulated as a cytogenetic biomarker of genotoxic damage associated to occupational exposure to BTX.

Our findings are consistent with previous reports in which increased chromosomal abnormalities in PBLs were associated with occupational exposure to benzene [3, 9, 35, 36]. However although most studies have mostly shown positive results, others have not found any association [52, 53].

Additionally, it is important to emphasize that increased genotoxic damage and, therefore a higher risk to develop cancer, have also been associated with other specific job occupations. For instance, a higher risk to develop hematologic diseases was observed in benzene exposed oil refinery workers [9], workers exposed to low levels of formaldehyde [35, 54], gas station attendants [36], painters [55] and petroleum refinery workers [56]. Further, an increased risk of laryngeal cancer was also reported in production-related workers, transport equipment operators, miners, tailors, blacksmith and toolmakers, painters, bricklayers and carpenters [57].

In our study, there was a significant increase in DNA-DI, evidenced by the comet assay, in exposed in comparison to the unexposed group. Comet assay has been used as a sensitive biomarker that reveals DNA damage caused either directly by reactive oxidant agents, or indirectly by substances that can generate free radicals [58, 59]. These findings are consistent with previous studies [55, 56, 60, 61] and allow us to confirm that occupational exposure to BTX induce genotoxic damage at both DNA and chromosomal level. However, we also note that smoking habit had no significant effect on DNA-DI among exposed and unexposed groups, which could be due to low cigarette consumption among the workers (1–3 cigarettes per day). Lack of association between DNA-DI and smoking habit in PBLs of individuals occupationally exposed to aromatic hydrocarbons, have been also indicated by several studies [55, 62–67].

**Table 6** Chromosomal breaks (chrb) (A) and chromatid breaks (chtb) (B) more frequently observed in the exposed and unexposed groups

| chrb | Exposed % | Unexposed % | p |
|---|---|---|---|
| A) | | | |
| chrb(6)(q11) | 16.6 | 0 | 0.0001** |
| chrb(9)(q12) | 12.5 | 0 | 0.0002** |
| B) | | | |
| chtb(1)(p11) | 12.5 | 4 | 0.03* |
| chtb(3)(p12) | 8 | 0 | 0.006** |

*Statistically significant difference relative to unexposed group at $p \leq 0.05$ (Fisher's exact test)
**Statistically significant difference relative to unexposed group at $p \leq 0.01$ (Fisher's exact test)

**Table 7** Evaluation of DNA damage index (DNA-DI) through Comet assay

| Groups | DNA-DI |
|---|---|
| Exposed ($n = 24$) | 235.70 ± 29.23** |
| Smokers ($n = 3$) | 211.66 ± 31.56 |
| No Smokers ($n = 21$) | 239.14 ± 28.00 |
| Alcohol Drinkers ($n = 21$) | 231.85 ± 29.19 |
| No Alcohol Drinkers ($n = 3$) | 262.66 ± 7.50 |
| Unexposed ($n = 24$) | 193.79 ± 22.22 |
| Smokers ($n = 3$) | 197.33 ± 16.66 |
| No Smokers ($n = 21$) | 193.28 ± 23.23 |
| Alcohol Drinkers ($n = 17$) | 193.88 ± 25.25 |
| No Alcohol Drinkers ($n – 7$) | 193.57 ± 13.89 |

The values are expressed as mean ± SD. **Statistically significant difference relative to unexposed group. $p \leq 0.000$ (Student's *t*-test)

In summary, our results demonstrated that occupational exposure to BTX is significantly associated with chromosomal and DNA damage in car paint shops workers and are indicative of high chromosomal instability (CIN). CIN, defined as a state of continuous formation of novel chromosome mutations at a rate higher than in normal cells, could predispose cells to further mutations and by that to an increased risk of malignant transformation [68, 69]. In fact, several prospective cancer studies have shown a linear trend between CAs in PBLs and subsequent cancer risk [35–37, 54, 70–73].

## Conclusions

BTX occupational exposure of car paints workers represents a relevant risk factor for the development of diseases associated with genetic damage. The high frequency of CAs and the high DNA-DI observed in this study indicate an urgent need of intervention not only to prevent the increased risk of developing cancer but also the application of strict health control and motivation to the use of appropriate protecting devices during work.

### Abbreviations

BTX, benzene, toluene and xylene; CAs, chromosomal alterations; chrtb/chrb, chromosome breaks and chromatid breaks; CIN, chromosomal instability; CYP450, cytochrome P450 enzymes; DNA-ID, DNA damage index; FRA, fragilities; IARC, international agency for research on cancer; MN, micronuclei; NCAs, numerical; PBLs, peripheral blood lymphocytes; ROS, reactive oxygen species; SCAs, Structural chromosomal alterations; SCE, sister-chromatid exchanges; SD, standard deviation

### Acknowledgements

We thank the Universidad del Rosario, Bogotá DC, Colombia, and the National Institute of Health of Colombia for their support for this research.

### Funding

This work was funded by Universidad del Rosario, Bogotá DC, Colombia.

### Authors' contributions

All authors made substantial contributions to the conception and design, analysis and interpretation of data, and critical review of the manuscript. LC, MS and MRL, conceived the study. MRL and MV performed the experiments and coordinated the data acquisition and analysis. MRL analyzed and interpreted the data and wrote the manuscript. LC, MS and MV participated to interpretation of data. All authors read and approved the final manuscript.

### Competing interests

The authors declare that they have no competing interests.

### References

1. Schnatter R. Petroleum worker studies and benzene risk assessment. J Toxic Environ Health A. 2000;61(5-6):433–7. doi:10.1080/00984100050166451.
2. WHO-IARC. Painting, firefighting, and shifwork/IARC monographs on the evaluation of the carcinogenic risks of chemicals to humans. Occupational exposure as a painter. 2010.
3. Kim SY, Choi JK, Cho YH, Chung EJ, Paek D, Chung HW. Chromosomal aberrations in workers exposed to low levels of benzene: association with genetic polymorphisms. Pharmacogenetics. 2004;14(7):453–63.
4. Ross D. The role of metabolism and specific metabolites in benzene-induced toxicity: evidence and issues. J Toxic Environ Health A. 2000;61(5-6):357–72. doi:10.1080/00984100050166361.
5. Kacew S, Lemaire I. Recent developments in benzene risk assessment. J Toxic Environ Health A. 2000;61(5-6):485–98.
6. Gad-el-Karim MM, Ramanujam VM, Ahmed AE, Legator MS. Benzene myeloclastogenicity: a function of its metabolism. Am J Ind Med. 1985;7(5-6):475–84.
7. Bird MG, Wetmore BA, Letinski DJ, Nicolich M, Chen M, Schnatter AR, et al. Influence of toluene co-exposure on the metabolism and genotoxicity of benzene in mice using continuous and intermittent exposures. Chem Biol Interact. 2010;184(1-2):233–9. doi:10.1016/j.cbi.2010.01.012.
8. Murata M, Tsujikawa M, Kawanishi S. Oxidative DNA damage by minor metabolites of toluene may lead to carcinogenesis and reproductive dysfunction. Biochem Biophys Res Commun. 1999;261(2):478–83. doi:10.1006/bbrc.1999.1041.
9. Tompa A, Jakab MG, Major J. Risk management among benzene-exposed oil refinery workers. Int J Hyg Environ Health. 2005;208(6):509–16. doi:10.1016/j.ijheh.2005.01.029.
10. Celi KA, Akbas E. Evaluation of sister chromatid exchange and chromosomal aberration frequencies in peripheral blood lymphocytes of gasoline station attendants. Ecotoxicol Environ Saf. 2005;60(1):106–12. doi:10.1016/j.ecoenv.2003.10.008.
11. Joo WA, Kang MJ, Son WK, Lee HJ, Lee DY, Lee E, et al. Monitoring protein expression by proteomics: human plasma exposed to benzene. Proteomics. 2003;3(12):2402–11. doi:10.1002/pmic.200300616.
12. Zhang L, Eastmond DA, Smith MT. The nature of chromosomal aberrations detected in humans exposed to benzene. Crit Rev Toxicol. 2002;32(1):1–42. doi:10.1080/20024091064165.
13. Major J, Jakab M, Megyesi A, Tompa A. Follow-up cytogenetic investigation of benzene-exposed workers: dose-related changes in chromosome aberration yields. Central Eur J Occupat Environ Med. 1996;2:2.
14. Major J, Jakab MG, Tompa A. Genotoxicological monitoring of 175 subjects living in the green belts, inner town or near chemical industrial estates in Greater Budapest agglomeration, Hungary. Mutat Res. 1998;412(1):9–16.
15. Costa C, Pasquale RD, Silvari V, Barbaro M, Catania S. In vitro evaluation of oxidative damage from organic solvent vapours on human skin. Toxicol In Vitro. 2006;20(3):324–31. doi:10.1016/j.tiv.2005.08.007.
16. Lan Q, Zhang L, Li G, Vermeulen R, Weinberg RS, Dosemeci M, et al. Hematotoxicity in workers exposed to low levels of benzene. Science. 2004; 306(5702):1774–6. doi:10.1126/science.1102443.
17. Smith MT, Rothman N. Biomarkers in the molecular epidemiology of benzene-exposed workers. J Toxic Environ Health A. 2000;61(5-6):439–45.
18. Mateuca RA, Decordier I, Kirsch-Volders M. Cytogenetic methods in human biomonitoring: principles and uses. Methods Mol Biol. 2012;817:305–34. doi:10.1007/978-1-61779-421-6_15.
19. Richmond ME. The Health Effects Institute's biomarker research in China. J Toxic Environ Health A. 2000;61(5-6):447–56. doi:10.1080/00984100050166479.
20. Carrano AV, Natarajan AT. International commission for protection against environmental mutagens and carcinogens. ICPEMC publication no. 14. Considerations for population monitoring using cytogenetic techniques. Mutat Res. 1988;204(3):379–406.
21. Natarajan AT, Boei JJ. Formation of chromosome aberrations: insights from FISH. Mutat Res. 2003;544(2-3):299–304.
22. Albertini RJ, Anderson D, Douglas GR, Hagmar L, Hemminki K, Merlo F, et al. IPCS guidelines for the monitoring of genotoxic effects of carcinogens in humans. International programme on chemical safety. Mutat Res. 2000;463(2):111–72.
23. White PA, Rasmussen JB. The genotoxic hazards of domestic wastes in surface waters. Mutat Res. 1998;410(3):223–36.
24. Hartmann A, Agurell E, Beevers C, Brendler-Schwaab S, Burlinson B, Clay P, et al. Recommendations for conducting the in vivo alkaline comet assay. 4th international comet assay workshop. Mutagenesis. 2003;18(1):45–51.
25. Collins AR. The comet assay: a heavenly method! Mutagenesis. 2015;30(1):1–4. doi:10.1093/mutage/geu079.
26. Singh NP, McCoy MT, Tice RR, Schneider EL. A simple technique for quantitation of low levels of DNA damage in individual cells. Exp Cell Res. 1988;175(1):184–91.
27. Collins AR. The comet assay for DNA damage and repair: principles, applications, and limitations. Mol Biotechnol. 2004;26(3):249–61. doi:10.1385/MB:26:3:249.
28. Pack SD, Stratakis CA. Chromosomes: Methods for Preparation. eLS. 2002. doi:10.1038/npg.els.0002709
29. Shaffer LG, McGowan-Jordan J, Schmid M. ISCN (2013): An international System for Human Cytogenetic Nomenclature. Basel: S. Karger; 2013
30. Collins AR, Dusinska M, Horska A. Detection of alkylation damage in human lymphocyte DNA with the comet assay. Acta Biochim Pol. 2001;48(3):611–4.
31. Moller P, Knudsen LE, Loft S, Wallin H. The comet assay as a rapid test in biomonitoring occupational exposure to DNA-damaging agents and effect of confounding factors. Cancer Epidemiol Biomark Prev. 2000;9(10):1005–15.
32. Swanepoel A. Evaluation of DNA damage and DNA repair by the comet assay in workers exposed to organic solvents: North-West University. 2004.
33. Lumley M, Barker H, Murray JA. Benzene in petrol. Lancet. 1990;336(8726):1318–9.
34. Tasaka T, Nagai M, Sasaki K, Murata M, Taoka T, Ikeda K, et al. Translocation (3;21) (q26.2;q22.1) found in a patient with myelodysplastic syndrome and long-term exposure to organic solvents. Br J Haematol. 1992;82(2):473–5.
35. Lan Q, Smith MT, Tang X, Guo W, Vermeulen R, Ji Z, et al. Chromosome-wide aneuploidy study of cultured circulating myeloid progenitor cells from workers occupationally exposed to formaldehyde. Carcinogenesis. 2015; 36(1):160–7. doi:10.1093/carcin/bgu229.
36. Santiago F, Alves G, Otero UB, Tabalipa MM, Scherrer LR, Kosyakova N, et al. Monitoring of gas station attendants exposure to benzene, toluene, xylene (BTX) using three-color chromosome painting. Mol Cytogenet. 2014;7(1):15. doi:10.1186/1755-8166-7-15.
37. Jang JE, Min YH, Yoon J, Kim I, Lee JH, Jung CW, et al. Single monosomy as a relatively better survival factor in acute myeloid leukemia patients with monosomal karyotype. Blood Cancer J. 2015;5:e358. doi:10.1038/bcj.2015.84.

38. Rowley JD. The critical role of chromosome translocations in human leukemias. Annu Rev Genet. 1998;32:495–519. doi:10.1146/annurev.genet.32.1.495.
39. Glover TW. Instability at chromosomal fragile sites. Recent results in cancer research Fortschritte der Krebsforschung Progres dans les recherches sur le cancer. 1998;154:185-99
40. Durkin SG, Glover TW. Chromosome fragile sites. Annu Rev Genet. 2007;41:169–92. doi:10.1146/annurev.genet.41.042007.165900.
41. Re A, Cora D, Puliti AM, Caselle M, Sbrana I. Correlated fragile site expression allows the identification of candidate fragile genes involved in immunity and associated with carcinogenesis. BMC Bioinf. 2006;7:413. doi:10.1186/1471-2105-7-413.
42. Arlt MF, Miller DE, Beer DG, Glover TW. Molecular characterization of FRAXB and comparative common fragile site instability in cancer cells. Genes Chromosomes Cancer. 2002;33(1):82–92.
43. Wang L, Paradee W, Mullins C, Shridhar R, Rosati R, Wilke CM, et al. Aphidicolin-induced FRA3B breakpoints cluster in two distinct regions. Genomics. 1997;41(3):485–8. doi:10.1006/geno.1997.4690.
44. Kotzot D, Martinez MJ, Bagci G, Basaran S, Baumer A, Binkert F, et al. Parental origin and mechanisms of formation of cytogenetically recognisable de novo direct and inverted duplications. J Med Genet. 2000;37(4):281–6.
45. Hellman A, Zlotorynski E, Scherer SW, Cheung J, Vincent JB, Smith DI, et al. A role for common fragile site induction in amplification of human oncogenes. Cancer Cell. 2002;1(1):89–97.
46. Glover TW, Stein CK. Induction of sister chromatid exchanges at common fragile sites. Am J Hum Genet. 1987;41(5):882–90.
47. Coquelle A, Pipiras E, Toledo F, Buttin G, Debatisse M. Expression of fragile sites triggers intrachromosomal mammalian gene amplification and sets boundaries to early amplicons. Cell. 1997;89(2):215–25.
48. Vincent-Salomon A, Benhamo V, Gravier E, Rigaill G, Gruel N, Robin S, et al. Genomic instability: a stronger prognostic marker than proliferation for early stage luminal breast carcinomas. PLoS One. 2013;8(10):e76496. doi:10.1371/journal.pone.0076496.
49. Debacker K, Kooy RF. Fragile sites and human disease. Human molecular genetics. 2007;16 Spec No. 2:R150-8. doi:10.1093/hmg/ddm136.
50. Popescu NC. Genetic alterations in cancer as a result of breakage at fragile sites. Cancer Lett. 2003;192(1):1–17.
51. Rondon M, Caicedo J, Robledo J. Establisment of chromosomic abnormalities and amplified DNA sequences in breast cancer. Revista Ciencias de la Salud. 2006;4(2):15.
52. Carere A, Antoccia A, Cimini D, Crebelli R, Degrassi F, Leopardi P, et al. Genetic effects of petroleum fuels: II. Analysis of chromosome loss and hyperploidy in peripheral lymphocytes of gasoline station attendants. Environ Mol Mutagen. 1998;32(2):130–8.
53. Lovreglio P, Maffei F, Carrieri M, D'Errico MN, Drago I, Hrelia P, et al. Evaluation of chromosome aberration and micronucleus frequencies in blood lymphocytes of workers exposed to low concentrations of benzene. Mutat Res Genet Toxicol Environ Mutagen. 2014;770:55–60. doi:10.1016/j.mrgentox.2014.04.022.
54. Costa S, Carvalho S, Costa C, Coelho P, Silva S, Santos LS, et al. Increased levels of chromosomal aberrations and DNA damage in a group of workers exposed to formaldehyde. Mutagenesis. 2015;30(4):463–73. doi:10.1093/mutage/gev002.
55. Moro AM, Brucker N, Charao M, Bulcao R, Freitas F, Baierle M, et al. Evaluation of genotoxicity and oxidative damage in painters exposed to low levels of toluene. Mutat Res. 2012;746(1):42–8. doi:10.1016/j.mrgentox. 2012.02.007.
56. Roma-Torres J, Teixeira JP, Silva S, Laffon B, Cunha LM, Mendez J, et al. Evaluation of genotoxicity in a group of workers from a petroleum refinery aromatics plant. Mutat Res. 2006;604(1-2):19–27. doi:10.1016/j.mrgentox. 2005.12.005.
57. Bayer O, Camara R, Zeissig SR, Ressing M, Dietz A, Locati LD, et al. Occupation and cancer of the larynx: a systematic review and meta-analysis. Eur Arch Otorhinolaryngol. 2016;273(1):9–20. doi:10.1007/s00405-014-3321-y.
58. Fairbairn DW, Olive PL, O'Neill KL. The comet assay: a comprehensive review. Mutat Res. 1995;339(1):37–59.
59. Fracasso ME, Perbellini L, Solda S, Talamini G, Franceschetti P. Lead induced DNA strand breaks in lymphocytes of exposed workers: role of reactive oxygen species and protein kinase C. Mutat Res. 2002;515(1-2):159–69.
60. Heuser VD, de Andrade VM, da Silva J, Erdtmann B. Comparison of genetic damage in Brazilian footwear-workers exposed to solvent-based or water-based adhesive. Mutat Res. 2005;583(1):85–94. doi:10.1016/j.mrgentox.2005. 03.002.
61. Heuser VD, Erdtmann B, Kvitko K, Rohr P, da Silva J. Evaluation of genetic damage in Brazilian footwear-workers: biomarkers of exposure, effect, and susceptibility. Toxicology. 2007;232(3):235–47. doi:10.1016/j.tox.2007.01.011.
62. Speit G, Witton-Davies T, Heepchantree W, Trenz K, Hoffmann H. Investigations on the effect of cigarette smoking in the comet assay. Mutat Res. 2003;542(1-2):33–42.
63. Ellahuene MF, Perez-Alzola LP, Farfan-Urzua M, Gonzalez-Hormazabal P, Garay M, Olmedo MI, et al. Preliminary evaluation of DNA damage related with the smoking habit measured by the comet assay in whole blood cells. Cancer Epidemiol Biomark Prev. 2004;13(7):1223–9.
64. Tovalin H, Valverde M, Morandi MT, Blanco S, Whitehead L, Rojas E. DNA damage in outdoor workers occupationally exposed to environmental air pollutants. Occup Environ Med. 2006;63(4):230–6. doi:10.1136/oem.2005.019802.
65. Fracasso ME, Doria D, Bartolucci GB, Carrieri M, Lovreglio P, Ballini A, et al. Low air levels of benzene: correlation between biomarkers of exposure and genotoxic effects. Toxicol Lett. 2010;192(1):22–8. doi:10.1016/j.toxlet.2009.04.028.
66. Andreoli C, Leopardi P, Crebelli R. Detection of DNA damage in human lymphocytes by alkaline single cell gel electrophoresis after exposure to benzene or benzene metabolites. Mutat Res. 1997;377(1):95–104.
67. Wojewodzka M, Kruszewski M, Iwanenko T, Collins AR, Szumiel I. Lack of adverse effect of smoking habit on DNA strand breakage and base damage, as revealed by the alkaline comet assay. Mutat Res. 1999;440(1):19–25.
68. Pikor L, Thu K, Vucic E, Lam W. The detection and implication of genome instability in cancer. Cancer Metastasis Rev. 2013;32(3-4):341–52. doi:10.1007/s10555-013-9429-5.
69. Zhang L, Lan Q, Guo W, Hubbard AE, Li G, Rappaport SM, et al. Chromosome-wide aneuploidy study (CWAS) in workers exposed to an established leukemogen, benzene. Carcinogenesis. 2011;32(4):605–12. doi:10.1093/carcin/bgq286.
70. Farkas G, Szekely G, Vass N, Kiss K, Gundy S. Rate of spontaneous numerical chromosome aberrations in Hungarian healthy population. Magyar onkologia. 2015;59(3):198–204.
71. Vodenkova S, Polivkova Z, Musak L, Smerhovsky Z, Zoubkova H, Sytarova S, et al. Structural chromosomal aberrations as potential risk markers in incident cancer patients. Mutagenesis. 2015;30(4):557–63. doi:10.1093/mutage/gev018.
72. Dillon LW, Burrow AA, Wang YH. DNA instability at chromosomal fragile sites in cancer. Curr Genet. 2010;11(5):326–37. doi:10.2174/138920210791616699.
73. Hagmar L, Bonassi S, Stromberg U, Brogger A, Knudsen LE, Norppa H, et al. Chromosomal aberrations in lymphocytes predict human cancer: a report from the european study group on cytogenetic biomarkers and health (ESCH). Cancer Res. 1998;58(18):4117–21.

# 18

# Clinical and molecular cytogenetic analyses of four patients with imbalanced translocations

Hong Yan Liu[1*], Jia Huang[1], Tao Li[1], Dong Wu[1], Hong Dan Wang[1], Yue Wang[2], Tao Wang[1], Liang Jie Guo[1], Qian Nan Guo[1], Fei Fei Huang[1], Rui Li Wang[3] and Ying Tai Wang[1]

**Abstract**

**Background:** Chromosomal abnormalities that result in genomic imbalances are main causes of congenital and developmental anomalies including intellectual disability and multiple congenital malformations. In this report we describe four patients from three families with imbalanced translocations. Only a small percentage of imbalanced translocation individuals can be born to live, most of them were aborted in embryonic period. It is of great significances to precisely analysis the chromosome variation to study the relationship between genotype and phenotype.

**Results:** Four patients showed common clinical manifestations including delayed growth, intellectual disability, language barrier and facial dysmorphisms. In addition to the above features, lower limbs dysplasia and both foot eversion were found in patient 1, brachydactylic hand, cerebellar ataxia and congenital heart defects were also found in patient 4. Conventional karyotype analysis revealed abnormal karyotypes 46, XX, der (6) t (6: 10) (p23; q24), 46, XX, der (20) t (3; 20) (p23; p13) and 46, XX, der (22) t (3; 22) (q27; q13.3) in the four patients, respectively. Array-CGH analyses confirmed 23.6 Mb duplication on 10q25.1-q26.3 and 0.9 Mb deletions on 6p25.3, 19.9 Mb duplication on 3p24.3-p26.3 and 0.25 Mb deletion on 20p13 and 12.5 Mb duplication on 3q27.2-q29 and 1.9 Mb deletions on 22q13.2-q13.33 in the four patients, respectively.

**Conclusion:** Parents with balanced translocation are passed the imbalanced chromosome to patient, and the partial monosomy and partial trisomy lead to multiple congenital malformations of four patients.

**Keyword:** Imbalanced translocation, Intellectual disability, Delayed growth, Language barrier, Chinese

## Background

Chromosomal abnormalities that result in genomic imbalances are main cause of congenital and developmental anomalies including intellectual disability and multiple congenital malformations. The abnormal chromosomes of parents can be passed to next generation, particularly for parents carrying a balanced translocation or inversion. Balanced chromosomal translocations are often identified as a cause of infertility [1], owing to meiotic impairment can lead to gamete formation problems, in man can cause failure of spermatogenesis [1, 2]. Research found that most breakpoint of balanced chromosome translocation was at or near the localization of segmental duplications which contribute to genomic instability [3], so the genetic disorders may increase of the offspring. Theoretically, for balanced translocation carriers, the chance of passing the imbalanced chromosome to child is 16/18, whereas passing a normal chromosome and balanced chromosome is 1/18, respectively. The former case will lead to either a spontaneous miscarriage or a live born child with intellectual disability and/or multiple congenital malformations. The reported live births rate of couple with balanced translocations ranges from 14 to 19.5 % [4, 5], and more than 80 % of fertilized eggs were spontaneous abortion because of aneuploidy, polyploidy, imbalanced translocation and other reasons [5]. In clinic, half of these babies

* Correspondence: liuhongyanqhhy@126.com
[1]Department of Medical Genetics Institute, People's Hospital of Zhengzhou University (Henan Provincial People's Hospital), Zhengzhou 450003, Henan, China
Full list of author information is available at the end of the article

with chromosome abnormalities were inherited from a parent carrying balanced translocation or inversion [6].

Precise characterization of the chromosomal rearrangements and identification of the associated genes are important for syndrome recognition and genetic risk assessment. Array-CGH is a powerful tool for the accurate detection of genomic imbalances. It enables identification of the genes that cause mental retardation when abnormal copy numbers exist [7]. In this report we present three families with imbalanced translocation. All families had offspring with mental retardation who carried imbalanced translocation. We provided detailed analysis of the genotype-phenotype correlation and discussed possible candidate genes.

## Methods

### Participants

Four Patients were from three Chinese families without family history of congenital malformations. Patients showed common clinical manifestations, such as delayed growth, intellectual disability, language barrier and facial dysmorphisms. Parents of these patients went to Medical Genetics Institute for genetic consulting. Routine clinical examination was performed on four patients. Detailed birth, medical and clinical manifestations were collected after informed consent was obtained. The pedigree of three families was shown in Fig. 1.

All examinations were performed according to the guidelines of the "declaration of Helsinki". Ethical approval was obtained from the People's Hospital of Henan Provincial Ethics Committee.

### Karyotyping and array-CGH analyses

Five milliliter peripheral venous blood was collected from four patients and their parents; 20 ml amniotic fluid was collected from mother of patient 4.

Karyotyping on GTG-banded chromosomes from patients and their parents was performed on cultured lymphocytes (patient 1 to 4 and their parents) and cultured amniocytes (family 3 II2) according to standard protocols.

To precisely determine the cytogenetic variation, a high-resolution chromosomal analysis was performed using a whole-genome oligonucleotide CGH microarray. Genomic DNA from four patients was extracted from peripheral blood lymphocytes using Qiagen blood kit (QIAGEN, Germantown, MD, USA).

Array-CGH was performed using an Agilent SurePrint G3 Human CGH Microarray Kit, 8x60K G4450A whole-genome oligonucleotide microarray (41 kb average probe spacing; 33 kb in Refseq genes). Digestion, ligation, PCR, Cy5-dUTP and Cy3-dUTP labeling, hybridization of test and reference DNA were performed according to the manufacturer's recommendations (Agilent Technologies, Santa Clara, California, USA). Slides were scanned using an Agilent SureScan Microarray Scanner, and analyzed using Agilent CytoGenomics 2.9. Significant copy-number changes were identified by at least three consecutive aberrant probes. Reference human genome was GRCh36/hg18.

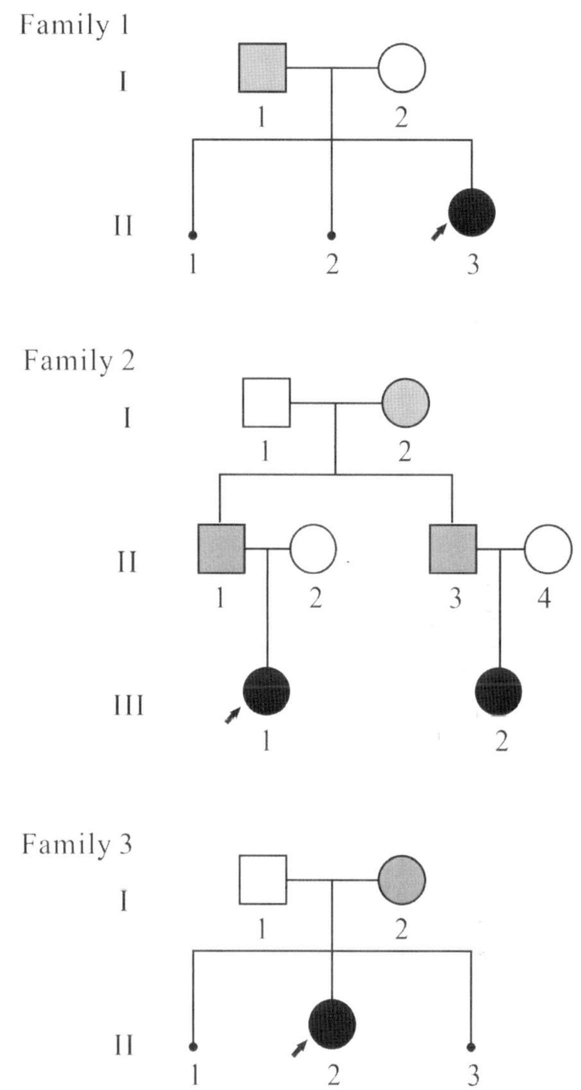


**Fig. 1** Pedigree of three families reported in this study. *Black symbols* indicate imbalanced translocation individuals; *grey symbols indicate* balanced translocation individuals; *black spot* indicate abortion

## Results

### Family 1

The patient 1 (family 1: II3) is a 3 years old female. She was from the third pregnancy of healthy and nonconsanguineous young parents. Her mother had a history of two miscarriages. The physical examination revealed that patient 1 presented with multiple congenital anomalies. She had significant facial dysmorphic features, including depressed nasal bridge, anteverted nostrils, long philtrum, downturned angles of mouth and thin upper lips, carp-shaped mouth, high arched palate, micrognathia, low set ears and low anterior hairline. Developmental evaluations showed delayed growth with short stature (85 cm, <3rd centile) and low weight (9.5 kg, <3rd centile). She walked without assistance at 2 years and 3 month of age, presented with walking instability. Limbs dysplasia included slim lower limbs and foot eversion on both sides. Neurological exam revealed muscular hypotonia, nerve reflex insensitivity, intellectual disability and language barrier. Feeding difficulty was present in early infancy. The patient has no history of seizure activity and congenital heart defect. Hearing, vision, and hands were normal.

The patient karyotyping was performed on peripheral blood lymphocytes. The report revealed abnormal karyotype 46, XX, der (6) t (6: 10) (p23; q24) (Fig. 2a). A similar protocol was followed for her parents' chromosome preparation. The report revealed normal mother with 46, XX pattern, but the father had balanced translocation with 46, XY, t (6; 10) (p23; q24) pattern. This chromosomal abnormality was a balanced translocation between 6 and 10 (Fig. 2b).

Array-CGH analysis was performed on lymphocytes DNA of this patient and detected a 23.6 Mb duplication at 10q25.1-q26.3 (chr10:111770926–135404523) and a 0.9 Mb deletion at 6p25.3 (chr6:170426–1106808) (Fig. 3a).

**Family 2**

In this family, two female cousins (patient 2 and 3) were found with delayed growth, intellectual disability and language barrier. Although with normal weight, their heights were lower than peers. The older cousin (patient 2), a 9 years old girl, also showed facial dysmorphic features, including depressed nasal bridge, ocular hypertelorism, broad nose, thin upper lip, round face with full cheeks and facial expression impairment. She could express some simple language, and have learning difficulties. She had normal motor system with good coordination and could play freely. The patient 2 had no history of seizures and cardiomyopathy. She had normal hearing and vision, as well as normal finger nails. The younger cousin (patient 3), a 4 years old girl, has facial dysmorphic features, including open mouth, thin upper lip and facial expression impairment. She could not speak any meaningful words. Other clinical manifestations were same as her older cousin.

Conventional karyotype analysis showed that two female cousins carried 46, XX, der (20) t (3; 20) (p23; p13) (Fig. 2c and d). The old cousin parents accepted the subsequent karyotyping with the report revealing normal 46, XX pattern of her mother, but the father had balanced translocation 46, XY, t (3; 20) (p23; p13) (Fig. 2e). The younger cousin parents and grandmother were also

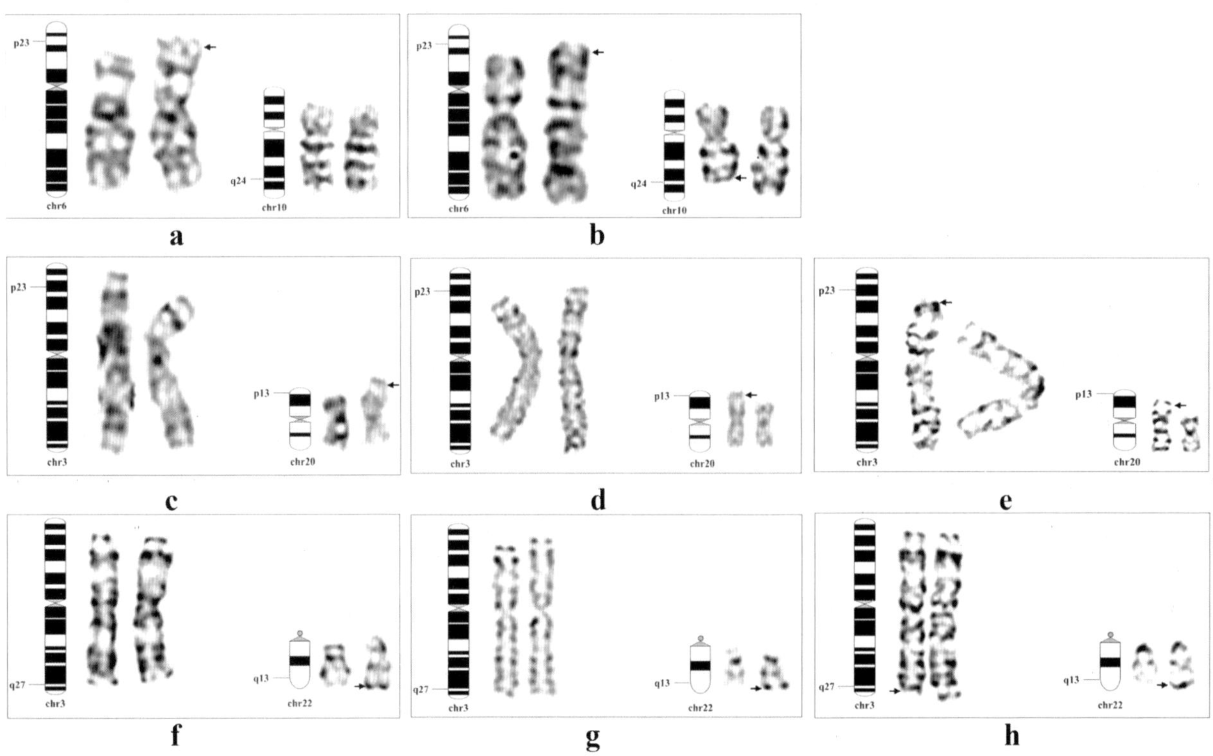


**Fig. 2** GTG-banding karyotype analysis image of patients and their parents. Family 1 was shown in upper panel. **a** and **b** were patient 1 and father, respectively; Family 2 was shown in middle panel. **c**, **d** and **e** were patient 2, 3 and father, respectively; Family 3 was shown in lower panel. **f**, **g** and **h** were patient 4, fetus and mother, respectively

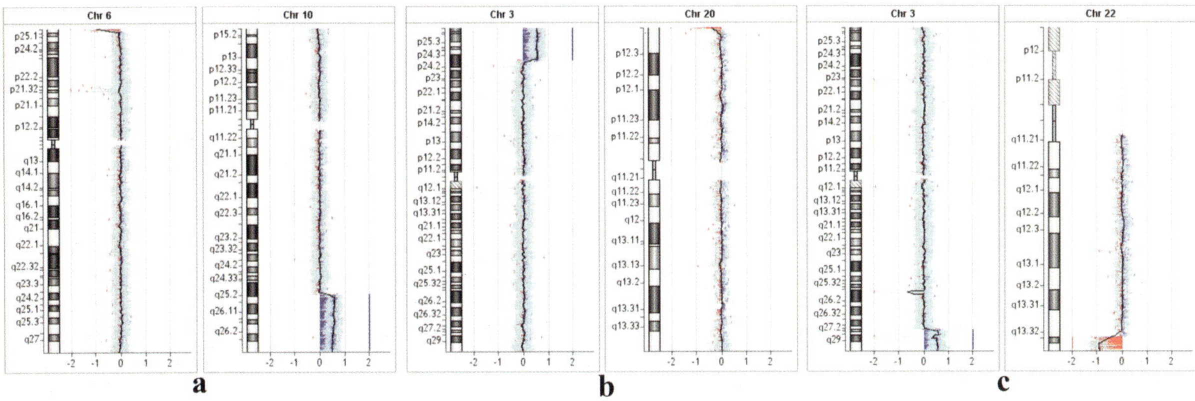

**Fig. 3** Array-CGH analysis showed telomeric rearrangements on two different chromosomes in four patients (**a**: patient 1; **b**: patient 2 and 3; **c**: patient 4). The log ratio was reported (log2 intensity of [Cy5 fluorochrome/Cy3 fluorochrome)] on the X-axis. Expected values were from −0.7 to −1 for a deletion (*red color*), 0 for normal (*black line*), and +0.5 to +1 for a duplication (*blue color*)

karyotyped. The report showed balanced translocation of 46, XX/XY, t (3; 20) (p23; p13) in the father and grandmother. Their GTG-banding images were not available.

Array-CGH analysis was performed in two female cousins to further characterize the rearrangement. This analysis identified that two female cousins have same abnormality rearrangement with a 19.9 Mb duplication at 3p24.3-p26.3 (chr3:93949–19992330) and 0.25 Mb deletion at 20p13 (chr20: 121521–373182) (Fig. 3b).

### Family 3

In this family, the healthy and nonconsanguineous young couples experienced three pregnancies history. After one miscarriage, they had a baby girl (family3: II2) at term by cesarean section. The couples went to our institution for genetic consulting, when pregnancy again, because their 5 years old daughter showed delayed growth, intellectual disability and language barrier. The girl also had facial expression dementia, paratrichosis (long eyelashes, bushy eyebrows and hair), brachydactylic hand, hypoplasia of distal phalanges, single palmar crease bilaterally, and thumb flat abduction of 90°. She walked independent at 3 years of age, but presented with cerebellar ataxia and walking instability. The girl could not finish fine motor coordination. She was not able to express simple language, speak slowly and ambiguously, and could only call mom and dad. Neurological exam revealed muscular hypotonia, nerve reflex insensitivity. She suffered congenital patent ductus arteriosus which was surgically cured at 2 years old. The hearing and vision was normal. Prenatal ultrasonography examination for the new pregnancy showed that fetus had bilateral multiple choroid plexus cyst with a larger size (3.3 * 3.3 mm) on the right side. The diameter of right renal pelvis was 4.5 mm. Thickening of the placenta and single umbilical artery was also present.

Karyotype analysis showed that the girl and fetus had same karyotyped 46, XX, der (22) t (3; 22) (q27; q13.3) (Fig. 2f and g). Their parents were also karyotyped with the report showing normal 46, XY in the father, but abnormal 46, XX, t (3; 22) (q27; q13.3) in the mother (Fig. 2h).

Array-CGH analysis on the peripheral blood DNA from the girl showed a 12.5 Mb duplication at chromosome 3q27.2-q29 (chr3:185307872–197840339), and a 1.9 Mb deletion at 22q13.2-q13.33 (chr22: 49286759–51178264) (Fig. 3c).

## Discussion

In this work, we report three families with balanced translocation. They all have imbalanced translocation offspring with delayed growth, intellectual disability and language barrier. The complex phenotypic manifestation of patients was contributed jointly by monosomy and trisomy of the two chromosomes. Generally, phenotypes associated with deletions are more severe than those associated with duplications. However, because the maximum tolerance in living organisms was different, it is very difficult to justify the predominant factors. By reviewing the published literatures, the prominent phenotypic features of these patients were not classified as some specific syndrome.

The same karyotype has been reported in one patient of India [8]. Conventional karyotype shows patient with 46, XY, der (6) t (6; 10) (p23; q24) pattern which is the same as patient 1. However, genitalia malformation, malformed ears, atrial septal defect and so forth features of India patient were not found in the patient 1. The lower limbs dysplasia was prominent in patient 1, but not reported in India patient. The facial features were similar in the two patients. The different breakpoint may be one of the main reasons that lead to the distinguished characteristics. One patient with 10q25.1-10q26.3 duplication reported by Carter et al. [9] has craniofacial dysmorphia, such as depressed nasal bridge, high arched palate, low set ears and low anterior hairline were same as patient 1, however, skeletal anomalies were present in this patient, including hip dysplasia and mild scoliosis, which were not found in patient 1. Hand anomaly and wide space between the first and second toes (sandal gap) were found in India patient and Carter's patient, but was not found in patient 1, foot eversion was only present in patient 1. Hearing loss was found in India patient and Carter's patient, while patient 1 with normal hearing. They all had delayed growth, Intellectual disability and language barrier. We summarized Table 1 for comparison of the clinical features of this patient with similar segmental duplication and/or deletion chromosome. The *FGFR2* was localized in this segmental duplication and was reported to be associated with many syndromes [10]. *FGFR2* is a member of the fibroblast growth factor receptor family and encodes a receptor tyrosine kinase important for osteogenesis. Patients with *FGFR2* missense mutation were mainly manifested as craniofacial and limb abnormalities. Duplication of *FGFR2* may be responsible for the craniofacial features and skeletal anomalies in the above patient. We summarized OMIM gene associated with phenotype localized in this duplicated segment 10q25.1-q26.3 (chr10:111770926–135404523) (Additional file 1). SMC3 mutation have been reported in subjects with Cornelia de Lange syndrome 3 [11], and these patients presented with craniofacial dysmorphia and mental retardation. *SFXN4* mutation was relevant to growth retardation, hypotonia, and speech delay [12]. *BBIP1* and *SHOC2* mutation can lead to mental retardation [13, 14]. Delayed growth, language barrier and neurocognitive developmental impairment may be a result of duplication of these genes.

One 40-year-old female with 6p25.3 -p25.2 (chr6: 203,722 - 2,740,501) deletion [15], extensive white matter changes is the main clinical feature, normal cognition and intelligence. Patient 1 with 6p25.3 (chr6:170426–1106808) deletion contain 3 Refseq gene, only one OMIM gene (*IRF4*) was associated with Skin/hair/eye pigmentation. Patient 1 was only 3 years old have not presentation these symptoms. Therefore, duplication of 10q25.1-q26.3 was leading role in contribute to the clinical findings seen in patient 1.

Partial trisomy 3p syndrome is characterized by multiple congenital abnormalities, delayed speech, intellectual deficiency and so forth [16]. The clinical manifestations are quite varied, depending on the amount of 3p genomic content in the trisomic state.

Patient 2 and 3 with 19.9 Mb (chr3:93949–19992330) duplication of the 3p24.3-p26.3, main clinical features are development delay, intellectual disability, language impairment and learning impairment. One 5 years old boy with pure 3p26.2-p24.1 duplication reported by Natera-de Benito et al. [17] and one 9 years old boy with pure 3p26.2-p25.3 duplication reported by Bittel et al. [18] share the above clinical malformations. Two genes located in the common segmental duplication of four patients, SUMF1 mutations result in defective post-translational modification of sulfatases, and show association with mental retardation, neurological deterioration, hydrocephalus and so on [19]. Loss of function mutation in SETD5 was associated with mental retardation, intellectual disability, delayed speech and so forth [20]. Duplication of tow genes may be account for development delay and cognitive impairment. Interestingly, the clinical feature of round face with full cheeks was found in patient 2 and two boy patients reported by Natera-de Benito et al. and Bittel et al., and the 9 years old boy presented with central obesity. *GHRL* located in the common segmental duplication of four patients, was known to be associated with obesity [21]. For patient 2 and 3, we will be extraordinarily watchful the possible onset of obesity. It is worth noting that the clinical feature of hand/foot anomaly and genital malformation were not found in patient 2 and 3, however, two boy patients reported by Natera-de Benito et al. and Bittel et al. were presented with above clinical features.

There are reports of individuals with deletion at 20p13 [22–24], we found that the similarly clinical features of these patients are developmental delay and intellectual disability. Patient 2 and 3 with 0.25 Mb (chr20: 121521–373182) deletion of the 20p13, at this segmental deletion contain 10 Refseq genes, not found OMIM gene associated with phenotype, of which two candidate gene (*SOX12* and *NRSN2*) was identified as nervous system expressing genes that may be associated with developmental delay [24].

The clinical manifestations of the 3q syndrome include typical facial features, growth and mental retardation, and frequent congenital heart defects [25]. Patient 4 presented with congenital patent ductus arteriosus, whereas other patient showed ventricular septal defect [25]. Patient 4 had long eyelashes and bushy eyebrows, which was also found in other family with 3q duplication [25, 26]. Patient 4 showed prominent cerebellar ataxia symptom, but the symptom was absence in other family with 3q duplication [25–27]. The feature of hand/foot anomaly was found in Patient 4 and other patients [25–27]. *TP63* located in the common segmental duplication of above patients, and was known to be associated with many syndromes. The clinical features of patient with *TP63* mutation were major presented with hand/foot anomaly and ectodermal

**Table 1** The clinical features of patient with similar segmental duplication and/or deletion chromosome

| | Patient 1 | [8] | [9] | [15] | Patient 2 | Patient 3 | [16] | [17] | [22] | [23] patient 2 | Patient 4 | [25] | [27] | [30] | [31] |
|---|---|---|---|---|---|---|---|---|---|---|---|---|---|---|---|
| Segmental duplication/ deletion | dup 10q25.1-10q26.3; del 6p25.3 | dup 10q24-10qter; del 6p23-6pter | dup 10q25.1-10q26.3[a] | del 6p25.3 -p25.2[b] | dup 3p26.3-p24.3; del 20p13 | dup 3p26.3-24.3; del 20p13 | dup 3p26.2-p24.1[c] | dup 3p26.2-p25.3 | del 20p13[d] | 20p13-pter | dup 3q27.2-3q29; del 22q13.32-22q13.33 | dup 3q26.3-qter | dup 3q27-qter[e], del4p16.3[f] | del 22q13.31–q13.33[g] | del 22q13.3[h] |
| Sex | F | M | F | F | F | F | M | M | F | F | F | M | F | M | F |
| Age at last follow up (years) | 3y | 1 m | 7y | 40y | 9y | 4y | 5y | 9y | 9y | 15y | 5y | 11 m | 4y | 5y | 14y |
| Development delay | + | + | + | - | + | + | + | + | + | + | + | + | + | + | + |
| Craniofacial features | | | | | | | | | | | | | | | |
| Ocular hypertelorism | - | + | - | - | + | - | + | - | - | - | - | - | + | - | - |
| Epicanthic folds | - | + | + | - | - | - | - | - | - | - | - | - | + | + | - |
| Depressed nasal bridge | + | + | + | - | + | - | + | - | - | - | - | Wide | Wide | - | - |
| Anteverted nostrils | + | - | - | - | - | - | - | - | - | - | - | + | - | - | - |
| Long philtrum | + | Broad | Flat | - | - | - | - | - | Flat | - | - | Prominent | + | - | - |
| Carp-shaped mouth | + | + | - | - | - | - | - | - | - | - | - | - | - | - | - |
| Thin upper lips | + | - | + | - | + | + | - | - | + | - | - | + | - | - | - |
| High arched palate | + | + | + | - | - | - | - | - | + | + | - | - | - | - | - |
| Micrognathia | + | + | - | - | - | - | - | - | - | - | - | + | - | - | - |
| Low set ears | + | + | + | - | - | - | - | - | - | + | - | + | - | - | - |
| Malformed ears | - | + | - | - | - | - | prominent ears | - | - | + | - | - | - | - | - |
| Low anterior hairline | + | - | + | - | - | - | - | - | + | - | - | + | high frontal hairline | - | - |
| Long eyelashes | - | - | - | - | - | - | - | - | - | - | + | + | - | - | - |
| Bushy eyebrows | - | - | - | - | - | - | - | - | - | - | + | + | - | - | - |
| Facial expression anomaly | - | - | - | - | + | + | - | - | - | - | + | - | - | - | - |
| Microcephaly | - | - | - | - | - | - | + | - | - | - | - | - | - | - | + |
| Cognitive development | | | | | | | | | | | | | | | |
| Intellectual disability | + | + | + | - | + | + | +(mild) | – | + | + | + | + | + | + | + |
| Language impairment | + | + | + | - | + | + | + | + | - | - | + | N.A | + | + | + |
| Learning impairment | + | N.A | + | - | + | + | + | + | + | + | + | N.A | N.A | N.A | N.A |
| Heart defect | - | + | - | - | - | - | - | - | - | - | + | + | - | - | - |
| Hearing loss | - | + | + | + | - | - | - | - | - | - | - | - | - | - | - |

**Table 1** The clinical features of patient with similar segmental duplication and/or deletion chromosome *(Continued)*

| | | | | | | | | | | | | | | | |
|---|---|---|---|---|---|---|---|---|---|---|---|---|---|---|---|
| Hand and foot | | | | | | | | | | | | | | | |
| Hand anomaly | - | + | + | + | - | - | + | + | + | + | + | + | + | + | - |
| Foot anomaly | + | + | + | - | - | - | + | - | + | - | - | + | - | - | - |
| Single palmar crease | - | + | - | - | - | - | + | - | - | - | + | - | - | - | - |
| Skeletal anomalies | | | | | | | | | | | | | | | |
| Limbs | + | - | - | - | - | - | - | - | - | - | - | - | - | - | - |
| Scoliosis | - | - | + | - | - | - | - | - | - | - | - | - | - | - | - |
| Hip dysplasia | - | - | + | - | - | - | - | - | - | - | - | + | - | - | - |
| Other | | | | | | | | | | | | | | | |
| Muscular hypotonia | + | - | + | - | - | - | + | - | - | - | + | - | + | + | + |
| Cerebellar ataxia | - | - | - | - | - | - | - | - | - | - | + | - | - | - | - |
| Genital malformation | - | + | - | - | - | - | + | + | - | - | - | - | - | - | - |
| Short neck | + | + | + | - | - | - | + | - | + | - | - | + | - | - | - |
| Epilepsy | - | - | - | - | - | - | + | - | - | + | - | - | - | + | + |
| Round face with full cheeks | - | - | - | - | + | - | + | + | - | - | - | - | - | - | - |
| Central obesity | - | - | - | - | - | - | - | + | - | - | - | - | - | - | - |

*F* female, *M* male, *y* years, *m* month, + presence of trait, − absence of trait, *N.A* not available, a: chr 10: 108 299 681–133 745 613, b: chr6: 203,722 - 2,740,501, c: chr3:3943808–29668053, d: chr20:1–1150000, e: chr3:183097052–198295559, f: chr4:1–769191, g: chr22:46,204,739–51,178,264, h: chr22:49,389,829–51,178,264

dysplasia. *TP63* duplication may be contributed to hand/foot anomaly of these patients. Development delay and cognitive impairment were also found in Patient 4 and other patients [25–27]. Interestingly, the clinical feature of cerebellar ataxia was only found in patient 4. Mutation in *KIAA0226* causes spinocerebellar ataxia [28] with patients presenting progressive incoordination of gait and poor co-ordination of hands, speech and eye movements, and cerebellar ataxia in early childhood and delayed motor development, as well as dysarthria and hyporeflexia. *KIAA0226* may be a candidate gene for ataxia of patient 4.

The 22q13.3 deletion syndrome, also known as Phelan-McDermid syndrome, this syndrome is characterized by neurological deficits which include global developmental delay, moderate to severe intellectual impairment, absent or severely delayed speech, and neonatal hypotonia. In addition, more than 50 % of patients show autism or autistic-like behavior, and therefore it can be classified as a syndromic form of autism spectrum disorders (ASD) [29], some patients also have seizure manifestations [30, 31], but patient 4 absence of autism and seizure manifestations, cerebellar ataxia is the prominent characteristic different from other patient with the deletion of 22q13.3 [30, 31]. Development delay and cognitive impairment were common features of patient 4 and other patients [30, 31]. *SHANK3* located in the segmental deletion, the *SHANK3* mRNA is localized to proximal and distal dendrites, and is highly expressed the hippocampus, cerebellar granular cells, caudate putamen and thalamic nuclei. It is a key part of normal neuron morphology and connectivity, and play an important role in synaptic formation and function, promote synaptic plasticity, and is critical for learning and memory [32]. Haploinsufficiency of *SHANK3* may be contributed to the development delay and cognitive impairment. *ARSA* encodes the lysosomal enzyme arylsulfatase A, mutation in this gene was reported in metachromatic leukodystrophy, characterized by progressive demyelination, gait disturbances, ataxias, optical atrophy, dementia, seizures, and spastic tetraparesis [33]. *ARSA* may be a candidate gene for ataxia of patient 4.

## Conclusion

The monosomy and trisomy of the two chromosomes lead to complex phenotypic manifestation of patients. These genes (Additional file 1) located in the region of rearrangement chromosome might promote abnormal clinical features of patients. We speculate that other genes may also be involved and multiple factors may play important role in the development of the abnormal features observed in our patients.

## Consent

Written informed consent was obtained from patient's parents.

### Competing interests

The authors declare that they have no competing interests.

### Authors' contributions

H-YL designed the study and subject recruitment. DW, TL, JH and H-DW performed DNA extraction, array-CGH analysis and interpretation of the data. TW, L-JG and F-FH performed GTG-banding karyotype analysis. H-YL, Q-NG, YW, R-LW, and Y-TW participated in disease diagnose. The manuscript was drafted by H-YL and JH, all authors contributed to the final draft. All authors read and approved the final manuscript.

### Acknowledgement

We thank our patients and their family member participation in this study.

### Funding

This study is supported in part by the Young Scientists Foundation of China (NO. 8501336), Foundation and Cutting-edge Research Projects of Henan Province Science and Technology Department (No. 122300410400), Oversea Training Projects for medical academic leaders of Henan Province (No. 2014089), Medical Science and Technology research projects of Henan Provincial Health Bureau (No. 201403180), Scientific and Technological projects of the Technology Bureau of Jinshui District (No. 38).

### Author details

[1]Department of Medical Genetics Institute, People's Hospital of Zhengzhou University (Henan Provincial People's Hospital), Zhengzhou 450003, Henan, China. [2]Department of Gynaecology and Obstetrics, People's Hospital of Zhengzhou University (Henan Provincial People's Hospital), Zhengzhou 450003, Henan, China. [3]Department of Ultrasonography, People's Hospital of Zhengzhou University (Henan Provincial People's Hospital), Zhengzhou 450003, Henan, China.

### References

1. Zhang HG, Wang RX, Li LL, Sun WT, Zhang HY, Liu RZ. Male carriers of balanced reciprocal translocations in Northeast China: sperm count, reproductive performance, and genetic counseling. Genet Mol Res. 2015;14(4):18792–8.
2. Dijkhuizen T, van Essen T, van der Vlies P, Verheij JB, Sikkema-Raddatz B, van der Veen AY, et al. FISH and array-CGH analysis of a complex chromosome 3 aberration suggests that loss of CNTN4 and CRBN contributes to mental retardation in 3pter deletions. Am J Med Genet A. 2006;140(22):2482–7.
3. Kara M, Sen A, Cetin ES, Kargun K. Chromosomal translocation t (10; 19) (q11.2;q13.4) in an infertile male. Eurasian J Med. 2014;46(3):220–3.
4. Manvelyan M, Schreyer I, Höls-Herpertz I, Köhler S, Niemann R, Hehr U, Belitz B, et al. Forty-eight new cases with infertility due to balanced chromosomal rearrangements: detailed molecular cytogenetic analysis of the 90 involved breakpoints. Int J Mol Med. 2007;19(6):855–64.
5. Stephenson MD, Sierra S. Reproductive outcomes in recurrent pregnancy loss associated with a parental carrier of a structural chromosome rearrangement. Hum Reprod. 2006;21(4):1076–82.
6. Kochhar PK, Ghosh P. Reproductive outcome of couples with recurrent miscarriage and balanced chromosomal abnormalities. J Obstet Gynaecol Res. 2013;39(1):113–20.
7. Goddijn M, Leschot NJ. Genetic aspects of miscarriage. Baillieres Best Pract Res Clin Obstet Gynaecol. 2000;14(5):855–65.
8. Ganguly BB, Kadam V, Kadam NN. Clinical expression of an inherited unbalanced translocation in chromosome 6. Case Rep Genet. 2011;2011: 396450. doi:10.1155/2011/396450.

9. Carter MT, Dyack S, Richer J. Distal trisomy 10q syndrome: phenotypic features in a child with inverted duplicated 10q25.1-q26.3. Clin Dysmorphol. 2010;19(3):140–5.
10. Ibrahimi OA, Zhang F, Eliseenkova AV, Itoh N, Linhardt RJ, Mohammadi M. Biochemical analysis of pathogenic ligand-dependent FGFR2 mutations suggests distinct pathophysiological mechanisms for craniofacial and limb abnormalities. Hum Mol Genet. 2004;13(19):2313–24.
11. Deardorff MA, Kaur M, Yaeger D, Rampuria A, Korolev S, Pie J, et al. Mutations in cohesin complex members SMC3 and SMC1A cause a mild variant of cornelia de Lange syndrome with predominant mental retardation. Am J Hum Genet. 2007; 80(3):485–94.
12. Hildick-Smith GJ, Cooney JD, Garone C, Kremer LS, Haack TB, Thon JN, et al. Macrocytic anemia and mitochondriopathy resulting from a defect in sideroflexin 4. Am J Hum Genet. 2013;93(5):906–14.
13. Scheidecker S, Etard C, Pierce NW, Geoffroy V, Schaefer E, Muller J, et al. Exome sequencing of Bardet-Biedl syndrome patient identifies a null mutation in the BBSome subunit BBIP1 (BBS18). J Med Genet. 2014;51(2):132–6.
14. Cordeddu V, Di Schiavi E, Pennacchio LA, Ma'ayan A, Sarkozy A, Fodale V, et al. Mutation of SHOC2 promotes aberrant protein N-myristoylation and causes Noonan-like syndrome with loose anagen hair. Nat Genet. 2009;41(9):1022–6.
15. Vernon HJ, Bytyci Telegrafi A, Batista D, Owegi M, Leigh R. 6p25 microdeletion: white matter abnormalities in an adult patient. Am J Med Genet A. 2013;161A(7):1686–9.
16. Rodovalho-Doriqui MJ, Freitas PL, Pinho JD, Cavalli LR, Pereira SR. 3p partial trisomy and 13q partial monosomy with congenital malformations and psychomotor developmental delay. Genet Mol Res. 2013;12(3):2562–6.
17. Natera-de Benito D, García-Pérez MA, Martínez-Granero MÁ, Izquierdo-López L. A patient with a duplication of chromosome 3p (p24.1p26.2): a comparison with other partial 3p trisomies. Am J Med Genet A. 2014;164A(2):548–50.
18. Bittel DC, Kibiryeva N, Dasouki M, Knoll JH, Butler MG. A 9-year-old male with a duplication of chromosome 3p25.3p26.2: clinical report and gene expression analysis. Am J Med Genet A. 2006;140(6):573–9.
19. Schlotawa L, Ennemann EC, Radhakrishnan K, Schmidt B, Chakrapani A, Christen HJ, et al. SUMF1 mutations affecting stability and activity of formylglycine generating enzyme predict clinical outcome in multiple sulfatase deficiency. Eur J Hum Genet. 2011;19(3):253–61.
20. Grozeva D, Carss K, Spasic-Boskovic O, Parker MJ, Archer H, Firth HV, et al. De novo loss-of-function mutations in SETD5, encoding a methyltransferase in a 3p25 microdeletion syndrome critical region, cause intellectual disability. Am J Hum Genet. 2014;94(4):618–24.
21. Wortley KE, del Rincon JP, Murray JD, Garcia K, Iida K, Thorner MO, et al. Absence of ghrelin protects against early-onset obesity. J Clin Invest. 2005;115(12):3573–8.
22. Jezela-Stanek A, Kucharczyk M, Pelc M, Gutkowska A, Krajewska-Walasek M. 1.15 Mb microdeletion in chromosome band 20p13 associated with moderate developmental delay-additional case and data's review. Am J Med Genet A. 2013;161A(1):172–8.
23. McGill AK, Pastore MT, Herman GE, Alliman S, Rosenfeld JA, Weaver DD. A tale of two deletions: a report of two novel 20p13 -> pter deletions. Am J Med Genet A. 2010;152A(4):1000–7
24. An Y, Amr SS, Torres A, Weissman L, Raffalli P, Cox G, et al. SOX12 and NRSN2 are candidate genes for 20p13 subtelomeric deletions associated with developmental delay. Am J Med Genet B Neuropsychiatr Genet. 2013;162(8):832–40.
25. Faas BH, De Vries BB, Van Es-Van Gaal J, Merkx G, Draaisma JM, Smeets DF. A new case of dup (3q) syndrome due to a pure duplication of 3qter. Clin Genet. 2002;62(4):315–20.
26. Abreu-González M, García-Delgado C, Cervantes A, Aparicio-Onofre A, Guevara-Yáñez R, Sánchez-Urbina R, et al. Clinical, Cytogenetic, and Biochemical Analyses of a Family with a t(3;13)(q26.2;p11.2): Further Delineation of 3q Duplication Syndrome. Case Rep Genet. 2013;2013: 895259. doi:10.1155/2013/895259.
27. Grossmann V, Müller D, Müller W, Fresser F, Erdel M, Janecke AR, et al. "Essentially" pure trisomy 3q27 -> qter: further delineation of the partial trisomy 3q phenotype. Am J Med Genet A. 2009;149A(11):2522–6.
28. Assoum M, Salih MA, Drouot N, H'Mida-Ben Brahim D, Lagier-Tourenne C, AlDrees A, et al. Rundataxin, a novel protein with RUN and diacylglycerol binding domains, is mutant in a new recessive ataxia. Brain. 2010;133(Pt8):2439–47.
29. Phelan K, McDermid HE. The 22q13.3 Deletion Syndrome (Phelan-McDermid Syndrome). Mol Syndromol. 2012;2(3–5):186–201.
30. Ishikawa N, Kobayashi Y, Fujii Y, Yamamoto T, Kobayashi M. Late-onset epileptic spasms in a patient with 22q13.3 deletion syndrome. Brain Dev. 2016;38(1):109–12.
31. Figura MG, Coppola A, Bottitta M, Calabrese G, Grillo L, Luciano D, et al. Seizures and EEG pattern in the 22q13.3 deletion syndrome: clinical report of six Italian cases. Seizure. 2014;23(9):774–9.
32. Costales JL, Kolevzon A. Phelan-McDermid Syndrome and SHANK3: Implications for Treatment. Neurotherapeutics. 2015;12:620–30. doi:10.1007/s13311-015-0352-z.
33. Eng B, Nakamura LN, O'Reilly N, Schokman N, Nowaczyk MM, Krivit W, et al. Identification of nine novel arylsulfatase a (ARSA) gene mutations in patients with metachromatic leukodystrophy (MLD). Hum Mutat. 2003;22(5):418–9.

# 19

# Genomic organization of repetitive DNAs highlights chromosomal evolution in the genus *Clarias* (Clariidae, Siluriformes)

Nuntiya Maneechot[1], Cassia Fernanda Yano[2], Luiz Antonio Carlos Bertollo[2], Nuntaporn Getlekha[1], Wagner Franco Molina[3], Sukhonthip Ditcharoen[1], Bundit Tengjaroenkul[4,6*], Weerayuth Supiwong[5], Alongklod Tanomtong[1,6] and Marcelo de Bello Cioffi[2]

**Abstract**

**Background:** The genus *Clarias* (Clariidae, Siluriformes) contains at least 61 species naturally spread over vast regions of Asia, India and Africa. However, *Clarias* species have also been introduced in many different countries and represent the most widespread catfishes in the world. These fishes are also known as "walking catfishes" due to their ability to move over land. A large degree of chromosomal variation has been previously found in this family, mainly using conventional cytogenetic investigations, with diploid chromosome numbers ranging between 48 and 100. In this study, we analyzed the karyotype structure and distribution of four repetitive DNA sequences (5S and 18S rDNAs and $(CA)_{15}$ and $(GA)_{15}$ microsatellites) in three *Clarias* species (*C. batrachus, C. gariepinus, C. macrocephalus*), as well as in a probable natural hybrid of the two latter species from different Thailand river basins.

**Results:** *Clarias gariepinus* and *C. macrocephalus* had 2n = 56 and 2n = 54, respectively, as well as karyotypes composed mainly by metacentric and submetacentric chromosomes. Their karyotypes differed in the number and location of 5S and 18S rDNA sites and in the degree of microsatellite accumulation. An intermediate chromosomal pattern incorporating those of the parental species was found in the probable hybrid, confirming its interspecific origin. *Clarias batrachus* had 2n = 104 chromosomes and its karyotype was dominated by mainly acrocentric elements, indicating that unusual multiple centric fissions were involved in its karyotype differentiation. The karyotype of this species presented an unexpected dispersion of ribosomal DNAs, possessing 54 and 12 sites of 5S and 18S rDNAs, respectively, as well as a high accumulation and differential distribution of both microsatellite repeats, representing 'hot spots' for chromosomal rearrangement.

**Conclusion:** Both conventional and molecular cytogenetic markers were useful tools for demonstrating remarkable evolutionary dynamism and highlighting multiple chromosomal rearrangements and hybridization events correlated with the notable karyotypic diversity of these walking catfishes.

**Keywords:** Chromosomal rearrangements, FISH, Karyotype evolution, Molecular cytogenetics, Centric fission

* Correspondence: btengjar@kku.ac.th
[4]Department of Veterinary Clinical Medicine, Faculty of Veterinary Medicine, Muang, Khon Kaen 40002, Thailand
[6]Toxic Substances in Livestock and Aquatic Animals Research Group, Khon Kaen University, Muang, Khon Kaen 40002, Thailand
Full list of author information is available at the end of the article

## Background

The catfish family Clariidae comprises 14 genera and more than 115 species found in India, Syria, Southern Turkey, Southeast Asia and Africa, with the highest species diversity found in the latter [1]. The genus *Clarias* Scopoli, 1763, comprises at least 57 species and is widely distributed across Africa and Southeast Asia [2, 3]. These fishes are known as "walking catfishes" because they have an accessory air-breathing organ that allow them to survive for months in oxygen-poor water or even completely out of water [4]. Moreover, some species are able to migrate over land using wriggling movements. These characteristics and behaviour may affect the dispersal, speciation and genetic parameters of the population, potentially altering the processes from those commonly recognized in other obligatory freshwater fishes. In *Clarias* species examined to date, diploid chromosome numbers range between 2n = 48 and 2n = 56, with the exception of *C. pachynema* (2n = 66) and one population of C. *batrachus* (2n = 100) (Table 1). However, all chromosomal data were obtained by conventional Giemsa-stained chromosomes and molecular cytogenetic studies are still virtually absent.

The molecular organization and cytogenetic mapping of repetitive DNA elements, including satellites, multigene families and microsatellite repeats, have been analyzed in a large number of species and have demonstrated enormous potential for expanding our understanding of karyotype differentiation in fishes (reviewed in [5]). In fact, the correlation between the presence of high amounts of repetitive sequences and the higher number of chromosomal rearrangements has been widely demonstrated, since the accumulation of repetitive DNAs in particular genomic regions may prompt chromosome breakages, deletions, inversions and amplifications [6].

In this study, we analyzed the karyotype structure and distribution of four repetitive DNA sequences [5S and 18S rDNAs and $(CA)_{15}$ and $(GA)_{15}$ microsatellites] in three *Clarias* species (*C. gariepinus*, *C. macrocephalus* and *C. batrachus*) and in a probable natural hybrid of *C. gariepinus* and *C. macrocephalus* from different Thailand river basins with the aim of investigating their chromosomal differentiation and relationships. We observed remarkable chromosomal dynamism and karyotype characteristics that confirmed the hybridization of *C. gariepinus* x *C. macrocephalus*.

## Results

### Karyotypes

No differences between male and female karyotypes were observed in any species. *Clarias gariepinus* showed a chromosome number of 2n = 56 (18 m + 20 sm + 18 st/a) and a fundamental number (NF) equal to 94. *Clarias macrocephalus* showed 2n = 54 (18 m + 20 sm + 16 st/a) and a NF of 92. The probable natural hybrid of *C. gariepinus* x *C. microcephalus* had a 2n between the two species (55) with a karyotype composed of 18 m + 20 sm + 17 st/a, and a NF equal to 91 (Fig. 1). *Clarias batrachus* showed a 2n = 104 (2 m + 4 sm + 98 st/a), with the NF equal to 110 (Fig. 2).

### Chromosome mapping of 5S and 18S rDNA sequences

The 18S rDNA probe hybridized to the subtelomeric/telomeric region of one medium-sized sm chromosomal pair in *C. gariepinus* and in one large st/a pair in *C. macrocephalus.* The 5S rDNA sequences were located in two small st/a pairs in *C. gariepinus* and in only one st/a pair in *C. macrocephalus.* Accordingly, the supposed hybrid of *C. gariepinus* x *C. microcephalus* had the intermediate number for both rDNA probes, with two 18S rDNA sites present in non-homologous chromosomes, in addition to three 5S rDNA sites (Fig. 1).

However, *C. batrachus* showed a surprising increase in the number of both rDNA classes, with six chromosomal pairs harbouring 18S rDNA sites and 27 chromosomal pairs harbouring 5S rDNA sites, including a syntenic condition in one pair (Fig. 2).

### Chromosome mapping of microsatellite sequences

In *C. gariepinus*, faint hybridization signals were found for these sequences across all chromosomes. However, in *C. macrocephalus* and *C. batrachus*, both $(CA)_{15}$ and $(GA)_{15}$ microsatellites were highly accumulated along all chromosomes. Significantly, the likely interspecific hybrid had the exact intermediate pattern of *C. gariepinus* and *C. macrocephalus*, with 27 chromosomes presenting a strong hybridization pattern, and the other 28 presenting weak accumulation of these sequences (Figs. 2 and 3).

## Discussion

### Karyotype variability among Clarias species

Clariidae is a very well defined monophyletic family based on the presence of a unique arborescent suprabranchial organ that enables the species to breathe atmospheric oxygen [4]. Nevertheless, Clariidae species are remarkable for the considerable variation in their external morphology [7–9]. Therefore, the chromosomal divergence among *Clarias* species (Table 1) also parallels the morphological differentiation of the clariid catfishes. In fact, the remarkable variability of the 2n and NF values in different *Clarias* species indicates that distinct chromosomal rearrangements occur during the evolution of their karyotypes. Karyotypes and other chromosomal characteristics of the three species in this study confirmed the patterns found for other *Clarias* species, except C. *batrachus* (2n = 104). However, *Clarias* and related cytogenetic parameters warrant deeper discussion.

The walking catfish *C. batrachus* is native to Southeast Asia, but has been introduced outside its native range,

**Table 1** Review of available data on 2n, karyotypes and sex systems in the genus *Clarias*

| Species | 2n | NF | Karyotype | Sex system | Locality | Reference |
|---|---|---|---|---|---|---|
| *C. albopunctatus* | 48 | 75 | 4 m + 23sm + 21a | ZW | Nigeria | [19] |
| *C. albopunctatus* | 48 | 74 | 4 m + 22sm + 22a | ZZ | Nigeria | [19] |
| *C. anguillaris* | 56 | 91 | 8 m + 27sm + 21a | ZW | Nigeria | [19] |
| *C. anguillaris* | 56 | 90 | 8 m + 26sm + 22a | ZZ | Nigeria | [19] |
| *C. anguillaris* | 48 | – | 27 m + 10sm + 3st + 8 t | – | Nigeria | [53] |
| *C. anguillaris* | 56 | – | 33 m + 12sm + 2st + 9 t | – | Nigeria | [53] |
| *C. batrachus* | 100 | 111 | 4 m + 7sm + 77a + 12mc | XY | Thailand | [54] |
| *C. batrachus* | 56 | – | – | | China | [55] |
| *C. batrachus* | 100 | 110 | 4 m + 6sm + 78a + 12mc | XX | Thailand | [54] |
| *C. batrachus* | 50 | 88 | 16 m + 8sm + 14st + 12a | | India | [56] |
| *C. batrachus* | 50 | 96 | 18 m + 20sm + 8st + 4a | | India | [57] |
| *C. batrachus* | 54 | – | | | | [58] |
| *C. batrachus* | 50 | 89 | 16 m + 11sm + 5st + 1at | ZW | India | [59] |
| *C. batrachus* | 50 | 88 | 16 m + 10sm + 6st + 18a | ZZ | India | [59] |
| *C. batrachus* | 51 | 89 | 16 m + 11sm + 5st + 18a + 1B-chromosome | ZW | India | [59] |
| *C. batrachus* | 51 | 88 | 16 m + 10sm + 6st + 18a + 1B-chromosome | ZZ | India | [59] |
| *C. batrachus* | 50 | 96 | 12 m + 18sm + 10st + 10 t | – | India | [60] |
| *C. batrachus* | 50 | 90 | 11 m + 7sm + 2st + 34a | – | Malaysia | [61] |
| *C. batrachus* | 54 | 74 | 12 m + 18sm + 10st + 14 t | – | India | [62] |
| C. batrachus | 104 | – | 2 m + 4sm + 98st/a | - | Thailand | Present study |
| *C. camerunensis* | 54 | – | – | – | Africa | [63] |
| *C. camerunensis* | 56 | – | 22 m + 20sm + 9st + 5 t | - | Nigeria | [53] |
| *C. ebriensis* | 50 | – | – | – | Africa | [63] |
| *C. ebriensis* | 48 | 77 | 6 m + 23sm + 19a | ZW | Nigeria | [19] |
| *C. ebriensis* | 48 | 76 | 6 m + 22sm + 20a | ZZ | Nigeria | [19] |
| *C. fuscus* | 56 | 106 | 18 m + 24sm + 8st + 6a | XX | China | [54] |
| *C. fuscus* | 56 | 106 | 19 m + 23sm + 8st + 6a | XY | China | [54] |
| *C. fuscus* | 56 | 106 | 20 m + 22sm + 8st + 6a | XX | China | [64] |
| *C. fuscus* | 56 | 106 | 20 m + 22sm + 8st + 6a | XY | China | [64] |
| *C. fuscus* | 56 | 102 | 18 m + 14sm + 14st + 10a | XX,XY | China | [65] |
| *C. fuscus* | 56 | 88 | 32 m/sm + 24st/a | – | Japan | [63] |
| *C. gariepinus* | 56 | 89 | 8 m + 25sm + 23a | ZW | Africa, Israel | [37, 66, 67] |
| *C. gariepinus* | 56 | 88 | 8 m + 24sm + 24a | ZZ | Africa, Israel | [37, 58, 67] |
| *C. gariepinus* | 56 | 87 | 14 m + 17sm + 25a | ZW | Egypt | [60] |
| *C. gariepinus* | 56 | 88 | 14 m + 18sm + 24a | ZZ | Egypt | [60] |
| *C. gariepinus* | 56 | 102 | 20 m + 16sm + 10st + 10a | – | India | [60] |
| *C. gariepinus* | 56 | 89 | 8 m + 25sm + 23a | ZW | Nigeria | [19] |
| *C. gariepinus* | 56 | 88 | 8 m + 24sm + 24a | ZZ | Nigeria | [19] |
| *C. gariepinus* | 56 | 96 | 21 m + 14sm + 5st + 16a | – | Malaysia | [61] |
| *C. gariepinus* | 56 | – | 25 m + 14sm + 14st + 3 t | – | Nigeria | [53] |
| *C. gariepinus* | 56 | 100 | 28 m + 6sm + 10a + 12 t | – | Turkey | [68] |
| *C. gariepinus* | 56 | 100 | 24 m + 10sm + 10a + 12 t | – | Turkey | [68] |
| *C. gariepinus* | 54 | 98 | 34 m + 10sm + 10 t | – | Nigeria | [69] |
| *C. gariepinus* | 56 | 102 | 6 m + 12sm + 28st + 10a | – | Nigeria | [70] |

**Table 1** Review of available data on 2n, karyotypes and sex systems in the genus *Clarias* *(Continued)*

| | | | | | | |
|---|---|---|---|---|---|---|
| *C. gariepinus* | 56 | 98 | 30 m + 6sm + 6st + 14 t | – | Thailand | [71] |
| *C. gariepinus* | 56 | 110 | 18 m + 20sm + 16st + 2a | – | Thailand | Present study |
| *C. jaensis* | 54 | – | 22 m + 12sm + 5st + 15 t | – | Nigeria | [53] |
| *C. macrocephalus* | 54 | 104 | 24 m + 20sm + 6st + 4a | | Thailand | [54] |
| *C. macrocephalus* | 54 | 98 | 22 m + 18sm + 4st + 10a | – | Malaysia | [61] |
| *C. macrocephalus* | 54 | 104 | 22 m + 16sm + 12st + 4a | – | Thailand | Present study |
| *C. macromystax* | 49 | – | 27 m + 10sm + 11st + 1 t | – | Nigeria | [53] |
| *C. platycephalus* | 54 | – | – | | Africa | [63] |
| *C. pachynema* | 66 | – | 30 m + 10sm + 16st + 10 t | – | Nigeria | [53] |

where it is considered an invasive species responsible for invading aquaculture farms and preying on fish stocks [10, 11]. Indeed, *C. batrachus* has type locality in Java [12], while the populations from Indochina either represent introduced stocks or belong to other *Clarias* species, as a number of different species have been recently identified both in Indochina and in the Sunda islands [13]. Accordingly, cytogenetic data also point to very distinct karyotypes for this species: i) 2n = 50 in Malaysia, ii) 2n = 50–54 in India, iii) 2n = 56 in China and 2n = 100–104 in Thailand, in addition to sex and B chromosomes in some of these populations (Table 1). This brief overview of species suggests that the *C. batrachus* in Thailand, with 2n = 104 and a karyotype dominated by one-armed chromosomes, may represent a different unnamed species.

The hypothetical 2n for Siluriformes, as described in studies of different species of this order, was proposed to be 2n = 56, with a karyotype composed mainly by m-sm chromosomes [14–16]. Chromosomal studies of species in the group Heteropneustidae, which is phylogenetically considered a sister-group to Clariidae [17], report that most of its members also have 2n = 56 [18]. *Clarias gariepinus*, with 2n = 56 chromosomes, as well as a higher number of two-armed chromosomes and few acrocentric chromosomes, retains the karyotype considered basal for Siluriformes. These data support the phylogeny proposed

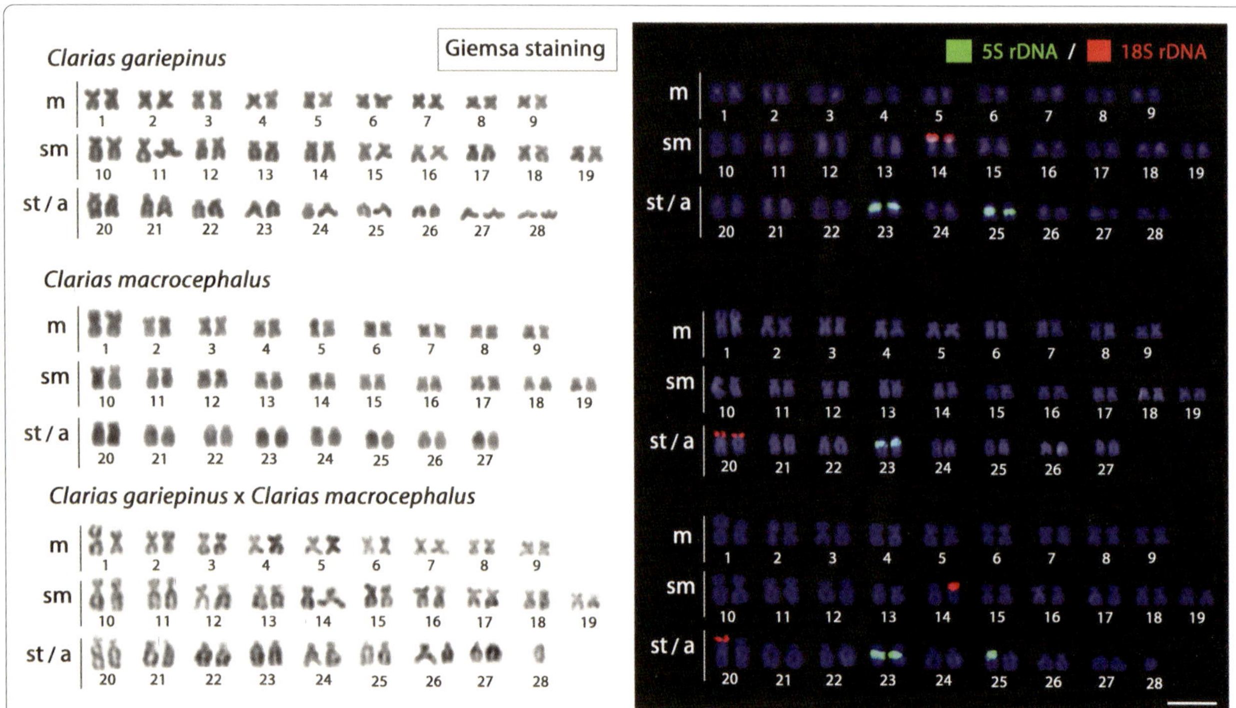


**Fig. 1** Karyotypes arranged from metaphase chromosomes of *Clarias gariepinus* (2n = 56), *Clarias macrocephalus* (2n = 54) and the natural hybrid of these species (2n = 55) after Giemsa staining and FISH with 18S rDNA (red) and 5S rDNA (green) probes. Note the intermediate level of distribution of the ribosomal sites in the hybrid specimen compared to the parental species. Scale bar = 5 μm

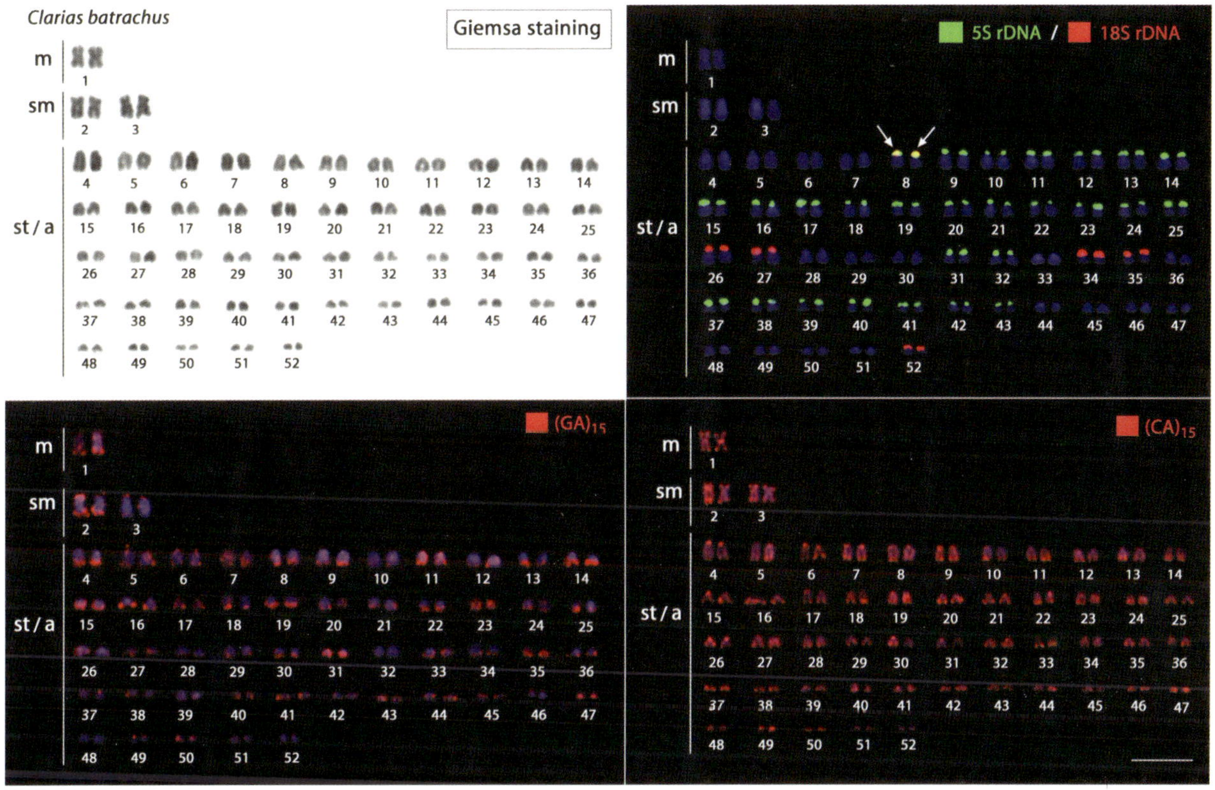


**Fig. 2** Karyotypes arranged from metaphase chromosomes of *Clarias batrachus* (2n = 104) after Giemsa staining and FISH with 18S rDNA (red), 5S rDNA (green), and $(GA)_{15}$ and $(CA)_{15}$ microsatellite probes. Note the high dispersion of 5S rDNA sites in the karyotype. Scale bar = 5 μm

for this family based on mtDNA analysis [9], in which *C. gariepinus* is placed together with *C. anguillaris,* as both species contain 2n = 56 chromosomes [19]. The decrease in the 2n of other Clariidae species (such as *C. macrocephalus* - Fig. 2), suggests that chromosomal fusions also participated in the karyotypic differentiation in the family.

Phylogenetically the species *C. batrachus* shows a derived position in the family [9]. In the present study, this species presented an unusual 2n = 104 and a karyotype dominated by acrocentric chromosomes. The occurrence of such a high 2n could be indicative of a polyploidization event. However, when considering the large number of acrocentric chromosomes and their relatively small size compared to the chromosomes found in the other *Clarias* species, the present data suggest that multiple centric fissions are, in fact, the most plausible explanation for karyotype diversification in this species. A similar process culminating in an increased 2n number has also been reported for species of the genus *Potamorhina*. One species - *P. altamazonica* - with a 2n = 102, diverged from the most frequent 2n (54) found in other congeneric species through a process of multiple centric fissions. In that case, meiotic analysis showed only bivalents at metaphase I and confirmed a large scale occurrence of extensive chromosomal fissions [20]. Additionally, extensive centric fission and heterochromatinization have been proposed in the karyotype diversification of the Alaska black fish (*Dallia pectoralis*) [21].

The chromosomal distribution of repetitive DNA elements revealed remarkable differences among the analyzed species. Both *C. gariepinus* and *C. macrocephalus* presented two 18S rDNA sites but were located in distinct chromosomal pairs, while four 5S rDNA sites were present in *C. gariepinus* and only two in *C. macrocephalus.* In addition, analysis of *C. batrachus* revealed six chromosomal pairs harbouring 18S rDNA sites and 27 chromosomal pairs harbouring 5S rDNA sites, including a synteny case. Though rDNAs are among the most conservative components of the eukaryotic genome, undergoing minimal changes over hundreds of millions of years, this conservatism appears to be a powerful source for genome instability [22]. Due to high similarity among clusters, chromosomes that carry extended rDNA arrays could be involved in heterologous synapses and recombination [23], providing variations of these sites inside the karyotypes.

Hypervariability in the number and location of rDNA loci, as presently reported in *C. batrachus,* has been previously described for several groups [24–26]. Variability in the number and position of rDNA sites suggested that

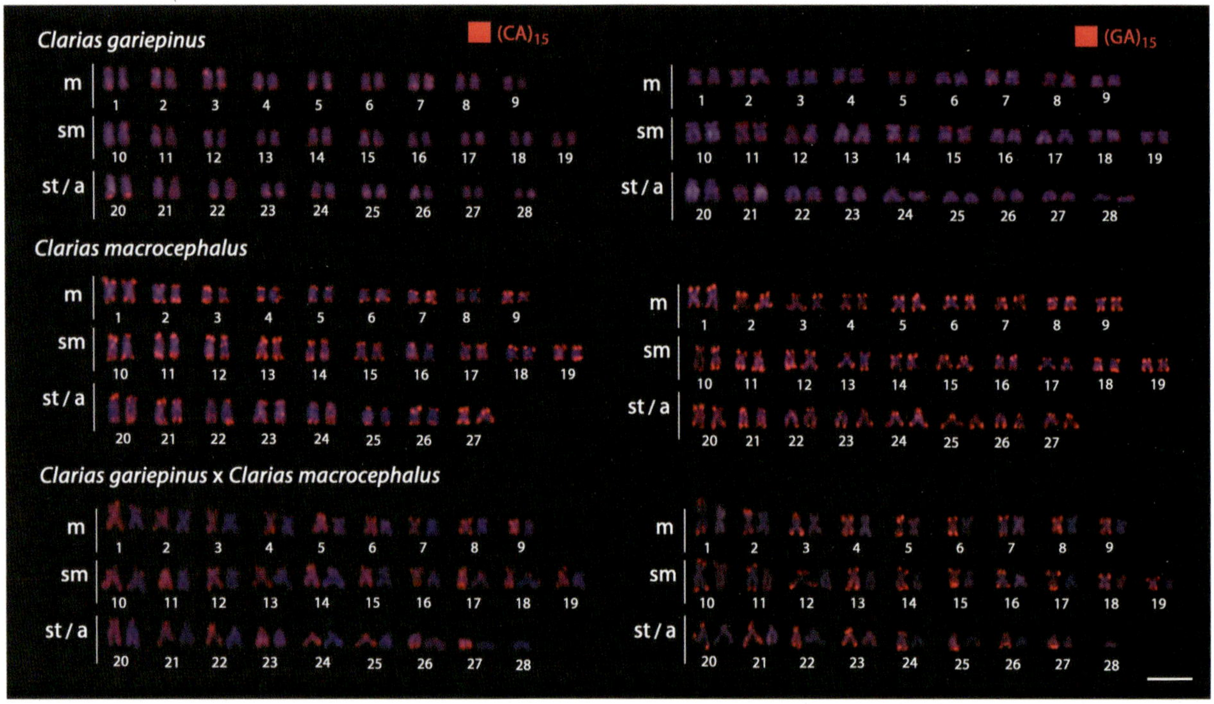


**Fig. 3** Karyotypes arranged from metaphase chromosomes of *Clarias gariepinus* (2n = 56), *Clarias macrocephalus* (2n = 54) and the natural hybrid of these species (2n = 55) after FISH with $(GA)_{15}$ and $(CA)_{15}$ microsatellite probes. Note the weak distribution of both microsatellites in *C. gariepinus*, their strong accumulation in *C. macrocephalus* and the intermediate distribution pattern in the hybrid specimen. Scale bar = 5 μm

chromosomal rearrangements played a role in the speciation of the plant *Sideritis dendrochahorra* [6]. This species possesses a large number of acrocentric chromosomes and multiple terminal 45S rDNA sites in most of its chromosomes. It has been suggested that in some groups, structural changes may be induced by selective pressures from ecological or environmental stresses [6, 27]. Among fishes, the spreading of rDNA has reportedly affected the recombination rates of two coexisting salmonid species, *Coregonus albula* and *C. fontanae*, leading to rapid genomic divergence and faster ecological speciation [28]. In some cases, transposable elements have been reported to play an important role in spreading rDNA sequences over the genome [24, 25]. Some classes of transposons appear to be able to "capture" entire genes and move them to other parts of the genome [29, 30]. Alternatively, several satellite DNA repeats may have originated from rDNA sequences and thus facilitate their dispersal into different genomic regions. For example in the fish *Hoplias malabaricus*, a highly amplified satellite repeat (5S*Hind*III-DNA) with sequence sharing similarity with 5S rDNA have been reported to exist in the centromeric region of several chromosomes [31, 32]. However, the reasons for the higher number of rDNA sites in *C. batrachus* still need to be clarified.

**Repetitive DNAs as a powerful tool for Clarias hybrids identification**

Cultured catfishes are one of the most important commodities in Thailand's domestic freshwater fish market, where *C. macrocephalus* is always preferred for consumption due to its better taste [33]. However, this species has a very slow growth rate and low disease resistance. At the end of 1980s, hybrid catfish production increased, with the most produced fish derived by crossing the Asian catfish (*C. macrocephalus*) and the African catfish (*C. gariepinus*) [34]; fast growth and high disease resistance made these species attractive to farmers [33, 35]. However, this hybrid form is currently abundant in all Thailand's rivers, threatening wild catfish populations due to competition, predation, and genetic introgression [34, 36]. In fact, these hybrids are potentially able to interbreed with the parental species, which can lead to gene pool introgression, as has been reported for *C. macrocephalus* [33].

Karyotype similarity, such as that which exists between *C. gariepinus* and *C. macrocephalus*, enhances the success of hybridization and back cross of many species [37]. In nature, the occurrence of chromosome numbers around the modal values of the clariid species may suggest that speciation within this group is related to a high rate of hybridization that results from common spawning [19].

However, when hybrids and individuals from parental species have similar karyotype structures, the use of differential cytogenetic techniques is required to provide distinguishable chromosomal markers [38]. Indeed, several known hybrids can be precisely identified and clearly distinguished from their parental species using cytogenetic markers [38–40]. For example, conventional staining helped in the precise identification of the parental chromosomal types of the artificial hybrid resulted from the cross between *Colossoma macropomum* and *Piaractus brachypomus* [41]. In the present work, repetitive DNAs proved to be informative and allowed for precise characterization of the hybridization process. The hybrid *C. gariepinus* x *C. macrocephalus* had two 18S rDNA sites in non-homologous chromosomes in addition to three 5S rDNA sites; these were the exact intermediate numbers present in the parental species. In addition to the rDNA markers, microsatellites were highly useful for confirming the hybrid nature of the fish. These ubiquitous repeated sequences are present in all eukaryotic genomes, either in euchromatin or in heterochromatin, inside coding regions of structural genes or between other repetitive sequences [42]. In the current analyzed species, *C. gariepinus* presented faint hybridization signals of $(CA)_{15}$ and $(GA)_{15}$ at subtelomeric regions, while in *C. batrachus* and *C. macrocephalus* these sequences were highly accumulated in all chromosomes. Notably, the *C. gariepinus* x *C. macrocephalus* hybrid showed 27 chromosomes with the strong hybridization pattern, characteristic of *C. macrocephalus* chromosomes and the other 28 elements presenting a weak accumulation, found in *C. gariepinus*.

However, what are the genomic and ecological consequences of such hybrid unbalance? Interspecific hybrids not only led to diversification and speciation but also have important ecological consequences [43]. Some hybrids appear prevalent in nature, suggesting an evolutionary advantage for having different sets of chromosomes for adaptation and development [44]. It is known, for example, that hybridization can promote the activation of mobile elements and rapid genomic changes [45, 46]. Among fishes, interspecific hybrids between the red crucian carp (*Carassius auratus*) × common carp (*Cyprinus carpio*) showed faster genomic changes compared to the parental species, facilitated by intron gains and losses, homologous recombination and the formation of novel genes [47]. This 'genomic shock' has also been reported in many allopolyploid plants, translating as gene loss, chromosome mispairing, retrotransposon activation, altered methylation or rearrangements between parental genomes that could lead to novel gene sequences or differential homologous gene expression in hybrids throughout evolution [48].

## Conclusions

This study demonstrated that both conventional and molecular cytogenetics were useful tools in highlighting the remarkable chromosomal diversification that characterizes evolution in the genus *Clarias*. The distribution of repetitive DNA sequences on chromosomes identified: i) a high variability in the number and position of rDNA sites, ii) multiple chromosomal rearrangements, including an unusual number of centric fissions, iii) a high dispersion of ribosomal sites in *C. batrachus* and iv) the natural hybridization of *C. gariepinus* x *C. macrocephalus*. In the latter case, the hybrid genome was fully identified by the distinctive patterns of microsatellites sequences found in both parental species. Concerning conservation issues, these data stressed that successful natural hybridizations are not limited by low variations in diploid number or conspicuous divergences in microsatellites distribution among species.

## Methods

### Materials

Individuals of both sexes of three *Clarias* species collected from different river basins of Thailand were analyzed: *C. batrachus* (8 ♂ and 8 ♀), *C. gariepinus* (8 ♂ and 8♀) and *C. macrocephalus* (9 ♂ and 8 ♀); also collected were those from a probable natural hybrid between *C. gariepinus* x *C. microcephalus* (7 ♂ and 9 ♀) (Fig. 4). The specimens were caught using a hand-net, placed in sealed plastic bags containing oxygen and clean water, and transported to the laboratory. Experiments were performed in accordance with ethical protocols, and anaesthesia using clove oil was administered prior to sacrificing the animals to minimize suffering. The process was approved by the Ethics Committee of Khon Kaen University and by the RGJ committee under no. PHD/K0081/2556. Mitotic chromosomes were obtained from cell suspensions of the anterior kidney using the conventional air-drying method [49]. The specimens were deposited in the fish collection of the Cytogenetic Laboratory, Department of Biology Faculty of Science, Khon Kaen University.

### Chromosome probes and FISH experiments

Two tandem-arrayed DNA sequences isolated from the genome of an Erythrinidae species, *Hoplias malabaricus*, were used as probes. The first probe contained a 5S rDNA repeat copy and included 120 base pairs (bp) of the 5S rRNA transcribed gene and 200 bp of the non-transcribed spacer (NTS) sequence [31]. The second probe corresponded to a 1,400 bp segment of the 18S rRNA gene obtained from nuclear DNA using PCR [32]. The 5S and 18S rDNA probes were cloned into plasmid vectors and propagated in DH5α *Escherichia coli* competent cells (Invitrogen, San Diego, CA, USA).

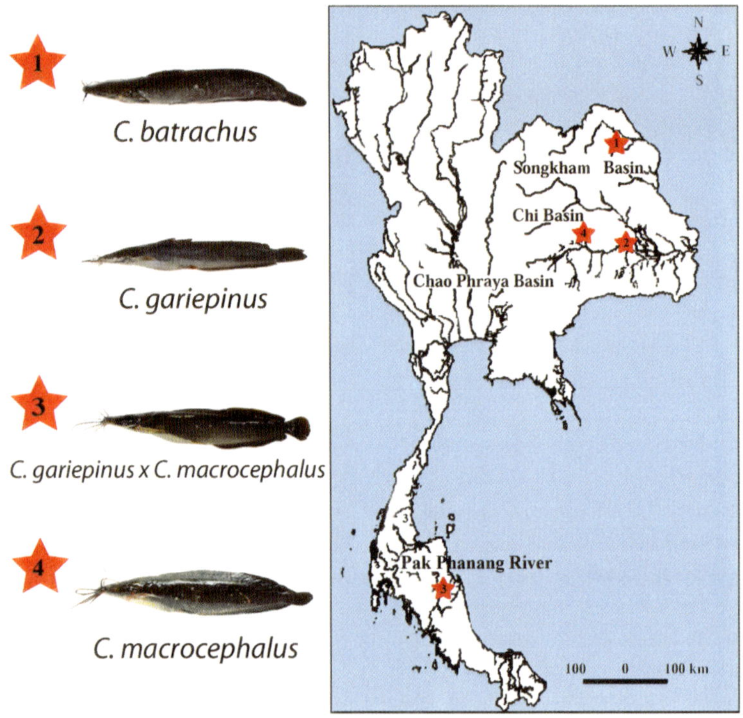


**Fig. 4** Collection sites of *Clarias* species from Thailand analyzed in the present study

The 18S and 5S rDNA probes were labelled with Spectrum Orange-dUTP and Spectrum Green-dUTP, respectively, using nick translation according to the manufacturer's recommendations (Roche, Mannheim, Germany).

The microsatellites $(CA)_{15}$ and $(GA)_{15}$, were used as probes and were synthesized as described by Kubat et al. [50]. These sequences were directly labelled with Cy3 at the 5' terminus during synthesis by Sigma (St. Louis, MO, USA).

Fluorescence *in situ* hybridization (FISH) was performed in highly stringent conditions on mitotic chromosome spreads [51]. Metaphase chromosome slides were incubated with RNAse (40 μg/ml) for 1.5 h at 37 °C. After denaturation of the chromosomal DNA in 70 % formamide/2× SSC, pH 7.0, at 70 °C for 4 min, the hybridization mixture (2.5 ng/μl probes, 2 μg/μl salmon sperm DNA, 50 % deionized formamide, 10 % dextran sulphate) was dropped on the slides. The hybridization was performed overnight at 37 °C in a moist chamber containing 2× SSC. The first post-hybridization wash was performed with 2× SSC for 5 min at 65 °C, and a final wash was performed at room temperature in 1× SSC for 5 min. Finally, the slides were counterstained with DAPI and mounted in an antifade solution (Vectashield from Vector Laboratories).

### Image processing

At least 30 metaphase spreads were analyzed to confirm the diploid chromosome number, karyotype structure and FISH results. Images were captured using an Olympus BX50 microscope (Olympus Corporation, Ishikawa, Japan) with CoolSNAP and Image Pro Plus 4.1 software (Media Cybernetics, Silver Spring, MD, USA). Chromosomes were classified as metacentric (m), submetacentric (sm), subtelocentric (st) or acrocentric (a) according to Levan et al. [52].

### Abbreviations

2n: diploid number; a: acrocentric chromosome; DAPI: 4',6-diamidino-2-phenylindole; dUTP: 2'-Deoxyuridine-5'-Triphosphate; FISH: fluorescence *in situ* hybridization; FN: fundamental number; m: metacentric chromosome; NTS: Non-transcribed spacer; PCR: polymerase chain reaction; rDNA: ribosomal DNA; rRNA: ribosomal RNA; sm: submetacentric chromosome; st: subtelocentric chromosome.

### Competing interests

The authors declare that they have no competing interests.

### Authors' contributions

NM carried out the cytogenetic analysis and drafted the manuscript, MBC helped in the cytogenetic analysis, drafted and revised the manuscript, CFY and NG carried out the molecular cytogenetic analysis, drafted and revised the manuscript, LACB. SD, WS and WFM drafted and revised the manuscript. AT and BT coordinated the study, drafted and revised the manuscript. All authors read and approved the final version of the manuscript.

**Acknowledgments**

This research was funded by the Research Group on Toxic Substances in Livestock and Aquatic Animals, Faculty of Veterinary Medicine and Royal Thai Government scholarship National Science and Technology Development Agency (NSTDA) for financial support and by the Brazilian agencies FAPESP and CNPq.



**Author details**

[1]Department of Biology, Faculty of Science, Khon Kaen University, Muang District, Khon Kaen, Thailand. [2]Departamento de Genética e Evolução, Universidade Federal de São Carlos, São Carlos, São Paulo, Brazil. [3]Departamento de Biologia Celular e Genética, Centro de Biociências, Universidade Federal do Rio Grande do Norte, Natal, RN, Brazil. [4]Department of Veterinary Clinical Medicine, Faculty of Veterinary Medicine, Muang, Khon Kaen 40002, Thailand. [5]Faculty of Applied Science and Engineering, Khon Kaen University, Nong Khai Campus, Muang, Nong Khai 43000, Thailand. [6]Toxic Substances in Livestock and Aquatic Animals Research Group, Khon Kaen University, Muang, Khon Kaen 40002, Thailand.


**References**


1. Nelson JS. Fishes of the world. 4th ed. New York: John Wiley and Sons, Inc. press; 2006.
2. Skelton PH. A complete guide to the freshwater fishes of southern Africa. 2nd ed. Cape Town, South Africa: Struik Publishers; 2001.
3. Ng HH, Kottelat M. *Clarias serniosus*, a new walking catfish (Teleostei: Clariidae) from Laos. Zootaxa. 2014;3884(5):437–44.
4. Teugels GG, Adriaens D. Taxonomy and phylogeny of Clariidae: an overview. In: Arratia G, Kapoor BG, Chardon M, Diogo R, editors. Catfishes. NH: Science Publishers Inc, Enfield; 2003. p. 465–87.
5. Cioffi MB, Bertollo LAC. Chromosomal distribution and evolution of repetitive DNAs in fish. In: Garrido R, editor. Repetitive DNAs genome dynamics. Basel: Karger; 2012. p. 197–221.
6. Raskina O, Barber JC, Nevo E, Belyayev A. Repetitive DNA and chromosomal rearrangements: speciation related events in plant genomes. Cytogenet Genome Res. 2008;120:351–57.
7. Boulenger GA. A revision of the African silurid fishes of the subfamily Clariinae. Proceedings of the Zoological Society of London. 1907;1908b: 1062–97.
8. Eyo JE. Congeneric discrimination of morphometric characters among members of the Pisces Genus *Clarias* (Clariidae) in Anambra River, Nigeria. The Zoologist. 2013;1:1–17.
9. Agnese JF, Teugels GG. Insight into the phylogeny of African Clariidae (Teleostei: Siluriformes): implications for their body shape evolution, biogeography and taxonomy. Mol Phylogenet Evol. 2005;36:546–53.
10. Teugels GG. The nomenclature of African *Clarias* species used in aquaculture. Aquaculture. 1984;38(4):373–4.
11. Teugels GG. A systematic revision of the African species of the genus *Clarias* (Pisces; Clariidae). Ann Mus Roy Afr Centr Sci Zool. 1986;247:1–199.
12. Kottelat M. The fishes of the inland waters of Southeast Asia: a catalogue and core bibliography of the fishes known to occur in freshwaters, mangroves and estuaries. Raffles Bull Zool. 2013;27:1–663.
13. Ng HH, Kottelat M. The identity of *Clarias batrachus* (Linnaeus, 1758), with the designation of a neotype (Teleostei: Clariidae). Proceedings of the Linnaean Society of London. 2008;153:725–32.
14. Ráb P. Karyotype of European catfish *Silurus glanis* (Siluridae, Pisces), with remarks on cytogenetics of siluroid fishes. Folia Zool Brno. 1981;32(2):271–86.
15. LeGrande WH. Chromosomal evolution in North American catfishes (Siluriformes, Ictaluridae) with particular emphasis on the madtoms, *Noturus*. Copeia. 1981;1:33–52.
16. Oliveira C, Gosztonyi AE. A cytogenetic study of *Diplomystes mesembrinus* (Teleostei, Siluriformes, Diplomystidae) with a discussion of chromosome evolution in Siluriforms. Caryologia. 2000;53:31–7.
17. Diogo R. Higher-level phylogeny of Siluriformes: an overview. In: Arratia G, Kapoor BG, Chardon M, Diogo R, editors. Catfishes Science. Publishers: Inc Enfield; 2003. p. 353–84.
18. Malla TM, Ganesh N. Cytogenetic and tissue toxicity by synthetic sindoor in freshwater catfish. Biomed Pharmacol J. 2009;2:885–9.
19. Eyo JE. Cytogenetic variations in *Clarias* species (Clariidae: Siluriformes) of the Anambra river using leucocytes culture tecniques. Anim Res Int. 2005;2(1):275–86.
20. Feldberg E, Porto JIR, Bertollo LAC. Karyotype evolution in Curimatidae (Teleostei, Characiformes) of the Amazon region. 1. Studies on the genera *Curimata, Psectrogaster, Steindachnerina* and *Curimatella*. Rev Brasil Genet. 1992;15(2):369–83.
21. Crossman EJ, Ráb P. Chromosome-banding study of the Alaska blackfish, *Dallia pectoralis* (Euteleostei: Esocae) with implications for karyotype evolution and relationships of esocoid fishes. Can J Zool. 1996;74:147–56.
22. Rebordinos L, Cross I, Merlo A. High Evolutionary Dynamism in 5S rDNA of Fish: State of the Art. Cytogenet Genome Res. 2013;141:103–13.
23. Raskina O, Belyayev A, Nevo E. Quantum speciation in *Aegilops*: molecular cytogenetic evidence from rDNA cluster variability in natural populations. Proc Natl Acad Sci USA. 2004;101:14818–23.
24. Cioffi MB, Martins C, Bertollo LAC. Chromosome spreading of associated transposable elements and ribosomal DNA in the fish *Erythrinus erythrinus*. Implications for genome change and karyoevolution in fish. BMC Evol Biol. 2010;10:271.
25. Symonová R, Majtánová Z, Sember A, Staaks GBO, Bohlen J, Freyhof J, et al. Genome differentiation in a species pair of coregonine fishes: an extremely rapid speciation driven by stress - activated retrotransposons mediating extensive ribosomal DNA multiplications. BMC Evol Biol. 2013;13:42.
26. Cioffi MB, Bertollo LAC, Villa MA, Oliveira EA, Tanomtong A, Yano CF, et al. Genomic organization of repetitive DNA elements and its implications for the chromosomal evolution of channid fishes (Actinopterygii, Perciformes). Plos One. 2015;10(6):e0130199.
27. Cox AV, Abdelnour GJ, Bennett MD, Leitch IJ. Genome size and karyotype evolution in the *Slipper orchids* (Cypripedioideae: Orchidaceae). Am J Bot. 1998;85:681–7.
28. Pereira CS, Pazian MF, Ráb P, Collares-Pereira MJ. Dynamics of Rex3 in the genomes of endangered Iberian Leuciscinae (Cyprinidae) and their natural hybrids. Mol Cytogenet. 2015;8:81.
29. Jiang N, Bao Z, Zhang X, Eddy SR, Wessler SR. Pack-MULE transposable elements mediate gene evolution in plants. Nature. 2004;431:569–73.
30. Lai J, Li Y, Messing J, Dooner HK. Gene movement by Helitron transposons contributes to the haplotype variability of maize. Proc Natl Acad Sci USA. 2005;102:9068–73.
31. Martins C, Ferreira IA, Oliveira C, Foresti F, Galetti Jr PM. A tandemly repetitive centromeric DNA sequence of the fish *Hoplias malabaricus* (Characiformes: Erythrinidae) is derived from 5S rDNA. Genetica. 2006;127:133.
32. Cioffi MB, Martins C, Centofante L, Jacobina U, Bertollo LAC. Chromosomal variability among allopatric populations of Erythrinidae fish *Hoplias malabaricus*: mapping of three classes of repetitive DNAs. Cytogenet Genome Res. 2009;125:132–41.
33. Senanan W, Kapuscinski AR, Na-Nakorn U, Miller LM. Genetic impacts of hybrid catfish farming (*Clarias macrocephalus* × *C. gariepinus*) on native catfish populations in central Thailand. Aquaculture. 2004;235:167–84.
34. Na-Nakorn U. "Pla Duk": breeding and farming. Thailand: Reo See Keaw Printing; 1994.
35. Ingthamjitr S. Hybrid catfish *Clarias* catfish seed production and marketing in Central Thailand and experimental testing of seed quality. Ph.D. Dissertation. Bangkok: Asian Institute of Technology; 1997.
36. Campton DE. Natural hybridization and introgression in fishes. In: Ryman N, Utter F, editors. Population genetics and fishery management. Washington Sea Grant Program. Seattle: University of Washington Press; 1987. p. 161–92.
37. Teugels GG, Guyomard R, Legendre M. Enzymatic variation in African clariid catfishes. J Fish Biol. 1992;40:87–96.
38. Porto-Foresti F, Hashimoto DT, Alves AL, Almeida RBC, Senhorini JA, Bortolozzi J, et al. Cytogenetic markers as diagnoses in the identification of the hybrid between piauçu (*Leporinus macrocephalus*) and piapara (*Leporinus elongatus*). Genet Mol Biol. 2008;31:195–202.
39. Almeida-Toledo LF, Foresti F, Toledo-Filho AS, Bernardino G, Ferrari W, Alcantara RCG. Cytogenetic studies in *Colossoma macropomum, Colossoma mitrei* and their interespecific hybrids. In: Klaustiews K, editor. Selection, hybridization and genetic engineering in aquaculture vol 1. Berlin: Heenemann Gm BH & Company; 1987. p. 190–5.
40. Brinn MNA, Porto JIR, Feldberg E. Karyological evidence for interspecific hybridization between *Cichla monoculus* and *C. temensis* (Perciformes, Cichlidae) in the Amazon. Hereditas. 2004;141:252–7.

41. Nirchio M, Fenocchio AS, Swarça AC, Pérez JE, Granado A, Estrada A, Ron E: Cytogenetic characterization of hybrids offspring between *Colossoma macropomum* (Cuvier, 1818) and *Piaractus brachypomus* (Cuvier, 1817) from Caicara del Orinoco, Venezuela, Caryologia. 2003;56:4, 405-411
42. Tautz D, Renz M. Simple sequences are ubiquitous repetitive components of eukaryotic genomes. Nucl Acids Res. 1984;12:4127–38.
43. Lewis WH. Polyploidy in species populations. In: Lewis WH, editor. Polyploidy: biological relevance. New York: Plenum; 1980. p. 103–44.
44. Mallet J. Hybrid speciation. Nature. 2007;446:279–83.
45. McClintock B. The significance of responses of the genome to challenge. Science. 1984;226:792–801.
46. Wang J, Ye LH, Liu QZ, Peng LY, Liu W, Yi XG, et al. Rapid genomic DNA changes in allotetraploid fish hybrids. Heredity. 2015;114:601–9.
47. Cox MP, Dong T, Shen G, Dalvi Y, Scott DB, Ganley ARD. An interspecific fungal hybrid reveals cross-kingdom rules for allopolyploid gene expression patterns. PLoS Genet. 2014;10:e1004180.
48. Bertollo LAC, Cioffi MB, Moreira-Filho O. Direct chromosome preparation from Freshwater Teleost Fishes. In: Ozouf-Costaz C, Pisano E, Foresti F, Almeida Toledo LF, editors. Fish cytogenetic techniques *(Chondrichthyans and Teleosts)*. CRC Press: Enfield USA; 2015. p. 21–6.
49. Kubat Z, Hobza R, Vyskot B, Kejnovsky E. Microsatellite accumulation in the Y chromosome of *Silene latifolia*. Genome. 2008;51:350–56.
50. Pinkel D, Straume T, Gray J. Cytogenetic analysis using quantitative, high sensitivity, fluorescence hybridization. Proc Natl Acad Sci USA. 1986;83:2934.
51. Levan A, Fredga K, Sandberg AA. Nomenclature for centromeric position on chromosomes. Hereditas. 1964;52(2):201.
52. Ifeoluwa OT, Adeogun AO, Bakare AA, Sowumi AA, Agwumba, Ugwumba OA. Karyotypic description of six species of *Clarias* (Siluriformes: Clariidae) from South West, Nigeria. J Anim Vet Adv. 2011;3(4):264–73.
53. Wu GM, Xin CB, Chen YL. A comparative study on the karyotypes of four species of catfish. Acta Genet Sinica. 1986;3(3):213–20.
54. Cui JX, Ren XH, Yu QX. Nuclear DNA content variation in fishes. Cytologia. 1991;56:425–9.
55. Rishi KK. Chromosomal homogeneity in two Indian catfishes. Geobios. 1978;5:121–3.
56. Prasad R. Clarias batrachus. In: Ponniah AG, John G, editors. Fish chromosome atlas. National Bureau of Fish Genetic Resources: Lucknow, India; 1998. p. 214–5.
57. Hinegardner R, Rosen DE. Cellular DNA content and the evolution of teleostean fishes. Amer Natur. 1972;106:621–44.
58. Pandey N, Lakra WS. Evidence of female heterogamety, B-chromosome and natural tetraploidy in the Asian catfish, *Clarias batrachus*, used in aquaculture. Aquaculture. 1997;149:31–7.
59. Nagpure NS, Kushwah B, Srivastava SK, Ponniah AG. Comparative Karyomorphology of African catfish *Clarias gariepinus* (Burchell) and Asian catfish *Clarias batrachus* (Linn.). Chromosome sci. 2000;4:57–9.
60. Siraj SS, Sukardi R, Phaik Imm CC, Mei KH, Vellasamy S, Panandam JM, et al. Chromosome analysis of walking catfish, *Clarias* spp. J Malaysian Soc Appl Biol. 2009;38(1):61–4.
61. Yaqoob S, Tahir Mohi-uddin T, Swaleha. Karyotypic analysis of walking catfish *Clarias batrachus* (Linnaeus, 1758). Researcher. 2012;4(5):46–8.
62. Ozouf-Costaz C, Parrent M, Teugels GG, Van der Berg E. Further karyological data on African clariid catfishes (Ostariophysi, Siluroidei). Abstr. VIII Congr. Soc Europ Ichthyol. 1994;1:56.
63. Luo JL, Wang ZX, Lin SP, Yang JH. Studies on the karyotype of *Clarias fuscus*. J Fish China. 1986;10:441–6.
64. Yu XJ, Zhou T, Li YC, Li K, Zhou M. Chromosomes of Chinese freshwater fishes. Beijing: Science Press; 1989.
65. Arai R, Hirano H. First record of the clariid catfish, *Clarias fuscus*, from Japan. Japan J Ichthyol. 1974;21:53–60.
66. Ozouf-costaz C, Teugels GG, Legendre M. Karyological analysis of three strains of the African catfish, *Clarias gariepinus* (Clariidae), used in Aquaculture. Aquaculture. 1990;87:271–7.
67. Karahan A, Ergene S. Chromosomal differentiation between populations of *Clarias gariepinus* (Burchell, 1822) from the Goksu Delta and Orontes River (Turkey). Turk J Biol. 2011;35:79–87.
68. Omotayo F. Karyological analysis of the African catfish, *Clarias gariepinus* (Burchell, 1822). Wudpecker J Agric Res. 2012;1(11):674–7.
69. Awodiran MO, Majolagbe FA, Komolafe OO, Adewumi AA, Oyebola OO, Oyewole RO. Cytogenetic study and serum protein characterization of *Clarias gariepinus* (Burchell, 1822) and *Heterobranchus bidorsalis* (Geoffroy Saint-Hillaire, 1809) in South western Nigeria. Int J Biol Chem. 2014;8(6):2377–86.
70. Donsakul T, Magtoon W. A karyotype of two clariid catfishes, *Clarias gariepinus* and interspecific hybridization between *C. gariepinus* and *C. macrocephalus*. In: The 17th Congress on science and technology of Thailand B-038. 1992. p. 406–7.

20

# Genome wide array-CGH and qPCR analysis for the identification of genome defects in Williams' syndrome patients

I. R. Hussein[1*], A. Magbooli[2†], E. Huwait[3†], A. Chaudhary[1,4†], R. Bader[5†], M. Gari[1,4†], F. Ashgan[1†], M. Alquaiti[1†], A. Abuzenadah[1,4†] and M. AlQahtani[1,2,4†]

**Abstract**

**Background:** Williams-Beuren Syndrome (WBS) is a rare neurodevelopmental disorder characterized by dysmorphic features, cardiovascular defects, cognitive deficits and developmental delay. WBS is caused by a segmental aneuploidy of chromosome 7 due to heterozygous deletion of contiguous genes at the long arm of chromosome 7q11.23. We aimed to apply array-CGH technique for the detection of copy number variants in suspected WBS patients and to determine the size of the deleted segment at chromosome 7q11.23 in correlation with the phenotype. The study included 24 patients referred to the CEGMR with the provisional diagnosis of WBS and 8 parents. The patients were subjected to conventional Cytogenetic (G-banding) analysis, Molecular Cytogenetic (Fluorescent In-Situ Hybridization), array-based Comparative Genomic Hybridization (array-CGH) and quantitative Real time PCR (qPCR) Techniques.

**Results:** No deletions were detected by Karyotyping, however, one patient showed unbalanced translocation between chromosome 18 and 19, the karyotype was 45,XX, der(19) t(18;19)(q11.1;p13.3)-18. FISH technique could detect microdeletion in chromosome 7q11.23 in 10/24 patients. Array-CGH and qPCR confirmed the deletion in all samples, and could detect duplication of 7q11.23 in three patients and two parents. Furthermore, the size of the deletion could be detected accurately by both array-CGH and qPCR techniques. Three patients not showing the 7q11.23 deletion were diagnosed by array-CGH to have deletion in chr9p13.1-p11.2, chr18p11.32-p11.21 and chr1p36.13.

**Conclusion:** Both FISH and array-CGH are reliable methods for the diagnosis of WBS; however, array-CGH has the advantage of detection of genome deletions/ duplications that cannot otherwise be detected by conventional cytogenetic techniques. Array-CGH and qPCR are useful for detection of deletion sizes and prediction of the interrupted genes and their impact on the disease phenotype. Further investigations are needed for studying the impact of deletion sizes and function of the deleted genes on chromosome 7q11.23.

**Keywords:** Williams Syndrome, Array-CGH, FISH, qPCR, Congenital heart defects

* Correspondence: irhussein@gmail.com
[†]Equal contributors
[1]Centre of Excellence in Genomic Medicine Research (CEGMR), King Abdulaziz University, Jeddah 21589, KSA, Saudi Arabia
Full list of author information is available at the end of the article

## Background

Congenital heart defects (CHDs) are major pediatric health problem in Saudi Arabia (SA). A prevalence of CHDs ranging between 2.1 and ~10.7/1000 live births was reported [1, 2], with the highest prevalence found in the Southwestern and the Northern Provinces [3]. A community-based National prevalence study of symptomatic CHDs reported a prevalence of 2.1/1000 children [4]. CHDs associated with other malformations present a challenging problem in clinical diagnosis and genetic counseling. Williams's syndrome (WS) or Williams-Beuren syndrome (WBS) (OMIM 194050) is a contiguous gene syndrome caused by hemizygous deletion of chromosome 7q11.23 and is often associated with a CHD. Affected children have distinctive facial features, congenital heart defects mainly supra valvular aortic stenosis, cognitive deficits, unique personality characteristics and infantile hypercalcemia [5, 6]. Other features included stellate iris pattern, elfin facial features, coordination problems, developmental delay, short stature, and friendly personality [7, 8]. The disease occurrence is mostly sporadic with an estimated prevalence ranging between 1/7500 and 1/25,000 [9, 10].

Most cases of WBS occur as random event during formation of reproductive cells (eggs or sperm) in a parent of an affected individual. In a small percentage of cases patients inherit the chromosomal deletion from a parent with the condition [9, 11].

Accurate diagnosis is essential for providing optimal medical care and proper genetic counselling and estimation the risk of recurrence in future pregnancies. The disease is not easily detectable using conventional cytogenetic analysis due to limited resolution of (<5 Mb) and is usually detected by Fluorescent in-Situ Hybridization (FISH). The development of more recent techniques such as quantitative Real-Time Polymerase Chain Reaction (qPCR), and microarray-based Comparative Genomic Hybridization (array-CGH) has allowed for more accurate diagnosis [11].

Common deletion size causing WBS spans 1.5 to 1.8 million base pair (Mb) which contains more than 25 genes and it is believed that loss of several of these genes probably contributes to the characteristic features of this disorder [12]. The deleted region is flanked by three large low copy-repeat sequences (LCR) (320 Kb) known as LCR blocks A, B, and C which share high similarity of nucleotide sequences leading to non-allelic homologous recombination (NAHR) conferring liability to mispairing and unequal crossing over leading to deletions and duplications [13]. Smaller or larger deletions have been reported and a phenotypic variability was identified to correlate with the size of deletion in the WBS region [14]. The use of qPCR has allowed the precise definition of the deletion size and more accurate identification of genotype /phenotype correlation in patients with WBS [15, 16]. More recently, array-CGH technique has been applied for the accurate diagnosis of the deleted genes causing the typical and atypical phenotypes in WBS [17, 18].

Patients with WBS are not easily diagnosed early in neonatal life until characteristic personality and phenotypic features become apparent later in childhood. Furthermore, the phenotype becomes variable with advancing age which imposes more challenge for clinical diagnosis. To our knowledge no previous studies for the molecular diagnosis of WBS have been reported in Saudi Arabia. Therefore, we aimed to investigate the clinical utility of array-CGH technique for the early diagnosis of WBS, and investigate the impact of size of deletion on the phenotype.

### Subjects & methods

Twenty four patients suspected for WBS and 8 parents were referred from the Pediatric Cardiology Clinic, King Abdulaziz University Hospital (KAUH), to the Center of Excellence in Genomic Medicine Research (CEGMR) for genetic diagnosis. They were 11 M: 13 F, their ages ranged between 1 and 18 years old (mean = 5.52). Besides, samples from 20 normal subjects were used as controls. Peripheral blood samples were obtained on Sodium heparin for chromosomal and FISH analysis, and another sample was taken on EDTA for DNA extraction. All samples were subjected to conventional cytogenetic analysis using GTG-banding and (FISH) technique, as well as array-CGH and real time qPCR techniques. Peripheral blood samples were obtained from patients after taking informed consent from the patients or their parents or patient's guardian. This study was approved by the Institutional Review Board and Ethical Committee of the (CEGMR), as part of a project funded by the KACST, King Abdulaziz University (KAU) (Code # 016-CEGMR-ETH).

## Methods

Conventional GTG-banding technique was applied for the chromosomal analysis of all patients as a routine procedure in the DGMU lab.

### Fluorescent In situ hybridization (FISH)

We used Vysis LSI ELN Probe, which is 180 kb Spectrum Orange directly labeled fluorescent DNA probe specific for the William's region locus (7q11.23-) and LSI D7s probe which is 108 kb Spectrum Green directly labeled fluorescent DNA probe specific for the region located in the (7q31). The probe tests the presence or absence of ELN and LIMK1 genes on chromosome 7q, control loci D7S613 genes were involved in "William's region" for validation of the reaction. All steps of hybridization and washing procedure were done following the manufacturer instructions (Vysis).

### Array-CGH technique

We applied the high resolution oligonucleotide-based 2x400 array-CGH technique using the Agilent platform. The SurePrint G3 Human CNV 2x400K Oligo Microarray kit (complete coverage of known CNVs) was used according to a modified protocol of Agilent's procedures. Briefly, genomic DNA was isolated and amplified, then purified using QIA-Miniprep_ Kit (QIAGEN) following manufacturer's instructions and quantified using Nano_-Drop Spectrophotometer. The DNA was labeled with Cy3-dUTP, the reference DNA, sex matched human genomic DNA was labeled with Cy5-dUTP. The labeled test and reference DNA were combined and purified, and then loaded onto the chips and hybridized according to manufacturer's instructions. Images of the array were acquired with Agilent scanner G2505C (HD) and analyzed with Feature Extraction Software v3.0.5.1 (Agilent Technology, Santa Clara, CA, USA) under designed parameters: Genome: hg 18, Aberration Filters: min Probes = 3, DNA min Avg Abs Log Ratio = 0.25 and max Aberrations = 100,000 and per cent penetrance = 0. Finally Cyto Report file was created and the Cytogenomics software (Agilent Cytogenomics v3.0.6.6) was used for data analysis. Several online genetic data bases were referred to during analysis of the results: the Database of Genomic Variants (DGVs), UCSC Genome browser on human Feb 2009 (GRCh 37/hg19 Assembly), and Database of Chromosomal Imbalance and Phenotype in Humans using Ensemble Resources (DECIPHER).

### Quantitative real time PCR (qPCR)

qPCR was performed on 25 samples (20 patients and 5 parents) using quantitative analysis and standard curve method [16]. We used SYBR Green Gene Expression Assays to detect the deletion on chromosome 7q11.23. The starting copy number of the unknown samples was determined using the comparative Ct method as previously described [19]. PCR primers' sequences for amplification of microsatellite markers were selected from the USCS database sequences of chromosome 7 from position 71.449.000 to 73.925.000 as previously described [16]. Twelve PCR primer pairs are generating amplified fragments in 100–300 kb intervals along the WBS deletion region covering 2.5 Mb. The SOX9 gene on chromosome 17 or the B2M2 genes were used as reference gene (s) for confirmation of the array-CGH results. PCR was carried out using an ABI StepOne Plus (Applied Biosystems) in a 96-well optical plate with a final reaction volume of 10 μl. All primers were prepared at 100 pmol/μl and all DNA samples were diluted at 10 ng/μl. PCR master mix consisted of the appropriate volumes of KAPA SYBR® FAST qPCR Master Mix (2X), High ROX, primers, template DNA and RNase-grade water up to 10 μl. Thermal cycling conditions consisted of initial denaturation at 95 °C for 3 min, followed by 40 cycles of 95 °C for 15 s, 60 °C for 30 s and 72 °C for 1 min. The fractional cycle-number (Ct) of a probe, where the measured fluorescence reaches a fixed threshold is directly related to the amount of input DNA. Melting curve analysis was performed to identify the presence of primer-dimers and the specificity of the reaction. Analysis of the results was done by using StepOne™ Software V2.3 (Applied Biosystems). A higher or lower starting copy-number of input DNA as a sign for a deletion or a duplication will result in an earlier or later increase of fluorescence. Quantification of target sequence is normalized and relative copy number (RCN) determined on the basis of comparative ΔΔCt method with a normal control DNA as the calibrator. The ΔΔCt is calculated as follow: ΔΔCt = (ΔCt unknown sample-ΔCt control sample). Normalized copy number = $2^{-\Delta\Delta Ct}$ A 0.5-fold RCN is used for deletion and 1.5-fold for duplication [19].

## Results

Cytogenetic analysis using GTG-banding revealed no deletion in chromosome 7q11.23 in all samples, except one sample had translocation chromosomes 18;19 the karyotype was45,XX,der(19)t(18;19) (q11.1;p13.3)-18. FISH Analysis has shown the deletion on chromosome 7q11.23 in 10/24 (41.6 %) patients, but no deletion was observed in the parents. Example of a normal chromosome (7q) and deletion in chromosome 7q11.23 is shown in Fig. 1. Array-CGH technique has shown deletion in 8/22 patients (36 %), however, three patients and two parents have shown duplication in chromosome7q11.23 critical region for WBS. Five samples had approximate similar deletion sizes: sample (No.bl-680-11; bl-1787; and bl-858-14) have deletion size (1.42 Mb), samples bl-320 and bl-272 have deletion size (1.41 Mb), and (1.40 Mb) respectively. However, samples No. bl-1071-11; bl-232-15, and bl-402-15 had a larger deletion size (1,44 Mb) and (1.63 Mb) respectively. The size of deletion was confirmed by qPCR. Patients (bl-664-10) and bl-1190) did not have enough DNA for array-CGH analysis and were detected by qPCR only, their sizes were (1.8 Mb) and (1.40 Mb) respectively. Patient (680–11) has shown deletion in chromosome 7q11.23 (72359696–73780263) (Fig. 2) and duplication in chromosome 22q11.21 (17031614–19362298) (2330 Mb) (Fig. 3), inherited from her mother who had the same duplication variant at chromosome22q11.21 (17274835–19327233) (2.052 Mb). Patient (320–12) had dup22q13.1 (35944612–37522778) (1578 Mb) inherited

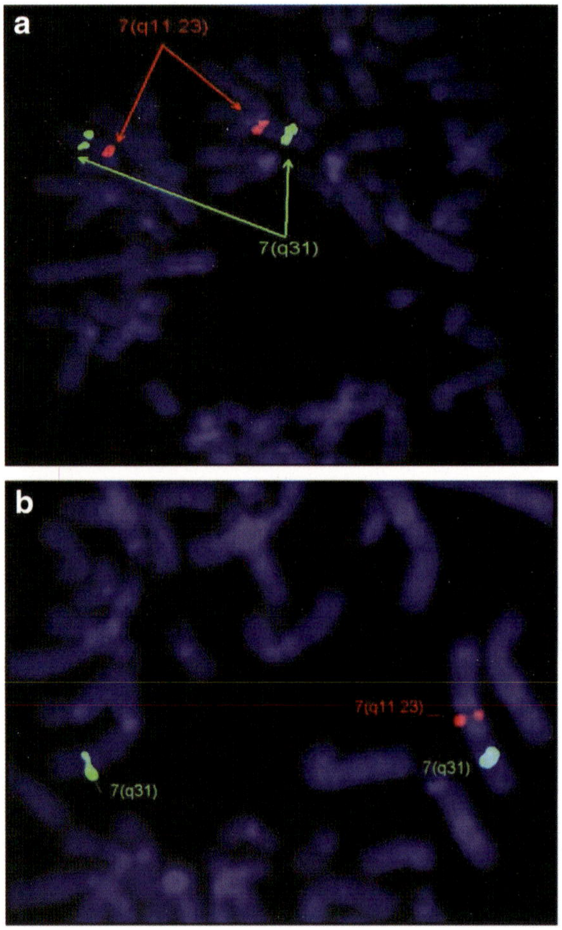


**Fig. 1** **a** FISH image shows no deletion in chr7q11.23. ELN probe showed two red signals on both chromosomes 7q11.23. **b** FISH image is showing the deletion of chr7q11.23. ELN probe showed only one red signal on one chromosome and absent signal on the other chromosome indicating deletion of 7q11.23

from her mother who had dup 22q12.3-q13.1 (34759898–38422701) (3662 Mb) Other Copy Number Variants (CNVs) such as microdeletions or micro duplications were detected in other chromosomes, a summary of the CNVs observed in patients and their parents are listed in (Table 1). Figure 4 presents the sizes of deletions in chromosome 7q11.23 in all samples.

Three patients had no deletion by FISH analysis; however, array-CGH has shown duplication in chromosome 7q11.23. Patient (bl-718-10) had dup7q11.23 (72635638–75885557) (3.249 Mb) (Fig. 5), patient (bl-889-12) had dup 7q11.22-11.23 (71073911–75851988) (4.77 Mb), and patient (bl-289-13) had dup 7q11.23 (70573442–75877956) (5.304 Mb). The mother of case (bl-320-12) had duplication 7q11.23 (72635638–75982676) (3.347 Mb), and the mother of case bl-1071 has dup 7q11.23 (76,271,711-76,321,898) (150 kb).

Three patients not showing deletion at chromosome 7q WBS critical region had shown deletion in other chromosomes such as case (bl-663) has deletion chr18p11.32- p11.21 (14.859 Mb), case (bl-1127) has del 1p36.13, and case (bl-1810) has del 9 p13.1-p11.2 (38758232–45359386) (6601 Mb). Patient (bl-663) has translocation between chromosomes (18, 19) which could not be detected by array-CGH; the deletion in chr18p11 was reported differently by array-CGH and GTG-banding with (different breakpoints), because there are no probes at the centromeric region in array-CGH scanning (no probes at the position 18q11.1). Table 2 summarizes the clinical data, results of FISH analysis, array-CGH and qPCR techniques.

Five mothers and three fathers were available for array-CGH analysis, no deletion in chr7q was observed in all samples; however, qPCR has shown interrupted regions of deletions in one father and one mother which was not observed by array-CGH analysis.

### Q-PCR technique

The deletion in chromosome 7q11.23 was confirmed by qPCR: Six samples (sample No.Bl-680, bl-320, bl-1787, bl-1071, bl-272 and bl-1190) had common deletion sizes range between 1.40 and 1.44 Mb starting from markers WBS1016 to WBS2447. Larger deletion (1.61 Mb and 1.80 Mb) was identified in sample (bl-402-15 and Bl-664-10) starting from STS marker WBS2447 to WBS522. Figure 6 illustrates graphic representation of chromosome 7q11.23 presenting variable sizes of deletions found in the patients and the corresponding markers and their positions on the chromosome.

## Discussion

WBS is reliably detected by FISH technique, however, no deletions on chromosome 7q could be detected by conventional GTG banding [20]. Although visible deletion could be detected by high resolution technique [21] FISH technique is more sensitive to detect small changes on one chromosome. Specific probes using ELN and LIMKI genes, the most common genes involved in WBS are designed for detection of deletion on metaphase and interphase chromosomes to confirm the clinical diagnosis. Elcioglu [22] reported deletion in 12 out of 14 patients of WBS using FISH analysis, two patients did not have deletions for the ELN gene [22]. Tassabehji [23] used cosmids containing LIMK1, ELN and syntaxin 1A (STXIA). They detected deletion of LIMK1 in all subjects, while ELN was deleted in two patients but not the other subjects suggesting that the gene was either not deleted or only partially deleted. One drawback for FISH is that it cannot cover the whole deleted region

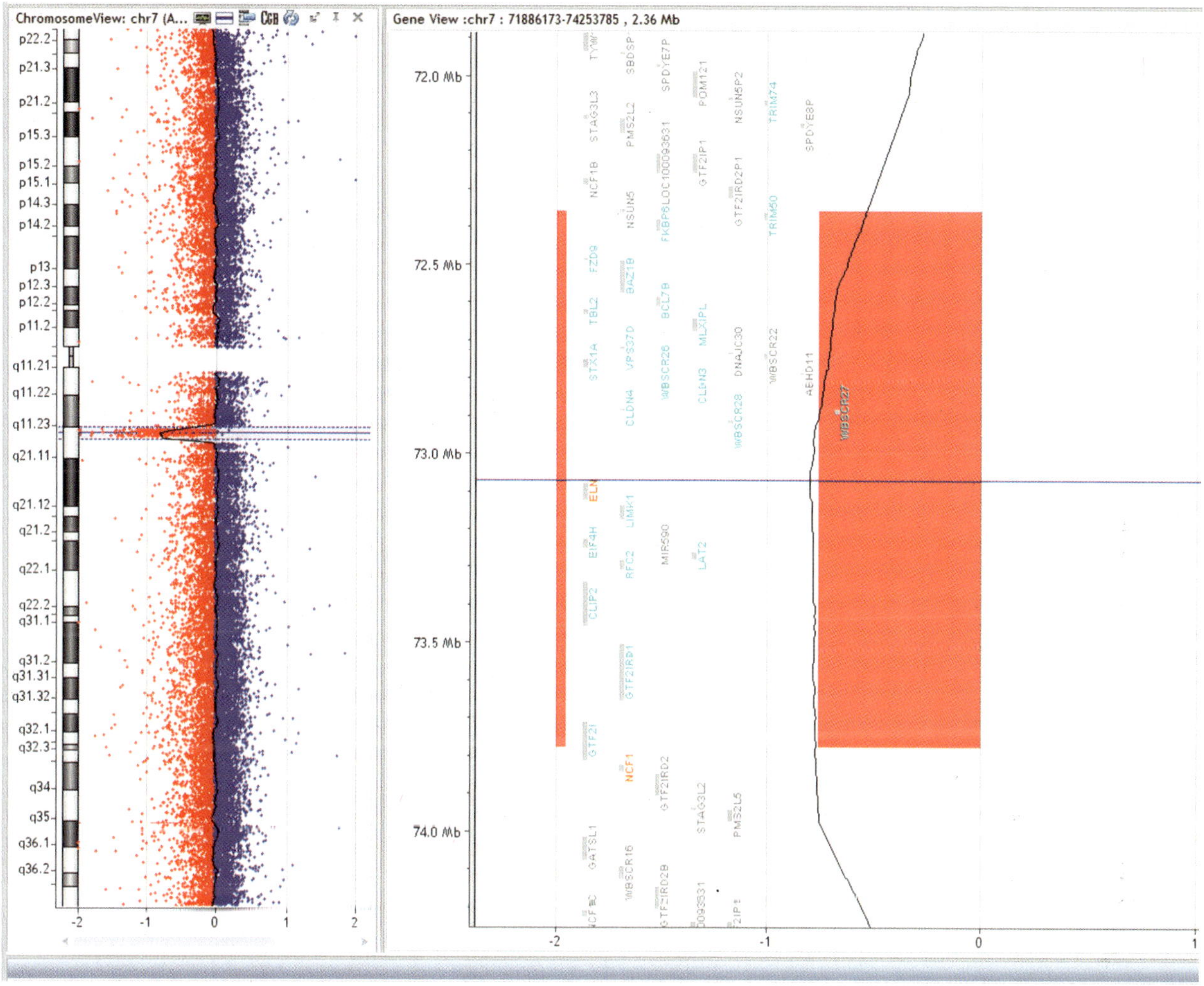


**Fig. 2** Array-CGH for chromosome7q (Agilent 2X400) showing deleted segment in chromosome 7q11.23 in patient (bl- 680–11), size of deletion 1.42 Mb, the deleted genes are shown within the deleted region

on chromosome 7q11.23 [24] ranging in deleted lengths from patient to patient. Whereas qPCR proved to be useful for detection of the deletion size in WBS region with resolution of 100- to 300-Kb intervals [16]. Twelve pair of primers covering the deleted segment on 7q11.23 allowed for the detection of deletion size. This is probably due to the high sensitivity and the specificity of qPCR which can detect small copy number changes that cannot be detected by FISH. Deletion sizes in our patients ranged between 1.40 Mb and 1.44 Mb (80 %), while two samples had larger deletions (1.61 and 1.80 Mb). Schubert & Laccone [16] used qPCR to scan 2.5 Mb of the WBS deletion region at a resolution of 100-300Kb. They found that 21/65 (32 %) patients had deletion in the WBS region, (38 %) of patients had deletion size of (1.4 Mb) and (33 %) displayed (1.7 Mb) deletion and three others have a 1.8 Mb while one patient had a 200Kb deletion and another one has the large 2.5 Mb deletion [16].

Several studies reported that the most common deletion size is 1.55 Mb which is present in >95 % of individuals diagnosed as WBS due to mis-pairing between the B-centromeric and B-medial LCR blocks [25, 26]. Bayes et al. [12] reported two common deletion regions, 1.5 Mb deletion in 95 % of patients, while 5 % showed a larger deletion (1.8 Mb) due to abnormal recombination between block Ac and Am [12]. However, smaller deletion of about 850Kb was observed by Botta et al., [27] in two patients showing the full spectrum of WBS phenotype. Dutra et al., [28, 29] used microsatellite DNA markers and MLPA technique for detection of deletion size. They found the 1.55 Mb deletion in (90.5) and (89 %) of patients,

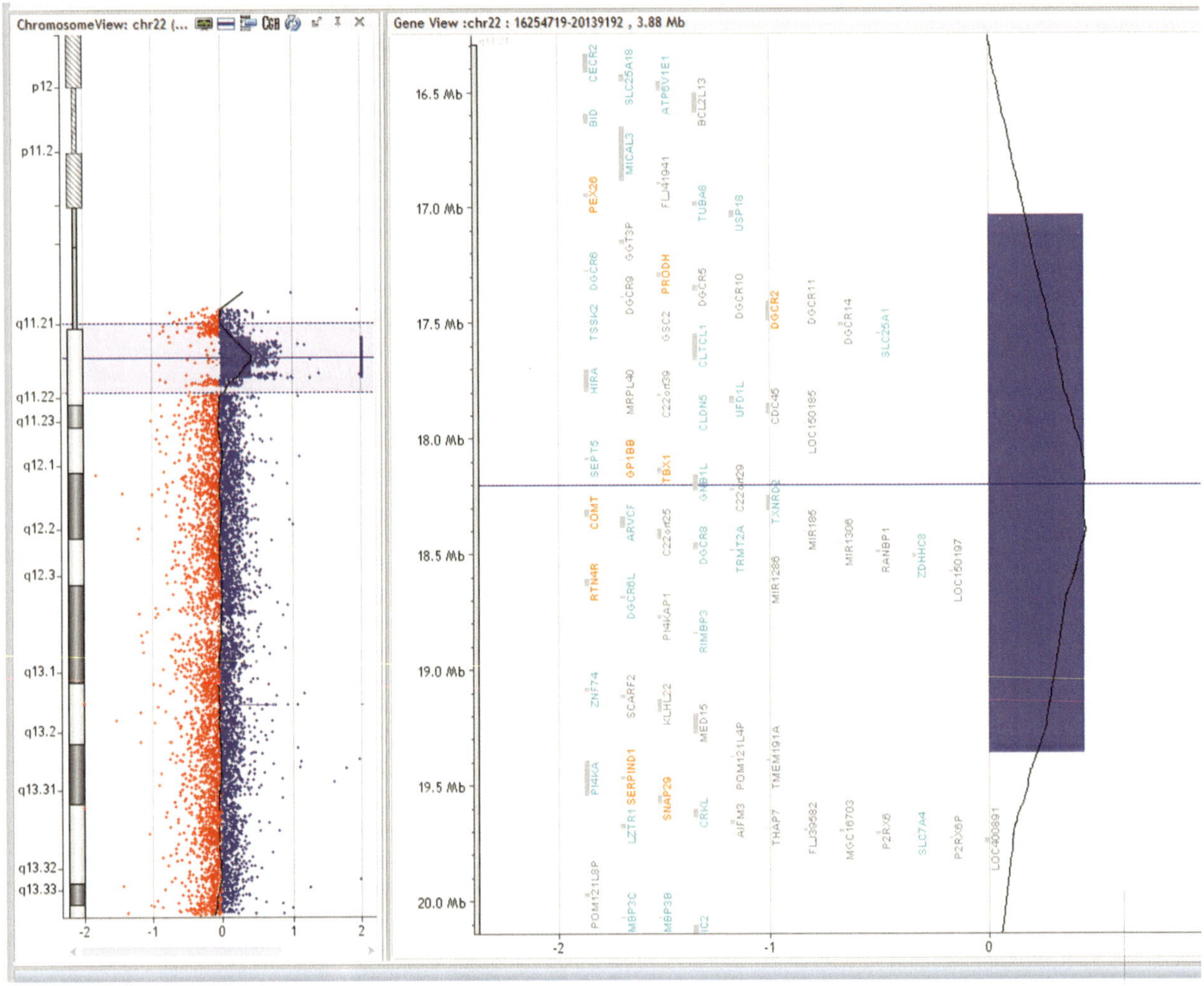


**Fig. 3** Array-CGH for chromosome 22 showing segmental duplication in the long arm of chromosome 22 (22q11.21) in case (bl-680-11) (inherited), the same duplication was found in both patient and her mother

and the 1.84 Mb deletion in (9.5) and (10.9 %) patients respectively.

Microarray—based CGH technique proved to be a reliable technique for dosage detection of genome variants. We could detect duplication of the WBS critical region in three patients and two mothers that could not be detected by FISH. The patients were referred to our Centre for the confirmation or/exclusion of WBS diagnosis. One patient (bl-718) (2 years' old, female) presented with dysmorphic features, failure to thrive, congenital hypocalcemia, left vocal cord paralysis, seizures, delayed speech and dilated cardiomyopathy. The other patient (bl-889) had supravalvular aortic stenosis, left pulmonary stenosis and dysmorphic features. The third patient (bl-289-13) presented with developmental delay, speech delay, microcephaly, low set ears, epilepsy and pulmonary stenosis. It is interesting to note that the first case of Dup7q11.23 was accidentally found in a child referred for evaluation of velocardiofacial syndrome [30]. Torniero et al. [31] reported a patient with duplication reciprocal to the WBS critical region on chr7q11.23 with dysmorphic features, speech delay, pachygyria and epilepsy, and proposed that at least one gene in the WBS critical region can impair neuronal migration. Beunders et al. [32] described the reciprocal duplication in 27 families, and triplication in another patient with speech delay, behavioral problems, dysmorphism, and suggested that amplification of the WBS region is disease causing with incomplete penetrance. More recent reports documented 7q11.23 duplication syndrome as a genetic disorder associated with speech/language delay, characteristic features, hypotonia and developmental delay [33, 34]. Our results confirmed that duplication of 7q WBS critical region

**Table 1** Summary of CNVs detected by array-CGH among Patients with Williams Syndrome

| Sample | Relation | Del/ Dup cytoband | Start-stop (bp) | Del/dup size (bp) | |
|---|---|---|---|---|---|
| BL-680-11 | WBS | Del 7q11.23 | 72359696–73780263 | 1,420,568 | De Novo |
| | | Dup 22q11.21 | 17031614–19362298 | 2,330,685 dup | Maternal |
| | | Del 10q11.21–q11.22 | 45489823–46532996 | 1,043,174 del | – |
| | | Del 15q11.2 | 18741716–20060120 | 1,318,405 | Maternal |
| Bl–744–10 | Mo. Of 680 | Dup 22q11.21 | 17274835–19327233 | 2,052,398 | – |
| | | Dup 15q11.2 | 18741716–20042737 | 1,301,022 | |
| BL-320–12 | WBS | Del 7q11.23 | 72367665–73777326 | 1,409,662 | De novo |
| | | Dup 7q11.23 | 75025883–75856615 | 830,733, | Mat |
| | | Dup 16p11.2 | 27875036–30927847 | 3,052,812 | Mat. |
| | | Dup 22q13.1 | 35944612–37522778 | 1,578,167 | Mat. |
| Bl-1771–10 | Mo of 320-12 | Dup 7q11.23 | 72635638–75982676 | Dup 3.34 Mb | |
| | | Dup 16p11.2 | 28110613–31427854 | 3,317,242 | |
| | | Dup 22q12.3–q13.1 | 34759898–38422701 | 3,662,804 | |
| BL-1810–10 | CHD | Del 9p13.1–p11.2 | 38758232–45359386 | 6,601,155 | De novo |
| | | Dup10q11.22 | 46388078–47970570 | 1,582,493 | |
| | | Del15q11.2 | 18818949–20308073 | 1,489,125 | |
| BL-1787–10 | WBS | Del 7q11.23 | 72359696–73780263 | 1,420,568 | De novo |
| | | Dup 10q11.22 | 46388078–47165895 | 777,818 | |
| | | Del 14q32.33 | 105403001–15594248 | 191,248 | |
| | | Del 15q11.2 | 18818949–19806019 | 987,071 | |
| Bl-272-14 | WBS | Del 7q11.23 | 72382983–73780263 | 1,397 | De novo |
| | | Dup 16p13.3 | 1961653–3066630 | 1,105 Mb | – |
| | | Dup 11p15.4 | 200300–2917590 | 2,717 Mb | |
| | | Del 22q11.23 | 22677959–22725353 | 47 Kb | |
| BL-1071-11 | WBS | Del 7q11.23 | 72338350–73780263 | 1,442 Mb | De Novo |
| | | Dup 7q11.23 | 76271711–76421898 | 150 Kb | – |
| | | Dup 15q11.2 | 19537035–20366729 | 830 Kb | Mat. |
| BL-402–15 | WBS | Del 7q11.23 | 72730855–74339044 | 1.608 Mb | De Novo |
| | | Dup 22q11.22 | 23056562–23245888 | 189 Kb | |
| Bl-1072-11 | Mo. of 1071-11 | Del 7q34 | 141413352–141438563 | 25 Kb | – |
| | | Dup 15q11.2 | 19465359–20418384 | 953 Kb | |
| Bl–858-14 | WBS<br>Lt. Pulm. St | Del 7q11.23 | 72721408–74139390 | 1,418 | De Novo |
| | | Dup22q11.22 | 23056562–23245888 | 189 Kb | |
| BL-718-10 | CHD | Dup 7q11.23 | 72635638–75885557 | 3,25 Mb | – |
| Bl-889-12 | Dysmorphic<br>Pulm .St | Dup7q11.22–q11.23 | 71073911–75851988 | 4,778 Mb | – |
| | | Del 7q34 | 141396899–141438563 | 41,665 Kb | – |
| | | Del 15q11.2 | 18741716–20335946 | 1,594 Mb | |
| BL-289-13 | Pulm. St | Dup 7q11.22–q11.23 | 70573442–75877956 | 5,304,515 | – |

is disease causing and patients are mainly presented with dysmorphic features, speech delay, intellectual disability, and congenital heart defects.

We observed dup7q11.23 in the mother of case (bl-320), the presence of duplication on chromosome 7q11.23 in the mother of a case with chr 7q11.23 deletion was previously observed by Torniero [31]. They reported the presence of duplication (7q11.23) in parents of probands with deletion or duplication in WBS critical region. The parents did not have any speech or cognitive impairment. Structural variants can increase the risk of secondary rearrangements causing disease in the offspring, Other studies [26, 35] suggested that segmental duplication (Dup 7q11.23) or inversion in the WBS critical region (WBS inv-1 variant) confer an increased risk factor for WBS deletion mediated by misalignment and non-allelic homologous recombination [26].

The impact of the deleted genes on the phenotype can be explained from other studies of gene functions. The most common deletion size (1.40 Mb-1.55 Mb) involved approximately 25–28 genes. The mostly described morbid genes were ELN, LIMK1. Elastin (ELN) gene (MIM 130160) was described to have a role in arterial development; it was shown that interruption of ELN expression leads to profound arterial thickening and increased risk of obstructive vascular disease [36], furthermore,

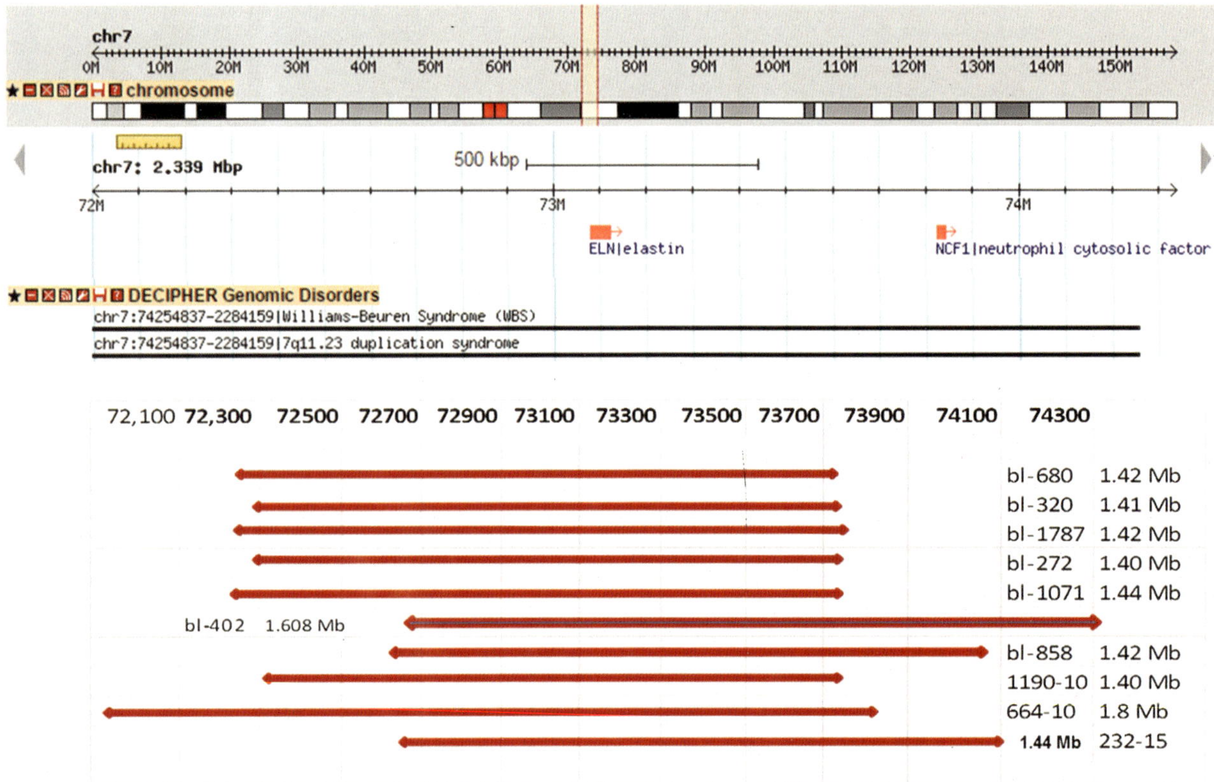


**Fig. 4** Map of chromosome 7q11.23 WBS critical region (http://www. Database of Genomic Variants) showing schematic representation of the deletions in ten patients. Six samples show typical deletion (1.40 - 1.44 Mb). Sample bl- 664-10 and bl-402 show larger deletions (1.8 and 1.6 Mb), samples bl-858 and bl-232 show different breakpoints but typical deletion size 1.42 and 1.44 Mb

ELN gene mutation is causative for isolated supravalvular aortic stenosis (SVAS), and can cause autosomal dominant SVAS [37, 38]. LIMK1 gene is expressed in the central nervous system during embryogenesis, including the inner nuclear layer of the retina, the cortex, the developing spinal cord, and dorsal root ganglia; it was identified as a strong candidate for the neurologic features of WBS [39].

Other commonly deleted genes are the WBSCR22 gene; its protein is predicted to have methyltransferase activity. Hemizygous deletion of this gene might contribute to the growth retardation, the myopathy or the premature aging effects in the pathogenesis of WBS [40]. The CLDN3 and CLDN4 belong to the CLAUDINS family; they are components of epithelial cell tight junctions and may play a role in internal organ development and function during pre- and postnatal life.

Variability in the deletion size may affect different number of genes, larger deletion was observed in two patients patient bl-402 has a deletion (1.63 Mb) involving (31) genes, the extra genes are (NCF1, GTF2IRD2, STAG3L2, PMS2P5) genes. The NCF1 gene, a NAD(P)H oxidase subunit, was shown to be involved in the generation of oxidative stress and can modify vascular stiffness observed in WBS patients [41]. Further studies on mouse model have linked haplo-insufficiency including elastin gene to increased vascular stiffness and hypertension [42]. It was observed that extension of the WBS deletion size to involve NCF1 gene was associated with protection from vascular stiffness and hypertension in WBS patients [41, 43]. This observation is useful for management of WBS patients by using anti- hypertensive and agents inhibiting oxidative stress for the protection from these illnesses [43]. Dutra et al. [28] indicated that SVAS as well as ocular and urinary abnormalities were more common in patients with a large deletion. Several studies reported no relationship between the size of the deletion and clinical features [28, 44, 45], and no difference in the frequency of maternal or paternal deletions, or the effect of the origin of deletion on the phenotype [28]. However, others suggested a parent of origin effect on microcephaly and growth retardation [46, 47]. Deletions in all of our samples are de novo; therefore no effect of parent of origin could be implicated in this study.

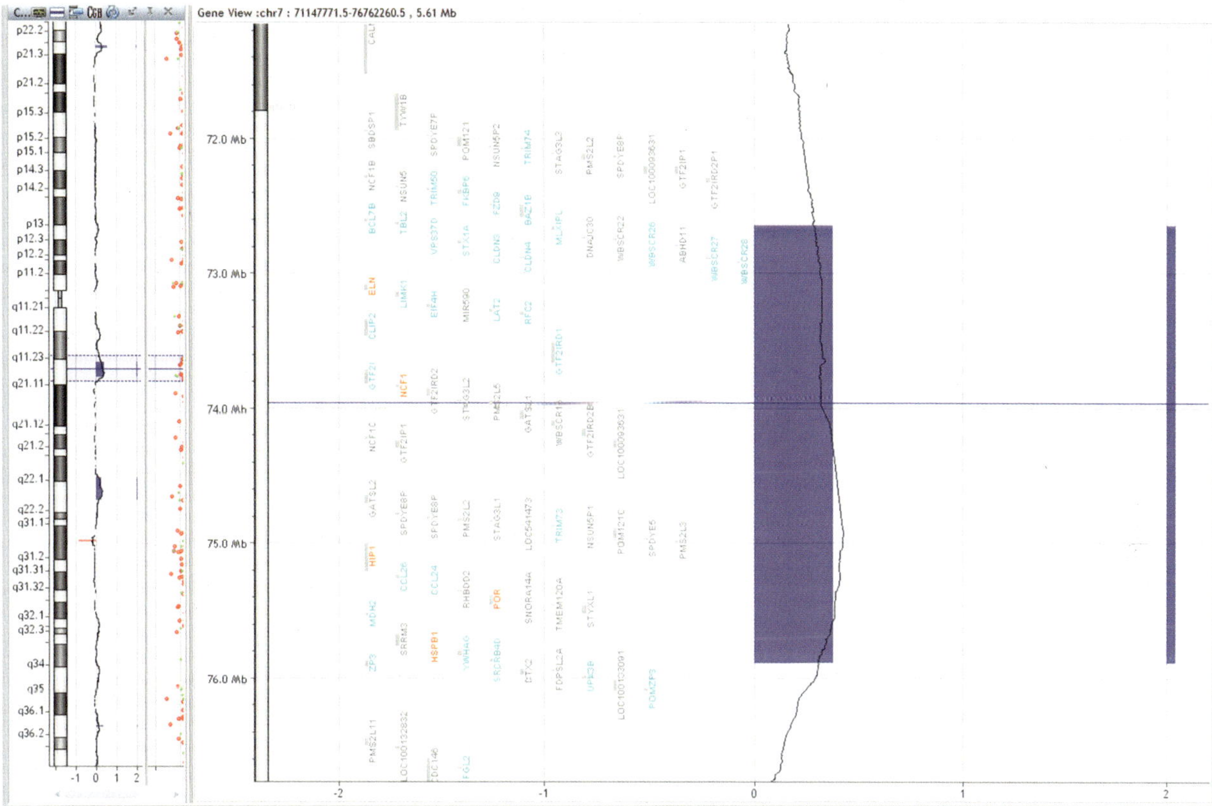


**Fig. 5** Chromosome 7 profile of the 2X400 array-CGH (Agilent) showing segmental duplication of chr 7q11.23 found in patient (bl-718-10), the genes included in the region (from 72635638 to 75885557) (3.249 Mb) are shown in the duplicated region

We observed that two patients who had no deletion by FISH or array-CGH, showed deletion of sporadic regions on chromosome 7q11.23 using qPCR. It was suggested that partial microdeletion can lead to false negative result by FISH probes. [27, 28, 48]. These patients do not have typical features of WBS and could be caused by deletion/or mutations in other genes which require further analysis.

Two patients (bl-680-11) and (bl-320) had duplication in chromosome 22q11.2 that was inherited from maternal side, the two mothers were apparently normal. Previous reports confirmed that micro duplication of 22q11.2 is frequently inherited and the majority of parents with 22q11.2 duplication showed no or minor abnormalities [49, 50]. It was observed that chromosome 22q11.2 contains multiple region-specific low copy repeats (LCR) which mediate genomic rearrangement during meiosis resulting into variable phenotypes [49], however, the size of the inherited duplication might be slightly different (e.g. case 680 and her mother). This could be a technical limitation in the array-CGH scanning, (the CNV calling algorithm is calling the ends of the duplication differently between the two samples due to probe density or type of probe used and the actual breakpoints are the same) [51].

Previous studies indicated the difficulty in clinical diagnosis of some patients presenting with overlapping features with other syndromes and not having typical heart defects characteristic of WBS and highlighted the importance of microarray analysis in the clinical diagnosis of these complex genetic conditions [52]. Three patients in our study were found to have deletion in other chromosomes: 1p36.13, 18p11.32p11.21, and 9p13.1-p11.2. Congenital heart defects associated with DD, mental retardation and other dysmorphic features were reported in 1p36 deletion syndrome [53], and partial monosomy18p [54], however, no cardiac defects were reported in deletion 9p11.2-p13.1.

## Conclusions

We can conclude that FISH and array-CGH are reliable and efficient methods for diagnosis of WBS. However, Array-CGH has the advantage of scanning the whole genome for regions of duplication /or deletion in cases with syndromic CHDs not clearly identified as WBS, allowing for the early management and better prognosis

**Table 2** Summary of the clinical data, results of FISH, array-CGH and qPCR analysis in patients with WBS

| | Age/ Sex | Dysmorphic features | CHD | MR | Dental Anomalies | Hyper calcemia | FISH | Array-CGH del. size |
|---|---|---|---|---|---|---|---|---|
| 680-11 | 8 yr/ F | + | SVAOS | + | + | No | Del 7 (q11.23) | Del 7q<br>1.42 Mb |
| BI-744-10 | 35 yr/F | Mother of case No. 680-11 | – | – | – | – | – | Dup 22q11.21 |
| 664-10 | 6 yr/M | + features of WBS | SVAOS | + | + | | Del 7 (q11.23) | Del 7q (qPCR)<br>1.8 Mb |
| 1190-10 | 9 yr/F | SVAOS,<br>Medullary nephrocalcinosis | SVAOS, AoCo, mild valvular Pul. st | + | + | No, high phosph | Del ch.7 (q11.23) | Del 7q (qPCR)<br>1.40 Mb |
| 1071-11 | 18 yr/F | Characteristic features of WBS | SVAOS | + | + | yes | Del 7q<br>(q11.23) | Del 7q<br>1.44 Mb |
| 320-12 | 3 yr/F | Dysmorphic<br>Mild LPA stenosis | SVAOS | + | + | No | Del 7q<br>(q11.23) | Del 7q<br>1.41 Mb |
| 1771-10 | 29 yr/ F | Mother of case No. 320-12 | – | – | – | – | No del | Dup 7q11.23<br>3.347 Mb |
| 1787-10 | 4 yr/F | +<br>Inguinal hernia | Congenital Pul. valve stenosis | + | + | No.<br>High phosph | Del 7q<br>(q11.23) | Del 7q<br>1.42 Mb |
| 272-14 | 2 yr/M | +<br>Inguinal hernia, short stature | Pul. St, ASD, VSD | + | + | | Del 7q<br>(q11.23) | Del 7q<br>1.39 Mb |
| 858-14 | 5y/ F | + features of WBS | Pulm. St, PFO | + | + | + | Del 7q11.23 | Del 7q 1.42 Mb |
| 663-10 | 14 yr/F | Dysmorphic, speech delay, MR | Aortic stenosis | + | – | – | 45,XX, der (19) t(18:19), (q11.1;p13.3 | Del 18p11.32–p11.21 (14.859 Mb) |
| 1140-11 | 7 yr/F | Squint, bulbous nose, flat nasal bridge, wide mouth, periorbital fullness, MR | VSD | + | + | No | Not done | Del 7q<br>0.2 Mb by qPCR |
| 718-10 | 2 yr/F | dil. Cardiomyopath seizure, failure to thrive, left vocal cord paralysis | Trivial mitral regurge, trivial pulmonary. insufficiency | + | – | Cong. Hypo- calcemia | No del | Dup 7q11.23<br>(3.249 Mb) |
| 889-12 | 1.1 yr/ F | dysmorphic | Supra valvular Ao. St.,<br>Lt pulmon.st | | – | – | No del | Dup 7q11.23 |
| 289-13 | 1.5 yr F | DD, microcephaly, low set ears, epilepsy, semian crease | Pulm. St. | – | – | – | No del 7q | Dup7q11.22–q11.23<br>– |

*Abbreviations*: *Del* deletion, *Chr* chromosome, *der* derivative, *q* long arm, *p* short arm, *F* female, *M* male, *yr* year, *ND* not done, *Pul. St.* pulmonary stenosis, *SVAOS* supra valvular Aortic stenosis

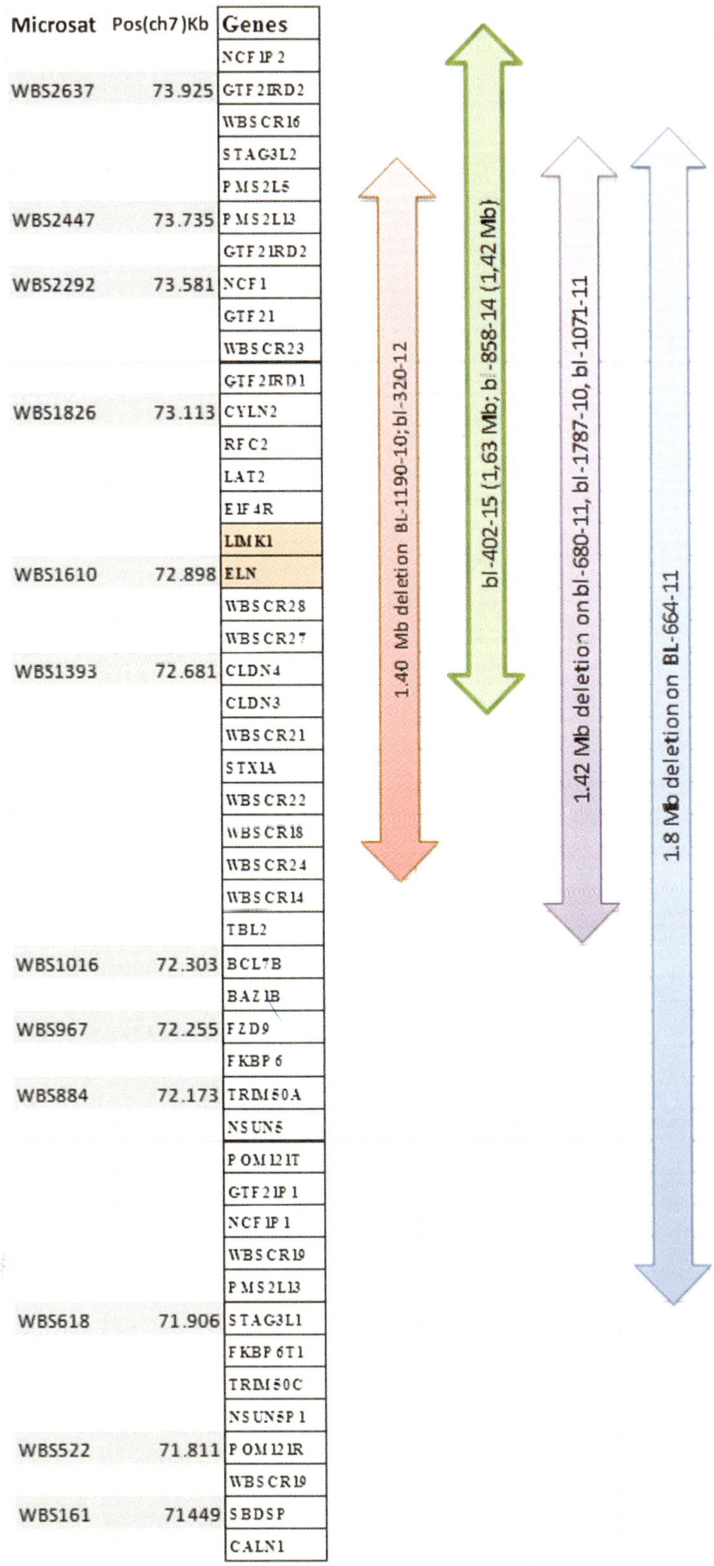


**Fig. 6** Graphic illustration of chromosome 7q11.23 showing the deleted regions of Williams-Beuren syndrome (with magnification of the region from nucleotides 71449–73.925) is showing the twelve microsatellite markers as grey bars that were assessed by qPCR. The vertical bars at the right side of the figure indicate the deleted regions of different sizes in our patients (adapted from Schubert and Laccone, 2006) [16]

of affected cases. Furthermore, both array-CGH and qPCR are useful for detection of the break points on the chromosome and can identify the genes that are interrupted on the deleted region and their impact on the disease phenotype.

### Abbreviations

Array-CGH, array-comparative genomic hybridization; CHDs, congenital heart defects; WBS, Williams –Beuren syndrome; WS, Williams' syndrome; FISH, Fluorescent in-Situ Hybridization; qPCR, quantitative real-time polymerase chain reaction; LCR, low copy repeat; CEGMR, Center of Excellence in Genomic Medicine Research; KAU, King AbdulAziz University; KAUH, King Abdulaziz University Hospital; DGMU, Diagnostic Genomic Medicine Unit; DGVs, Database of Genomic Variants; DECIPHER, Database of Chromosomal Imbalance and Phenotype in Humans using Ensemble Resources; PCR, polymerase chain reaction; RCN, relative copy number; CNVs, copy number variants; SA, Saudi Arabia; SVAS, supravalvular aortic stenosis

### Acknowledgement

The authors would like to thank King Abdulaziz City for Science and Technology (KACST), King Abdulaziz University, for funding this study as part of the project (P-L-11-0556). We also thank all the patients and their families who participated in this study for donating their blood samples.

### Funding

The study was part of a project funded by King Abdulaziz City for Science and Technology (KACST), KSA, Project No. (P-L-11-0556). The research team declares that the copyrights are reserved to the KACST and that all views, scientific findings, conclusions, and recommendations mentioned in the study represent the sole opinion of the research team and do not in any way reflect KACST views.

### Authors' contribution

IRH conceived of the study, participated in its design, interpreted the molecular results, and drafted the manuscript, MQ and FA carried out the array-CGH analysis, A M carried out the FISH and qPCR analysis, EH participated in the design of the study, R B carried out the echocardiography for the patients, AC participated in design of the study and coordination, MG and AA helped to draft the manuscript, MHQ supervised the cytogenetic studies and helped to draft the manuscript. All authors read and approved the final manuscript.

### Competing interest

The authors declare that they have no competing interests.

### Author details

[1]Centre of Excellence in Genomic Medicine Research (CEGMR), King Abdulaziz University, Jeddah 21589, KSA, Saudi Arabia. [2]Diagnostic Genomic Medicine Unit (DGMU), King Abdulaziz University, Jeddah, KSA, Saudi Arabia. [3]Faculty of Science, King Abdulaziz University, Jeddah, KSA, Saudi Arabia. [4]Faculty of Medical Sciences, King Abdulaziz University, Jeddah, KSA, Saudi Arabia. [5]Pediatric Cardiology Department, King Abdulaziz University, Jeddah, KSA, Saudi Arabia.

### References

1. Alabdulgader AA. Congenital heart disease in 740 subjects: epidemiological aspects. Ann Trop Paediatr. 2001;21(2):111–8.
2. Fida NM, Al-Aama J, Nichols W, Nichols W, Alqahtani M. A prospective study of congenital malformations among live born neonates at a University Hospital in Western Saudi Arabia. Saudi Med J. 2007;28(9):1367–73.
3. Greer W, Sandridge AL, Al-Menieir M, Al Rowais A. Geographical distribution of congenital heart defects in Saudi Arabia. Ann Saudi Med. 2005;25(1):63–9.
4. Alqurashi M, Mouzan ME, Herbish AA, Salloum AA, Omer[Double Dagger] AA. Symptomatic congenital heart disease in the Saudi children and adolescents project. Ann Saudi Med. 2007;27(6):442–4.
5. Williams JC, Barratt-Boyes BG, Lowe JB. Supravalvular aortic stenosis. Circulation. 1961;24:1311–8.
6. Beuren AJ, Apitz J, Harmjanz D. Supravalvular aortic stenosis in association with mental retardation and a certain facial appearance. Circulation. 1962;26:1235–40.
7. Preus M. The Williams syndrome: objective definition and diagnosis. Clin Genet. 1984;25(5):422–8.
8. Martin ND, Snodgrass GJ, Cohen RD. Idiopathic infantile hypercalcaemia–a continuing enigma. Arch Dis Child. 1984;59(7):605–13.
9. Morris CA, Thomas IT, Greenberg F. Williams syndrome: autosomal dominant inheritance. Am J Med Genet. 1993;47(4):478–81.
10. Stromme P, Bjornstad PG, Ramstad K. Prevalence estimation of Williams syndrome. J Child Neurol. 2002;17(4):269–71.
11. Shaffer LG, Lupski JR. Molecular mechanisms for constitutional chromosomal rearrangements in humans. Annu Rev Genet. 2000;34:297–329.
12. Bayes M, Magano LF, Rivera N, Flores R, Perez Jurado LA. Mutational mechanisms of Williams-Beuren syndrome deletions. Am J Hum Genet. 2003;73(1):131–51.
13. Valero MC, de Luis O, Cruces J, Perez Jurado LA. Fine-scale comparative mapping of the human 7q11.23 region and the orthologous region on mouse chromosome 5G: the low-copy repeats that flank the Williams-Beuren syndrome deletion arose at breakpoint sites of an evolutionary inversion(s). Genomics. 2000;69(1):1–13.
14. Karmiloff-Smith A, Grant J, Ewing S, Carette MJ, Metcalfe K, Donnai D, Read AP, Tassabehji M. Using case study comparisons to explore genotype-phenotype correlations in Williams-Beuren syndrome. J Med Genet. 2003;40(2):136–40.
15. Tassabehji M. Williams-Beuren syndrome: a challenge for genotype-phenotype correlations. Hum Mol Genet. 2003;12(Spec No 2):R229–37.
16. Schubert C, Laccone F. Williams-Beuren syndrome: determination of deletion size using quantitative real-time PCR. Int J Mol Med. 2006;18(1107-3756 (Print)):799–806.
17. Rothlisberger B, Hoigne I, Huber AR, Brunschwiler W, Capone Mori A. Deletion of 7q11.21-q11.23 and infantile spasms without deletion of MAGI2. Am J Med Genet A. 2010;152A(2):434–7.
18. Antonell A, Del Campo M, Magano LF, Kaufmann L, de la Iglesia JM, Gallastegui F, Flores R, Schweigmann U, Fauth C, Kotzot D, et al. Partial 7q11.23 deletions further implicate GTF2I and GTF2IRD1 as the main genes responsible for the Williams-Beuren syndrome neurocognitive profile. J Med Genet. 2010;47(5):312–20.
19. Vanguilder HD, Vrana KE, Freeman WM. Twenty-five years of quantitative PCR for gene expression analysis. Biotechniques. 2008;44(5):619–26.
20. Lowery MC, Morris CA, Ewart A, Brothman LJ, Zhu XL, Leonard CO, Carey JC, Keating M, Brothman AR. Strong correlation of elastin deletions, detected by FISH, with Williams syndrome: evaluation of 235 patients. Am J Hum Genet. 1995;57(1):49–53.
21. Wu YQ, Nickerson E, Shaffer LG, Keppler-Noreuil K, Muilenburg A. A case of Williams syndrome with a large, visible cytogenetic deletion. J Med Genet. 1999;36(12):928–32.
22. Elcioglu N, Mackie-Ogilvie C, Daker M, Berry AC. FISH analysis in patients with clinical diagnosis of Williams syndrome. Acta Paediatr. 1998;87(1):48–53.
23. Tassabehji M, Metcalfe K, Karmiloff-Smith A, Carette MJ, Grant J, Dennis N, Reardon W, Splitt M, Read AP, Donnai D. Williams syndrome: use of chromosomal microdeletions as a tool to dissect cognitive and physical phenotypes. Am J Hum Genet. 1999;64(1):118–25.
24. Nickerson E, Greenberg F, Keating MT, McCaskill C, Shaffer LG. Deletions of the elastin gene at 7q11.23 occur in approximately 90 % of patients with Williams syndrome. Am J Hum Genet. 1995;56(5):1156–61.

25. Meng X, Lu X, Li Z, Green ED, Massa H, Trask BJ, Morris CA, Keating MT. Complete physical map of the common deletion region in Williams syndrome and identification and characterization of three novel genes. Hum Genet. 1998;103(5):590–9.
26. Merla G, Brunetti-Pierri N, Micale L, Fusco C. Copy number variants at Williams-Beuren syndrome 7q11.23 region. Hum Genet. 2010;128(1):3–26.
27. Botta A, Novelli G, Mari A, Novelli A, Sabani M, Korenberg J, Osborne LR, Digilio MC, Giannotti A, Dallapiccola B. Detection of an atypical 7q11.23 deletion in Williams syndrome patients which does not include the STX1A and FZD3 genes. J Med Genet. 1999;36(6):478–80.
28. Dutra RL, Pieri Pde C, Teixeira AC, Honjo RS, Bertola DR, Kim CA. Detection of deletions at 7q11.23 in Williams-Beuren syndrome by polymorphic markers. Clinics (Sao Paulo). 2011;66(6):959–64.
29. Dutra RL, Honjo RS, Kulikowski LD, Fonseca FM, Pieri PC, Jehee FS, Bertola DR, Kim CA. Copy number variation in Williams-Beuren syndrome: suitable diagnostic strategy for developing countries. BMC Res Notes. 2012;5:13.
30. Somerville MJ, Mervis CB, Young EJ, Seo EJ, del Campo M, Bamforth S, Peregrine E, Loo W, Lilley M, Perez-Jurado LA, et al. Severe expressive-language delay related to duplication of the Williams-Beuren locus. N Engl J Med. 2005;353(16):1694–701.
31. Torniero C, Dalla Bernardina B, Novara F, Cerini R, Bonaglia C, Pramparo T, Ciccone R, Guerrini R, Zuffardi O. Dysmorphic features, simplified gyral pattern and 7q11.23 duplication reciprocal to the Williams-Beuren deletion. Eur J Hum Genet. 2008;16(8):880–7.
32. Beunders G, van de Kamp JM, Veenhoven RH, van Hagen JM, Nieuwint AW, Sistermans EA. A triplication of the Williams-Beuren syndrome region in a patient with mental retardation, a severe expressive language delay, behavioural problems and dysmorphisms. J Med Genet. 2010;47(4):271–5.
33. Velleman SL, Mervis CB. Children with 7q11.23 Duplication Syndrome: Speech, Language, Cognitive, and Behavioral Characteristics and their Implications for Intervention. Perspect Lang Learn Educ. 2011;18(3):108–16.
34. Mohan S, Nampoothiri S, Yesodharan D, Venkatesan V, Koshy T, Paul SF, Perumal V. Reciprocal Microduplication of the Williams-Beuren Syndrome Chromosome Region in a 9-Year-Old Omani Boy. Lab Med. 2016;47(2):171–5.
35. Cusco I, Corominas R, Bayes M, Flores R, Rivera-Brugues N, Campuzano V, Perez-Jurado LA. Copy number variation at the 7q11.23 segmental duplications is a susceptibility factor for the Williams-Beuren syndrome deletion. Genome Res. 2008;18(5):683–94.
36. Li DY, Brooke B, Davis EC, Mecham RP, Sorensen LK, Boak BB, Eichwald E, Keating MT. Elastin is an essential determinant of arterial morphogenesis. Nature. 1998;393(6682):276–80.
37. Li DY, Toland AE, Boak BB, Atkinson DL, Ensing GJ, Morris CA, Keating MT. Elastin point mutations cause an obstructive vascular disease, supravalvular aortic stenosis. Hum Mol Genet. 1997;6(7):1021–8.
38. Park S, Seo EJ, Yoo HW, Kim Y. Novel mutations in the human elastin gene (ELN) causing isolated supravalvular aortic stenosis. Int J Mol Med. 2006;18(2):329–32.
39. Tassabehji M, Metcalfe K, Fergusson WD, Carette MJ, Dore JK, Donnai D, Read AP, Proschel C, Gutowski NJ, Mao X, et al. LIM-kinase deleted in Williams syndrome. Nat Genet. 1996;13(3):272–3.
40. Doll A, Grzeschik KH. Characterization of two novel genes, WBSCR20 and WBSCR22, deleted in Williams-Beuren syndrome. Cytogenet Cell Genet. 2001;95(1–2):20–7.
41. Del Campo M, Antonell A, Magano LF, Munoz FJ, Flores R, Bayes M, Perez Jurado LA. Hemizygosity at the NCF1 gene in patients with Williams-Beuren syndrome decreases their risk of hypertension. Am J Hum Genet. 2006;78(4):533–42.
42. Campuzano V, Segura-Puimedon M, Terrado V, Sanchez-Rodriguez C, Coustets M, Menacho-Marquez M, Nevado J, Bustelo XR, Francke U, Perez-Jurado LA. Reduction of NADPH-oxidase activity ameliorates the cardiovascular phenotype in a mouse model of Williams-Beuren Syndrome. PLoS Genet. 2012;8(2), e1002458.
43. Kozel BA, Danback JR, Waxler JL, Knutsen RH, de Las Fuentes L, Reusz GS, Kis E, Bhatt AB, Pober BR. Williams syndrome predisposes to vascular stiffness modified by antihypertensive use and copy number changes in NCF1. Hypertension. 2014;63(1):74–9.
44. Wang MS, Schinzel A, Kotzot D, Balmer D, Casey R, Chodirker BN, Gyftodimou J, Petersen MB, Lopez-Rangel E, Robinson WP. Molecular and clinical correlation study of Williams-Beuren syndrome: No evidence of molecular factors in the deletion region or imprinting affecting clinical outcome. Am J Med Genet. 1999;86(1):34–43.
45. Pober BR. Williams-Beuren syndrome. N Engl J Med. 2010;362(3):239–52.
46. Perez Jurado LA, Peoples R, Kaplan P, Hamel BC, Francke U. Molecular definition of the chromosome 7 deletion in Williams syndrome and parent-of-origin effects on growth. Am J Hum Genet. 1996;59(4):781–92.
47. Brondum-Nielsen K, Beck B, Gyftodimou J, Horlyk H, Liljenberg U, Petersen MB, Pedersen W, Petersen MB, Sand A, Skovby F, et al. Investigation of deletions at 7q11.23 in 44 patients referred for Williams-Beuren syndrome, using FISH and four DNA polymorphisms. Hum Genet. 1997;99(1):56–61.
48. Heller R, Rauch A, Luttgen S, Schroder B, Winterpacht A. Partial deletion of the critical 1.5 Mb interval in Williams-Beuren syndrome. J Med Genet. 2003;40(8):e99.
49. Ou Z, Berg JS, Yonath H, Enciso VB, Miller DT, Picker J, Lenzi T, Keegan CE, Sutton VR, Belmont J, et al. Microduplications of 22q11.2 are frequently inherited and are associated with variable phenotypes. Genet Med. 2008;10(4):267–77.
50. Wentzel C, Fernstrom M, Ohrner Y, Anneren G, Thuresson AC. Clinical variability of the 22q11.2 duplication syndrome. Eur J Med Genet. 2008;51(6):501–10.
51. Scherer SW, Lee C, Birney E, Altshuler DM, Eichler EE, Carter NP, Hurles ME, Feuk L. Challenges and standards in integrating surveys of structural variation. Nat Genet. 2007;39(7 Suppl):S7–S15.
52. Honeywell C, Gardin L, Jimenez-Rivera C, Allanson J. Array CGH ends diagnostic odyssey for infant with features of Williams and Alagille syndrome. Am J Med Genet A. 2009;149A(5):1102–3.
53. Battaglia A, Hoyme HE, Dallapiccola B, Zackai E, Hudgins L, McDonald-Mcginn D, Bahi-Buisson N, Romano C, Williams CA, Brailey LL, et al. Further delineation of deletion 1p36 syndrome in 60 patients: a recognizable phenotype and common cause of developmental delay and mental retardation. Pediatrics. 2008;121(2):404–10.
54. Schmidt B, Udink Ten Cate F, Weiss M, Koehler U. Cardiac malformation of partial trisomy 7p/monosomy 18p and partial trisomy 18p/monosomy 7p in siblings as a result of reciprocal unbalanced malsegregation—and review of the literature. Eur J Pediatr. 2012;171(7):1047–53.

21

# Comparative deletion mapping at 1p31.3-p32.2 implies *NFIA* responsible for intellectual disability coupled with macrocephaly and the presence of several other genes for syndromic intellectual disability

Jonathan D. J. Labonne[1,2], Yiping Shen[3], Il-Keun Kong[4], Michael P. Diamond[1], Lawrence C. Layman[1,2,5] and Hyung-Goo Kim[1,2*]

**Abstract**

**Background:** While chromosome 1 is the largest chromosome in the human genome, less than two dozen cases of interstitial microdeletions in the short arm have been documented. More than half of the 1p microdeletion cases were reported in the pre-microarray era and as a result, the proximal and distal boundaries containing the exact number of genes involved in the microdeletions have not been clearly defined.

**Results:** We revisited a previous case of a 10-year old female patient with a 1p32.1p32.3 microdeletion displaying syndromic intellectual disability. We performed microarray analysis as well as qPCR to define the proximal and distal deletion breakpoints and revised the karyotype from 1p32.1p32.3 to 1p31.3p32.2. The deleted chromosomal region contains at least 35 genes including *NFIA*. Comparative deletion mapping shows that this region can be dissected into five chromosomal segments containing at least six candidate genes (*DAB1*, *HOOK1*, *NFIA*, *DOCK7*, *DNAJC6*, and *PDE4B*) most likely responsible for syndromic intellectual disability, which was corroborated by their reduced transcript levels in RT-qPCR. Importantly, one patient with an intragenic microdeletion within *NFIA* and an additional patient with a balanced translocation disrupting *NFIA* display intellectual disability coupled with macrocephaly.

**Conclusion:** We propose *NFIA* is responsible for intellectual disability coupled with macrocephaly, and microdeletions at 1p31.3p32.2 constitute a contiguous gene syndrome with several genes contributing to syndromic intellectual disability.

**Keywords:** 1p microdeletion, Intellectual disability, Delayed psychomotor development, Craniofacial anomalies, *DAB1*, *HOOK1*, *NFIA*, *DOCK7*, *DNAJC6*, *PDE4B*

* Correspondence: hkim@gru.edu
[1]Department of Obstetrics & Gynecology, Augusta University, 1120 15th Street, Augusta, GA 30912, USA
[2]Department of Neuroscience and Regenerative Medicine, Medical College of Georgia, Augusta University, 1120 15th Street, Augusta, GA 30912, USA
Full list of author information is available at the end of the article

## Background

Interstitial microdeletions of the short arm of chromosome 1 are rare and to date at least 19 cases have been reported [1–17] (Table 1). It is thought that many genes, which are critical for early development, reside within the short arm of chromosome 1 [4]. These heterozygous deletions, in some cases, might have resulted in the eventual death of the affected individuals [3, 7, 9, 11]. Patients with 1p interstitial microdeletions display a number of clinical features including intellectual disability, craniofacial anomalies, seizures, tooth abnormalities, urinary tract anomalies, and skeletal, cardiac as well as limb defects [3, 4, 7, 12, 16, 17].

Revisiting CNV (copy number variation) cases reported during the pre-microarray era is uncommon, because the patients are deceased or lost to follow-up. Re-evaluation of earlier cases using microarray analysis, however, provides more accurate information on the candidate genes contained within the CNV regions. Furthermore, it also allows monitoring of any changes in the patient's clinical features over time [18]. More than a decade ago, an apparent interstitial microdeletion at 1p32.1p32.3 was reported in a 10-year old girl with delayed psychomotor development and facial dysmorphism. This *de novo* structural chromosomal rearrangement was detected by karyotype analysis alone followed by fluorescent *in situ* hybrization (FISH) without defining the exact size and location of the microdeletion [10]. Here we revisited this proband to revise the karyotype and to define the size of this microdeletion by molecular analysis. From molecular dissection of our case with six published cases of microdeletions, a balanced translocation, and seven unpublished DECIPHER cases [23], we propose that there are at least six chromosomal segments within this region, and each segment harbors at least one candidate gene for intellectual disability. We also determined the transcript levels of six candidate genes (*DAB1, HOOK1, NFIA, DOCK7, DNAJC6* and *PDE4B*) for syndromic intellectual disability.

## Methods

### Case presentation

The proband (DGDP005) is a 23-year-old female with a history of developmental delay and intellectual disability. In infancy, developmental milestones were delayed and she exhibited impaired motor skills (Table 2). The patient displayed craniofacial anomalies including macrocephaly (Fig. 1a, b, d-g), frontal bossing (Fig. 1b) and low-set ears (Fig. 1d). She was diagnosed with attention deficit hyperactivity disorder (ADHD), obsessive compulsive disorder (OCD), ocular hypertension (OHT), and developmental encephalopathy with cognitive impairment (Table 2).

At age 10, her grades were Bs and Cs, but school challenges warranted special education. She also had difficulty falling asleep and she took nightly melatonin. She was diagnosed with ADHD, hypertonia, and possible sensory integration difficulties (further details on her phenotype up to age10 can be found in Zinner and Batanian (2003) [10]).

At 14 years of age, she took the Stanford Binet Intelligence Scales-Fifth edition (SB5). She had difficulty staying on a task requiring redirection. Her general cognitive ability was estimated to be in the low average range with a full scale intelligence quotient (FSIQ) score of 83 (95 % confidence interval 79–87), suggesting intellectual disability. She received a score of 79 in the nonverbal reasoning abilities, which is in the borderline range, and higher than only 8 % of her peers. In verbal reasoning abilities, she scored 88, which is in the low average, and just above ~12 % of her peers. Her ability to solve verbal and nonverbal problems using inductive or deductive reasoning was average. Her overall thinking and reasoning was worse than ~87 % of children of her age. She scored in the low average range for general information gathering, attention span, and concentration. Her ability to see patterns, relationships, and spatial orientations among diverse pieces of visual display, as well as her ability with numbers and numerical problem solving with word problems or with picture relationships were borderline.

At age 16, she was found to display OHT and ADHD, language disability in written language expression as well as in math calculation and math reasoning. She passed the vision test scoring 20/10 and 20/20 for the right and left eye respectively. Her hearing was adequate for the classroom functioning. She showed significant difficulties in fine motor functions with soft neurological signs. Overall, the assessment showed that she continued to be a student with intellectual disability and ADHD.

When she was 18, the patient was re-evaluated by the child neurology services. She was diagnosed with developmental encephalopathy with cognitive impairment, OCD and ADHD. She was treated with fluoxetine and Adderall for OCD and ADHD, respectively. Some of her facial dysmorphisms became more evident at age 18, such as her prominent forehead, narrow nose, and thin lips (Fig. 1). She still displayed low-set ears (Fig. 1d). At the age of 22, she was admitted to the hospital and diagnosed with subarachnoid as well as intraventricular hemorrhage with layering in the posterior fossa. She was also diagnosed with a right anterior communicating artery aneurysm and continued to show developmental delay, OCD and ADHD.

### Cell culture

Lymphocytes were isolated from the patient's blood samples by density gradient centrifugation as we have done

**Table 1** Patients with 1p interstitial microdeletions

| Patient | Karyotype | Source | Phenotype | Methods and coordinates |
|---|---|---|---|---|
| 1 | del(1)(p21p32) | [1][a]1979 | Severe psychomotor retardation, craniofacial and skeletal anomalies, short stature, overweight. | Karyotyping |
| 2 | del(1)(p22.1p31.2) | [2][a]1987 | Psychomotor retardation, craniofacial and limb anomalies. | Karyotyping |
| 3 | del(1)(p22.1p31.2) | [3][a]1991 Pt 1 | Developmental delay, intellectual disability, craniofacial anomalies. | Karyotyping |
| 4 | del(1)(p22.3p31.3) | [3][a]1991 Pt 2 | Developmental delay, seizures craniofacial and limb anomalies. | Karyotyping |
| 5 | del(1)(p32.3p34.1) | [4][a]1991 | Mental and motor developmental delay, craniofacial and limb anomalies, hypotonia. | Karyotyping |
| 6 | del(1)(p36.1p36.2) | [5][a]1993 | Developmental delay, craniofacial anomalies, neuroblastoma. | Karyotyping |
| 7 | del(1)(p32.1p32.3) | [6][a]1995 | Developmental delay, craniofacial and limb anomalies. | Karyotyping |
| 8 | del(1)(p21p22.3) | [7][a]1997 | Craniofacial and limb anomalies, congenital heart disease, rib abnormalities. | Karyotyping |
| 9 | del(1)(p34.1p34.3) | [8][a]1999 Pt 1 | Severe learning disability, attention deficit disorder (ADD), craniofacial anomalies. | Karyotyping and FISH with probes specific for chromosome 1 (COATA-SOME™1, p5205-DG.5) |
| 10 | del(1)(p34.1p34.3) | [8][a]1999 Pt 2 | Attention deficit hyperactivity disorder (ADHD), craniofacial anomalies, disturbed behaviors. | Karyotyping and FISH with probes specific for chromosome 1 (COATA SOME™1, p5205-DG.5) |
| 11 | del(1)(p32.1p32.3) | [9][a] 2002 Pt 1 | Global developmental delay, craniofacial anomalies, absence of corpus callosum, type I Chiari malformation, tethered cord. | Karyotyping and FISH with probes specific for whole chromosome painting |
| 12 | del(1)(p32.1p32.3) | [9][a]2002 Pt 2 | Intraventricular hemorrhage, seizures, thin corpus callosum, limb anomalies | Karyotyping and FISH with probes specific for whole chromosome painting |
| 13 | del(1)(p32.1p32.3) | [10][a]2003 | Delayed psychomotor development, craniofacial anomalies | Karyotyping and FISH using whole chromosome 1 painting probe (wcp1) |
| 14 | del(1)(p36) | [11][a]2004 | Craniofacial anomalies, moderate intellectual disability, seizures. | FISH with TelVysion 1p (Vysis), P5124 (Oncor), a YAC 273d11 (CEPH) |
| 15 | del(1)(p31.3p32.2) | [12] 2010 | Craniofacial anomalies, hypoplasia of corpus callosum, ventriculomegaly, hypotonia | 105K Oligoarray CGH & BAC array CGH, 4.93 Mb deletion, 1p32.2p31.3 (chr1:58,193,565-63,125,273)X1 *dn*, hg19 |
| 16 | del(1)(p36.3) | [13][a] 2010 | Prader-Willi like features. | MLPA, FISH with BAC probes, real-time q-PCR |
| 17 | del(1)(p31.1p32.2) | [14] 2014 | Craniofacial anomalies, partially hypoplastic corpus callosum, mild ventriculomegaly, intraparenchymal hemorrhages, cerebral palsy. | SNP- microarray (SNP-CMA), 22.9 Mb deletion (chr1:55,113,975-77,992,492)X1, hg19 |
| 18 | del(1)(p36.3) | [16] 2008 | Developmental delay, facial dysmorphisms, neuroblastoma | MLPA, 244 K oligo microarray, a deletion of 1.59 Mb at 1p36.3 and a duplication of 3.26 Mb at 1p36.3 (1,741,058-5,004,693)X3, hg18, FISH with Vysis 1p36 and BACs |
| 19[b] | del(1)(p31.3p32.1) | [17] 2007 | Abnormal corpus callosum, Ventriculomegaly, developmental tethered spinal cord, Chiari I malformation | array Comparative genomic hybridization (aCGH) |
| 20 | del(1)(p32.1p32.3) | [22] 2015 | Microcephaly, urogenital anomalies, hearing loss, choanal atresia. | SNP microarray, 6.4 Mb deletion (chr1:54,668,618-61,113,264)X1, hg19, FISH with BACs |
| DCP274057 | partial C-terminal duplication of *NFIA* | DECIPHER | 90 kb duplication at 1p31.3, global developmental delay | |
| DCP260253 | intragenic deletion of *NFIA* | DECIPHER | 117 kb deletion at 1p31.3, phenotype not available | |

**Table 1** Patients with 1p interstitial microdeletions *(Continued)*

| | | | |
|---|---|---|---|
| DCP285169 | intragenic duplication of *NFIA* | DECIPHER | 419 kb duplication paternally inherited at 1p31.3, additional 2.07 Mb maternal deletion at 15q13, delayed fine motor development, expressive language delay, impaired social interactions, receptive language delay |
| DCP288170 | intragenic *NFIA* deletion | DECIPHER | 229 kb deletion at 1p31.3, intellectual disability, macrocephaly |
| DCP300407 | del(1)p32.1 | DECIPHER | 281 kb deletion at 1p32.1, cognitive impairment |
| DCP264827 | del(1)p31.3 | DECIPHER | 5.43 Mb deletion at 1p31.3, abnormally folded helix, ADHD, constipation, flat forehead, global developmental delay, hypothyroidism, malar flattening |
| DCP276512 | del(1)p31.3p32.1 | DECIPHER | 8.83 Mb deletion at 1p31.3-1p32.1, delayed speech and language |

[a] Microdeletions without genomic coordinates reported in the pre-microarray era. Pt denotes patient
[b]Pt 19 has additionally a chromosomal translocation 46,XY,t(1;3)(p22;q21)dn

previously [19]. Lymphoblastoid cell line (LCL) was generated from the patient's blood in order to determine the transcript levels of genes of interests.

### Genomic DNA extraction and microarray

Genomic DNA was extracted from the patient's blood samples using a standard phenol-chloroform protocol with minor modifications. The human genome 244 K array (Agilent technologies, G4411B) was used to detect copy number variation as described previously in Miller et al. (2012) [20].

### Real-Time genomic qPCR and RT-qPCR

Primers targeting regions encompassing the proximal and distal deletion breakpoints were designed for qPCR. Primer pairs were first evaluated by determining the primer efficiency using a serial dilution of genomic DNA as template.

Primers were also designed against exonic regions of genes of interests for RT-qPCR. Total RNA was isolated from cell lines established from patient DGDP005 using the RNeasy Plus Mini kit (Qiagen) following the manufacturer's instructions. cDNA was synthesized from 1 μg of total RNA using the RevertAid First cDNA Synthesis Kit (Thermo Scientific) according to the manufacturer's protocol. All Real-Time qPCR reactions were carried out using 2 μl of sample, 10 ml of Fast Essential DNA Green Master (Roche) and 2.5 μM primers in a total reaction volume of 20 μl.

## Results

### Microarray

Microarray performed on genomic DNA derived from patient DGDP005 revealed a 9.45 Mb microdeletion at 1p31.3p32.2 (chr1: 57,633,718- 67,087,056, GRCh38/hg38). The deleted chromosomal region contains at least 35 genes, including *NFIA* (Fig. 2).

### Comparative deletion mapping

We compared all clinical features displayed by DGDP005 with five previously reported microdeletion cases namely, Campbell et al. (2002) [9], Koehler et al. (2010) [12], Ji et al. (2014) [14], Lu et al. (2007) [17], Rao et al. (2014) [21], Kehrer et al. (2015) [22] at 1p31.1p32.2 overlapping our microdeletion at 1p31.3p32.2, as well as one translocation case involving the *NFIA* gene in Lu et al. (2007) [17] (Table 3). We also compared the microdeletion in DGDP005 to seven cases from the DECIPHER database [24] (Fig. 2, Table 1). The refined candidate gene region represented by DCP300407 and proximal breakpoint of DCP276512 was depicted in two orange lines (Fig. 2), while two vertical black lines depict narrowed candidate region among 5 small CNVs including 4 DCP cases and a microdeletion of Rao et al. (2014) [21]. We examined the functions of all genes involved in the microdeletion by reviewing the literature to highlight candidate genes that could contribute to phenotypes observed in DGDP005 (Table 4). Patient DGAP174 of Lu et al. (2007) was not included in determining genotype-phenotype relationships (Table 3), because of an accompanying chromosomal translocation t(1;3)(p31.1; q25.1) [17].

### Real-Time qPCR

We performed qPCR to refine the flanking coordinates of the deletion breakpoints. qPCR assays using primers designed from the *DAB1* gene revealed that the distal deletion breakpoint is located between *DAB1* exon 1 and its 5′-UTR. The *SLC35D1* gene was found to be completely deleted as predicted by microarray (Figs. 2

**Table 2** Timescale of DGDP005's medical evaluations as well as her clinical features

| Age | Evaluation | Clinical features |
|---|---|---|
| <5 years | Pediatrician | - Crawling, sitting, walking and attaining language milestones delayed |
| | | - Craniofacial anomalies including macrocephaly |
| | | - Problematic motor skills. |
| ~10 years | Developmental pediatrician | - Special education implemented in curriculum |
| | | - Difficulty falling asleep and treatment with melatonin |
| | | - ADHD |
| | | - Hypertonia. |
| | | - Possible sensory motor difficulties. |
| 14 years | Standford Binet Intelligence Scales-Fifth edition (SB5) | - Difficulty staying on the task and needed to be redirected from time to time |
| | | - Overall thinking and reasoning at ~13 percentile. |
| | | - Borderline nonverbal reasoning abilities |
| | | - Verbal reasoning at ~12 percentile |
| | | - Verbal and nonverbal problem solving at ~ 58 percentile |
| | | - Ability to gather information at ~ 18 percentile |
| | | - Numerical problem solving at ~7 percentile. |
| | | - Borderline visual display abilities |
| | | - Ability to maintain attention at ~13 percentile. |
| | | - Full scale quotient of 83 (95 % confidence interval 79-87) suggesting intellectual disability. |
| 16 years | Individualized education program review team | - OHT |
| | | -ADHD |
| | | - Language disability in written language expression |
| | | - Disability in math calculation and reasoning |
| | | - Difficulties in fine graph motor functions with soft neurological signs. |
| | | - Continues to be a student with disability |
| 18 years | Child neurology services | - Developmental encephalopathy |
| | | - Cognitive impairment |
| | | - OCD as well as ADHD |
| | | -Treatment with fluoxetine (aka Prozac10 mg) and Adderall (15 mg) |
| | | - More pronounced facial dysmorphisms including prominent forehead, low-set ears, narrow nose thin lips |
| 22 years | Admitted to emergency | - Diagnosed with intraventricular hemorrhage with layering in the posterior fossa. |
| | | - Right anterior communicating artery aneurysm |
| | | - Developmental delay, OCD and ADHD |

and 3). The proximal deletion breakpoint was found to reside in the intergenic region between gene *SLC35D1* and uncharacterized gene *C1orf141* (Figs. 2 and 3).

### RT-qPCR

Expression analysis of six genes of interest by RT-qPCR revealed that the transcript levels of *NFIA*, *DAB1* and *DNAJC6* were markedly reduced in the patient relative to a healthy white female control (Fig. 4). Transcripts derived from *HOOK1* and *DOCK7* were reduced approximately by half, while *PDE4B* transcripts decreased moderately (Fig. 4).

## Discussion

The female patient (DGDP005) examined in this study was first reported as a 10-year old girl possessing a rare 1p32.1p32.3 microdeletion [10]. Characterization of the microdeletion in the patient by microarray allowed the refinement of the microdeletion from 1p32.1p32.3 to 1p31.3p32.2. The health condition of DGDP005 has

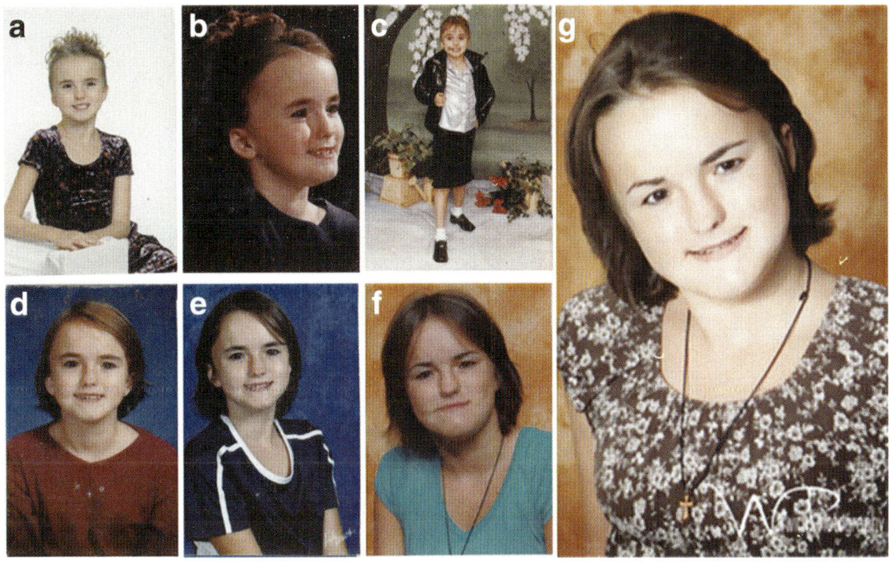


**Fig. 1** Phenotypic features of DGDP005. **a** Facial and head appearance including macrocephaly and upper body picture at 4 years (**b**) Lateral facial feature of 4 years of age showing frontal bossing (**c**) Full body picture as a 7 years old (**d**) upper body and head appearance presenting with macrocephaly at 12 (**e**) 13 (**f**) 16 and (**g**) 18 years of age

been monitored regularly since the first few months of her life. Psychomotor delay and craniofacial anomalies were apparent since infancy [10]. During the follow-up, she has continued to display developmental delay and as a result, special education has been implemented in her curriculum. Craniofacial anomalies such as macrocephaly and frontal bossing became more pronounced over time, suggesting the involvement of culprit gene(s) in continuous skull development since infancy [10]. Additional features such as OCD and intraventricular hemorrhage were also observed after the age of ten, emphasizing the importance of follow-up.

We have now determined the size of the deletion in DGDP005 by microarray and refined the locations of the flanking deletion breakpoints by qPCR (Figs. 2 and 3). The deleted region is at least 9.45 Mb encompassing more than 35 annotated genes including *NFIA* [17]. Only four smaller-sized heterozygous microdeletions (Rao 2014, Lu 2007, Koehler 2010 and Kehrer 2015) have been reported so far within this interval (Fig. 2). The patient of Koehler et al. (2010) [12] had a 1p31.3p32.2 microdeletion while another patient DGAP174 of Lu et al. (2007) had a deletion at 1p31.3p32.1 with additional translocation, 46,XY, t(1;3)(p31.1;q25.1) [17]. The patient of Rao et al. (2014) had a small microdeletion spanning exons 4–9 within *NFIA* [21]. The distal part of the microdeletion of Kehrer overlaps with the proximal part of DGDP005 and the more refined candidate region is represented by DCP300407. Two larger microdeletions of two half siblings (DGAP205-1 and DGAP205-1S) (Table 3) reported in Campbell et al. (2002) and a patient described in Ji et al. (2014) encompassing the whole chromosomal region deleted in DGDP005, have also previously been published [9, 14] (Fig. 2).

Haploinsufficiency of the *NFIA* gene is expected to cause an abnormal corpus callosum, ventriculomegaly or hydrocephalus, developmental delay, tethered spinal cord, Chiari I malformation, seizures, urinary tract defects, and craniofacial anomalies [17, 21]. Furthermore, disruption of *nfia* in mouse results in severe developmental defects including agenesis of corpus callosum, severe communicating hydrocephalus, female subfertility, and male sterility [24]. Five CNV cases (DCDP274057, DCP260253, DCP285169, DCP288170, Rao 2014) only had *NFIA* disrupted (Fig. 2). Among these five DECIPHER cases, DCP288170 with an intragenic deletion within *NFIA*, displayed intellectual disability. Although, this phenotype was not emphasized in Lu et al. (2007) [17], DGAP104 with a balanced translocation of t(1;20)(p31.3;q13.31) disrupting *NFIA* at 1p31.3 breakpoint (Table 3) also displayed intellectual disability (global IQ score of 52). Patient DCP274057 presents with global developmental delay while DCP285169 displays expressive and receptive language delay. The patient reported in Rao et al. (2014) with a deletion involving exons 4–9 of *NFIA* was only 8 years-old, and had not yet been evaluated intellectual disability [21]. The aforementioned patients clearly suggest that disruption of *NFIA* is likely to cause intellectual disability, or cognitive deficits. Indeed, the *NFIA* transcript levels were

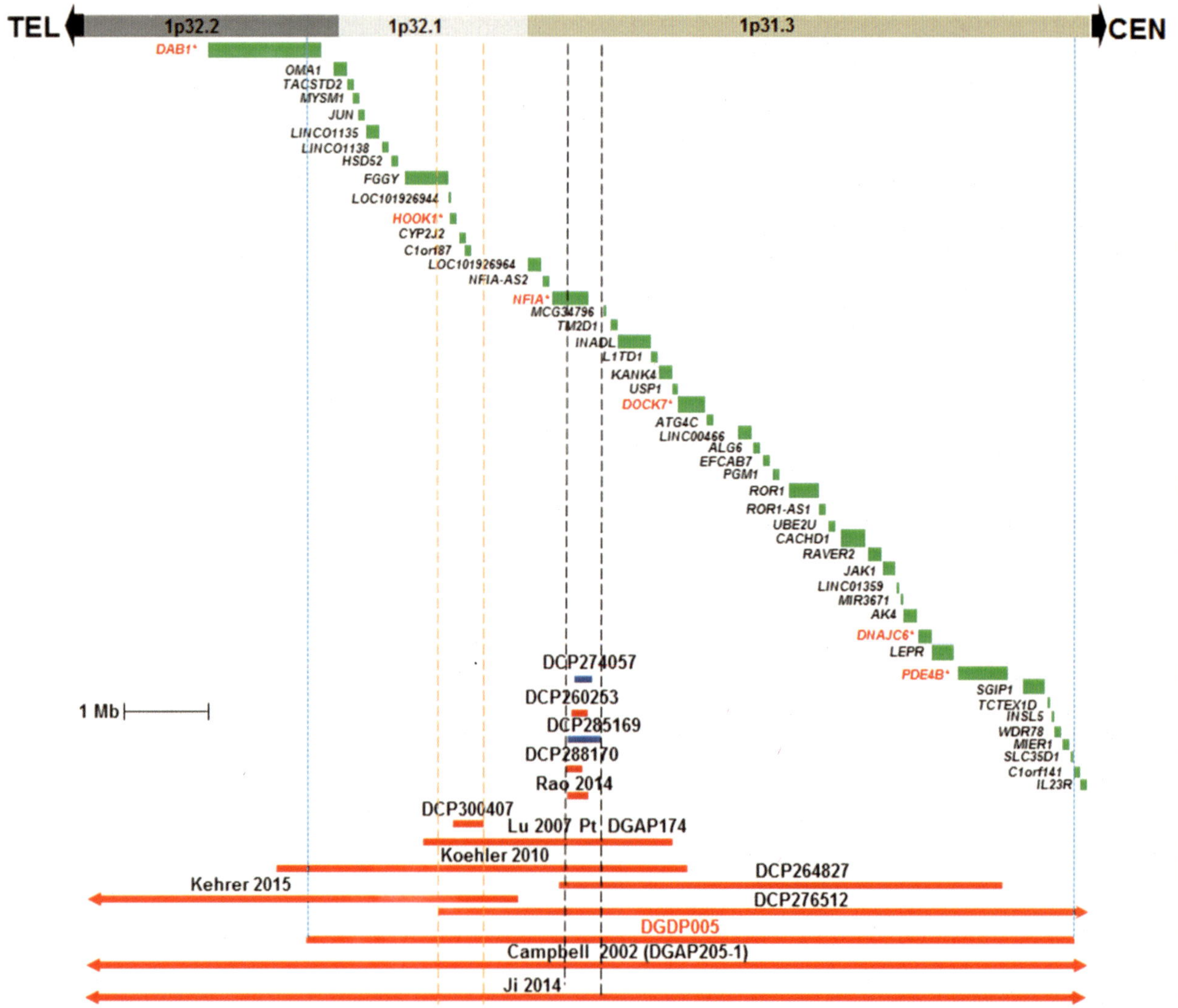


**Fig. 2** Comparative deletion mapping of patients with CNVs at 1p31.3p32.2. The genes located within this interval are displayed. Microdeletions are represented by solid red bars while microduplications are displayed in blue. Patients with CNVs from the DECIPHER database (Firth et al., 2009) are denoted by 'DCP' followed by the reference number. The sizes of the deleted regions in Rao 2014, Lu 2007 (DGAP174), Koehler 2010, Kehrer 2015, Campbell 2002 (DGAP205-1), Ji 2014 and seven DECIPHER cases relative to our patient (DGDP005) are displayed. Four CNVs (DCPP274057, DCP260253, DCP288170, Rao 2014) have only *NFIA* disrupted implying that it is causative gene in all four patients. Patient DCP285169 with a 419 kb duplication including the second half of *NFIA* presents with language delay, impaired social interactions, and delayed motor development. But he also has an additional 2.07 Mb microdeletion at 15q13. The microdeletion in patient DCP300407 does not include *NFIA*, yet the patient displays cognitive impairment, suggesting the likely contribution of *HOOK1*. Two microdeletions (Ji 2014 and Campbell 2002) extend beyond the 1p32.2 and 1p31.3 interval. Vertical lines in blue represent the proximal and distal boundaries of the microdeletion in DGDP005. Two orange lines are refined candidate gene region overlapping eight microdeletions including DCP300407. Two vertical black lines depict narrowed candidate region among 5 small CNVs [4 DCP cases and patient of Rao et al. (2014)]. Asterisk denotes candidate genes in this region

markedly reduced in DGDP005 (Fig. 4) suggesting that *NFIA* may be contributing to syndromic intellectual disability.

Notably, four microdeletion patients namely Campbell et al., 2002 [9], Koehler et al., 2010 [12], Ji et al., 2014 [14] and DGDP005 had in common macrocephaly (Table 3). Importantly, a balanced translocation patient DGAP104, in whom *NFIA* is disrupted at 1p31.3 [17] also had macrocephaly. Furthermore, the patient reported in Rao et al. (2014) [21] with a smaller microdeletion within *NFIA* also had macrocephaly (Fig. 2 and Tables 1 and 3). Collectively, these findings underscore that the haploinsufficiency of NFIA is sufficient to cause intellectual disability and macrocephaly, two of the core phenotypic features of del (1)(p31.3p32.2) microdeletion syndrome.

**Table 3** Clinical features of DGDP005 along with five additional microdeletion cases and a balanced translocation t(1;20)(p31.3;q13.31)*dn* disrupting the *NFIA* gene

| Clinical features | DGDP005 del(1)p31.3 p32.2 | Koehler et al. 2010 del(1)p31.3 p32.2 | Campbell et al. 2002 DGAP205-1 & DGAP205-1S del(1)p31.3 p32.3 | Ji et al.2014 del(1)p31.1 p32.2 | Rao et. al 2014 del(1) p31.3 | Lu et al., 2007 DGAP174[a] del(1)(p31.3 p32.1) | Lu et al., 2007 DGAP104 Balanced translocation t(1;20) (p31.3;q13.31)*dn* |
|---|---|---|---|---|---|---|---|
| Developmental delay | + | + | + | + | + | + | + |
| Intellectual disability | + | NS | + | NS | NS | + | + |
| Macrocephaly | + | + | + | + | + | + | + |
| Frontal bossing | + | - | + | NS | NS | NS | NS |
| Developmental encephalopathy | + | - | - | - | - | - | - |
| OHT | + | - | - | - | - | - | - |
| Intraventricular hemorrhage | + | - | + | + | - | - | - |
| Impaired motor skills | + | NS | + | NS | NS | + | + |
| Attention deficit disorder | + | NS | - | NS | NS | + | + |
| Hypertonia | + | NS | NS | NS | NS | - | NS |
| OCD | + | - | + | - | NS | - | - |
| Seizures | - | - | + | + | - | NS | NS |
| Abnormal corpus callosum | NS | + | + | + | + | + | + |
| Ventriculomegaly | - | + | + | + | + | + | - |
| Tethered spinal cords | - | - | + | - | - | + | + |
| Chiari I malformation | - | NS | + | - | - | + | + |
| Urinary tract defects | - | - | + | + | + | NS | - |

NS: Not Stated; Pt: Patient
[a]DGAP174 also has an additional chromosome translocation, 46,XY, t(1:3)(p31.1;q25.1)*dn*

**Table 4** Functions of candidate genes possibly contributing to clinical phenotypes observed in patient DGDP005

| Gene name | Gene symbol | Age | Association with neuro-developmental features | Remarks |
|---|---|---|---|---|
| Nuclear factor I/A | *NFIA* | [16] ~2 yrs<br>[21] 8 yrs | Abnormal corpus callosum, ventriculomegaly, hydrocephalus, developmental delay, tethered spinal cord, chiari I malformation, and urinary track defect | Disruption of *Nfia* in mice result in severe developmental defects including agenesis of the corpus callosum, severe communicating hydrocephalus, neurological defects, male sterility, female subfertility [24] |
| Dab, reelin signal transducer homolog 1 | *DAB1* | [37] ~7.5 yrs | Autism | |
| Hook homolog 1(Drosophila) | *HOOK1* | [23] 5 yrs | Cognitive impairment (DCP300407) | Cytosolic protein possessing a conserved N-terminal domain that binds to microtubules. Interacts with CLN3, the causative gene for autosomal recessive Batten disease. |
| Dedicator of cytokinesis 7 | *DOCK7* | [38] 5–7 yrs | Epileptic encephalopathy, dysmorphic features and intellectual disability | *DOCK7* plays a role in neural development |
| DnaJ (Hsp40) homolog, C, member 6 | *DNAJC6* | [31] 17–44 yrs | Parkinson disease Subfamily | - |
| Phosphodiesterase 4B, cAMP-specific | *PDE4B* | [35] NS | Schizophrenia | - |

NS; Not stated

While comparing the clinical features of our patient with the two half-siblings [9] who have a larger microdeletion including *NFIA*, we found that DGDP005 does not manifest ventriculomegaly, tethered spinal cord, Chiari I malformation, or urinary tract defects. Similarly, the patient having a smaller microdeletion encompassing *NFIA* [12] displayed only three of the clinical features as a result of *NFIA* deletion, namely abnormal corpus callosum, ventriculomegaly and developmental delay. Incomplete penetrance may partly explain why all phenotypes expected from *NIFA* disruption are not manifested in the patients with an *NFIA* deletion (Table 3 and Fig. 2) [25]. We have not included DGAP174 [17] in the comparison because he had a *de novo* translocation t(1;3)(p31.1; q25.1)*dn* in addition to a 2.2 Mb interstitial deletion at 1p31.3-p32.1 (Table 3).

Reviewing phenotypes displayed by patients with microdeletions at 1p31.3-1p32.2 enabled identification of at least 17 clinical features seen across all patients (Table 3). Because of the putative chromosomal segments with corresponding candidate genes for cognitive impairment within this region, it is obvious that not all phenotypes observed can be attributed to *NFIA* alone. It is likely that genes including *NFIA* in this region are haploinsufficient thereby contributing to the 17 clinical features observed across all patients (Table 3) [17]. It supports the idea that the 1p31.3p32.2 microdeletion may constitute a "chromosome syndrome" postulated in Zinner and Batanian

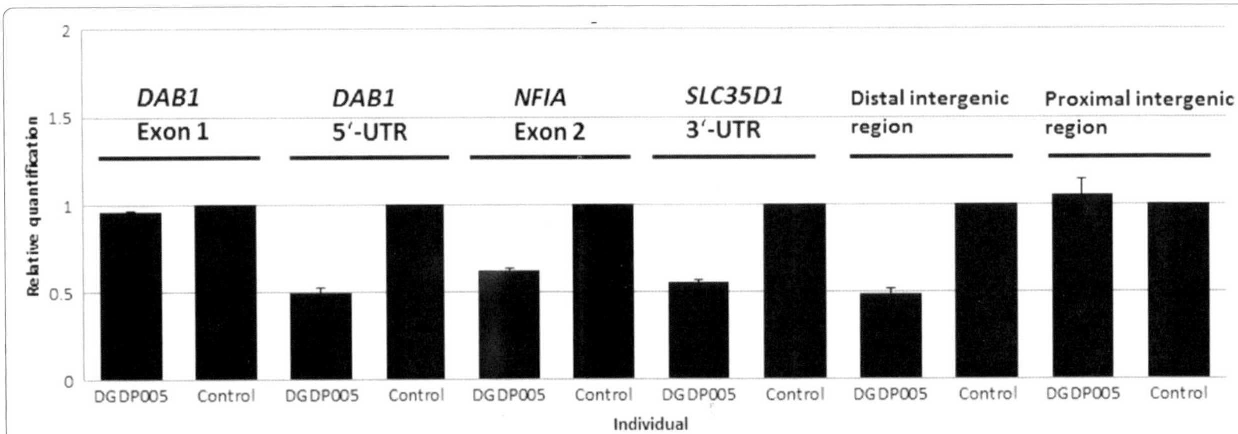


**Fig. 3** Refining the deletion breakpoints in DGDP005 by qPCR. The 5′-UTR of the *DAB1* gene is deleted while its first exon is intact indicating that the distal deletion breakpoint lies between *DAB1* exon 1 and the 5′-UTR. The *NFIA* gene and *SLC35D1* are both completely deleted in our patient. Two separate loci located in the proximal and distal intergenic region between *SLC35D1* and *C1orf141* were also assayed by qPCR. The distal intergenic region residing closer to *SLC35D1* was found to be contained in the microdeletion, while the proximal intergenic region was intact. A value close to 1 indicates that the locus is not deleted, while a value near 0.5 shows deletion on another allele

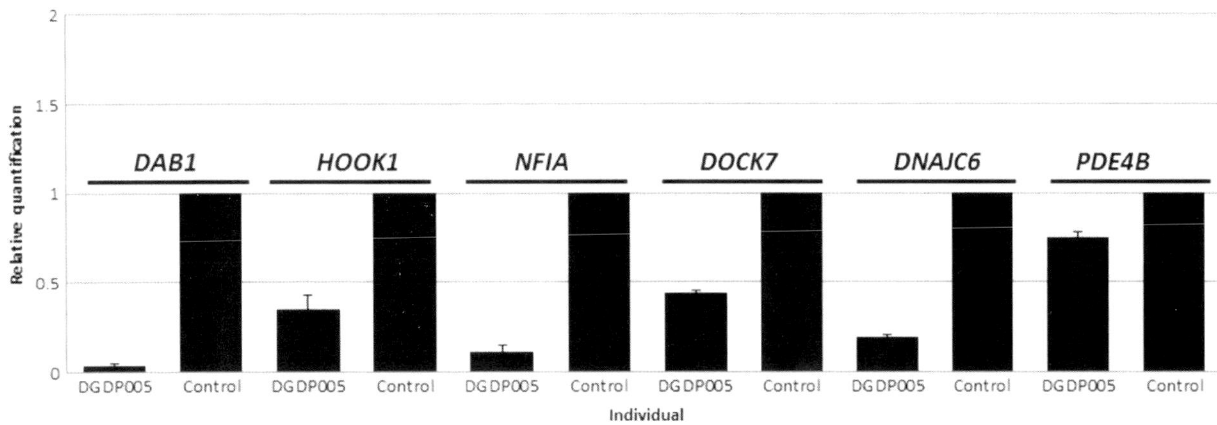


**Fig. 4** Transcript levels of six candidate genes involved in CNVs were determined by RT-qPCR. The level of transcripts of *DAB1*, *NFIA* and *DNAJC6* were markedly reduced in DGDP005 relative to the healthy white female control. Transcripts derived from *HOOK1* and *DOCK7* were reduced approximately by half, while *PDE4B* transcripts decreased moderately

(2003) [10], which meant to be contiguous gene deletion syndrome [26]. Recently, Ji et al. (2014) [14] also postulated the possible involvement of genes other than *NFIA*. We have reviewed the functions of all genes within the 1p31.3p32.2 microdeletion in DGDP005. Molecular dissection of this region suggests the presence of at least five chromosomal segments, with six candidate genes for intellectual disability. Each segment contains *DAB1*, *HOOK1*, *NFIA*, *DOCK7*, and *DNAJC6* as well as *PDE4B*, respectively. We propose six candidate genes (*DAB1*, *HOOK1*, *DOCK7*, *DNAJC6*, *PDE4B*, and *NFIA*) for the clinical features such as intellectual disability and OCD observed in DGDP005, because each of these genes is involved directly or indirectly in neurological disorders (Table 4).

While HOOK1 interacts with CLN3, the causative gene for the autosomal recessive Batten disease characterized by visual impairment, gait anomalies, seizures, dementia and sometimes mental deterioration [27–30], *DNAJC6* has been shown to be implicated in Parkinson disease [31]. It is noteworthy that Batten disease is also characterized by progressive neurodegeneration and impaired motor skills [32] like Parkinson disease [33, 34]. Furthermore, patient DCP300407 with only *HOOK1*, *CYP2J2* and *C1orf87* deleted (Fig. 2) displays cognitive impairment [24]. Additionally, *PDE4B* is implicated in schizophrenia [35], whereas *DAB1* truncated in our patient is required for synaptic function as well as associative learning in mice [36], and has been shown to be associated with autism [37].

Recently, mutation in *DOCK7* has been found to be associated with epileptic encephalopathies, dysmorphic features and intellectual disability [38]. Interestingly, DGDP005 displays some of the phenotypes expected from *DOCK7* mutation indicating that *DOCK7* may also contribute to intellectual disability and craniofacial anomalies in our patient. As is the case for *DOCK7*, cognitive impairment is an overlapping clinical feature also produced by disruption in *NFIA*. This further supports the hypothesis that deletion at 1p31.3p32.2 constitutes a contiguous gene deletion syndrome. As expected, the transcript levels of *DOCK7* and *HOOK1* was reduced approximately by half. The level of transcripts of *DAB1*, *DNAJC6* and *PDE4B* were also reduced in our patient relative to a healthy white female control (Fig. 4). The significant reduction of transcripts of *NFIA* and two additional genes (*DAB1* and *DNAJC6*) suggests an allele-specific expression pattern (Fig. 4). This may be due to a loss of the allele actively transcribed in the microdeletion. It is unclear whether the causative effect of each candidate gene is stoichiometrically contributing to the manifestation of the phenotype or an effect of one gene is masked by the effect of other gene when more than one candidate gene is deleted in a microdeletion. If some of the candidate genes participate in overlapping molecular pathways leading to cognitive impairment, the effect of one gene may be masked by another.

## Conclusion

Revisiting patient DGDP005 has allowed us to refine the flanking proximal and distal breakpoints, enabling us to compare the clinical phenotypes of DGDP005 to reported cases and unpublished DECIPHER cases. Comparative deletion mapping showed that there are at least six candidate genes including, *NFIA*, *HOOK1*, *DOCK7*, *DAB1*, *DNAJC6*, and *PDE4B*, that could contribute to the syndromic or non-syndromic intellectual disability. Most importantly, the genomic and clinical delineation result implies *NFIA* responsible for intellectual disability coupled with macrocephaly. Smaller-sized microdeletions across this interval and rare point mutations in the genes should reveal a better understanding of the pathological role of individual gene residing within this region. Additionally, expression studies including haploinsufficiency of aforementioned candidate genes in this interval will provide more insights both on the number of candidate genes and their impact on this contiguous gene syndrome.

## Consent

This study was approved by the Institutional Review Board of Augusta University and written informed consent was obtained from the mother of DGDP005 for the publication of this report and accompanying images.

#### Abbreviations

qPCR: quantitative polymerase chain reaction; DAB1: DISABLED, DROSOPHILA, HOMOLOG OF, 1; HOOK1: HOOK, DROSOPHILA, HOMOLOG OF, 1; NFIA: NUCLEAR FACTOR I/A; DOCK7: DEDICATOR OF CYTOKINESIS 7; DNAJC6: DNAJ/HSP40 HOMOLOG, SUBFAMILY C, MEMBER 6; PDE4B: PHOSPHODIESTERASE 4B, cAMP-SPECIFIC; CNV: copy number variation; FISH: fluorescent in situ hybridization; RT-qPCR: reverse-transcriptase quantitative polymerase chain reaction; ADHD: attention deficit hyperactivity disorder; ADD: attention deficit disorder; OCD: obsessive compulsive disorder; OHT: ocular hypertension; SB5: Stanford binet intelligence scales-fifth edition; FSIQ: full-scale intelligence quotient; DCP: DECIPHER; SLC35D1: SOLUTE CARRIER FAMILY 35 (UDP-GLUCURONIC ACID/UDP-N-ACETYLGALACTOSAMINE DUAL TRANSPORTER), MEMBER D1; C1orf141: Homo sapiens chromosome 1 open reading frame 141.

#### Competing interest

The authors declare that they have no competing interests.

#### Authors' contributions

JL generated data and wrote the manuscript. HGK conceived the project, analyzed and interpreted the data of comparative deletion mapping, and wrote the manuscript. Microarray was performed by YS. LL, MD, IKK revised the manuscript. All authors read and approved the final manuscript.

#### Acknowledgements

We would like to thank the patient who kindly consented to participate in our study. We wish to thank Lynn Chorich and Megan Sullivan. We also extend our thanks to Paul Browne. The present study makes use of data generated by the DECIPHER community. A full list of centres who contributed to the generation of the data is available from http://decipher.sanger.ac.uk and via email from decipher@sanger.ac.uk. Funding for the DECIPHER project was provided by the Wellcome Trust. This study was undertaken following the guidelines established by the Institutional Review Board at AU.

#### Author details

[1]Department of Obstetrics & Gynecology, Augusta University, 1120 15th Street, Augusta, GA 30912, USA. [2]Department of Neuroscience and Regenerative Medicine, Medical College of Georgia, Augusta University, 1120 15th Street, Augusta, GA 30912, USA. [3]Department of Neurology, Massachusetts General Hospital, Harvard Medical School, Boston, MA 02114, USA. [4]Department of Animal Science, Division of Applied Life Science (BK21plus), Institute of Agriculture and Life Science, Gyeongsang National University, Jinju, Gyeongsangnam-do, Korea. [5]Neuroscience Program, Medical College of Georgia, Augusta University, Augusta, GA 30912, USA.

#### References

1. Bene M, Duca-Marinescu A, Ioan D, Maximilian C. De novo interstitial deletion del(1)(p21p32). J Med Genet. 1979;16:323–7.
2. Petersen MB, Warburg M. Interstitial deletion 1p in a 30 year old woman. J Med Genet. 1987;24:229–31.
3. Lai MM, Robards MF, Berry AC, Fear CN, Hart C. Two cases of interstitial deletion 1p. J Med Genet. 1991;28:128–30.
4. Yoshino M, Watanabe Y, Harada N, Abe K. De novo interstitial deletion of 1p (pter——p34.1::p32.3——qter). J Med Genet. 1991;28:539–40.
5. Biegel JA, White PS, Marshall HN, Fujimori M, Zackai EH, Scher CD, Brodeur GM, Emanuel BS. Constitutional 1p36 deletion in a child with neuroblastoma. Am J Hum Genet. 1993;52:176–82.
6. Barton JS, O'Loughlin J, Howell RT, L'E OR. Developmental delay and dysmorphic features associated with a previously undescribed deletion on chromosome 1. J Med Genet. 1995;32:636–7.
7. Stockton DW, Ross HL, Bacino CA, Altman CA, Shaffer LG, Lupski JR. Severe clinical phenotype due to an interstitial deletion of the short arm of chromosome 1: a brief review. Am J Med Genet. 1997;71:189–93.
8. Martinez JE, Tuck-Muller CM, Gasparrini W, Li S, Wertelecki W. 1p microdeletion in sibs with minimal phenotypic manifestations. Am J Med Genet. 1999;82:107–9.
9. Campbell CG, Wang H, Hunter GW. Interstitial microdeletion of chromosome 1p in two siblings. Am J Med Genet. 2002;111:289–94.
10. Zinner SH, Batanian JR. Second reported patient with del(1)(p32.1p32.3) and similar clinical features suggesting a recognizable chromosomal syndrome. Am J Med Genet A. 2003;122A:164–7.
11. Neumann LM, Polster T, Spantzel T, Bartsch O. Unexpected death of a 12 year old boy with monosomy 1p36. Genet Couns. 2004;15:19–26.
12. Koehler U, Holinski-Feder E, Ertl-Wagner B, Kunz J, von Moers A, von Voss H, Schell-Apacik C. A novel 1p31.3p32.2 deletion involving the NFIA gene detected by array CGH in a patient with macrocephaly and hypoplasia of the corpus callosum. Eur J Pediatr. 2010;169:463–8.
13. Xu F, Cheng DH, Di YF, Tan K, Li LY, Lu GX, Tan YQ. Identification of a cryptic 1p36.3 microdeletion in a patient with Prader-Willi-like syndrome features. Zhonghua Yi Xue Yi Chuan Xue Za Zhi. 2010;27:524–9.
14. Ji J, Salamon N, Quintero-Rivera F. Microdeletion of 1p32-p31 involving NFIA in a patient with hypoplastic corpus callosum, ventriculomegaly, seizures and urinary tract defects. Eur J Med Genet. 2014;57:267–8.
15. Nyboe D, Kreiborg S, Kirchhoff M, Hove HB. Familial craniosynostosis associated with a microdeletion involving the NFIA gene. Clin Dysmorphol. 2015;24:109–12.
16. Isidor B, Le Cunff M, Boceno M, Boisseau P, Thomas C, Rival JM, David A, Le Caignec C. Complex constitutional subtelomeric 1p36.3 deletion/duplication in a mentally retarded child with neonatal neuroblastoma. Eur J Med Genet. 2008;51:679–84.
17. Lu W, Quintero-Rivera F, Fan Y, Alkuraya FS, Donovan DJ, Xi Q, Turbe-Doan A, Li QG, Campbell CG, Shanske AL, Sherr EH, Ahmad A, Peters R, Rilliet B, Parvex P, Bassuk AG, Harris DJ, Ferguson H, Kelly C, Walsh CA, Gronostajski RM, Devriendt K, Higgins A, Ligon AH, Quade BJ, Morton CC, Gusella JF, Maas R. L. NFIA haploinsufficiency is associated with a CNS malformation syndrome and urinary tract defects. PLoS Genet. 2007;3, e80.
18. Jun KR, Ullmann R, Khan S, Layman LC, Kim HG. Interstitial microduplication at 2p11.2 in a patient with syndromic intellectual disability: 30-year follow-up. Mol Cytogenet. 2014;7:52.
19. Nishimoto HK, Ha K, Jones JR, Dwivedi A, Cho HM, Layman LC, Kim HG. The historical Coffin-Lowry syndrome family revisited: identification of two novel mutations of RPS6KA3 in three male patients. Am J Med Genet A. 2014;164A:2172–9.
20. Miller DT, Shen Y, Wu BL. Oligonucleotide microarrays for clinical diagnosis of copy number variation and zygosity status.Curr Protoc Hum Genet. 2008;58:8.12.1– 8.12.17.
21. Rao A, O'Donnell S, Bain N, Meldrum C, Shorter D, Goel H. An intragenic deletion of the NFIA gene in a patient with a hypoplastic corpus callosum, craniofacial abnormalities and urinary tract defects. Eur J Med Genet. 2014;57:65–70.
22. Kehrer M, Schaferhoff K, Bonin M, Jauch A, Bevot A, Tzschach A. Interstitial 1p32.1p32.3 deletion in a patient with multiple congenital anomalies. Am J Med Genet A. 2015;167:2406–10.
23. das Neves L, Duchala CS, Tolentino-Silva F, Haxhiu MA, Colmenares C, Macklin WB, Campbell CE, Butz KG, Gronostajski RM. Disruption of the murine nuclear factor I-A gene (Nfia) results in perinatal lethality, hydrocephalus, and agenesis of the corpus callosum. Proc Natl Acad Sci U S A. 1999;96:11946–51.
24. Firth HV, Richards SM, Bevan AP, Clayton S, Corpas M, Rajan D, Van Vooren S, Moreau Y, Pettett RM, Carter NP. DECIPHER: Database of Chromosomal

Imbalance and Phenotype in Humans Using Ensembl Resources. Am J Hum Genet. 2009;84:524–33.
25. Cooper DN, Krawczak M, Polychronakos C, Tyler-Smith C, Kehrer-Sawatzki H. Where genotype is not predictive of phenotype: towards an understanding of the molecular basis of reduced penetrance in human inherited disease. Hum Genet. 2013;132:1077–130.
26. Schmickel RD. Contiguous gene syndromes: a component of recognizable syndromes. J Pediatr. 1986;109:231–41.
27. Spalton DJ, Taylor DS, Sanders MD. Juvenile Batten's disease: an ophthalmological assessment of 26 patients. Br J Ophthalmol. 1980;64:726–32.
28. Santavuori P. Neuronal ceroid-lipofuscinoses in childhood. Brain Dev. 1988; 10:80–3.
29. Luiro K, Yliannala K, Ahtiainen L, Maunu H, Jarvela I, Kyttala A, Jalanko A. Interconnections of CLN3, Hook1 and Rab proteins link Batten disease to defects in the endocytic pathway. Hum Mol Genet. 2004;13:3017–27.
30. Mole SE, Williams RE, Goebel HH. Correlations between genotype, ultrastructural morphology and clinical phenotype in the neuronal ceroid lipofuscinoses. Neurogenetics. 2005;6:107–26.
31. Koroglu C, Baysal L, Cetinkaya M, Karasoy H, Tolun A. DNAJC6 is responsible for juvenile parkinsonism with phenotypic variability. Parkinsonism Relat Disord. 2012;19:320–4.
32. Cotman SL, Staropoli JF. The juvenile Batten disease protein, CLN3, and its role in regulating anterograde and retrograde post-Golgi trafficking. Clin Lipidol. 2012;7:79–91.
33. Klein C, Schlossmacher MG. The genetics of Parkinson disease: Implications for neurological care. Nat Clin Pract Neurol. 2006;2:136–46.
34. Beitz JM. Parkinson's disease: a review. Front Biosci (Schol Ed). 2014;6:65–74.
35. Millar JK, Pickard BS, Mackie S, James R, Christie S, Buchanan SR, Malloy MP, Chubb JE, Huston E, Baillie GS, Thomson PA, Hill EV, Brandon NJ, Rain JC, Camargo LM, Whiting PJ, Houslay MD, Blackwood DH, Muir WJ, Porteous DJ. DISC1 and PDE4B are interacting genetic factors in schizophrenia that regulate cAMP signaling. Science. 2005;310:1187–91.
36. Trotter J, Lee GH, Kazdoba TM, Crowell B, Domogauer J, Mahoney HM, Franco SJ, Muller U, Weeber EJ, D'Arcangelo G. Dab1 is required for synaptic plasticity and associative learning. J Neurosci. 2013;33:15652–68.
37. Li J, Liu J, Zhao L, Ma Y, Jia M, Lu T, Ruan Y, Li Q, Yue W, Zhang D, Wang L. Association study between genes in Reelin signaling pathway and autism identifies DAB1 as a susceptibility gene in a Chinese Han population. Prog Neuropsychopharmacol Biol Psychiatry. 2013;44:226–32.
38. Perrault I, Hamdan FF, Rio M, Capo-Chichi JM, Boddaert N, Decarie JC, Maranda B, Nabbout R, Sylvain M, Lortie A, Roux PP, Rossignol E, Gerard X, Barcia G, Berquin P, Munnich A, Rouleau GA, Kaplan J, Rozet JM, Michaud JL. Mutations in DOCK7 in individuals with epileptic encephalopathy and cortical blindness. Am J Hum Genet. 2014;94:891–7.

# 22

# Identification of mosaic and segmental aneuploidies by next-generation sequencing in preimplantation genetic screening can improve clinical outcomes compared to array-comparative genomic hybridization

Hsing-Hua Lai[1], Tzu-Hsuan Chuang[1], Lin-Kin Wong[1], Meng-Ju Lee[1], Chia-Lin Hsieh[1], Huai-Lin Wang[1] and Shee-Uan Chen[2*]

**Abstract**

**Background:** Chromosomal mosaicism is observed as the presence of both euploid and aneuploid cells in a particular blastocyst. Recent studies have reported that the implantation rate of mosaic embryo transfer is remarkably lower than the euploid embryos. The superior capability of next-generation sequencing (NGS) to detect chromosomal mosaicism in preimplantation genetic screening (PGS) remains controversial, and several data displayed similar implantation and pregnancy rates using NGS or array comparative genomic hybridization (aCGH).

**Results:** In this study, the main inconsistency of aneuploidy detection and clinical performance between the NGS and aCGH were assessed. The phase I consisted of a parallel comparison in 182 blastocysts from 45 selected PGS patients for both the NGS and aCGH platforms. The phase II retrospectively compared the clinical outcomes of 90 patients with NGS-screened euploid embryo transfer to that of 129 patients with aCGH-screened euploid embryo transfer. The parallel comparison showed that the inconsistency of embryo euploidy was 11.8% ($p = 0.01$). Chromosomal mosaicism (10.7% with NGS *vs.* 3.9% with aCGH) and segmental aneuploidy (10.7% with NGS *vs.* 6.7% with aCGH) contributed to the discrepancy mainly. The chromosomally mosaic embryos (20%–50% of aneuploidy) and several embryos with segmental aneuploidy (≥10 Mbp) were hard to distinguish using the aCGH platform, but could be clearly identified using the NGS platform. After the first euploid embryo cryotransfer, the β-HCG(+) rate and implantation rate significantly increased in the PGS/NGS patients (HCG[+] rate: 73.3% in PGS/NGS *vs.* 60.5% in PGS/aCGH, $p = 0.048$; implantation rate: 53.2% in PGS/NGS *vs.* 45.0% in PGS/aCGH, $p = 0.043$). The clinical and ongoing pregnancy rates appeared higher in the NGS group, but did not reached statistical significance.

**Conclusions:** The results demonstrated that the NGS platform can identify embryos with chromosomal mosaicism and segmental aneuploidy more precisely than the aCGH platform, and the following clinical performance of NGS was more favorable.

**Keywords:** Preimplantation genetic screening/chromosome mosaicism/segmental aneuploidy/next-generation sequencing

* Correspondence: sheeuan@ntu.edu.tw
[2]Department of Obstetrics and Gynecology, National Taiwan University Hospital and College of Medicine, Taipei, Taiwan
Full list of author information is available at the end of the article

## Background

During the early stage of embryo development, chromosomal abnormalities (aneuploidies) often lead to growth arrest, repeated implantation failure, or recurrent miscarriage [1–3]. Embryonic aneuploidy is one of the main factors affecting the success rates of in vitro fertilization (IVF), and it originates from either a meiotic or a post-zygotic error. Increased maternal age is the primary cause of most meiotic errors, which occur during oogenesis. Other contributions to embryonic aneuploidy are the errors that arise after fertilization; even embryos produced by fertile couples could be aneuploid due to random mitotic flaws. Nonetheless, the aneuploid rate is comparatively higher for the couples undergoing IVF than for the fertile couples. In IVF-produced embryos, post-zygotic chromosomal abnormalities happen more frequently than the meiotic errors [4].

The presence of two or more distinct cell lines that exist in the same embryo is known as mosaicism, which is mainly caused by mitotic errors [5, 6]. Improper segregation of chromosomes in the first three cleavage divisions is reported to have the highest tendency toward mosaicism [7]. The three main mechanisms by which chromosomal mosaicism occurs, leading to a gain or loss of chromosomes, include anaphase lagging [8, 9], endoreplication [10], and non-disjunction [11]. Compared with the cleavage-stage embryos created by IVF, chromosomal mosaicism persists but occurs to a lesser extent in the blastocyst stage [12], in which these mosaic blastocysts have varying degrees of mosaicism. According to Fragouli et al [13], most mosaic blastocysts have different abnormalities in every cell (chaotic), but around 10% of these mosaics contain both diploid and aneuploid cells.

Because the embryonic aneuploidy affects IVF outcomes, selection of embryos without chromosomal aneuploidy for transfer using reliable comprehensive chromosome screening (CCS) techniques is a critical issue in the field of preimplantation genetic screening (PGS) [14–16]. Advances in CCS/PGS led to the development of array-comparative genomic hybridization (aCGH), which has become a widely-used method to analyze the whole chromosome copy numbers [17–19]. The aCGH platform is employed to analyze the chromosomal aneuploidy in metaphase II (MII) oocytes, cleavage stage embryos, and blastocysts [20, 21], and it indeed improved the clinical outcomes of IVF patients [22]. However, some limitations of the worldwide aCGH platform restrict it from detecting low-rate aneuploidy (chromosomal mosaicism) and segmental aneuploidy in biopsied trophectoderm (TE) samples. The narrow dynamic range for interpretation, human errors during the manipulation process, or inconclusive results caused by biological effects may introduce natural or artificial bias, which hampers the detection of chromosomal mosaicism and segmental aneuploidy in the embryos (A technical guide to aneuploidy calling with 24sure V3, Illumina).

Recently, next-generation sequencing (NGS) was introduced in the reproductive medicine as a new methodology for CCS [23–25]. Compared to the aCGH platform, NGS is a sequencing-based analysis technique and thus has higher resolution (about 2 mega base pairs, Mbp) and broader dynamic range (copy-number scale) for interpretation [23, 24]. Intriguingly, the consistency reported by several studies displayed the same efficiency in comprehensive aneuploidy screening between the aCGH and NGS platforms [26–28], and the author also observed that the identification of chromosomal mosaicism by NGS could be more sensitive than aCGH [27]. Still, there is no well-designed study to compare these two CCS platforms in a double-blind fashion by two independent laboratories.

According to the recent report released by the European Society of Human Reproduction and Embryology (ESHRE), the implantation rate of mosaic embryo transfer is significantly lower than that of euploid embryos [29]. Although a few mosaic embryos have the capacity of implantation or even live birth, the success rate is low [30]. Therefore, we performed a parallel comparison between the aCGH and NGS platforms to investigate the main cause of inconsistent results, and then compared the clinical outcomes of euploid embryo transfer by PGS/NGS with those by PGS/aCGH. We hypothesized that the main contribution to the inconsistency of the two CCS platforms was mosaic embryo identification, and clinical outcomes could be improved after excluding mosaic embryo transfer by screening with NGS.

## Methods

### Study design

This study was a retrospective analysis involving women with an indication for PGS in their IVF programs between 2014 and 2015. The study was approved by the appropriate ethics reviewing committee of National Taiwan University Hospital (Institutional Review Board Number: 201510127RIND). All patients were from the outpatient department of a fertility center (Hsinchu, Taiwan), and counseled by fertility specialists regarding the PGS. Consistency between the NGS and well-validated aCGH was assessed in the selected samples of 45 patients (182 blastocysts). In phase I, the embryos in the parallel comparison between NGS and aCGH were processed for TE biopsy, which was followed by whole genome amplification (WGA) and whole chromosome screening. The results of two platforms were compared for consistency. In phase II, the clinical outcomes of 90 women with PGS/NGS screened embryo transfers in 2015 were compared to those with 129 PGS/aCGH screened embryo transfers in 2014.

### Study objects

In the parallel comparison, 45 women were 21–42 years of age (mean age: 35.5 years). The patients with severe male infertile factors, advanced maternal age (≥36 years), history of repeated implantation failure, or using donated oocytes for single embryo transfer, and planned to undergo PGS in their IVF cycles were included. The patients underwent a complete consultation involving the possible advantages, previously reported success rates, and risks of misdiagnosis of the aCGH and NGS. In the comparison of clinical outcomes, 90 patients with PGS/NGS screened embryo transfers in 2015 and 129 patients with PGS/aCGH screened embryo transfers in 2014 displayed similar demographics. Written informed consents were obtained from all the couples included in the study.

### IVF and embryo biopsy procedure

The patients were treated with individualized stimulation protocols [31], following with oocyte retrieval operation. The MII oocytes were fertilized and cultured at 37 °C, 6.0% $CO_2$, 5.0% $O_2$. Embryos were cultured in groups, and droplets of one-step human embryo culture media (Global, LifeGlobal, USA) under mineral oil were used. A hole in the zona pellucida was made by laser (Saturn 5, Research Instrument, UK) in most 4-day-old embryos to assist embryo hatching. On day 5, the blastocysts with inner-cell mass (ICM) grading ≥ B [32] and a distinct cellular TE were biopsied. The other blastocysts that did not meet the criteria on day 5 were evaluated again on day 6 and day 7 for the possibility of biopsy.

In the biopsy procedure, around 5–10 TE cells were aspirated using a biopsy pipette (Origio, Måløv, Denmark) and then removed by shearing force between the biopsy pipette and holding pipette. The procedure was performed with micromanipulation equipment in droplets of PGD Biopsy medium (Global, LifeGlobal, USA). The biopsied TE cells were washed in sterile 1x phosphate-buffered saline (PBS) solution (Cell Signaling Technology, Cell Signaling Technologies, USA) containing 1% polyvinylpyrrolidone (PVP) solution (Sigma, Sigma-Aldrich, USA) twice. The washed cells were gently expelled into a 0.2-ml PCR tube with 2.5 μl of PBS/PVP to the following amplification, and then the blastocysts were vitrified. Details of the procedure can be found in Chang et al., 2013 [33].

### Whole-genome amplification, and DNA quantification

The biopsied cells were lysed, and the released genomic DNA was fragmented. The fragmented DNAs were amplified according to the manufacturer's procedures for the Sureplex WGA system (Sureplex, Illumina, USA). Succinctly, the biopsied cells were lysed by Sureplex cell extraction buffer and cell extraction master mix. Then they were incubated at 75 °C for 10 min followed by 95 °C for 4 min. The released genomic DNAs were randomly fragmented in Sureplex pre-amplification cocktail and incubated according to the following program: 1 cycle of 95 °C for 2 min, and 12 cycles of 95 °C for 15 s, 15 °C for 50 s, 25 °C for 40 s, 35 °C for 30 s, 65 °C for 40 s, 75 °C for 40 s, and holding at 4 °C. Finally, Sureplex amplification cocktail was added and the final program was as: 14 cycles of 95 °C for 15 s, 65 °C for 1 min, 75 °C for 1 min, and holding at 4 °C. The dsDNA High-Sensitivity (HS) Assay Kit (Qubit®, Life Technologies, USA) was used to quantify the concentration of amplified DNAs. After biopsy, the sample was treated with WGA. The amplification products from the 45 patients of the first phase were divided into two portions for the following aCGH and NGS analyses.

### aCGH analysis

The amplified WGA products were assessed by aCGH testing with 24sure V3 microarray (Illumina, Inc.) at the Genesis Genetic Asia Laboratory (Taiwan, Taipei). The products and reference DNAs were labeled with Cy3 and Cy5 fluorophores using random primers for 2–4 h. Then the labeling mixes were combined and co-precipitated with COT Human DNA in preparation for hybridization. Labeled DNAs were re-suspended in a dexsulphate hybridization buffer and hybridized onto the 24sure chip for 12 h. Thereafter, the chips were washed and dried. A laser scanner was used to read the resulting images, and BlueFuse Multi Software (Illumina, Inc.) was used to analyze the scan data. More details of aCGH testing procedure can be found in Huang et al., 2013 [34]. Once a specific amplification was observed, autosomal profiles were analyzed for gain or loss whole chromosomal ratios, using a 3 x SD assessment, greater than ± 0.3log2 ratio call, or both. For hybridization quality control, female samples hybridized with a male reference (sex mismatch) had to show a consistent gain of chromosome X and a consistent loss of chromosome Y [35].

### NGS analysis

The same WGA product of each sample was processed to prepare DNA libraries at the PGS laboratory of Stork Fertility Center (Hsinchu, Taiwan), by following the manufacturer's guidelines for VeriSeq PGS (Illumina, Inc). The diluted DNA (0.2 ng/μl, 1 ng total) was tagged and fragmented ("tagmented") using the Nextera XT transposome (Amplicon Tagmentation Mixture and Tagmentation DNA Buffer) through a limited-cycle PCR reaction. Then the index sequences were added to the samples to enable dual-indexed sequencing (2 x 36 bp). The tagmented DNAs with added indexes were amplified using the Nextera PCR Master Mix (NPM) through a PCR program: 1 cycle of 72 °C for 3 min, and 12 cycles of 95 °C for 10 s, 55 °C for 30 s, 72 °C for 30 s, 1 cycle at 72 °C for 5 min, and holding at 4 °C.

The PCR products were cleaned using the AMPure XP beads (A63881, Beckam Coulter, USA), providing a size selection from the population. After processing, the purified libraries were washed with 80% ethanol solution, then they were eluted by Nextera XT Resuspension Buffer. The purified DNA libraries were then normalized to equalize the quantity of each sample in the final pooling using the Library Normalization Additive and beads. Then, the normalized samples with equal volumes were pooled, denatured, and then sequenced. The Miseq Reagent Kit v.3 (Illumina, Inc) was used on a Miseq System (Illumina, Inc). The generated bioinformatics data was also analyzed by BlueFuse Multi Software (Illumina, Inc). Embryos were identified if they displayed a median chromosomal copy number deviated from the default copy number, and a possible trisomy or monosomy of autosomal chromosomes was seen as a copy number > 2 or < 2, respectively. Details of preparation procedures and the determination principles of automated copy number for each chromosome on BlueFuse Multi Software (Illumina, Inc.) were described in Fiorentino et al., 2014 [26].

#### Mosaicism identification

The detection sensitivity to chromosomal mosaicism on both CCS platforms were determined by a mixing experiment (Fiorentino, 2014 ESHRE abstract) [36]. The sample with whole chromosome loss/gain (100% of monosomy/trisomy) were serial diluted with euploid sample (50%, 40%, 30%, 20%, 10% of aneuploidy), and then were tested on the two CCS platforms. With aCGH system, the X-separation was used to distinguish mosaic embryos [28]. If the absolute $\log_2$ value of an aneuploidy was higher than half of the X-separation, this aneuploidy was determined as "pure," since the all tested cells in the fraction were like with this aneuploidy. In contrast, if the absolute $\log_2$ value of an aneuploidy was lower than half of the X-separation, it would be determined as mosaic, since this fraction could contain both euploid and aneuploid cells. With the NGS system, samples with ≥ 50% aneuploidy (>2.5 or < 1.5 copy number) could be distinguished clearly, and samples with aneuploidy between 20% and 50% (2.0 ± 0.2–0.5 copy number) could be observed only under the finest background (overall noise < 0.20). According to Greco et al., 2015 [30], the live births has been reported only in the transfers of mosaic embryo with under 50% of aneuploidy, and thus the embryos with aneuploid percentage between 20% and 50% was classified as mosaic (low-rate aneuploid). The embryos with aneuploid percentage under 20% was classified as euploid, and with aneuploid percentage over 50% as aneuploid.

#### Clinical outcomes and definition

The serum β-hCG was measured 2 weeks after cryotransfer of one or two euploid blastocysts, and if positive, transabdominal ultrasonography was performed at 7 weeks gestation. Once the gestational sac and fetal heartbeat were detected, the patient was considered to have achieved a clinical pregnancy. In contrast, the absence of an identifiable gestational sac was defined as "chemical pregnancy." After 16 weeks of gestation, the patient was included in the ongoing pregnancy group. The number of fetal heartbeat-positive pregnancies per transferred blastocyst was defined as the implantation rate (shown as a percentage). The miscarriage rate was defined as the number of 16-week pregnancies lost per cryotransfer (shown as a percentage).

#### Statistical analysis

The count data were presented as percentages, and the continuous data as averages with standard deviations (SDs). Multiple parameters compared between the groups were analyzed using the Student *t* test or Manny-Whitney *U* test, depending on the population distribution. Comparisons of percentage distribution between the groups were analyzed by Chi-square test. Significant differences were defined as two-sided *p*-value <0.05. All the analyses were generated using scientific GraphPad software (Prism, GraphPad Software, USA).

### Results

#### Patient profile

Forty-five patients (mean age = 35.5 years, range 21–42) selected from the study cohort undergoing PGS were involved in this parallel comparison of NGS and aCGH (Table 1). The causes of infertility included severe male factor (5/45, 11.1%), advanced maternal age (≥36 year, 20/45, 44.4%), repeated implantation failure (14/45, 31.1%), donated-oocyte recipients (6/45, 13.3%). Among all patients, 182 blastocysts were harvested and biopsied. Excluding the samples that failed to amplify, 178 embryos were screened by the NGS and aCGH.

#### Parallel comparison

Table 2 showed the results of double-blind interpretation of NGS and aCGH screening in 178 blastocysts obtained from the 45 patients. In the consistency assessment of embryo ploidy, aneuploid (51.1% with NGS *vs.* 46.1% with aCGH) and mosaic embryos (10.7% with NGS *vs.* 3.9% with aCGH) identified were both higher with NGS than aCGH. The percentage of embryos diagnosed as abnormal (aneuploid and mosaic) by NGS was 61.8%, while the percentage for aCGH was 50.0%. The overall inconsistency of embryo euploidy between the two CCS platforms was 11.8% (21/178, $p = 0.01$).

In the consistency assessment of aneuploid embryos, NGS detected 26 embryos with complex aneuploidy (≥3 variations), but 2 embryos in them were identified as merely monosomy and segmental aneuploidy, respectively, with the aCGH. An aneuploid embryo with both the ch.18

**Table 1** Patient profile of parallel comparison

| | |
|---|---|
| Patient number | 45 |
| Mean female age (years) | 35.5 (21–42) |
| Baseline AMH(ng/mL)[a] | 4.0 ± 3.7 |
| Antral follicle count[a] | 8.9 ± 4.4 |
| Indications[b] | |
| Severe male factor | 5 (11.1%) |
| Advanced female age (≧36 years) | 20 (44.4%) |
| Repeated implantation failure | 14 (31.1%) |
| Donated-oocyte recipient for single embryo transfer | 6 (13.3%) |
| Number of embryos biopsied (≧ grade BC) | 182 |
| Number of embryos with WGA failure | 4 |
| Number of embryos screened by PGS | 178 |

*AMH* anti-Mullerian hormone, *WGA* whole genome amplification, *PGS* preimplantation genetic screening
[a]Data are presented as mean ± SD
[b]Data are presented as the number of the class (percentage of the class)

**Table 2** Parallel comparisons between NGS and aCGH

| | NGS | aCGH | *P*-value |
|---|---|---|---|
| Patient number | 45 | | |
| No. of embryo screened | 178 | | |
| Euploid (%) | 68 (38.2%) | 89 (50.0%) | 0.01* |
| Aneuploid (%) | 91 (51.1%) | 82 (46.1%) | |
| Mosaic (%) | 19 (10.7%) | 7 (3.9%) | |
| Inconsistency of embryo euploidy[a] | 21 (11.8%) | | |
| Aneuploidy assessment | | | |
| No. of aneuploid embryo | 91 | 82 | |
| Complex aneuploidy (%) | 26 (28.5%) | 24 (30.5%) | 0.78 |
| Trisomy (%) | 14 (15.4%) | 13 (14.6%) | |
| Monosomy (%) | 32 (35.2%) | 33 (40.2%) | |
| Segmental aneuploidy (≥10 Mbp) (%)[b] | 19 (20.9%) | 12 (14.6%) | |
| Inconsistency of embryo aneuploidy[c] | 9 (5.1%) | | |
| Mosaicism assessment | | | |
| No. of mosaic embryo | 19 | 7 | |
| Whole chromosomal mosaicism | 16 (84.2%) | 5 (71.4%) | 0.59 |
| Segmental chromosomal mosaicism | 3 (15.8%) | 2 (28.6%) | |
| Inconsistency of chromosomal mosaicism[d] | 12 (6.7%) | | |

*NGS* next-generation sequencing, *aCGH* array-comparative genomic hybridization
**P*-values <0.05 are defined as statistically significant, and they are calculated by Chi-square analysis
[a]The number of euploid embryos were different on the two platforms
[b]The segmental aneuploidy was defined as the variation length reaching 10 Mbp by the both two laboratories
[c]The number of aneuploid embryos were different on the two platforms
[d]The detected chromosomal mosaicism were different on the two platforms

trisomy and duplication of ch.7p23.3-p21.2 on the NGS was identified as a mosaic on ch.18 by the aCGH (Fig. 1a). Eight aneuploid embryos with segmental variations (mean length = 30.8 Mbp) identified with the NGS were not detected on the aCGH (6 euploids and 2 suspected mosaics, Fig. 1b). Thus, the overall inconsistency of chromosomal aneuploidy between the two platforms was 5.1% (9/178, $p = 0.78$); the main discrepancy was the detection of segmental aneuploidy (10.7% with NGS, 19/178 *vs.* 6.7% with aCGH, 12/178).

In the consistency assessment of chromosomal mosaicism in the mosaic embryos, 12 mosaic embryos with whole chromosomal mosaicism identified with the NGS (mean aneuploid percentage = 34.4%) were not found by the aCGH (12 euploids, Fig. 2a). Additionally, three mosaic embryos with segmental chromosomal mosaicism on NGS (mean aneuploid percentage = 33.3%; mean length = 73 Mbp) were not detected by the aCGH (3 euploids, Fig. 2b). Only four mosaic embryos with chromosomal mosaicism were identified by both the two screening platforms, and three mosaic embryos detected by aCGH were identified as aneuploid embryos by NGS (aneuploid percentage >50%). Therefore, the overall inconsistency of chromosomal mosaicism between the two platforms was 6.7% (12/178, $p = 0.59$), and mosaicism detection was the main cause of inconsistency between the two platforms (10.7% with NGS, 19/178 *vs.* 3.9% with aCGH, 7/178).

**Clinical outcomes**

Table 3 displayed the reproductive outcomes of the 90 patients with PGS/NGS-diagnosed embryo transfer in 2015 and the 129 patients with PGS/aCGH-diagnosed embryo transfer in 2014. Of the initial PGS results, the beginning number of patients undergoing PGS was 135 in the NGS group and 202 in the aCGH group; the number of PGS-screening embryos was 472 in the NGS group and 827 in the aCGH group, respectively. The detection rate of mosaicism was significantly higher in the NGS group of 5.3% (25/472) than in the aCGH group of 1.7% (14/827) ($p < 0.01$), while the rate of segmental aneuploidy showed no difference between the two groups (10.2% [48/472] *vs.* 9.6% [79/827], $p = 0.77$). The patients with euploid embryos were enrolled in this study for transfer, and the patients with no euploid embryos were excluded. The percentage of exclusion was 32.6% (44/135) in the NGS group, greater than 20.8% (42/202) in the aCGH group ($p = 0.02$). Of the comparisons of clinical outcomes, no significant differences were observed in the baseline characteristics of patients undergoing transfer(s), including the female age, infertility indication, anti-Müllerian hormone (AMH), antral follicle count (AFC), and mean endometrial thickness before transfer. The β-HCG positive rate and implantation rate after the first cryotransfer were significantly higher in the

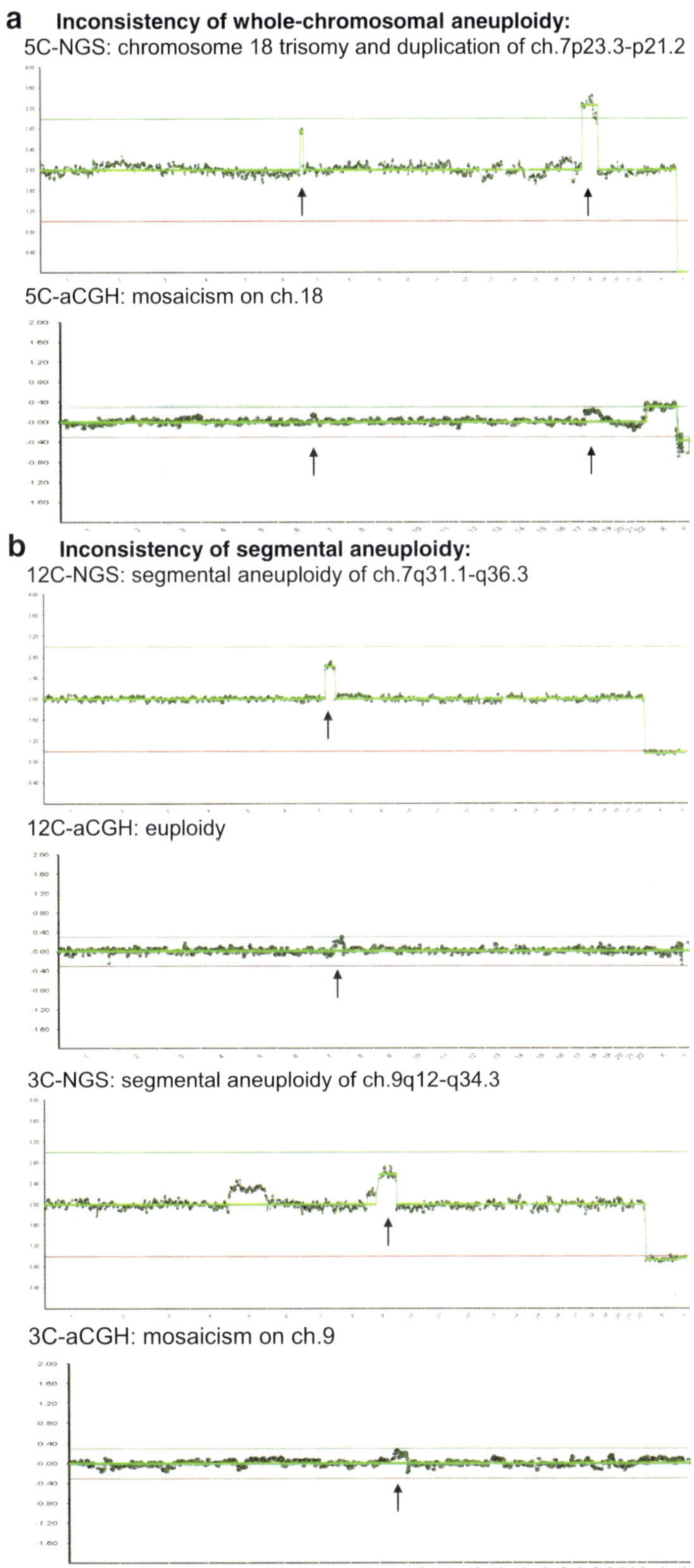


**Fig. 1** (See legend on next page.)

(See figure on previous page.)
**Fig. 1** Examples of inconsistent aneuploidy between the two chromosome screening platforms generated by the same amplification products. NGS, next-generation sequencing; aCGH, array-comparative genomic hybridization. **a** Embryo 5C was identified as aneuploid with trisomy 18 and duplication of ch.7p23.3-p21.2 using the NGS platform, but the aneuploidy was suspected as mosaicism at ch.18 using the aCGH platform. **b** Embryo 12C was identified as aneuploid with duplication of ch.7 q31.1-q36.3 using the NGS platform (47 Mbp), but the aneuploidy was not obvious with the aCGH platform. Embryo 3C was identified as aneuploid with duplication of ch.9q12-q34.3 using the NGS platform (83 Mbp), but the aneuploidy was suspected as mosaicism with the aCGH platform

NGS group than the aCGH group (HCG(+) rate: 73.3% *vs.* 60.5%, $p = 0.048$; implantation rate: 53.2% *vs.* 45.0%, $p = 0.043$). The clinical pregnancy rate and ongoing pregnancy rate appeared higher, and the miscarriage rate was lower in the NGS group than those in the aCGH group. However, the difference did not reach statistical significance. The average number of transferred embryos in both groups was 1.2 blastocysts.

## Discussion

The present analysis is the first study to demonstrate that the PGS/NGS platform can identify embryos with

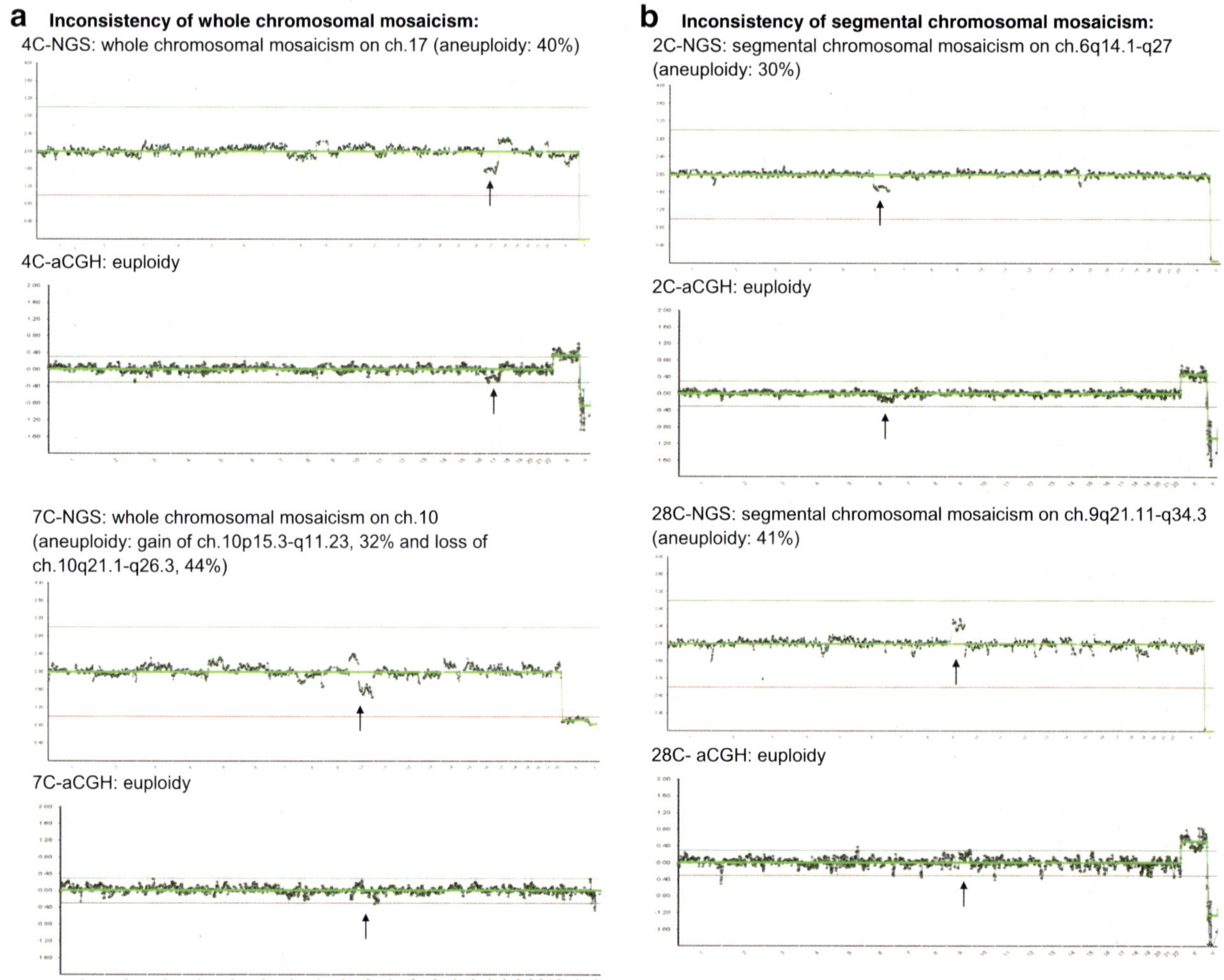


**Fig. 2** Examples of inconsistent mosaicism between the two chromosome screening platforms generated by the same amplification products. NGS, next-generation sequencing; aCGH, array-comparative genomic hybridization. **a** Embryo 4C was identified as mosaic with partial deletion of ch.17 (40% of aneuploidy) using the NGS platform, but the mosaicism was not obvious with the aCGH platform. Embryo 7C was identified as mosaic with both the partial duplication of ch.10p15.3-q11.23 (32% of aneuploidy) and partial deletion of ch.10q21.1-q26.3 (44% of the aneuploidy) using the NGS platform, but the mosaicism was not obvious with the aCGH platform. **b** Embryo 2C was identified as mosaic with partial deletion of ch.6q14.1-q27 using the NGS platform (30% of aneuploidy), but the segmental chromosomal mosaicism was not detected using the aCGH platform. Embryo 28C was identified as a mosaic with partial duplication of 9q21.11-q34.3 using the NGS platform (41% of aneuploidy), but the segmental chromosomal mosaicism was not detected using the aCGH platform

**Table 3** Clinical outcomes of patients undergoing NGS and aCGH

| | NGS | aCGH | *P*-value |
|---|---|---|---|
| Number of patients undergoing PGS | 135 | 202 | — |
| Number of embryos diagnose by PGS[a] | 472 | 827 | — |
| Euploid | 180 (38.1%) | 364 (44.0%) | 0.04* |
| Aneuploid | 219 (46.4%) | 370 (44.7%) | 0.60 |
| Mosaic | 25 (5.3%) | 14 (1.7%) | <0.01** |
| Segmental aneuploid | 48 (10.2%) | 79 (9.6%) | 0.77 |
| Number of patients with no euploid embryo to transfer[a] | 44 (32.6%) | 42 (20.8%) | 0.02* |
| Aneuploid | 23 (17.0%) | 32 (15.8%) | 0.77 |
| Mosaic | 6 (4.4%) | 0 (0%) | — |
| Segmental aneuploid | 15 (11.1%) | 10 (5.0%) | 0.05 |
| Number of transferred patients[a] | 90 (66.7%) | 129 (63.9%) | — |
| Mean female age (years)[b] | 37.5 ± 5.5 (27–53) | 37.2 ± 4.5 (27–51) | 0.68 |
| Indications[a] | | | |
| Severe male factor | 9 (10%) | 25 (19%) | 0.08 |
| Advanced female age (≥36 years) | 32 (36%) | 42 (33%) | |
| Repeated implantation failure | 32 (36%) | 47 (36%) | |
| Oocyte –donation cycle for SET | 17 (19%) | 15 (12%) | |
| Baseline AMH (ng/mL)[b] | 4.5 ± 3.7 | 4.9 ± 3.6 | 0.42 |
| Antral follicle count[b] | 11.0 ± 4.6 | 11.2 ± 4.7 | 0.82 |
| Mean endometrial thickness (mm)[b] | 9.3 ± 1.8 | 9.2 ± 1.4 | 0.72 |
| Clinical outcomes after the first cryotransfer[a] | | | |
| HCG(+) pregnancy | 66 (73%) | 78 (60%) | 0.048* |
| Implantation | 64 (53%) | 67 (45%) | 0.043* |
| Clinical pregnancy | 59 (66%) | 73 (57%) | 0.18 |
| Ongoing pregnancy | 51 (57%) | 59 (46%) | 0.11 |
| Multiple pregnancy | 3 (3%) | 4 (3%) | 1.00 |
| Miscarriage | 8 (9%) | 14 (11%) | 0.48 |
| Average transferred embryo per cryotransfer[b] | 1.2 ± 0.5 | 1.2 ± 0.4 | 0.11 |

*AMH* anti-Müllerian hormone, *NGS* next-generation sequencing, *aCGH* array-comparative genomic hybridization, *SET* single embryo transfer

**P*-values <0.05 indicates statistical significance, and they are calculated by either the Mann-Whitney *U* test or Chi-square test depending on the population

[a]Data are presented as the number of the class (percentage of the class)

[b]Data are presented as mean ± SD

chromosomal mosaicism and segmental aneuploidy more precisely than the PGS/aCGH platform. Furthermore, we showed that the clinical outcomes of patients with NGS-screened embryo transfer had significantly better results than those with aCGH-screened embryo transfer after excluding the transfers of mosaic and segmental aneuploid embryos.

The study included a parallel comparison and a clinical outcome comparison between the two CCS platforms. In the first parallel comparison, the amplified products of samples were analyzed with both the NGS and aCGH, which were produced by the same manufacture (Illumina, San Diego, USA). The analyses of raw data were conducted using the same software (BlueFuse Multi, Illumina, Inc.), and the final interpretations were determined by the two independent laboratories in a double-blind fashion. The inconsistency between the two CCS platforms was 11.8% ($p = 0.01$). This discrepancy was mainly due to the identification of mosaicism (10.7% with NGS *vs.* 3.9% with aCGH), including both whole chromosomal mosaicism (9.0% with NGS *vs.* 2.8% with aCGH), and segmental chromosomal mosaicism (1.7% with NGS *vs.* 1.1% with aCGH). The total percentage of mosaic embryos detected with NGS in the study (10.7%) was similar to that of Fragouli et al., 2011, around 10% [13]. The second cause of inconsistency was the detection of segmental aneuploidy (10.7% with NGS *vs.* 6.7% with aCGH). The reported incidences of segmental aneuploidy varied broadly between studies [28]. The total percentage of segmental-aneuploid embryos detected with NGS in this study was slightly higher than the past data, which the aCGH was used [37], around 6%–7%.

The robust detection power of NGS platform resulted in a more accurate screening of embryos with low-rate and segmental aneuploidies compared to aCGH, which reflected in the following comparison of clinical outcomes. Since the lower implantation rate and live births of mosaic embryo has been reported [29, 30], we excluded the patients with mosaic embryo transfer in the phase II comparison to assess the clinical performance in euploid embryos of two platforms. With similar patient demographics, the patients with NGS-screened embryo transfer achieved significantly higher HCG(+) rate (73.3% *vs.* 60.5%, $p = 0.048$) and implantation rate (53.2% *vs.* 45.0%, $p = 0.043$) than patients with aCGH-screened embryo transfer. Possibly due to the sample size, the clinical and ongoing pregnancy rates did not reach significant difference between two arms, and the NGS group displayed more favorable. We have concluded that NGS screened embryo transfer had significantly better results than aCGH after control the proportion of mosaic or segmental aneuploidy, which could influence the clinical outcome of IVF. The percentages of patients excluded for transfer due to mosaicism or segmental aneuploid in the NGS group appeared higher than those in the aCGH group, but no significance reached yet (mosaic: 4.4% *vs.* 0%; segmental aneuploid: 11.1% *vs.* 5.0%, $p = 0.05$). The results implied that the efficacy of single euploid embryo transfer may be effectively improved by the NGS screening due to the more rigorous identification of mosaic and segmental-aneuploid embryos, whose competency deserves further study to validate [25, 29, 30].

Accordingly, NGS possesses two advantages compared to aCGH for the identification of low-rate and segmental aneuploidies: a broader dynamic range for interpretation of low-rate aneuploidy (mosaicism) and increased chromosomal resolution of about 2 Mbp to detect segmental aneuploidy. Moreover, a library-based sample preparation could also decrease the background noise caused by artifacts, which may affect the final aneuploid results [26, 38]. Nonetheless, several data have reported that no significant differences were found in detection of mosaicism or segmental aneuploidy between the NGS and aCGH platforms in strict parallel comparisons [27, 28, 39]. In contrast, the present study showed that identification of both mosaicism and segmental aneuploidy differed significantly between the NGS and aCGH platforms when mosaicism was defined as an aneuploid rate between 20% and 50% (low-rate aneuploidy) [30], and segmental aneuploidy was defined as $\geq 10$ Mbp [40]. Since both the demographics of patients and sample size of parallel comparison in our study were very similar to those of Yang et al. in 2015 [27], the opposite results could be due to the different definitions used for data interpretation.

Chromosomal mosaicism is common during preimplantation development. It was once reported as 65% and 70% during the early mitotic stage [41, 42], and as 10% during the blastocyst stage [4]. The chromosomal mosaicism was also observed in the prenatal tests of non-IVF people, including chorionic villus (about 1.78%) and amniotic fluid (about 0.46%) [43]. The propagation of abnormal cell line(s) in the mosaic embryos had negative effect in the pregnancy, and the undetected mosaicism and aneuploidies in the PGS/aCGH was recently reported as a cause to the first trimester pregnancy loss [44]. However, the IVF patients with single mosaic embryo transfer could still achieve live births according to Greco el al., 2015 [30], and thus the competency of mosaic embryo remained uncertain. Additionally, the incidence of confined placental mosaicism (CPM) would also be a bias to the accuracy of PGS, which the trophectoderm samples were used [12]. According to our preliminary data during 2015 and 2016, two out of ten patients with NGS-diagnosed mosaic embryo transfer had normal reports of amniocentesis (both karyotyping and array screening) and then achieved live births (data not shown).

Although excluding mosaic and segmental aneuploid embryo transfer based on NGS identification led to significantly higher HCG(+) rate and implantation rate in this study, some patients with advanced maternal age may not have any euploid embryo to transfer and must consider mosaic embryo transfer instead. Thus both complete consultations before mosaic embryo transfer and appropriate prenatal testing after mosaic embryo transfer are mandatory in these patients. For mosaic embryos, we should counsel the possibility of discarding a competent embryo versus transferring an embryo that may have a lower implantation potential and possible adverse obstetrical and neonatal outcomes [45]. In this study, six out of 44 patients only had mosaic embryos to consider transfer in the NGS group, and none in the aCGH group. After complete consultation, all of them choose to transfer the unscreened embryos rather than transferring the mosaics [46].

The study is also restricted by its retrospective nature. Certainly, it is not known whether mosaic or segmental-aneuploid embryo transfers were actually involved in the outcomes of PGS/aCGH group, and it is only assumed that the reduced clinical outcomes of patients with aCGH-screened embryo transfer were due to the methodological limitation of chromosomal mosaic detection and segmental aneuploidy identification. In addition, there is a possibility for false positive rate with NGS testing, given the fact that certain level, different distribution, or the segmental size of aneuploidy of mosaicism could be harmless. The detection of mosaicism or small-size aneuploidy are still challenged by both the biological and technical biases, which include sampling bias, confined mosaicism, reciprocal errors, artifacts from whole-genome amplification, S-phase artifacts, or smoothing mask from algorithm [47, 48]. Two independent laboratories interpreted the data generated from the same amplified products on the two CCS platforms in this study. Although the interpretation would be made in a double-blind manner, the subjective decisions may be involved in samples without the finest overall backgrounds of CCS. The aCGH is a widely prevalent CCS platform in PGS. However, the accuracy is difficult to be defined merely based on the parallel comparison between aCGH and NGS, since their methodologies are completely different. The array system has been applied and verified in prenatal and postnatal diagnoses for years, other than higher resolution, but also for its efficiency on mosaicism and CNVs micro-deletion and micro-duplication detection. However, the aCGH for preimplantational testings and the arrays for prenatal/postnatal testings involved different probe designs and cell number, and thus with different resolutions. The widely-used aCGH for PGS in this study has broad coverage to the 24 chromosomes, but with comparatively lower resolution. The mosaicism with aneuploid ratio under 40% or segmental aneuploidy with length <5 Mbps are difficult to be detected in clinical application. Therefore, the inconsistency in this study seems to be more likely originated from the methodological limitations of aCGH itself.

Up to now, there is no consensus for the golden standard method in CCS. A future study with the third platform, such as oligo-array or single nucleotide polymorphism (SNP) array could be applied to evaluate the mosaicism and segmental aneuploidy detected with either aCGH or NGS platform. Furthermore, the examinations to samples from miscarriages with PGS-diagnosed mosaic or segmental aneuploid embryo transfer can also clarify the actual effect of detected abnormalities.

## Conclusions

Conclusively, this study demonstrated that the PGS/NGS platform identified the embryos with chromosomal mosaicism and segmental aneuploidy more clearly than that of PGS/aCGH. Upon excluding the transfer of mosaic and segmental-aneuploid embryos, the patients with NGS-screened embryo transfer achieved significantly higher HCG(+) and implantation rates than those with aCGH-screened embryo transfer. The clinical and ongoing pregnancy rates appeared higher, but did not reached statistical significance in the NGS group. A large randomized controlled clinical trial confirming the clinical effectiveness is needed to validate these findings before the extensive use of NGS-based PGS.

### Abbreviations

aCGH: Array comparative genomic hybridization; AFC: Antral follicle count; AMH: Anti-Müllerian hormone; CCS: Comprehensive chromosome screening; CPM: Confined placental mosaicism; ICM: Inner-cell mass; IVF: In vitro fertilization; MII: Metaphase II; NGS: Next-generation sequencing; PGS: Preimplantation genetic screening; SNP: Single nucleotide polymorphism; TE: Trophectoderm; WGA: Whole genome amplification

### Acknowledgements

The authors thank Jhih-Yuan Hsieh, scientist at the Department of Preimplantation Genetic Laboratory, Stork Fertility Center (Hsinchu, Taiwan), and John Chan, senior manager at the Genesis Genetics Asia Laboratory (Taipei, Taiwan) for conducting the two CCS analyses in the study.

### Funding

No external funding was obtained for this study.

### Authors' contributions

HL designed the study concept; TC analyzed the collected data and wrote the manuscript; LW collected the raw data; ML, CH, and HW recruited the patients; SC reviewed the manuscript, revised the final version, and approved the submitted version.

### Competing interest

The authors declare that they have no competing interests.

### Author details

[1]Stork Fertility Center, Stork Ladies Clinic, Hsinchu, Taiwan. [2]Department of Obstetrics and Gynecology, National Taiwan University Hospital and College of Medicine, Taipei, Taiwan.

### References

1. Voullaire L, Wilton L, McBain J, Callaghan T, Williamson R. Chromosome abnormalities identified by comparative genomic hybridization in embryos from women with repeated implantation failure. Mol Hum Reprod. 2002;8: 1035–41.
2. Rubio C, Simon C, Vidal F, Rodrigo L, Pehlivan T, Remohi J, et al. Chromosomal abnormalities and embryo development in recurrent miscarriage couples. Hum Reprod. 2003;18:182–8.
3. Hodes-Wertz B, Grifo J, Ghadir S, Kaplan B, Laskin CA, Glassner M, et al. Idiopathic recurrent miscarriage is caused mostly by aneuploid embryos. Fertil Steril. 2012;98:675–80.
4. Delhanty Joy DA. The origins of genetic variation between individual human oocytes and embryos: implications for fertility. Hum Fertil. 2013;16:241–5.
5. Delhanty JD, Harper JC, Ao A, Handyside AH, Winston RM. Multicolour FISH detects frequent chromosomal mosaicism and chaotic division in normal preimplantation embryos from fertile patients. Hum Genet. 1997;99:755–60.
6. Munné S, Sandalinas M, Escudero T, Màrquez C, Cohen J. Chromosome mosaicism in cleavage-stage human embryos: evidence of a maternal age effect. Reprod Biomed Online. 2002;4:223–32.
7. Katz-Jaffe MG, Trounson AO, Cram DS. Mitotic errors in chromosome 21 of human preimplantation embryos are associated with non-viability. Mol Hum Reprod. 2004;10:143–7.

8. Coonen E, Derhaag JG, Dumoulin JCM, van Wissen LCP, Bras M, Janssen M, et al. Anaphase lagging mainly explains chromosomal mosaicism in human preimplantation embryos. Hum Reprod. 2004;19:316–24.
9. Capalbo A, Bono S, Spizichino L, Biricik A, Baldi M, Colamaria S, et al. Sequential comprehensive chromosome analysis of polar bodies, blastomeres and trophoblast: insights into female meiotic errors and chromosomal segregation in the preimplantation window of embryo development. Hum Reprod. 2003;28: 509–18.
10. Fox DT, Duronio RJ. Endoreplication and polyploidy: insights into development and disease. Develop. 2013;140:3–12.
11. Bean CJ, Hassold TJ, Judi L, Hunt PA. Fertilization in vitro increases non-disjunction during early cleavage divisions in a mouse model system. Hum Reprod. 2002;17:2362–7.
12. Johnson DS, Cinnioglu C, Ross R, Filby A, Gemelos G, Hill M, et al. Comprehensive analysis of karyotypic mosaicism between trophectoderm and inner cell mass. Mol Hum Reprod. 2010;16:944–9.
13. Fragouli E, Escalona A, Gutierre-Mateo C, Tormasi S, Sepulveda S, Noriega L, et al. Comparative genomic hybridization of blastocysts with use of FISH, CHG, and aCGH: scientific data and technical evaluation. Hum Reprod. 2011;26:480–90.
14. Chen M, Wei S, Hu J, Quan S. Can Comprehensive Chromosome Screening Technology Improve IVF/ICSI Outcomes? A Meta-Analysis PLoS One. 2015; 10:e0140779.
15. Dahdouh EM, Balayla J, García-Velasco JA. Impact of blastocyst biopsy and comprehensive chromosome screening technology on preimplantation genetic screening: a systematic review of randomized controlled trials. Reprod Biomed Online. 2015;30:281–9.
16. SenGupta SB, Dhanjal S, Harper JC. Quality control standards in PGD and PGS. Reprod Biomed Online. 2016;32:263–70.
17. Yang Z, Salem SA, Liu X, Kuang Y, Salem RD, Liu J. Selection of euploid blastocysts for cryopreservation with array comparative genomic hybridization (aCGH) results in increased implantation rates in subsequent frozen and thawed embryo transfer cycles. Mol Cytogenet. 2013;6:32.
18. Feichtinger M, Stopp T, Göbl C, Feichtinger E, Vaccari E, Mädel U, et al. Increasing live birth rate by preimplantation genetic screening of pooled polar bodies using array comparative genomic hybridization. PLoS One. 2015;10:e0128317.
19. Sermon K, Capalbo A, Cohen J, Coonen E, De Rycke M, De Vos A, et al. The why, the how and the when of PGS 2.0: current practices and expert opinions of fertility specialists, molecular biologists, and embryologists. Mol Hum Reprod. 2016;22:845–57.
20. Fragouli E, Wells D, Thronhill A, Serhal P, Faed MJ, Harper JC. Comparative genomic hybridization analysis of human oocytes and polar bodies. Hum Reprod. 2006;21:2319–28.
21. Fragouli E, Lenzi M, Ross R, Katz-Jaffe M, Schoolcraft WB, Wells D. Comprehensive molecular cytogenetic analysis of the human blastocyst stage. Hum Reprod. 2008;23:2596–608.
22. Greco E, Bono S, Ruberti A, Lobascio AM, Greco P, Biricik A. Comprehensive genomic hybridization selection of blastocysts for repeated implantation failure treatment: a pilot study. Biomed Res Int 2014; https://doi.org/10.1155/2014/457913.
23. Wells D, Kaur K, Grifo J, Glassner M, Taylor JC, Fragouli E, et al. Clinical utilisation of a rapid low-pass whole genome sequencing technique for the diagnosis of aneuploidy in human embryos prior to implantation. J Med Genet. 2014;51:553–62.
24. Fiorentino F, Biricik A, Bono S, Spizzichino L, Cotroneo E, Cottone G, et al. Development and validation of a next-generation sequencing (NGS)-based protocol for 24-chromosome aneuploidy screening of embryos. Fertil Steril. 2014;101:1375–82.
25. Fan J, Wang L, Wang H, Ma M, Wang S, Liu Z, et al. The clinical utility of next-generation sequencing for identifying chromosome disease syndromes in human embryos. Reprod Biomed Online. 2015;31:62–70.
26. Fiorentino F, Bono S, Biricik A, Nuccitelli A, Cotroneo E, Cottone G, et al. Application of next-generation sequencing technology for comprehensive aneuploidy screening of blastocysts in clinical preimplantation genetic screening cycles. Hum Reprod. 2014;29:2802–13.
27. Yang Z, Lin J, Zhang J, Fong WI, Li P, Zhao R et al. Randomized comparison of next-generation sequencing and array comparative genomic hybridization for preimplantation genetic screening: a pilot study. BMC Med Genomics 2015; https://doi.org/10.1186/s12920-015-0110-4.
28. Vera-Rodríguez M, Michel CE, Mercader A, Bladon AJ, Rodrigo L, Kokocinski F, et al. Distribution patterns of segmental aneuploidies in human blastocysts identified by next-generation sequencing. Fertil Steril. 2016;105:1047–55.
29. Fragouli E, (2015 ESHRE). An investigation into the developmental potential of mosaic embryos. European Society of Human Reproduction and Embryology. Abstract.
30. Greco E, Minasi MG, Fiorentino F. Healthy Babies after Intrauterine Transfer of Mosaic Aneuploid Blastocysts. N Engl J Med. 2015;373:2089–90.
31. Wang HL, Lai HH, Chuang TH, Shih YW, Huang SC, Lee MJ, et al. A patient friendly corifollitropin alfa protocol without routine pituitary suppression in normal responders. Plos One. 2016;11:e0154123.
32. Gardner DK, Schoolcraft WB. Culture and transfer of human blastocysts. Curr Opin Obstet Gynecol. 1999;11:307–11.
33. Chang LJ, Huang CC, Tsai YY, Hung CC, Fang MY, Lin YC, et al. Blastocyst biopsy and vitrification are effective for preimplantation genetic diagnosis of monogenic diseases. Hum Reprod. 2013;28:1435–44.
34. Huang CC, Chang LJ, Tsai YY, Hung CC, Fang MY, Su YN, et al. A feasible strategy of preimplantation genetic diagnosis for carriers with chromosomal translocation: using blastocyst biopsy and array comparative genomic hybridization. J Formos Med Assoc. 2013;112:537–44.
35. Gutierez-Mateo C, Colls P, Sanchez-Garcia J, Escudero T, Prates R, Ketterson K, et al. Validation of microarray comparative genomic hybridization for comprehensive chromosome analysis of embryos. Fertil Steril. 2011;95:953–8.
36. Fiorentino F, (2014 ESHRE). Development, validation and clinical application of a NGS-based protocol for PGS of embryos. European Society of Human Reproduction and Embryology. Abstract.
37. Fragouli E, Alfarawati S, Spath K, Jaroudi S, Sarasa J, Enciso M, et al. The origin and impact of embryonic aneuploidy. Hum Genet. 2013;132:1001–13.
38. Ma GC, Chen HF, Yang YS, Lin WH, Tsai FP, Lin CF, Chiu C, Chen M. A pilot proof-of-principle study to compare fresh and vitrified cycle preimplantation genetic screening by chromosome microarray and next generation sequencing. Mol Cytogenet. 2016;9:25.
39. Ou J, Wang W, Feng T, Liao L, Meng Q, Zou Q, et al. Identification of small segmental translocations in patients with repeated implantation failure and recurrent miscarriage using next generation sequencing after in vitro fertilization/intracytoplasmic sperm injection. Mol Cytogenet. 2015;8:105.
40. Rodrigo L, Mateu E, Mercader A, Cobo AC, Peinado V, Milan M, et al. New tools for embryo selection: comprehensive chromosome screening by array comparative genomic hybridization. Biomed Res Int. 2014;517125.
41. Wells D, Delhanty JD. Comprehensive chromosomal analysis of human preimplantation embryos using whole genome amplification and single cell comparative genomic hybridization. Mol Hum Reprod. 2000;16:909–17.
42. Mertzanidou A, Wilton L, Cheng J, Spits C, Venneste E, Moreau Y, et al. Microarray analysis reveals abnormal chromosomal complements in over 70% of 14 normally developing human embryos. Hum Reprod. 2013;28:256–64.
43. Carey L, Scott F, Murphy K, Mansfield N, Barahona P, Leigh D, et al. Prenatal diagnosis of chromosomal mosaicism in over 1600 cases using array comparative genomic hybridization as a first line test. Prenat Diagn. 2014;34:478–86.
44. Maxwell SM, Colls P, Hodes-Wertz B, McCulloh DH, McCaffrey C, Wells D, et al. Why do euploid embryos miscarry? A case-control study comparing the rate of aneuploidy within presumed euploid embryos that resulted in miscarriage or live birth using next-generation sequencing. Fertil Steril. 2016;106:1414–9.
45. Munné S, Grifo J, Wells D. Mosaicism: "survival of the fittest" versus "no embryo left behind.". Fertil Steril. 2016;105:1146–9.
46. Besser AG, Mounts EL. Counselling considerations for chromosomal mosaicism detected by preimplantation genetic screening. Reprod Biomed Online. 2017; doi: 10.1016/j.rbmo.2017.01.003. [Epub ahead of print]
47. Treff NR, Franasiak JM. Detection of segmental aneuploidy and mosaicism in the human preimplantation embryo: technical considerations and limitations. Fertil Steril. 2017;107:27–31.
48. Scott RT, Galliano D. The challenge of embryonic mosaicism in preimplantation genetic screening. Fertil Steril. 2016;105:1150–2.

# 23

# A pilot proof-of-principle study to compare fresh and vitrified cycle preimplantation genetic screening by chromosome microarray and next generation sequencing

Gwo-Chin Ma[1,2,3,4†], Hsin-Fu Chen[5,6†], Yu-Shih Yang[5], Wen-Hsiang Lin[1,2], Feng-Po Tsai[7], Chi-Fang Lin[5], Chi Chiu[8] and Ming Chen[1,2,5,8,9,10*]

## Abstract

**Background:** Single embryo transfer (SET) has been utilized as a strategy to reduce the chance of multifetal gestations in in vitro fertilization (IVF) but lower pregnancy rate remains a concern. Recent studies showed that favorable outcome regarding SET can be achieved by selecting embryos with "more normal" genetic components. We explored the use of rapid array comparative genomic hybridization (aCGH) to select blastocysts for fresh SET and compared with the protocols adopting vitrified (ultrarapidly frozen) embryo transfer cycle. Validation of the rapid protocol of aCGH and comparison of the result with the regular protocol of aCGH and next generation sequencing (NGS) are also performed.

**Results:** First-time IVF patients with normal karyotype ($n = 21$) were enrolled for elective fresh SET cycle ($n = 8$, designated as fresh SET group) or vitrified embryo transfer cycle ($n = 13$; designated as vitrified ET group) coupling with comprehensive chromosomal screening by a 9-h rapid aCGH from Day 5 trophectoderm (TE) biopsy. In fresh SET group, 86 blastocysts (10.8 blastocysts/patient) were biopsied and analyzed. Aneuploidy was detected in 53.5 % (46/86) of the biopsied blastocysts. All patients had a single embryo transferred on the following day. The clinical pregnancy rate was 87.5 % (7/8) and the ongoing pregnancy rate was 62.5 % (5/8). In vitrified ET group, 58 blastocysts (4.5 blastocysts/patient) were biopsied and 56 blastocysts were analyzed. Aneuploidy was detected in 39.3 % (22/56) of biopsies. The patients accepted for SET or double embryos transfer (DET) in non-stimulated cycles. The clinical pregnancy rate and the ongoing pregnancy rate was 76.9 % (10/13) and 53.8 % (7/13) respectively. Spontaneous abortions occurred in both of the two patient groups. In the series of fresh SET group, no twin pregnancy was noted and at least one healthy baby had been born at gestational age (GA) $37^{+6}$ weeks when submission. The results of PGS by rapid aCGH, regular aCGH and NGS were comparable in most occasions.

**Conclusion:** This study evaluates the use of rapid aCGH to select blastocysts for fresh SET and demonstrates its feasibility in a real clinical IVF program. A successful livebirth is achieved and the favorable outcome is superior to the protocol adopting vitrified ET cycle in our own setting. Additional studies are needed to verify this pilot data and validate its application in large randomized trials.

**Keywords:** Chromosomal microarray, Aneuploidy, Fresh embryo transfer, SET, PGS

* Correspondence: mchen_cch@yahoo.com
†Equal contributors
[1]Department of Genomic Medicine and Center for Medical Genetics, Changhua Christian Hospital, Changhua, Taiwan
[2]Department of Genomic Science and Technology, Changhua Christian Hospital Healthcare System, Changhua, Taiwan
Full list of author information is available at the end of the article

## Background

Preimplantation genetic screening (PGS) has been considered a feasible strategy, by reducing the probability of transferring the aneuploid embryos during in vitro fertilization (IVF), in improving the implantation rate as well as the livebirth rate in the practice of artificial reproductive technology (ART) for decades [1]. However, a much wider acceptance by the academic community does not occur until recently, by some recent seminal studies which allowed us to have a more comprehensive understanding of the critical points in the whole IVF-PGS process [2–5]. The famous "Mastenbroek controversy" published in 2007 stating that for women with advanced maternal age, the livebirth rate of the PGS group was poorer than the non-PGS group did raise a huge concern for the validity of PGS and the traditional PGS by fluorescence in situ hybridization (FISH) was almost abandoned [6, 7]. However, more and more recent studies had made us known that the ironic outcome revealed by that randomized study may be due to the limitations of the genetic tool used for PGS itself (FISH), as well as the timing of the biopsy was set at the cleavage stage embryos (Day 3). The outcomes of PGS, especially the most important livebirth rate, are at least greatly affected by three critical parameters: the timing of biopsy, the genetic tools used for PGS, and to freeze or not to freeze the biopsied embryos [8–12]. After 2007, since the emergence of many new technologies available for genetic investigation, researchers are keen to verify and validate the new tools when being used in PGS [5, 13–15]. Nowadays it is a reality to use the latest technology such as array comparative genomic hybridization (aCGH) and next generation sequencing (NGS) platforms to screen the embryos because of the advancement of a critical technique called whole genome amplification (WGA). The aCGH and NGS had become accessible for PGS after WGA [15–19]. However, such amplification may also introduce errors and thereby other research groups had heartily advocated for WGA-free quantitative polymerase chain reaction (qPCR) based rapid diagnosis [8, 11, 20]. Excellent results were achieved by even using single embryo transfer (SET) in fresh cycle by the group led by Richard Scott Jr and Nathan Treff based in US [11], and even with a limited set of chromosomes being tested by our group [21].

It is now understood that the blastomere biopsy at Day 3 cleavage-stage embryos may impair the implantation potential while the trophectoderm (TE) biopsy at Day 5/6 blastocysts may not [3]. However, due to the sophistication of the genetic tools used to screen the developing embryos, it is not always feasible to have the report turnout time to be less than one day, since all embryos must not survive in vitro after 7 days post-fertilization unless being frozen. Therefore in before for all amplification-based technologies, including aCGH and NGS, it is not feasible to do fresh embryo transfer if the timing of the biopsy was set at Day 5/6. Earlier studies did report some cycles based upon PGS by aCGH on Day 3 embryos [10, 22–24], but very few at Day 5/6 because the protocol of aCGH usually needs at least 2–3 days, in which the time for analysis was not counted in [25]. To freeze the biopsied embryos sent for PGS, and to transfer the thawed euploid embryos in non-stimulated cycles, becomes the standard practice for most IVF-PGS centers. Recently, some researchers showed that the combination of PGS and embryo vitrification (ultrarapid freeze) can produce better clinical outcomes compared to non-PGS ET [26] while we considered fresh ET remains a preferred choice in routine IVF if a rapid PGS is feasible. Quite recently the newest protocol of rapid aCGH analyzes suited for PGS was available, and therefore, we conducted this pilot study to evaluate its feasibility in a real clinical setting: TE biopsy on Day 5, 9-h aCGH analysis, followed by fresh SET on Day6. Additionally, we compared the results with the protocols adopting vitrified ET cycle.

## Results

### Rapid PGS aCGH

A total of 21 patients were subjected to in IVF-rapid PGS aCGH treatment, including 8 patients with fresh SET (fresh SET group) and 13 patients with vitrified SET/DET (vitrified ET group) (Table 1). The average age of the patients was 36.0 years (range of 29–42 years), with a mean age of 33.6 years (range of 29–37 years) in fresh SET group and 37.5 years (range of 34–42 years) in vitrified ET group. In fresh SET group, 86 blastocysts (10.8 blastocysts/patient) were biopsied and analyzed. Euploidy was found in 46.5 % (40/86) of the embryos, whereas chromosome abnormalities were found in the remaining 53.5 % (46/86) of embryos (Table 1). Among the aneuploid blastocysts, 43.5 % (20/46) had single chromosomal abnormality [of which. 35.0 % (7/20) displayed single chromosome loss, 15.0 % (3/20) displayed single chromosome gain and 50.0 % (10/20) displayed single segmental aneuploidy with an aberration between 6.4 Mb and 85.9 Mb], 21.7 % (10/46) had dual chromosomal abnormalities and 34.8 % (16/46) had severe, compound genetic defects involving in three or more chromosomes (Table 2 and Fig. 1). Look at the single-chromosome level, 143 chromosome abnormalities, including 82 whole chromosome gain/loss and 61 segmental aneuploidies, were found in the 46 aneuploid embryos (Fig. 2a). In vitrified ET group, a total of 58 blastocysts (4.5 blastocysts/patient) were biopsied. Of which, two blastocysts failed with WGA and thus finally 56 blastocysts were analyzed. Euploidy and aneuploidy were detected in 60.7 % (34/56) and 39.3 % (22/56) of

**Table 1** Summary of rapid aCGH results for 86 embryos from 8 patients accepted for fresh single embryo transfer (SET) and 58 embryos from 13 patients choosing vitrified SET or double embryo transfer (DET)

| Case no. | Age of patient | No. of embryos for aCGH | | | | SET or DET | Chemical pregnancy (+hCG) | Outcome |
|---|---|---|---|---|---|---|---|---|
| | | Total | WGA failure | Euploid | Aneuploid | | | |
| I. Fresh SET | | | | | | | | |
| 1 | 29 | 10 | 0 | 1 | 9 | SET | Yes | Live birth[a] (at GA = $37^{+6}$ weeks) |
| 2 | 33 | 9 | 0 | 4 | 5 | SET | Yes | Abortion (at GA = 5 weeks) |
| 3 | 34 | 14 | 0 | 3 | 11 | SET | No | — |
| 4 | 34 | 14 | 0 | 6 | 8 | SET | Yes | Ongoing pregnancy (GA = 37 weeks) |
| 5 | 37 | 13 | 0 | 7 | 6 | SET | Yes | Ongoing pregnancy (GA = 13 weeks) |
| 6 | 34 | 9 | 0 | 5 | 4 | SET | Yes | Abortion (at GA = 4 weeks) |
| 7 | 37 | 9 | 0 | 8 | 1 | SET | Yes | Ongoing pregnancy (GA = 16 weeks) |
| 8 | 31 | 8 | 0 | 6 | 2 | SET | Yes | Ongoing pregnancy (GA = 7 weeks) |
| Overall | | 86 | 0 | 40 | 46 | | | |
| II. Vitrified ET | | | | | | | | |
| 1 | 41 | 3 | 0 | 1 | 2 | SET | Yes | Live birth (at GA = 39 weeks) |
| 2 | 40 | 4 | 0 | 1 | 3 | SET | Yes | Termination (acardiac monster) (at GA = $14^{+4}$ week) |
| 3 | 34 | 4 | 0 | 3 | 1 | SET | Yes | Ongoing pregnancy (GA = $19^{+4}$ week) |
| 4 | 39 | 5 | 0 | 1 | 4 | SET | Yes | Ongoing pregnancy (GA = 22 week) |
| 5 | 42 | 3 | 0 | 2 | 1 | DET | No | — |
| 6 | 37 | 6 | 0 | 5 | 1 | DET | Yes | Live birth (at GA = 38 weeks) |
| 7 | 36 | 5 | 0 | 4 | 1 | DET | Yes | Live birth (at GA = 37 weeks) |
| 8 | 37 | 5 | 0 | 2 | 3 | DET | Yes | Abortion (at GA = $8^{+3}$ weeks) |
| 9 | 42 | 5 | 0 | 2 | 3 | DET | No | — |
| 10 | 37 | 3 | 0 | 3 | 0 | DET | Yes | Ongoing pregnancy (GA = 16 week) |
| 11 | 34 | 5 | 0 | 5 | 0 | DET | No | — |
| 12 | 34 | 5 | 0 | 3 | 2 | DET | Yes | Abortion (at GA = $10^{+6}$ weeks) |
| 13 | 35 | 5 | 2 | 2 | 1 | DET | Yes | Ongoing pregnancy (GA = $12^{+3}$ weeks) |
| Overall | | 58 | 2 | 34 | 22 | | | |

[a]Single birth (3040 g; AS 8 > 9) by C-section due to breech presentation
*WGA* whole genome amplification, *GA* gestational age

biopsies respectively (Table 1). Among the aneuploid blastocysts, 59.1 % (13/22) had single chromosomal abnormality [of which. 30.8 % (4/13) displayed single chromosome loss, 15.4 % (2/13) displayed single chromosome gain and 53.8 % (7/13) displayed single segmental aneuploidy with an aberration between 12.3 Mb and 75.4 Mb], 13.6 % (3/22) had dual chromosomal abnormalities and 27.3 % (6/22) had severe, compound genetic defects involving in three or more chromosomes (Table 2). In the single-chromosome level, 51 chromosome abnormalities, including 20 whole chromosome gain/loss and 31 segmental aneuploidies, were found in the 22 aneuploid embryos (Fig. 2b). Overall, the aneuploidy rate of the 142 embryos examined was 47.9 % (68/142). Chromosome abnormalities were detected in all chromosomes where genetic defects involving chromosome 5, 15, 19, 22 and X were most frequently observed while errors in chromosome 2, 9, 12, 17, 20 and 21 seen relatively uncommon (Fig. 2c). The diagnostic results were validated by regular aCGH and NGS (see the *Methods* section and Fig. 3). The rate of correct diagnosis was 100 % in all embryos. The positive and negative predictive rates of rapid aCGH in our series were thus 100 %.

### Clinical outcome

In both of fresh SET and vitrified ET group, all patients had at least one euploid embryo available for fresh transfer on Day 6 (fresh SET group) or in non-stimulated cycles (vitrified ET group). Combining the data of rapid aCGH and blastocyst grading, the best-graded euploid embryo(s) were chosen for ET for each of the patients. In fresh SET group, the clinical pregnancy rate was 87.5 % (7/8) and the ongoing pregnancy rate was 62.5 % (5/8). Spontaneous abortions occurred in two patients at GA 5 and GA 4 weeks (the genetic analysis cannot be

**Table 2** Details of rapid aCGH results of aneuploid blastocysts derived from 8 patients for fresh SET and 13 patients for vitrified ET

| Case no. | Total no. of aneuploid blastocysts | Single chromosomal abnormality [Single chromosome loss/Single chromosome gain/Single segmental aneuploidy] | Dual chromosomal abnormality | Complex chromosomal abnormality |
|---|---|---|---|---|
| I. Fresh SET | | | | |
| 1 | 9 | 4 (44.4 %) [1/2/1] | 2 (22.2 %) | 3 (33.3 %) |
| 2 | 5 | 3 (60.0 %) [1/1/1] | 0 (0 %) | 2 (40.0 %) |
| 3 | 11 | 2 (18.2 %) [1/0/1] | 5 (45.5 %) | 4 (36.4 %) |
| 4 | 8 | 3 (37.5 %) [0/0/3] | 1 (12.5 %) | 4 (50.0 %) |
| 5 | 6 | 4 (66.7 %) [3/0/1] | 0 (0 %) | 2 (33.3 %) |
| 6 | 4 | 2 (50.0 %) [0/0/2] | 2 (50.0 %) | 0 (0 %) |
| 7 | 1 | 1 (100.0 %) [0/0/1] | 0 (0 %) | 0 (0 %) |
| 8 | 2 | 1 (50.0 %) [1/0/0] | 0 (0 %) | 1 (50.0 %) |
| Overall | 46 | 20 (43.5 %) [7/3/10] | 10 (21.7 %) | 16 (34.8 %) |
| II. Vitrified ET | | | | |
| 1 | 2 | 1 (50.0 %) [1/0/0] | 0 (0 %) | 1 (50.0 %) |
| 2 | 3 | 2 (66.7 %) [0/0/2] | 1 (33.3 %) | 0 (0 %) |
| 3 | 1 | 1 (100.0 %) [0/0/1] | 0 (0 %) | 0 (0 %) |
| 4 | 4 | 2 (50.0 %) [1/1/0] | 1 (25.0 %) | 1 (25.0 %) |
| 5 | 1 | 1 (100.0 %) [0/1/0] | 0 (0 %) | 0 (0 %) |
| 6 | 1 | 1 (100.0 %) [0/0/1] | 0 (0 %) | 0 (0 %) |
| 7 | 1 | 1 (100.0 %) [0/0/1] | 0 (0 %) | 0 (0 %) |
| 8 | 3 | 2 (66.7 %) [0/0/2] | 0 (0 %) | 1 (33.3 %) |
| 9 | 3 | 1 (33.3 %) [1/0/0] | 1 (33.3 %) | 1 (33.3 %) |
| 10 | 0 | 0 (0 %) [0/0/0] | 0 (0 %) | 0 (0 %) |
| 11 | 0 | 0 (0 %) [0/0/0] | 0 (0 %) | 0 (0 %) |
| 12 | 2 | 1 (50.0 %) [1/0/0] | 0 (0 %) | 1 (50.0 %) |
| 13 | 1 | 0 (0 %) [0/0/0] | 0 (0 %) | 1 (100.0 %) |
| Overall | 22 | 13 (59.1 %) [4/2/7] | 3 (13.6 %) | 6 (27.3 %) |

performed due to the spontaneous expulsion of the gestational tissue). No twin pregnancy was noted in this series and at least one healthy baby had been born at GA $37^{+6}$ weeks (Table 1). In vitrified ET group, the clinical pregnancy rate and the ongoing pregnancy rate was 76.9 % (10/13) and 53.8 % (7/13) respectively. Spontaneous abortions occurred in two patients at GA $8^{+3}$ and GA $10^{+6}$ weeks. One fetus was terminated at GA $14^{+4}$ weeks due to acardiac monster. Genetic analysis by aCGH for tissues from the aborted and terminated fetuses revealed no specific finding; all cases had a normal karyotype.

## Discussion

PGS has become a well-established tool in the practice of IVF nowadays with the development of many sophisticated tools used for investigating the genetic complements of the embryos before being transferred [14, 27]. However, the major difficulty in these genetic tools, such as the latest NGS, is the complexity of analytical pipelines [28]. Therefore to freeze the embryos to earn more time for the reliable analysis of the PGS results remains the mainstream in most PGS centers, especially those involving aCGH and NGS [19]. It is now known that the biopsy timing will be better at Day 5/6 blastocyst stage instead of Day 3 cleavage-stage embryos in regard to the implantation potential [3], and this new finding creates an even more difficulty: the time span of analysis if we want to do it in fresh transfer will be shortened from 3 days to 1 day, which rendered the analysis of aCGH and NGS almost impossible. Up to this submission, there are very few reports achieving this goal when using high-complexity-tool such as aCGH or NGS and also successfully conducted the fresh SET [25, 29].

In order to facilitate the analytical bioinformatics pipelines used in aCGH and NGS, some resolution was sacrificed for efficiency and also because of the process of WGA may introduce errors, and some leading groups

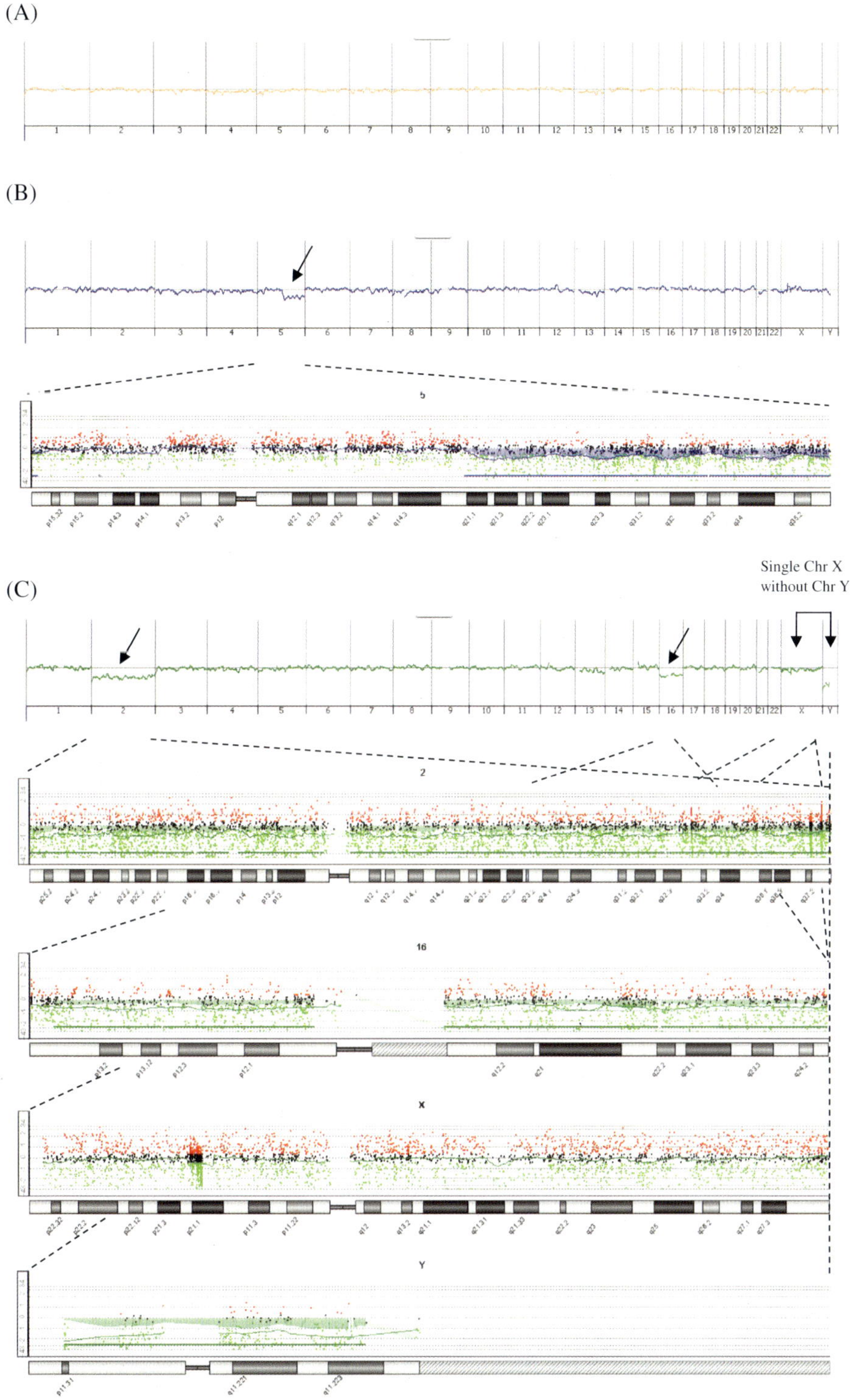


**Fig. 1** Representative rapid aCGH results of blastocysts obtained by trophectoderm biopsy at post-fertilization Day5 showed **a** euploid chromosomes [arr(1–22) × 2,(XY) × 1], **b** a segmental aneuploidy [arr 5q15q35.3(94,800,050-180,684,501) × 1] and **c** a complex chromosomal abnormality [arr(1,3-15,17-22) × 2,(2) × 1,(16) × 1,(X) × 1]. Arrow indicated the aneuploidy chromosome or chromosomal fragment. The reference DNA used for aCGH was whole genome amplification product of a normal male embryo DNA

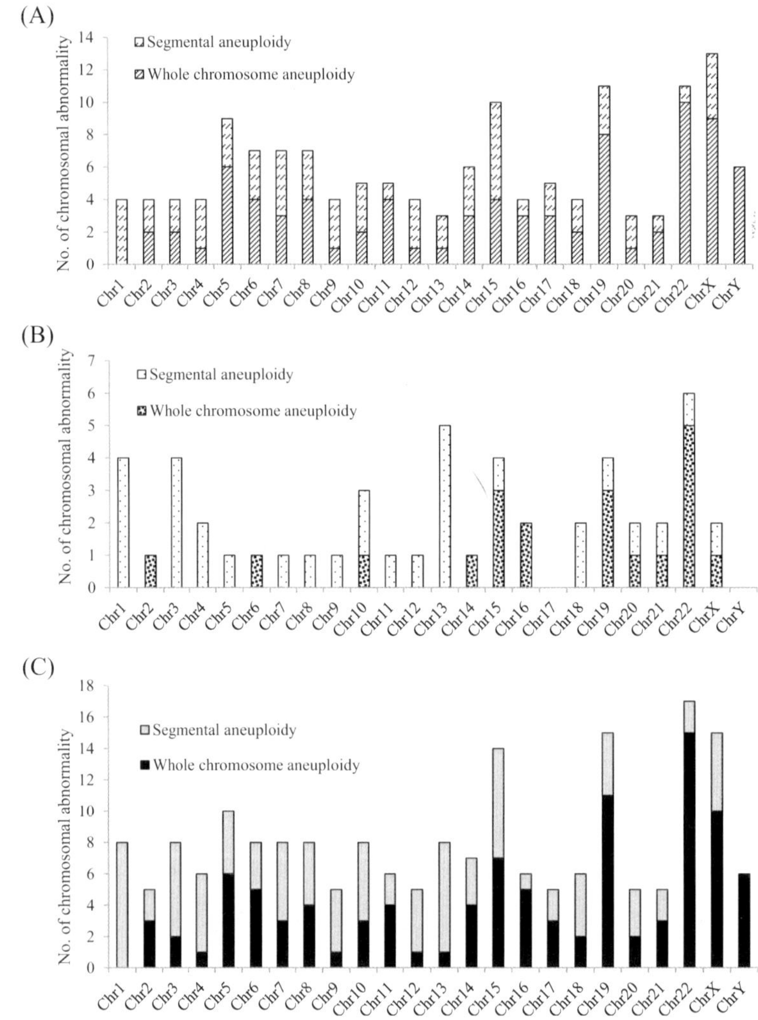


**Fig. 2** Chromosomal abnormalities, at the single-chromosome level, detected by rapid aCGH in **a** 86 embryos from 8 patients accepted for fresh SET, **b** 58 embryos from 13 patients choosing vitrified ET, and **c** all 144 embryos from the 21 patients. A total of 194 chromosome abnormalities (143 in in fresh SET group and 51 in vitrified ET group), including 102 whole chromosome gain/loss and 92 segmental aneuploidies, were found in 68 aneuploid embryos

admitted it is now available for PGS to use these fancy technologies in a "low-pass" strategy [18].

It is now well known that mosaicism is a common phenomenon in the development of early human embryos [30], and therefore whether the "best" embryo can really be selected with the most sophisticated genetic tools remains in doubt. Another group thus proposed for amplification-free quantitative polymerase chain reaction (qPCR) based PGS strategy, which only detects the copy number changes involving the whole chromosomal arm level, and surprisingly the result was excellent. They published a series of excellent data to demonstrate that by using qPCR, the accuracy was comparable to aCGH [8, 15, 20], the implantation rate and delivery rate were also excellent [2, 4], and such impression even was validated in a randomized trial concerning delivery rate and neonatal/obstetrical outcome (the BEST trial) [11].

Regarding the aneuploidies detected by rapid aCGH in this pilot study, the overall aneuploidy rate was 47.9 % (53.5 % in fresh SET group and 39.3 % in vitrified ET group), which is similar to a recent series comparing aCGH and NGS (which is around 60 %, see Yang et al., 2015 [19]), and was considered to be a result that both of the analyses included segmental aneuploidies greater than 5 Mb (in Yang's series, they reported a 42 Mb gain on 16q and a 16 Mb loss on 18q). The cytogenetic abnormalities distributed in all 24 chromosomes. However, in a recent validation study to compare NGS and aCGH to detect the cytogenetic abnormalities in the TE cells of human embryos, the resolution has been greatly enhanced to 1.19-3.89 Mb [31]. In theory the resolution of

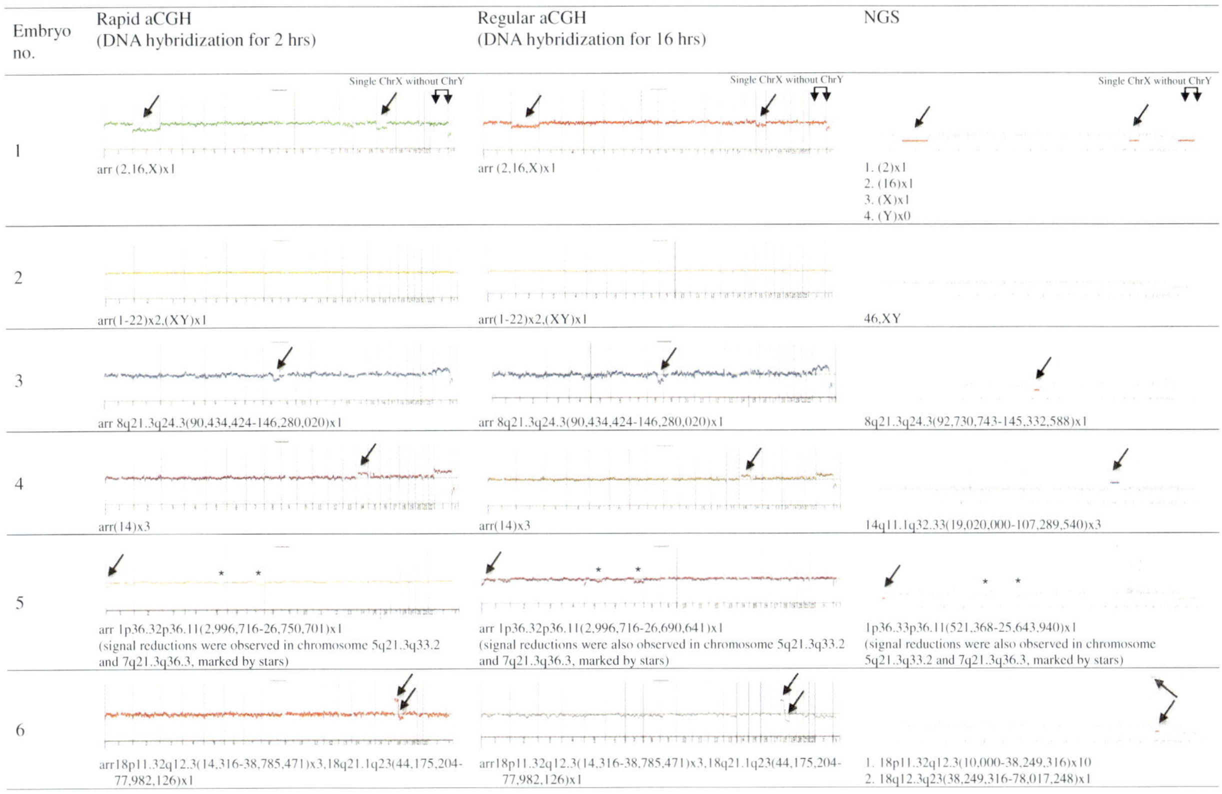


**Fig. 3** Exemplified PGS results by use of rapid aCGH (DNA hybridization for 2 h), regular aCGH (DNA hybridization for 16 h) and next generation sequencing (NGS) for the same WGA products. Rapid and regular aCGH were performed with CytoScan 60 K microarray chip (Agilent customer array, Changhua Christian Hospital, Taiwan) on a G4900DA SureScan microarray scanner (Agilent Technologies, CA, USA). NGS was performed using Ion PGM Hi-Q Sequencing Kit with Ion 316 chip (Life technologies, California, USA) on the Ion Torrent PGM Instrument (Life technologies) platform. Aneuploidy chromosomes or chromosomal fragments are indicated by arrows. Some atypical segmental gains and/or losses with copy number change < 1 but > 0.5 (a likely result of embryo mosaicism) were also classified as segmental aneuploidies and marked by stars. The results of rapid aCGH are comparable with that of regular aCGH and NGS

aCGH and NGS must be much higher than qPCR (which only detects aneuploidy in a chromosomal arm level and the aneuploidy rate was around 30 %, see Forman et al., 2014 [11]), however, it has been noted that aCGH may have a higher false positive rate than qPCR [20], in which some euploid embryos may be sacrificed and not transferred. Our report is one of the very few studies up to 2016 (and the first report from Taiwan) adopting Day 5 blastocysts biopsy, 9-h aCGH and fresh SET to achieve successful singleton livebirth. Furthermore, the favorable outcome in terms of the clinical pregnancy rate and the ongoing pregnancy rate is superior to the protocol adopting vitrified ET cycle (87.5 and 62.5 % in fresh SET group, and 76.9 % and 53.8 % in vitrified ET group). We admit the case number is very small ($n = 8$ in fresh SET group and $n = 13$ in vitrified ET group) and it is only a pilot study which needs further validation in a prospective, large-scale and better be randomized study to explore its real efficacy.

However, despite in theory the resolution of NGS should be much better than aCGH in picking up aberrations in genetic complements. The current "low-pass strategy" adopted by NGS made it only comparable to the aCGH platform when using in PGS [19, 31, 32]. With the advance of bioinformatics pipelines it can be expected that NGS can pick up more aneuploidies than aCGH, as well as the turn-around time for analysis should be greatly shortened, to make fresh embryo transfer feasible in the near future. When three competing PGS tools (qPCR, aCGH and NGS) can all produce results in one single day, then it is possible to conduct a real randomized trial to compare the efficacy and may further enhance our understanding of the early development of human embryos, and to improve the whole IVF-PGS process.

It is noteworthy that despite it was thought that freeze-thaw process might damage the embryos whereas a growing number of epidemiological studies had suggested otherwise: that an increased rate of adverse perinatal outcomes such as low birth weight was noted in fresh IVF cycles compared with frozen embryo transfer cycles. It is considered superovulation has a significant impact upon endometrial receptivity and therefore frozen embryo transfer cycles should be considered in those high-responders [33]. However, we considered that if in the future time constraint is no longer considered a problem when the advantage and safety of frozen ET cycles are well established [34], the effort should be placed upon improving the bioinformatics pipelines of NGS from "low-pass-strategy" into an algorithm with a better resolution that can better utilize the advantage of NGS technology itself.

## Methods

### Patient recruitment

During January of 2014 to December of 2015, 21 infertile couples visited the clinic center for their first-time IVF and elected either fresh SET ($n = 8$; designated as fresh SET group) or vitrified SET/DET ($n = 13$; designated as vitrified ET group) by conjugation with comprehensive chromosomal screening via a 9-h rapid PGS aCGH protocol for trophectoderm (TE) biopsy on Day 5. All the couples have a normal karyotype and the patients are expected to have a good prognosis (female age ≤ 42 years, no prior miscarriage and no remarkable personal and family history). After pre-treatment counseling was provided, all the 21 couples agreed to participate in this study and signed an informed consent prior to the sample collection and evaluation. The study was approved by the Ethics Committees of Changhua Christian Hospital, Changhua, Taiwan and adhered to the guidelines approved by the Institutional Review Board.

### Fertilization, embryo culture and TE biopsy

Intracytoplasmic sperm injection (ICSI) was performed following the removal of cumulus cells and the presence of two pronuclei and two polar bodies 16–18 h after injection was ascertained normal fertilization. Fertilized embryos were cultured in sequential media (Sage, CA, USA) to the blastocyst stage. On Day 3, a laser-created narrow channel was made in the zona pellucida of all embryos. On Day 5, fully differentiated embryos were biopsied using suction to gently extrude and pull 3–8 TE cells from blastocysts. The biopsied cells were washed in 1X PBS (catalog no. 70013–032) (Gibco by life technology, CA, USA) and collected into a microcentrifuge tube with 2.5 μl 1X PBS (Gibco by life technology). The cells were used directly for whole genome amplification (WGA).

### Rapid aCGH

The WGA was performed using REPLI-g Single Cell Kit (Qiagen, Hilden, Germany) and following the manufacturer's instructions. Amplified DNA was purified using the QIAamp DNA Blood Mini Kit (Qiagen). The DNA purities and concentrations were examined by Nanodrop 2000 spectrophotometer (Thermo Fisher Scientific, Delaware, USA). Approximately 1 μg of purified DNA was fluorescently labeled with Cy3 d-CTP or Cy5-dCTP using SureTag DNA Labeling Kit (Agilent Technologies, CA, USA) and then cleaned up by Microcon YM-30 centrifugal filter unit (Millipore, MA, USA). The yield DNA was hybridized with CytoScan 60 K microarray chip (Agilent customer array, Changhua Christian Hospital, Taiwan) at 65 °C for 2 h. The image on a chip was acquired with a G4900DA SureScan microarray scanner (Agilent Technologies, CA, USA) and analyzed with Agilent Genomic Workbench software (Agilent Technologies) for DNA gain or loss across all 24 chromosomes. Aberrations were detected by using default setting with an algorithm of z-score conjugated with a filter of a minimum of 5 Mb aberrations. All aCGH procedures were completed within 9 h, allowing rapid evaluation of the TE biopsies and providing a feasible opportunity for fresh embryo transfer on the following day, Day 6.

### Regular aCGH

To evaluate the reliability of rapid aCGH, WGA products of all the biopsied blastocysts were processed for the regular aCGH analysis. All procedures of regular aCGH analysis are the same as that described in rapid aCGH, except for the DNA-chip probes hybridization duration which was extended (from 2 h) to 16 h.

### NGS

WGA products of all the biopsied blastocysts were also processed for the NGS analysis in order to evaluate the reliability of rapid aCGH and compare the performances of difference platforms (i.e. rapid aCGH, regular aCGH and NGS). Approximately 1 μg of WGA DNA was used for library construction using Ion Xpress Plus gDNA Fragment Library Preparation Kit Set (Life technologies, California, USA) and following the manufacturer's instructions. The quantity of library was determined using Qubit dsDNA HS assay kits (Life technologies) with Qubit fluorometer (Life technologies). The template-positive Ion Sphere Particles (ISPs) were generated using Ion PGM Hi-Q Template Kits (Life technologies) with the Ion OneTouch 2 Instrument (Life technologies) and then enriched with the Ion OneTouch ES Instrument (Life technologies). Sequencing was performed on the Ion Torrent PGM Instrument (Life technologies) platform using the Ion PGM Hi-Q Sequencing Kit and Ion 316 chip (Life technologies). PGS analysis for aneuploidy detection was performed by the Ion Reporter Server System (https://ionreporter.thermofisher.com/ir/).

### Embryo selection for transfer

Only euploid blastocyst ascertained by rapid aCGH analysis was selected for transfer. When multiple euploid blastocysts are available, the best grade one was chosen for transfer. Embryo grading is based on the principle proposed in Sakkas and Gardner (2005) [35]. In brief, the blastocyst is given a grade based on three main components of the embryo: (1) expansion degree and hatching status, (2) the inner cell mass (ICM) development, and (3) the TE cell quality. The graded embryo is given a number grade (1–6), followed by a letter grade for the ICM and then the TE (A, B or C). All embryos, which were classified as aneuploid, were confirmed again by aCGH before discarded.

## Conclusions

In this study, we demonstrate the results of aCGH (including rapid and regular protocol) and NGS (regular protocol) being used for PGS are comparable to each other with high consistency. Furthermore, we also demonstrate the feasibility of using rapid protocol aCGH to select blastocysts for fresh SET in a real clinical IVF setting, in which at least one successful live-birth has already been achieved. Meanwhile, in terms of the clinical pregnancy rate as well as the ongoing pregnancy rate, PGS by aCGH followed by fresh cycle ET seems superior (or at least comparable) to PGS by aCGH coupled with vitrified cycle ET. Additional studies are needed to verify this pilot data and validate its clinical utility in large prospective randomized trials.

### Abbreviations

aCGH: array comparative genomic hybridization; ART: artificial reproductive technology; DET: double embryo transfer; ET: embryo transfer; FISH: fluorescence in situ hybridization; GA: gestation age; ICM: inner cell mass; ICSI: intracytoplasmic sperm injection; ISPs: ion Sphere Particles; IVF: in vitro fertilization; NGS: next generation sequencing; PGS: preimplantation genetic screening; qPCR: quantitative polymerase chain reaction; SET: single embryo transfer; TE: trophectoderm; WGA: whole genome amplification.

### Competing interests

The authors declared no competing interests.

### Authors' contributions

GCM, HFC, YSY, MC designed the study. FPT and MC recruited the patients. CFL, CC collected the clinical data. GCM, FPT, WHL, MC did the experiments and performed the analyses. GCM, WHL and MC wrote the paper. All authors read and approved the final manuscript.

### Acknowledgements

The study was supported by grants (103-CCH-IST-006) from Changhua Christian Hospital, Changhua, Taiwan and Poyuan Women Clinic, Changhua, Taiwan.

### Author details

[1]Department of Genomic Medicine and Center for Medical Genetics, Changhua Christian Hospital, Changhua, Taiwan. [2]Department of Genomic Science and Technology, Changhua Christian Hospital Healthcare System, Changhua, Taiwan. [3]Institute of Biochemistry, Microbiology and Immunology, Chung-Shan Medical University, Taichung, Taiwan. [4]Department of Medical Laboratory Science and Biotechnology, Central Taiwan University of Science and Technology, Taichung, Taiwan. [5]Department of Obstetrics and Gynecology, College of Medicine and Hospital, National Taiwan University, Taipei, Taiwan. [6]Graduate Institute of Medical Genomics and Proteomics, College of Medicine, National Taiwan University, Taipei, Taiwan. [7]Poyuan Women Clinic, Changhua, Taiwan. [8]Department of Medical Genetics, National Taiwan University Hospital, Taipei, Taiwan. [9]Department of Obstetrics and Gynecology, Changhua Christian Hospital, Changhua, Taiwan. [10]Department of Life Science, Tunghai University, Taichung, Taiwan.

### References

1. Handyside AH. 24-chromosome copy number analysis: a comparison of available technologies. Fertil Steril. 2013;100(3):595–602.
2. Scott Jr RT, Ferry K, Su J, Tao X, Scott K, Treff NR. Comprehensive chromosome screening is highly predictive of the reproductive potential of human embryos: a prospective, blinded, nonselection study. Fertil Steril. 2012;97(4):870–5.
3. Scott KL, Hong KH, Scott Jr RT. Selecting the optimal time to perform biopsy for preimplantation genetic testing. Fertil Steril. 2013;100(3):608–14.
4. Scott Jr RT, Upham KM, Forman EJ, Hong KH, Scott KL, Taylor D, et al. Blastocyst biopsy with comprehensive chromosome screening and fresh embryo transfer significantly increases in vitro fertilization implantation and delivery rates: a randomized controlled trial. Fertil Steril. 2013;100(3):697–703.
5. Lee HL, McCulloh DH, Hodes-Wertz B, Adler A, McCaffrey C, Grifo JA. In vitro fertilization with preimplantation genetic screening improves implantation and live birth in women age 40 through 43. J Assist Reprod Genet. 2015; 32(3):435–44.
6. Mastenbroek S, Twisk M, van Echten-Arends J, Sikkema-Raddatz B, Korevaar JC, Verhoeve HR, et al. In vitro fertilization with preimplantation genetic screening. New Engl J Med. 2007;357(1):9–17.
7. Mastenbroek S, Twisk M, van der Veen F, Repping S. Preimplantation genetic screening: a systematic review and meta-analysis of RCTs. Hum Reprod Update. 2011;17(4):454–66.
8. Treff NR, Tao X, Ferry KM, Su J, Taylor D, Scott Jr RT. Development and validation of an accurate quantitative real-time polymerase chain reaction-based assay for human blastocyst comprehensive chromosomal aneuploidy screening. Fertil Steril. 2012;97(4):819–24.
9. Braude P. Selecting the 'best' embryos: prospects for improvement. Reprod Biomed Online. 2013;27(6):244–53.
10. Rubio C, Rhodrigo L, Mir P, Mateu E, Peinado V, Milan M, et al. Use of array comparative genomic hybridization (array-CGH) for embryo assessment: clinical results. Fertil Steril. 2013;99(4):1044–8.
11. Forman EJ, Hong KH, Franasiak JM, Scott Jr RT. Obstetrical and neonatal outcomes from the BEST Trial: single embryo transfer with aneuploidy screening improves outcomes after in vitro fertilization without compromising delivery rates. Am J Obstet Gynecol. 2014;210(2):157. e1-6.
12. Mastenbroek S, Repping S. Preimplantation genetic screening: back to the future. Hum Reprod. 2014;29(9):1846–50.
13. Hens K, Dondrop WJ, Geraedts JP, de Wert GM. Comprehensive embryo testing. Experts' opinions regarding future directions: an expert panel study on comprehensive embryo testing. Hum Reprod. 2013;28(5):1418–25.
14. Brezina PR, Kutteh WH. Clinical application of preimplantation genetic screening. BMJ. 2015;350:g7611.
15. Treff NR, Levy B, Su J, Northrop LE, Tao X, Scott Jr RT. SNP microarray-based 24 chromosome aneuploidy screening is significantly more consistent than FISH. Mol Hum Reprod. 2010;16(8):583–9.
16. Schoolcraft WB, Treff NR, Stevens JM, Ferry K, Katz-Jaffe M, Scott Jr RT. Live birth outcome with trophectoderm biopsy, blastocyst vitrification, and single-nucleotide polymorphism microarray-based comprehensive chromosome screening in infertile patients. Fertil Steril. 2011;96(3):638–40.
17. Fiorentino F, Bono S, Biricik A, Nuccitelli A, Cotroneo E, Cottone G, et al. Application of next-generation sequencing technology for comprehensive aneuploidy screening of blastocysts in clinical preimplantation genetic screening cycles. Hum Reprod. 2014;29(12):2802–13.
18. Wells D, Kaur K, Grifo J, Glassner M, Taylor JC, Fragouli E, et al. Clinical utilisation of a rapid low-pass whole genome sequencing technique for the diagnosis of aneuploidy in human embryos prior to implantation. J Med Genet. 2014;51(8):553–62.

19. Yang Z, Lin J, Zhang J, Fong WL, Li P, Zhao R, et al. Randomized comparison of next-generation sequencing and array comparative genomic hybridization for preimplantation genetic screening: a pilot study. BMC Med Genomics. 2015;8:30.
20. Capalbo A, Treff NR, Cimadomo D, Tao X, Upham K, Ubaldi FM, et al. Comparison of array comparative genomic hybridization and quantitative real-time PCR-based aneuploidy screening of blastocyst biopsies. Eu J Hum Genet. 2015;23(7):901–6.
21. Yang YS, Chang SP, Chen HF, Ma GC, Lin WH, Tsai FP, et al. Preimplantation genetic screening of blastocysts by multiplex qPCR followed by fresh embryo transfer: validation and verification. Mol Cytogenet. 2015;8:49.
22. Liu J, Sillis ES, Yang Z, Salem SA, Rahil T, Collins GS, et al. Array comparative genomic hybridization screening in IVF significantly reduces number of embryos available for cryopreservation. Clin Exp Reprod Med. 2012; 39(2):52–7.
23. Sills ES, Yang Z, Walsh DJ, Salem SA. Comprehensive genetic assessment of the human embryo: can empiric application of microarray comparative genomic hybridization reduce multiple gestation rate by single fresh blastocyst transfer? Arch Gynecol Obstet. 2012;286(3):755–61.
24. Keltz MD, Vega M, Sirota I, Lederman M, Moshier EL, Gonzales E, et al. Preimplantation genetic screening (PGS) with Comparative genomic hybridization (CGH) following day 3 single cell blastomere biopsy markedly improves IVF outcomes while lowering multiple pregnancies and miscarriages. J Assist Reprod Genet. 2013;30(10):1333–9.
25. Grifo J, Adler A, Lee HL, Morin SJ, Smith M, Liu L, et al. Deliveries from trophectoderm biopsied, fresh and vitrified blastocysts derived from polar body biopsied, vitrified oocytes. Reprod Biomed Online. 2015;31(2):210–6.
26. Schoolcraft WB, Katz-Jaffe MG. Comprehensive chromosome screening of trophectoderm with vitrification facilitates elective single-embryo transfer for infertile women with advanced maternal age. Fertil Steril. 2013;100:615–9.
27. Gardner DK, Meseguer M, Rubio C, Treff NR. Diagnosis of human preimplantation embryo viability. Hum Reprod Update. 2015;21(6):727–47.
28. Gargis AS, Kaiman L, Bick DP, da Silva C, Dimmock DP, Funke BH, et al. Good laboratory practice for clinical next-generation sequencing informatics pipelines. Nat Biotechnol. 2015;33(7):689–93.
29. Yang Z, Liu J, Collins GS, Salem SA, Liu X, Lyle SS, et al. Selection of single blastocysts for fresh transfer via standard morphology assessment alone and with array CGH for good prognosis IVF patients: results from a randomized pilot study. Mol Cytogenet. 2012;5:24.
30. Vanneste E, Voet T, Le Caignec C, Ampe M, Konings P, Melotte C, et al. Chromosome instability is common in human cleavage-stage embryos. Nat Med. 2009;15(5):577–83.
31. Zheng H, Jin H, Liu J, Wang WH. Application of next-generation sequencing for 24- chromosome aneuploidy screening of humanpreimplantation embryos. Mol Cytogenet. 2015;8:38.
32. Wang L, Cram DS, Shen J, Wang X, Zhang J, Song Z, et al. Validation of copy number variation sequencing for detecting chromosome imbalances in human preimplantation embryos. Biol Reprod. 2014;91(2):37.
33. Weinerman R, Mainigi M. Why should we transfer frozen instead of fresh embryos: the translational rationale. Fertil Steril. 2014;102(1):10–8.
34. Zhang L, Yan L, Zhi X, Yan J, Qian J. Female fertility: is it safe to freeze? Chin Med J. 2015;128(3):390–7.
35. Sakkas D, Gardner DK. Noninvasive methods to assess embryo quality. Curr Opin Obstet Gynecol. 2005;17:283–8.

# Copy number variants prioritization after array-CGH analysis – a cohort of 1000 patients

Isabel Marques Carreira[1,2,3,4*], Susana Isabel Ferreira[1], Eunice Matoso[2,5], Luís Miguel Pires[1], José Ferrão[1], Ana Jardim[1], Alexandra Mascarenhas[1], Marta Pinto[1], Nuno Lavoura[1], Cláudia Pais[1], Patrícia Paiva[1], Lúcia Simões[1], Francisco Caramelo[6], Lina Ramos[6], Margarida Venâncio[3,7], Fabiana Ramos[3,7], Ana Beleza[7], Joaquim Sá[7], Jorge Saraiva[3,7] and Joana Barbosa de Melo[1,2,3,4]

**Abstract**

**Background:** Array-based comparative genomic hybridization has been assumed to be the first genetic test offered to detect genomic imbalances in patients with unexplained intellectual disability with or without dysmorphisms, multiple congenital anomalies, learning difficulties and autism spectrum disorders.
Our study contributes to the genotype/phenotype correlation with the delineation of laboratory criteria which help to classify the different copy number variants (CNVs) detected. We clustered our findings into five classes ranging from an imbalance detected in a microdeletion/duplication syndrome region (class I) to imbalances that had previously been reported in normal subjects in the Database of Genomic Variants (DGV) and thus considered common variants (class IV).

**Results:** All the analyzed 1000 patients had at least one CNV independently of its clinical significance. Most of them, as expected, were alterations already reported in the DGV for normal individuals (class IV) or without known coding genes (class III-B). In approximately 14 % of the patients an imbalance involving known coding genes, but with partially overlapping or low frequency of CNVs described in the DGV was identified (class IIIA). In 10.4 % of the patients a pathogenic CNV that explained the phenotype was identified consisting of: 40 class I imbalances, 44 class II *de novo* imbalances and 21 class II X-chromosome imbalances in male patients. In 20 % of the patients a familial pathogenic or potentially pathogenic CNV, consisting of inherited class II imbalances, was identified that implied a family evaluation by the clinical geneticists.

**Conclusions:** As this interpretation can be sometimes difficult, particularly if it is not possible to study the parents, using the proposed classification we were able to prioritize the multiple imbalances that are identified in each patient without immediately having to classify them as pathogenic or benign.

**Keywords:** Array comparative genomic hybridization (array-CGH), Copy number variation (CNV) classification, Intellectual disability, Multiple congenital anomalies, Learning difficulties, Autism spectrum disorders

## Background

Microarray-based comparative genomic hybridization (array-CGH), also called chromosomal microarray or molecular karyotyping, allows the possibility to screen the whole genome at once and with high resolution. It is currently assumed that array-CGH should be the first genetic test offered to detect genomic imbalances in patients with intellectual disability (ID) with or without dysmorphisms, multiple congenital anomalies (MCA), learning difficulties and autism spectrum disorders (ASD) [1, 2]. As array-CGH allows the detection of imbalances below the 5–10 Mb resolution level of conventional cytogenetics, the average diagnostic yield can be up to 10 % higher [3–7]. It also allows the detection of a large number of Copy Number Variants (CNVs) in these patients as well as in healthy individuals, which poses a great challenge in the interpretation of the results [8]. In

* Correspondence: citogenetica@fmed.uc.pt
Isabel Marques Carreira and Susana Isabel Ferreira shared first authorship
[1]Laboratório de Citogenética e Genómica – Faculdade de Medicina, Universidade de Coimbra, Pólo Ciências da Saúde, Sub-Unidade 1 - Piso 2, Azinhaga de Santa Comba, 3000-354 Coimbra, Portugal
[2]CIMAGO – Centro de Investigação em Meio Ambiente, Genética e Oncobiologia, Faculdade de Medicina, Universidade de Coimbra, Coimbra, Portugal
Full list of author information is available at the end of the article

addition to this increase in the detection of CNVs, the use of array-CGH in large cohorts of patients with ID, ASD and MCA has led to the identification of novel microdeletion and microduplication syndromes [9, 10].

In this study we report the frequency of imbalances, their inheritance and conclusions of a cohort of 1000 patients with ID, ASD, MCA and learning disabilities studied by array-CGH. We propose a classification of CNVs into five different classes as a way to prioritize the multiple imbalances detected in each patient, helping not only the organization and interpretation of the results, but also in those cases where parents were unwillingly to be tested or were unavailable, the elaboration of a more comprehensive report.

## Results

A cohort of a 1000 patients with ID, MCA and/or ASD was studied by array CGH using an oligonucleotide platform. After array analysis, detected CNVs were classified into 5 different classes (Table 1): class I - deletions or duplications in a region associated with a microdeletion or a microduplication syndrome; class II - deletions or duplications in a region not reported in the Database of Genomic Variants (DGV) and involving known coding genes; class IIIA- deletions or duplications reported in low frequency in DGV or that do not totally overlapped with the ones reported, involving known coding regions; class IIIB - deletions or duplications reported in low frequency in DGV or that do not totally overlapped with the ones reported, without involving known coding genes; class IV - deletions or duplications reported in normal subjects in DGV or that are considered common variants.

When a class I or class II CNV was found, the study of the parents was requested in order to ascertain its origin and delineate the strategy for family management and future prenatal diagnosis. For cases where a IIIA CNV was identified, decision whether or not to pursue with parental evaluation was left to the clinicians. For class IIIB and class IV CNVs no study of parents was needed, and a normal array-CGH result was issued. Since class IIIB CNVs at present do not have genes reported, no causality was attributed, but the information was included in a summary table in the report, to allow a future revision, if genes or regulatory regions are later described.

There were cases where the origin of the imbalances was not possible to determine, either because of unwillingness of both parents to be evaluated, in situations of adoption or in monoparental cases in which the available progenitor was not a carrier of the proband's CNVs.

In our cohort we identified at least one class IV CNV in each patient. As they are considered benign copy number variations present in normal individuals, like the results by Choucair and collaborators [11], class IV imbalances were disregarded for the frequency evaluation. In this study group, 489 patients only had class IV imbalances. Excluding class IV CNVs, we identified a total of 843 CNVs in the remaining 611 cases: 40 as class I (4.8 %), 452 as class II (53.6 %), 166 as class IIIA (19.7 %) and 185 as class IIIB (21.9 %) (Fig. 1).

The distribution of all the imbalances from the different classes according to genomic size was evaluated

**Table 1** Class definition of CNVs depending on its clinical significance

| | | |
|---|---|---|
| Class I | Deletion or duplication in a region associated with a microdeletion or a microduplication syndrome | Pathogenic |
| Class II | Deletion or duplication not reported in the DGV and involving known coding genes | Potentially Pathogenic |
| Class IIIA | Deletion or duplication reported in low frequency in the DGV or that do not totally overlap with the ones reported, involving known coding genes | Uncertain significance - Likely pathogenic |
| Class IIIB | Deletion or duplication reported in low frequency in the DGV or that do not totally overlap with the ones reported, without known coding genes | Uncertain significance - Likely benign |
| Class IV | Deletions or duplications reported in normal subjects in the DGV or that are considered common variants | Benign |

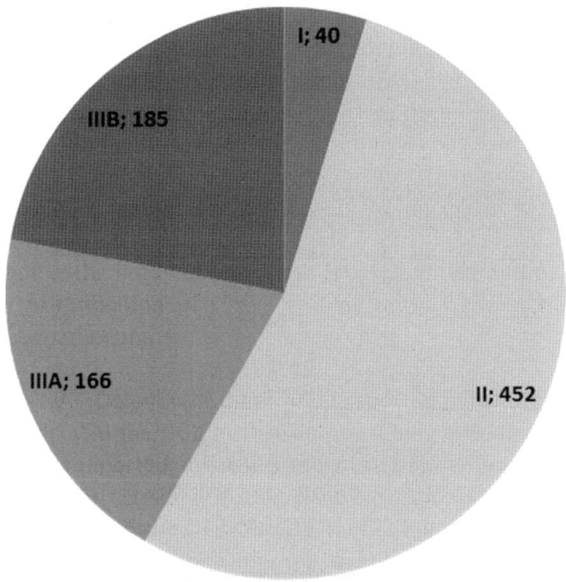


**Fig. 1** Distribution of the 843 CNVs identified in 611 of the 1000 cases by classes I to IIIA: 40 imbalances belong to class I (4.8 %), 452 to class II (53.6 %), 166 to class IIIA (19.7 %) and 185 to class IIIB (21.9 %)

(Fig. 2). From the figure analysis we can observe that as the genomic size of the imbalance increases, the probability to find imbalances from the four classes reduces. Above 3 Mb in size we only found imbalances belonging to class I and II. There is an association with statistical significance ($\chi^2(1) = 40.591$; $p < 0.001$) between class I and II and sizes above 3 Mb, and between class IIIA and IIIB and sizes below 3 Mb.

Class I imbalances (Table 2) were present in 40 patients: twenty-two deletions and sixteen duplications, a triple X and a Klinefelter syndrome which were confirmed without other clinical significant imbalances present. Fifteen imbalances were *de novo*, two maternal, four paternal and in nineteen cases the inheritance was not possible to determine. Table 3 contains the list of all the syndromes identified and the number of cases within each one. Of the 40 imbalances, 42.5 % had between 1–3 Mb in size, eleven cases (27.5 %) had a genomic size between 1-2 Mb and six (15 %) an imbalance with 2-3 Mb, with the remaining distributed by different genomic ranges (Fig. 2). The smallest class I imbalance detected corresponds to a 184 kb deletion in 8q22.2 involving Cohen syndrome gene, *COH1*, and the largest, disregarding the triple X and Klinefelter cases, corresponds to a 30 Mb deletion at the short arm of chromosome 5, involving the Cri du Chat region. In 38 % of the cases the imbalances were *de novo* and in 48 % it was not possible to ascertain the family inheritance. From the available data, it was shown that chromosome 3q29 deletion and the 17q12 duplication were similarly observed in the mothers, while the chromosomes 3q29 duplication syndrome, 16p11.2 deletion syndrome and 22q11.2 duplication and deletion syndromes were observed similarly in the male progenitors.

We detected 452 class II imbalances present in 340 cases, since some patients had multiple imbalances classified in this class. Of the 452 alterations, 191 were deletions (42.25 %), 255 duplications (56.42 %), two were X-chromosome triplications (0.44 %) and the remaining four were tetrasomies (0.89 %) (Table 4). Considering the

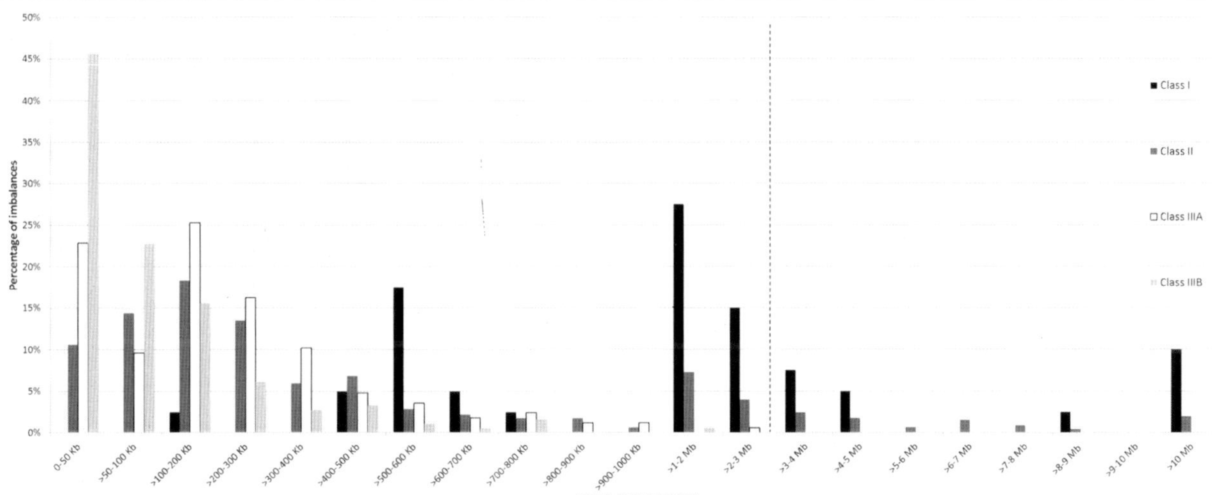


**Fig. 2** Distribution of all the imbalances according to the genomic size. As the genomic size of the imbalance increases, the number of imbalances from the four classes reduces. Above 3 Mb in size only imbalances belonging to classes I and II are observed. Class IV imbalances are not represented as they are considered benign copy number variations. There is an association with statistical significance ($\chi^2(1) = 40.591$; $p < 0.001$) between classes I and II and sizes above 3 Mb and between classes IIIA and IIIB and sizes below 3 Mb – dashed line

**Table 2** Class I imbalances distributed according to the type of imbalance and inheritance

| Imbalance / Inheritance | Deletion | Duplication | Klinefelter | Triple X | |
|---|---|---|---|---|---|
| *De novo* | 8 | 5 | 1 | 1 | 15 |
| Maternal | 1 | 1 | 0 | 0 | 2 |
| Paternal | 2 | 2 | 0 | 0 | 4 |
| Unknown | 11 | 8 | 0 | 0 | 19 |
| | 22 | 16 | 1 | 1 | 40 |

totality of class II imbalances, 70 % had a genomic size between 1.9 kb, that corresponds to the size of the smallest imbalance detected (a deletion), and 500 kb. 15 % of the cases had an imbalance between 1–5 Mb, with the remaining distributed by different genomic ranges, as observed in Fig. 2.

Analyzing class II imbalances in respect to inheritance pattern, there was a clear difference considering the distribution of inherited vs *de novo* imbalances: 82 % of the inherited CNVs had a genomic size ranging from 1.985 kb to 600 kb, against 28 % of the *de novo*, while 51 % of the *de novo* imbalances had a genomic size ranging from 1 to 5 Mb. The higher the genomic size of the imbalance, the lower the probability of being inherited (Fig. 3). Our data show a significant association ($\chi^2(1) = 44.456$; $p < 0.001$) between *de novo* imbalances and sizes above 500 kb and between inherited imbalances and sizes below 500 kb.

One hundred and sixty-six class IIIA imbalances were identified in 137 different patients: sixty deletions (36.15 %), 103 duplications (62.05 %) and three amplifications (1.8 %). To date, only one patient whose parents were studied revealed to have a *de novo* class IIIA imbalance. In the others there was a similar proportion of maternal and paternal inheritance (Table 5). The maximum genomic size of imbalances in this class was 2.5 Mb, with 84 % of the imbalances ranging from 1.9 kb and 400 kb (Fig. 2).

We identified 185 class IIIB imbalances, fifty-six deletions (30.3 %), thirty duplications (16.2 %) and ninety-nine variations (53.5 %), ranging from 284 bp to 1.4 Mb, with 84 % of them having between 284 bp-200 kb.

In the studied cohort of patients, we concluded that the great majority, 76 % of all the inherited CNVs identified were smaller than 500 kb, as Fig. 4 illustrates.

**Table 3** List of all the syndromes identified (class I imbalances) and the number of cases

| Syndrome | Chromosome | OMIM ID | Number of cases |
|---|---|---|---|
| Chromosome 1q21.1 deletion syndrome | 1q21.1 | 612474 | 3 na |
| Chromosome 1q21.1 duplication syndrome | 1q21.1 | 612475 | 1 na |
| Chromosome 3q29 deletion syndrome | 3q29 | 609425 | 1 mat |
| Chromosome 3q29 duplication syndrome | 3q29 | 611936 | 2 (1pat, 1na) |
| Wolf-Hirschhorn syndrome | 4p16.3 | 194190 | 1 dn |
| Cri du Chat syndrome | 5p | 123450 | 1 na |
| Williams-Beuren region duplication syndrome | 7q11.23 | 609757 | 2 (1dn, 1na) |
| Cohen syndrome | 8q22.2 | 216550 | 1 na |
| Chromosome 9p deletion syndrome | 9p | 158170 | 1 dn |
| Kleefstra syndrome | 9q34.3 | 610253 | 1 na |
| Chromosome15q11q13 duplication syndrome | 15q11q13 | 608636 | 1 na |
| Chromosome 15q13.3 deletion syndrome | 15q13.3 | 612001 | 1 na |
| Chromosome 16p11.2 deletion syndrome | 16p11.2 | 611913 | 5 (1pat, 2dn, 2na) |
| Chromosome 16p11.2 duplication syndrome | 16p11.2 | 614671 | 3 (1dn, 2na) |
| Smith –Magenis syndrome | 17p11.2 | 182290 | 1 na |
| Potocki-Lupski syndrome | 17p11.2 | 610883 | 2 dn |
| Chromosome 17q12 duplication syndrome | 17q11.2 | 614526 | 2 (1mat,1na) |
| Chromosome 19q13.11 deletion syndrome | 19q13.11 | 613026 | 1 dn |
| Chromosome 22q11.2 deletion syndrome, distal | 22q11.2 | 611867 | 5 (1pat, 3dn, 1na) |
| Chromosome 22q11.2 duplication syndrome | 22q11.2 | 608363 | 3 (1pat, 1dn, 1na) |
| Triple X | X | | 1dn |
| Klinefelter | X | | 1dn |

*mat* maternal origin, *pat* paternal origin, *dn de novo*, *na* inheritance not available

**Table 4** Class II imbalances distributed according to the type of imbalance and inheritance

| Imbalance / Inheritance | Deletion | Duplication | Triplication | Tetrasomy | |
|---|---|---|---|---|---|
| *De novo* | 30 | 13 | 0 | 1 | 44 |
| Maternal | 38 | 74 | 0 | 2 | 114 |
| Paternal | 38 | 48 | 0 | 0 | 86 |
| Maternal and paternal | 1 | 0 | 0 | 1 | 2 |
| Unknown | 84 | 120 | 2 | 0 | 206 |
| | 191 | 255 | 2 | 4 | 452 |

## Discussion

Array-CGH has proven to be an important tool not only in the detection of submicroscopic chromosomal imbalances and delineation of structural imbalances but also in the establishment of genotype/phenotype correlation. All of the 1000 cases studied in this cohort presented ID with or without dysmorphisms, learning difficulties, MCA or ASD. All of them had imbalances detected by array-CGH. Overall, there were 843 imbalances (class I-III) in 611 of the 1000 cases (Fig. 1). Imbalances classified as class IV are not discussed as they correspond to benign CNVs. In order to define the relevance of the identified imbalances and their correlation with the identified phenotypes we classified them into five classes:

### Class I - Deletion or duplication in a region associated with a microdeletion or a microduplication syndrome

Of the 1000 patients, forty (4 %) fitted into this category with more deletions compared to duplications. In a study by Shoukier and collaborators, in 342 patients, 42 (12 %) had an imbalance that corresponded to a known microdeletion or microduplication syndrome, with a higher proportion of deletions to duplications (33 vs 9) [12]. The most common findings in our cohort were imbalances involving 16p11.2 and 22q11.2 microdeletion/duplication syndromes region, interestingly the same result as recently reported by Ahn et al, 2013 [13]. In the cases where pattern of inheritance was studied, as expected, most of them were *de novo*. One of these cases had a *de novo* 19q13.11q13.12 deletion that provides evidence for

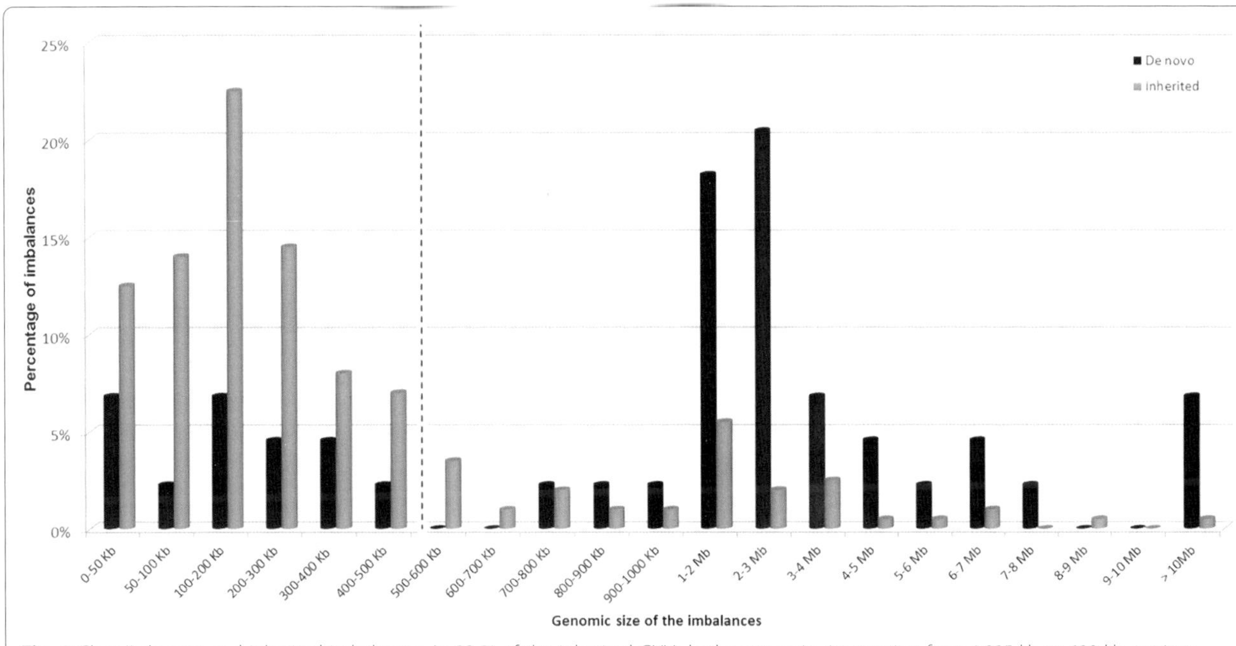


**Fig. 3** Class II *de novo* and inherited imbalances. In 82 % of the inherited CNVs had a genomic size ranging from 1.985 kb to 600 kb, against 28 % of the de novo, while 51 % of the de novo imbalances had a genomic size ranging from 1 to 5 Mb. The higher the genomic size of the imbalance, the lower the probability of being inherited. Our data show a significant association ($\chi^2(1) = 44.456$; $p < 0.001$) between *de novo* imbalances and sizes above 500 kb and between inherited imbalances and sizes below 500 kb – dashed line

**Table 5** Class IIIA imbalances distributed according to the type of imbalance and inheritance

| Imbalance | Deletion | Duplication | Amplification | |
|---|---|---|---|---|
| Inheritance | | | | |
| *De novo* | 0 | 1 | 0 | 1 |
| Maternal | 10 | 9 | 0 | 19 |
| Paternal | 10 | 6 | 0 | 16 |
| Unknown | 83 | 44 | 3 | 130 |
| | 103 | 60 | 3 | 166 |

the involvement of *UBA2* gene haploinsuffiency in cutis aplasia [14].

Of the six inherited imbalances, three were deletions in chromosomes 3q29, 16p11.2 and 22q11.2, and three were duplications, in 3q29, 17q12 and 22q11.2. The 3q29 deletion and the 17q12 duplication were maternally inherited, while the 3q29 and 22q11.2 duplications and the 16p11.2 and 22q11.2 deletions were paternal in origin. In the results by Shoukier and collaborators, half of the 42 imbalances were *de novo*, 9 were maternally inherited, with 4 imbalances on the X-chromosome, and in 12 inheritance was unknown [12].

Concerning inherited CNVs, the difficulties in interpretation are due to: 1) incomplete penetrance; 2) phenotypic variability; and 3) lack of clinical evaluation of the carrier progenitor. The chromosome 16p11.2 deletion was inherited from a healthy father, which is commonly reported in the literature and in agreement with the variable clinical outcome associated with this imbalance that can include a normal phenotype [12, 15]. Concerning chromosome 22q11.2 imbalances, the father with the 22q11.2 duplication is healthy, having however only completed the basic scholarship but is currently not able to read or write and his ID is similar to his daughter. The chromosome 22q11.2 deletion is inherited from the paternal grandmother, and the proband is the only one with phenotypic features. These cases clearly show the inter and intra-familial phenotypic variability associated with this imbalance [16]. The 3q29 deletion was inherited from the mother without ID but that had learning difficulties, and actually presents speech difficulties and psychiatric disease. The 3q29 duplication and the 17q12 duplication were inherited from healthy progenitors that have only completed basic scholarship.

The inherited cases posed a delicate problem, in terms of future pregnancies, in healthy parents that had an apparently normal phenotype, even though many of them had only completed basic schooling.

Class I imbalances are considered pathogenic and molecular/conventional cytogenetics-FISH study of the

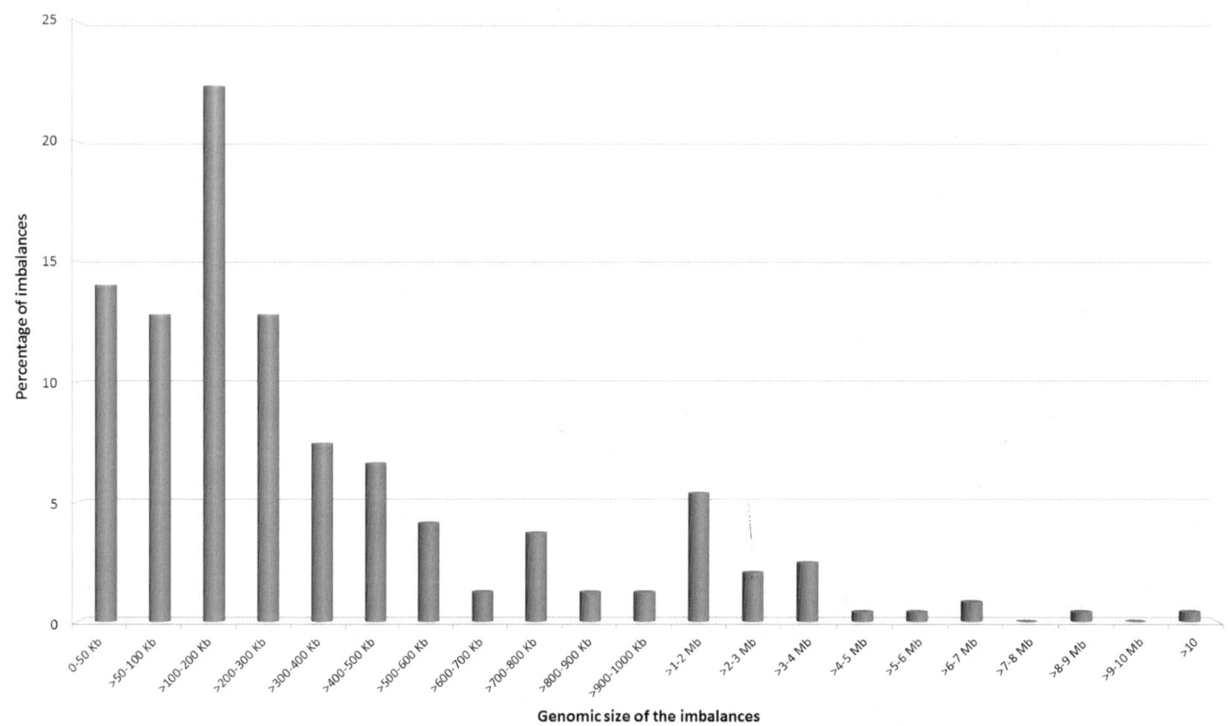


**Fig. 4** Inherited CNVs distribution according to genomic size. 76 % of all the inherited CNVs identified were smaller than 500 kb

progenitors is recommended, namely to exclude a balanced rearrangement (Table 1).

#### Class II - Deletion or duplication not reported in the DGV and involving known coding genes

In the studied cohort, 34 % of the patients demonstrated 452 class II imbalances (Fig. 1). This high percentage is most probably due to the fact that the first 250 cases of this cohort of patients were highly selected as they had a strong clinical phenotype, normal karyotype and most had a normal subtelomeric analysis by fluorescence *in situ* hybridization (FISH) or multiplex ligation-dependent probe amplification (MLPA). Patient selection is one of the factors that most influences the diagnostic yield, as stated by Shoukier and collaborators, whose cohort of patients had already performed conventional cytogenetics and subtelomere screening before array-CGH, similar to our first 250 patients [12].

Almost 50 % of the identified class II imbalances were inherited, making the genotype/phenotype correlation difficult to establish as most of the carrier progenitors had apparently normal phenotypes, although they have not been through a thorough clinical evaluation. As previously mentioned, larger inherited imbalances also had a phenotypic manifestation in the carrier progenitor. Smaller inherited imbalances can either not be the cause of the proband's phenotype or can have incomplete penetrance in the carrier progenitor. There are some exceptions, as for example the 12.5 Mb inherited imbalance that corresponds to an X-chromosome duplication in a boy, inherited from his healthy mother, which illustrates how X-chromosome inactivation in females can mask large imbalances. In the range of 8–9 Mb we identified a chromosome 4 maternal duplication in a girl with attention-deficit hyperactivity disorder whose mother presented learning difficulties at school [17]. In the 6–7 Mb range two imbalances were identified: in 18p11.32p11.31 with 6.9 Mb duplication and in 8p21.3p21.1 with 6.2 Mb duplication both inherited from affected fathers, one with ID and the other with learning difficulties, as he only completed basic school.

Class II imbalances have a spectrum that ranges from pathogenic, potentially pathogenic to uncertain significance but likely pathogenic (Table 1). In this type of imbalance, the study of parents is recommended and helps the prioritization of CNVs – if *de novo*, CNV is most likely pathogenic.

#### Class IIIA - Deletion or duplication reported in low frequency in the DGV or that do not totally overlap with the ones reported, involving known coding genes

Imbalances classified in this class corresponded to 20 % of all the identified CNVs (Fig. 1). These CNVs can be population CNVs with low representation in the public databases. This class includes imbalances of uncertain significance tending to be probably benign. In only one patient inheritance was determined to be *de novo*, and in this patient the imbalance might be considered of uncertain significance but likely pathogenic.

Class IIIA imbalances have uncertain significance, ranging from likely pathogenic to likely benign (Table 1). In this type of CNVs, the study of parents is optional and the management of the origin and its impact has to be evaluated in the clinical context.

#### Class IIIB - Deletion or duplication reported in low frequency in the DGV or that do not totally overlap with the ones reported, without known coding genes

In this cohort of patients, 22 % of the imbalances were classified as IIIB. Accordingly to the available data, as they do not include genes, these imbalances were not considered relevant for the phenotype. Nevertheless, they were included in a table attached to the report sent to the clinician, allowing these cases to be revisited and reclassified in the light of future knowledge.

Class IIIB imbalances have uncertain significance, but being likely benign (Table 1). The study of parents is not recommended.

## Conclusion

Array-CGH has revolutionized post natal cytogenetics diagnostic, increasing the detection rate and replacing conventional cytogenetics [1]. However, karyotyping cannot be completely abandoned and, in certain cases, both techniques should be performed in order to understand the biological mechanism involved in the origin of an imbalance and contribute, not only to identify the carriers, but also to do a correct evaluation of the recurrence risk in these families. The importance of the proposed CNVs prioritization arises, specially, when a preliminary report is done requesting parental studies. It was important for the clinical management of the family to have an indication of the relationship between the genotype and the phenotype. Classifying CNVs in different classes allowed us to establish the continuum pathogenic–benign and their final impact on the phenotype, after determining their origin. In classes I and II, parental blood samples were always requested to determine the origin of the imbalance either by array-CGH, MLPA, FISH or karyotype. Prenatal diagnosis was recommended in subsequent gestations to progenitors from classes I and II probands. In class IIIA imbalances it was left to clinicians' criteria, after the genetic counseling, the necessity to perform subsequent laboratory and familial studies. For classes IIIB and IV no parental blood samples were requested by the laboratory, but these results were sent to the clinician in a table attached to the report for future management.

This classification allowed a prioritization of the cases, particularly when a report had to be issued requesting parents study.

## Methods

### Patients

A cohort of 1000 unrelated patient samples was analyzed by oligoarray-CGH in our Cytogenetics and Genomics laboratory over a period of 3 years. The samples were provided by clinical geneticists and pediatricians from 3 national hospitals, as part of a common undertaking to determine the etiology of ID with or without dysmorphisms, learning difficulties, MCA and ASD. The levels of ID of our patients ranged from mild to moderate or severe as determined by the gold standard scales and the ASD patients were evaluated by ADI-R and ADOS. The study was approved by the Hospitals Ethics Committee.

Various techniques were used to confirm and characterize the imbalances identified by oligoarray-CGH, such as, high resolution conventional cytogenetics, FISH or MLPA, depending on the type and dimension of the imbalance and availability of FISH and MLPA probes in the laboratory. In order to determine the origin of the imbalances, parental blood samples were requested and, additionally to the previous mentioned techniques, array-CGH was also used in particular cases.

In 325 patients conventional cytogenetics had been previously performed. Fourteen patients with an abnormal karyotype were analyzed by array-CGH. Of those, five patients presented a deletion, two a duplication, two had apparently balanced translocations, one had a 47, XXY karyotype, three patients presented inversions and one had a derivative chromosome. These cases were analyzed by oligoarray-CGH to refine the breakpoints and the genomic content of the rearrangements, or to determine if there were genomic imbalances involved in apparently balanced translocations, as they can remain undetected [18], and inversions carriers, or even to clarify if there was an additional imbalance, like in the case of a Klinefelter patient, which could explain a severe phenotype.

### DNA extraction

Genomic DNA was extracted from peripheral blood lymphocytes using Jetquick blood and cell culture DNA Midi Spin kit according to the manufacturers' instructions (Genomed, Löhne, Germany). DNA concentration and purity were measured using a NanoDrop1000 Spectrophotometer (Thermo Scientific, Waltham, USA).

### Array-CGH

High-resolution whole genome analysis was performed using Agilent SurePrint G3 Human Genome microarrays. Although 180 K oligonucleotide microarray format (Agilent Technologies, Santa Clara, CA, USA) was the most used, the 60 K was requested for fifty-four cases. These microarrays contain approximately 180 000 and 60 000 sixty-mer probes with a 17 kb and 54 kb average probe spacing, respectively. Labeling was performed using Agilent Genomic DNA enzymatic labeling kit (Agilent Technologies, Santa Clara, CA, USA) and clean-up of labeled genomic DNA was performed using Amicon ultra 0.5 ml centrifugal filters according to manufacturers' instructions (Millipore, Billerica, MA, USA). Slides were scanned on an Agilent scanner and processed with Feature Extraction software (v10.7). Each patient DNA was labeled both in Cy3 and Cy5 and hybridized against the DNA of two phenotypically distinct patients according to the loop model [19]. Results were analyzed using Agilent Genomic Workbench (v6.0 and v6.5) software with the following settings: ADM2 as aberration algorithm, threshold of 6.0, moving average 2 Mb. The results are according to Human Genome build 19 and include imbalances with at least three consecutive probes with abnormal $\log_2$ ratios. All the imbalances were interpreted consulting the UCSC genome browser (http://genome.ucsc.edu), Decipher (Database of Chromosomal Imbalance and Phenotype in Humans Using Ensembl Resources - http://decipher.sanger.ac.uk/), ClinGen (Clinical Genome Resource - https://www.clinicalgenome.org/), OMIM (Online Mendelian Inheritance in Man - http://www.ncbi.nlm.nih.gov/omim) and DGV (http://projects.tcag.ca) databases.

### Statistical analysis

The statistical analysis was mainly conducted aiming to describe the proportions found in each group resorting to suitable figures and tables. Association hypotheses regarding nominal variables were tested using the chi-square test taking into account the Cochran rules for validity of the test. The level of significance adopted was 0.05 %.

#### Competing interests

The authors declare that they have no competing interests

#### Authors' contributions

IMC, JBM – have designed the study and drafted the manuscript. SIF – has been involved in array-CGH data acquisition, analysis and interpretation and drafted the manuscript. EM – has been involved in array-CGH data interpretation and critically revised the manuscript. LMP, JF – have been involved in array-CGH data acquisition and analysis. AJ, AM, MP, NL, CP, PP, LS – have performed conventional cytogenetics procedures, including karyotype and FISH analysis. FC- has performed statistical analysis to the results. LR, MV, FR, AB, JS, JS – have clinically evaluated the patients and their families, provided clinical information for the interpretation of results. All authors read and approved the final manuscript.

#### Acknowledgments

The authors wish to thank the patients and their families.

**Author details**
[1]Laboratório de Citogenética e Genómica – Faculdade de Medicina, Universidade de Coimbra, Pólo Ciências da Saúde, Sub-Unidade 1 - Piso 2, Azinhaga de Santa Comba, 3000-354 Coimbra, Portugal. [2]CIMAGO – Centro de Investigação em Meio Ambiente, Genética e Oncobiologia, Faculdade de Medicina, Universidade de Coimbra, Coimbra, Portugal. [3]Faculdade de Medicina, Universidade de Coimbra, Coimbra, Portugal. [4]CNC, IBILI – Faculdade de Medicina, Universidade de Coimbra, Coimbra, Portugal. [5]Laboratório de Citogenética, Hospital Pediátrico de Coimbra, Coimbra, Portugal. [6]Laboratório de Bioestatística e Informática Médica, IBILI – Faculdade de Medicina, Universidade de Coimbra, Coimbra, Portugal. [7]Serviço de Genética Médica, Hospital Pediátrico – Centro Hospitalar e Universitário de Coimbra, Coimbra, Portugal.

**References**

1. Miller DT, Adam MP, Aradhya S, Biesecker LG, Brothman AR, Carter NP, et al. Consensus statement: chromosomal microarray is a first-tier clinical diagnostic test for individuals with developmental disabilities or congenital anomalies. Am J Hum Genet. 2010;86:749–64.
2. Friedman JM, Baross A, Delaney AD, Ally A, Arbour L, Armstrong L, et al. Oligonucleotide microarray analysis of genomic imbalance in children with mental retardation. Am J Hum Genet. 2006;79:500–13.
3. Lu X, Shaw CA, Patel A, Li J, Cooper ML, Wells WR, et al. Clinical implementation of chromosomal microarray analysis: summary of 2513 postnatal cases. PLoS One. 2007;2, e327.
4. Rodríguez-Revenga L, Vallespín E, Madrigal I, Palomares M, Mur A, García-Miñaur S, et al. A parallel study of different array-CGH platforms in a set of Spanish patients with developmental delay and intellectual disability. Gene. 2013;521:82–6.
5. D'Arrigo S, Gavazzi F, Alfei E, Zuffardi O, Montomoli C, Corso B, Buzzi E, Sciacca FL, Bulgheroni S, Riva D, Pantaleoni C. The Diagnostic Yield of Array Comparative Genomic Hybridization Is High Regardless of Severity of Intellectual Disability/Developmental Delay in Children. J Child Neurol 2015.
6. Coutton C, Dieterich K, Satre V, Vieville G, Amblard F, David M, et al. Array-CGH in children with mild intellectual disability: a population-based study. Eur J Pediatr. 2015;174:75–83.
7. Nicholl J, Waters W, Mulley JC, Suwalski S, Brown S, Hull Y, et al. Cognitive deficit and autism spectrum disorders: prospective diagnosis by array CGH. Pathology. 2014;46:41–5.
8. Gijsbers AC, Schoumans J, Ruivenkamp CA. Interpretation of array comparative genome hybridization data: a major challenge. Cytogenet Genome Res. 2011;135:222–7.
9. Slavotinek AM. Novel microdeletion syndromes detected by chromosome microarrays. Hum Genet. 2008;124:1–17.
10. Shaffer LG, Bejjani BA, Torchia B, Kirkpatrick S, Coppinger J, Ballif BC. Theidentification of microdeletion syndromes and other chromosome abnormalities: Cytogenetic methods of the past, new technologies for the future. Am J Med Genet Part C Semin Med Genet. 2007;145:335–45.
11. Choucair N, Ghoch JA, Corbani S, Cacciagli P, Mignon-Ravix C, Salem N, et al. Contribution of copy number variants (CNVs) to congenital, unexplained intellectual and developmental disabilities in Lebanese patients. Mol Cytogenet. 2015;8:26.
12. Shoukier M, Klein N, Auber B, Wickert J, Schr¨oder J, Zoll B, et al. Array CGH in patients with developmental delay or intellectual disability: are there phenotypic clues to pathogenic copy number variants? Clin Genet. 2013;83:53–65.
13. Ahn JW, Bint S, Bergbaum A, Mann K, Hall RP, Ogilvie CM. Array CGH as a first line diagnostic test in place of karyotyping for postnatal referrals - results from four years' clinical application for over 8,700 patients. Mol Cytogenet. 2013;6:16.
14. Melo JB, Estevinho A, Saraiva J, Ramos L, Carreira IM. Cutis Aplasia as a clinical hallmark for the syndrome associated with 19q13.11 deletion: the possible role for *UBA2* gene. Mol Cytogenet. 2015;8:21.
15. Bijlsma EK, Gijsbers AC, Schuurs-Hoeijmakers JH, van Haeringen A, Fransen van de Putte DE, Anderlid BM, et al. Extending the phenotype of recurrent rearrangements of 16p11.2: deletions in mentally retarded patients without autism and in normal individuals. Eur J Med Genet. 2009;52:77–87.
16. Tan TY, Collins A, James PA, McGillivray G, Stark Z, Gordon CT, et al. Phenotypic variability of distal 22q11.2 copy number abnormalities. Am J Med Genet A. 2011;155:1623–33.
17. Matoso E, Melo JB, Ferreira SI, Jardim A, Castelo TM, Weise A, et al. Insertional translocation leading to a 4q13 duplication including the EPHA5 gene in two siblings with attention-deficit hyperactivity disorder. Am J Med Genet A. 2013;161:1923–8.
18. Di Gregorio E, Savin E, Biamino E, Belligni EF, Naretto VG, D'Alessandro G, et al. Large cryptic genomic rearrangements with apparently normal karyotypes detected by array-CGH. Mol Cytogenet. 2014;7:82.
19. Menten B, Maas N, Thienpont B, Buysse K, Vandesompele J, Melotte C, et al. Emerging patterns of cryptic chromosomal imbalance in patients with idiopathic mental retardation and multiple congenital anomalies: a new series of 140 patients and review of published reports. J Med Genet. 2006;43:625–33.

# Permissions

All chapters in this book were first published in MC, by BioMed Central; hereby published with permission under the Creative Commons Attribution License or equivalent. Every chapter published in this book has been scrutinized by our experts. Their significance has been extensively debated. The topics covered herein carry significant findings which will fuel the growth of the discipline. They may even be implemented as practical applications or may be referred to as a beginning point for another development.

The contributors of this book come from diverse backgrounds, making this book a truly international effort. This book will bring forth new frontiers with its revolutionizing research information and detailed analysis of the nascent developments around the world.

We would like to thank all the contributing authors for lending their expertise to make the book truly unique. They have played a crucial role in the development of this book. Without their invaluable contributions this book wouldn't have been possible. They have made vital efforts to compile up to date information on the varied aspects of this subject to make this book a valuable addition to the collection of many professionals and students.

This book was conceptualized with the vision of imparting up-to-date information and advanced data in this field. To ensure the same, a matchless editorial board was set up. Every individual on the board went through rigorous rounds of assessment to prove their worth. After which they invested a large part of their time researching and compiling the most relevant data for our readers.

The editorial board has been involved in producing this book since its inception. They have spent rigorous hours researching and exploring the diverse topics which have resulted in the successful publishing of this book. They have passed on their knowledge of decades through this book. To expedite this challenging task, the publisher supported the team at every step. A small team of assistant editors was also appointed to further simplify the editing procedure and attain best results for the readers.

Apart from the editorial board, the designing team has also invested a significant amount of their time in understanding the subject and creating the most relevant covers. They scrutinized every image to scout for the most suitable representation of the subject and create an appropriate cover for the book.

The publishing team has been an ardent support to the editorial, designing and production team. Their endless efforts to recruit the best for this project, has resulted in the accomplishment of this book. They are a veteran in the field of academics and their pool of knowledge is as vast as their experience in printing. Their expertise and guidance has proved useful at every step. Their uncompromising quality standards have made this book an exceptional effort. Their encouragement from time to time has been an inspiration for everyone.

The publisher and the editorial board hope that this book will prove to be a valuable piece of knowledge for researchers, students, practitioners and scholars across the globe.

# List of Contributors

**Pasakorn Saenjundaeng, Alongklod Tanomtong and Sumalee Phimphan**
Toxic Substances in Livestock and Aquatic Animals Research Group, Department of Biology, Faculty of Science, Khon Kaen University, Muang District, Khon Kaen, Thailand

**Marcelo de Bello Cioffi, Luiz Antonio Carlos Bertollo, Cassia Fernanda Yano and Terumi Hatanaka**
Departamento de Genética e Evolução, Universidade Federal de São Carlos, São Carlos, SP, Brazil

**Ezequiel Aguiar de Oliveira**
Departamento de Genética e Evolução, Universidade Federal de São Carlos, São Carlos, SP, Brazil
Secretaria de Estado de Educação de Mato Grosso - SEDUC-MT, Cuiabá, MT, Brazil

**Weerayuth Supiwong**
Faculty of Applied Science and Engineering, Khon Kaen University, Nong Kai Campus, Muang, Nong Kai, Thailand

**Maria João Collares-Pereira**
Faculdade de Ciencias, Centre for Ecology, Evolution and Environmental Changes, Universidade de Lisboa, Campo Grande, PT-1749-016 Lisbon, Portugal

**Petr Ráb and Alexandr Sember**
Laboratory of Fish Genetics, Institute of Animal Physiology and Genetics, Czech Academy of Sciences, Rumburská 89, 277 21 Liběchov, Czech Republic

**Thomas Liehr**
Institute of Human Genetics, Jena University Hospital, Am Klinikum 1, D-07747 Jena, Germany

**Birsen Karaman, Asadollah Ghanbari, Zehra Oya Uyguner, Güven Toksoy, Umut Altunoglu and Seher Basaran**
Department of Medical Genetics, Istanbul Medical Faculty, Istanbul University, Millet cad.34039 Capa, İstanbul, Turkey

**Hülya Kayserili**
Department of Medical Genetics, Istanbul Medical Faculty, Istanbul University, Millet cad.34039 Capa, İstanbul, Turkey
Medical Genetics Department and Genetic Diagnosis Center, Koç University School of Medicine, 34010 İstanbul, Turkey

**Agus Budi Setiawan, Shinji Kikuchi, Hidenori Sassa and Takato Koba**
Laboratory of Genetics and Plant Breeding, Graduate School of Horticulture, Chiba University, Matsudo, Chiba 271-8510, Japan

**Chee How Teo**
Center for Research in Biotechnology for Agriculture, University of Malaya, 50603 Kuala Lumpur, Malaysia

**Boris Zagradišnik, Danijela Krgović, Špela Stangler Herodež, Andreja Zagorac and Nadja Kokalj Vokač**
Laboratory of Medical Genetics, University Medical Centre Maribor, Ljubljanska 5, 2000 Maribor, Slovenia

**Bogdan Ćižmarević**
Department of Otorhinolaryngology, University Medical Centre Maribor, Ljubljanska 5, 2000 Maribor, Slovenia

**Yuan Tian, Linlin Zhang, Weifang Tian, Jinshuang Gao and Liting Jia**
Department of Clinical Laboratory, The Third Affiliated Hospital of Zhengzhou University, No. 7 Front Kangfu Street, Er'qi District, Zhengzhou 450052, China

**Shihong Cui**
Department of gynaecology and obstetrics, The Third Affiliated Hospital of Zhengzhou University, No. 7 Front Kangfu Street, Er'qi District, Zhengzhou 450052, China

**Irina S. Stepanova, Leonid S. Adonin, Florina M. Batalova, Vladimir N. Parfenov and Dmitry S. Bogolyubov**
Laboratory of Cell Morphology, Institute of Cytology, Russian Academy of Sciences, St. Petersburg 194064, Russia

**Artem M. Kiselev**
Laboratory of Cell Morphology, Institute of Cytology, Russian Academy of Sciences, St. Petersburg 194064, Russia
Federal Almazov North-West Medical Research Centre, St. Petersburg 197341, Russia
ITMO University, Institute of Translational Medicine, St. Petersburg 197101, Russia

**Olga I. Podgornaya**
Laboratory of Cell Morphology, Institute of Cytology, Russian Academy of Sciences, St. Petersburg 194064, Russia

Department of Cytology and Histology, Faculty of Biology, St. Petersburg State University, St. Petersburg 199034, Russia
Far Eastern Federal University, School of Biomedicine, Vladivostok 690950, Russia

**Thiago Vidotto**
Department of Genetics, Ribeirão Preto Medical School, University of São Paulo, Ribeirão Preto, Brazil

**Daniel Guimarães Tiezzi**
Deparment of Gynecology and Obstetrics, Clinical Hospital of Ribeirão Preto, Ribeirão Preto, Brazil

**Jeremy A. Squire**
Department of Genetics, Ribeirão Preto Medical School, University of São Paulo, Ribeirão Preto, Brazil
Department of Pathology and Legal Medicine, Ribeirão Preto Medical School, University of São Paulo, 3900 Bandeirantes Avenue, Monte Alegre, Ribeirão Preto, São Paulo 14040-900, Brazil
Department of Pathology and Molecular Medicine, Queen's University, Kingston, Canada

**Darinka Šumanović-Glamuzina and Zeljka Bilinovac**
Department of Pediatrics, University Hospital Mostar, Mostar, Bosnia and Herzegovina

**Bernarda Lozić**
Department of Pediatrics, University Hospital Centre Split, Split, Croatia

**Beata Stasiewicz-Jarocka, Barbara Panasiuk, Alina T. Midro and Piotr S. Iwanowski**
Department of Clinical Genetics, Medical University of Bialystok, Waszyngtona St. 13, PO Box 22, 15-089 Białystok, Poland

**Tatijana Zemunik**
Department of Medical Biology, School of Medicine Split, University of Split, Split, Croatia

**Steffi Urbschat, Christoph Sippl, Jana Engelhardt, Joachim Oertel and Ralf Ketter**
Department of Neurosurgery, Saarland University, 66421 Homburg/Saar, Germany

**Kai Kammers**
Division of Biostatistics and Bioinformatics, Department of Oncology, Sidney Kimmel Comprehensive Cancer Center, Johns Hopkins University School of Medicine, Baltimore, MD, USA

**Kaihui Zhang, Rui Dong, Ying Wang, Haiyan Zhang, Yufeng Zhang, Zhongtao Gai and Yi Liu**
Pediatric Research Institute, Qilu Children's Hospital of Shandong University, 23976 Jingshi Road, Jinan, Shandong 250022, China

**Yali Yang and Yan Huang**
Rehabilitation Center, Qilu Children's Hospital of Shandong University, 23976 Jingshi Road, Jinan, Shandong 250022, China

**Thomas Liehr, Kathleen Wilhelm, Moneeb A. K. Othman, Ahmed H. Al-Rikabi, Kristin Mrasek, Monika Ziegler, Stefanie Kankel, Katharina Kreskowski and Anja Weise**
Jena University Hospital, Institute of Human Genetics, Friedrich Schiller University, Postfach D-07740, Jena, Germany

**Isolde Schreyer**
Jena University Hospital, Institute of Human Genetics, Friedrich Schiller University, Postfach D-07740, Jena, Germany
Center for Ambulant Medicine, Jena University Hospital, Jena, Germany

**Alma Kuechler**
Institut für Humangenetik, Universitätsklinikum Essen, Essen, Germany

**Emmanouil Manolakos**
Access to Genome, ATG Labs, Athens, Greece

**Sylke Singer and Andreas Dufke**
Institut für Medizinische Genetik und angewandte Genomik, Tübingen, Germany

**Tereza Jančušková and Radek Čmejla**
Synlab czech s.r.o., synlab genetics s.r.o, Praha, Czech Republic

**Magdalena Koczkowska, Beata Stefania Lipska-Ziętkiewicz, Mariola Iliszko and Janusz Limon**
Department of Biology and Genetics, Medical University of Gdansk, 1 Debinki Street, 80-211 Gdansk, Poland

**Janusz Ryś, Agnieszka Harazin-Lechowska and Anna Kruczak**
Department of Tumor Pathology, M. Sklodowska-Curie Memorial Institute of Oncology, 11 Garncarska Street, 31-115 Krakow, Poland

**Markku Miettinen and Jerzy Lasota**
Laboratory of Pathology, National Cancer Institute, Building 10, Room B1B47, 10 Center Drive, Bethesda 20892, MD, USA

**Wojciech Biernat**
Department of Pathology, Medical University of Gdansk, 17 Smoluchowskiego Street, 80-214 Gdansk, Poland

**Benoît Ducourneau, Hervé Bisiau and Agnès Daudignon**
Service d'Hématologie-Immunologie-Cytogénétique, CH Valenciennes, Valenciennes, France

**Thomas Smol**
Service d'Hématologie-Immunologie-Cytogénétique, CH Valenciennes, Valenciennes, France
Université de Lille Nord de France, Lille, France
Institut de génétique médicale, Hôpital Jeanne de Flandre, CHRU Lille, Lille, France

**Annika Dufour and Christine Terré**
Laboratoire de Cytogénétique Hématologique, CH Versailles, Le Chesnay, France

**Sabine Tricot**
Service d'Hématologie Clinique, CH Valenciennes, Valenciennes, France

**Mathieu Wemeau**
Service d'Hématologie Clinique, CH Arras, Arras, France

**Laure Stalnikiewicz**
Service d'Hématologie Clinique, CH Lens, Lens, France

**Franck Bernardi**
Laboratoire de Biologie, CH Douai, Douai, France

**Peter Duesberg**
Department of Molecular and Cell Biology; Donner Laboratory, University of California at Berkeley, Berkeley, CA 94720, USA

**Mathew Bloomfield**
Department of Molecular and Cell Biology; Donner Laboratory, University of California at Berkeley, Berkeley, CA 94720, USA
Present address: Department of Natural Sciences and Mathematics, Dominican University of California, San Rafael, CA, USA

**Dongdong Xu, Yurong Zhang and Bao Lou**
Marine Fishery Institute of Zhejiang Province, Key Lab of Mariculture and Enhancement of Zhejiang Province, 316100 Zhoushan, Zhejiang Province, People's Republic of China

**Wagner Franco Molina**
Departamento de Biologia Celular e Genética, Centro de Biociências, Universidade Federal do Rio Grande do Norte, Campus Universitário, Lagoa Nova, 3000, Natal, RN 59078-970, Brazil

**Cassia Fernanda Yano and Marcelo de Bello Cioffi**
Departamento de Genética e Evolução, Universidade Federal de São Carlos, Rodovia Washington Luís, km 235, São Carlos, SP 13565-905, Brazil

**Ezequiel Aguiar de Oliveira**
Departamento de Genética e Evolução, Universidade Federal de São Carlos, Rodovia Washington Luís, km 235, São Carlos, SP 13565-905, Brazil
Secretaria de Estado de Educação de Mato Grosso – SEDUC-MT, Cuiabá, MT, Brazil

**Fang Liu, Xingxing Wang, Xinglei Cui, Zhongli Zhou, Chunying Wang, Xiaoyan Cai, Yuhong Wang and Kunbo Wang**
State Key Laboratory of Cotton Biology, Institute of Cotton Research of Chinese Academy of Agricultural Science, Anyang, Henan 455000, China

**Yuling Liu**
State Key Laboratory of Cotton Biology, Institute of Cotton Research of Chinese Academy of Agricultural Science, Anyang, Henan 455000, China
National Key Laboratory of Crop Genetic Improvement, Huazhong Agricultural University, Wuhan 430070, China

**Renhai Peng**
State Key Laboratory of Cotton Biology, Institute of Cotton Research of Chinese Academy of Agricultural Science, Anyang, Henan 455000, China
Anyang Institute of Technology, Anyang, Henan 455000, China

**Zhongxu Lin**
National Key Laboratory of Crop Genetic Improvement, Huazhong Agricultural University, Wuhan 430070, China

**Mónica Villalba-Campos, Lilian Chuaire-Noack and Magda Carolina Sánchez-Corredor**
Facultad de Ciencias Naturales y Matemáticas, Universidad del Rosario, Bogotá, DC, Colombia

**Milena Rondón-Lagos**
Facultad de Ciencias Naturales y Matemáticas, Universidad del Rosario, Bogotá, DC, Colombia
Department of Medical Sciences, University of Turin, Via Santena 7, 10126 Turin, Italy

**Hong Yan Liu, Jia Huang, Tao Li, Dong Wu, Hong Dan Wang, Tao Wang, Liang Jie Guo, Qian Nan Guo, Fei Fei Huang and Ying Tai Wang**
Department of Medical Genetics Institute, People's Hospital of Zhengzhou University (Henan Provincial People's Hospital), Zhengzhou 450003, Henan, China

**Yue Wang**
Department of Gynaecology and Obstetrics, People's Hospital of Zhengzhou University (Henan Provincial People's Hospital), Zhengzhou 450003, Henan, China

**Rui Li Wang**
Department of Ultrasonography, People's Hospital of Zhengzhou University (Henan Provincial People's Hospital), Zhengzhou 450003, Henan, China

**Nuntiya Maneechot, Nuntaporn Getlekha and Sukhonthip Ditcharoen**
Department of Biology, Faculty of Science, Khon Kaen University, Muang District, Khon Kaen, Thailand

**Alongklod Tanomtong**
Department of Biology, Faculty of Science, Khon Kaen University, Muang District, Khon Kaen, Thailand
Toxic Substances in Livestock and Aquatic Animals Research Group, Khon Kaen University, Muang, Khon Kaen 40002, Thailand

**Cassia Fernanda Yano, Luiz Antonio Carlos Bertollo and Marcelo de Bello Cioffi**
Departamento de Genética e Evolução, Universidade Federal de São Carlos, São Carlos, São Paulo, Brazil

**Wagner Franco Molina**
Departamento de Biologia Celular e Genética, Centro de Biociências, Universidade Federal do Rio Grande do Norte, Natal, RN, Brazil

**Bundit Tengjaroenkul**
Department of Veterinary Clinical Medicine, Faculty of Veterinary Medicine, Muang, Khon Kaen 40002, Thailand
Toxic Substances in Livestock and Aquatic Animals Research Group, Khon Kaen University, Muang, Khon Kaen 40002, Thailand

**Weerayuth Supiwong**
Faculty of Applied Science and Engineering, Khon Kaen University, Nong Khai Campus, Muang, Nong Khai 43000, Thailand

**I. R. Hussein, F. Ashgan and M. Alquaiti**
Centre of Excellence in Genomic Medicine Research (CEGMR), King Abdulaziz University, Jeddah 21589, KSA, Saudi Arabia

**M. AlQahtani**
Centre of Excellence in Genomic Medicine Research (CEGMR), King Abdulaziz University, Jeddah 21589, KSA, Saudi Arabia
Diagnostic Genomic Medicine Unit (DGMU), King Abdulaziz University, Jeddah, KSA, Saudi Arabia
Faculty of Medical Sciences, King Abdulaziz University, Jeddah, KSA, Saudi Arabia

**A. Chaudhary, M. Gari and A. Abuzenadah**
Centre of Excellence in Genomic Medicine Research (CEGMR), King Abdulaziz University, Jeddah 21589, KSA, Saudi Arabia
Faculty of Medical Sciences, King Abdulaziz University, Jeddah, KSA, Saudi Arabia

**A. Magbooli**
Diagnostic Genomic Medicine Unit (DGMU), King Abdulaziz University, Jeddah, KSA, Saudi Arabia

**E. Huwait**
Faculty of Science, King Abdulaziz University, Jeddah, KSA, Saudi Arabia

**R. Bader**
Pediatric Cardiology Department, King Abdulaziz University, Jeddah, KSA, Saudi Arabia

**Michael P. Diamond**
Department of Obstetrics and Gynecology, Augusta University, 1120 15th Street, Augusta, GA 30912, USA

**Jonathan D. J. Labonne and Hyung-Goo Kim**
Department of Obstetrics and Gynecology, Augusta University, 1120 15th Street, Augusta, GA 30912, USA
Department of Neuroscience and Regenerative Medicine, Medical College of Georgia, Augusta University, 1120 15th Street, Augusta, GA 30912, USA

**Lawrence C. Layman**
Department of Obstetrics and Gynecology, Augusta University, 1120 15th Street, Augusta, GA 30912, USA
Department of Neuroscience and Regenerative Medicine, Medical College of Georgia, Augusta University, 1120 15th Street, Augusta, GA 30912, USA
Neuroscience Program, Medical College of Georgia, Augusta University, Augusta, GA 30912, USA

**Yiping Shen**
Department of Neurology, Massachusetts General Hospital, Harvard Medical School, Boston, MA 02114, USA

**Il-Keun Kong**
Department of Animal Science, Division of Applied Life Science (BK21plus), Institute of Agriculture and Life Science, Gyeongsang National University, Jinju, Gyeongsangnam-do, Korea

**Hsing-Hua Lai, Tzu-Hsuan Chuang, Lin-Kin Wong, Meng-Ju Lee, Chia-Lin Hsieh and Huai-Lin Wang**
Stork Fertility Center, Stork Ladies Clinic, Hsinchu, Taiwan

**Shee-Uan Chen**
Department of Obstetrics and Gynecology, National Taiwan University Hospital and College of Medicine, Taipei, Taiwan

**Wen-Hsiang Lin**
Department of Genomic Medicine and Center for Medical Genetics, Changhua Christian Hospital, Changhua, Taiwan

Department of Genomic Science and Technology, Changhua Christian Hospital Healthcare System, Changhua, Taiwan

**Gwo-Chin Ma**
Department of Genomic Medicine and Center for Medical Genetics, Changhua Christian Hospital, Changhua, Taiwan
Department of Genomic Science and Technology, Changhua Christian Hospital Healthcare System, Changhua, Taiwan
Institute of Biochemistry, Microbiology and Immunology, Chung-Shan Medical University, Taichung, Taiwan
Department of Medical Laboratory Science and Biotechnology, Central Taiwan University of Science and Technology, Taichung, Taiwan

**Ming Chen**
Department of Genomic Medicine and Center for Medical Genetics, Changhua Christian Hospital, Changhua, Taiwan
Department of Genomic Science and Technology, Changhua Christian Hospital Healthcare System, Changhua, Taiwan
Department of Obstetrics and Gynecology, College of Medicine and Hospital, National Taiwan University, Taipei, Taiwan
Department of Medical Genetics, National Taiwan University Hospital, Taipei, Taiwan
Department of Obstetrics and Gynecology, Changhua Christian Hospital, Changhua, Taiwan
Department of Life Science, Tunghai University, Taichung, Taiwan

**Chi-Fang Lin and Yu-Shih Yang**
Department of Obstetrics and Gynecology, College of Medicine and Hospital, National Taiwan University, Taipei, Taiwan

**Hsin-Fu Chen**
Department of Obstetrics and Gynecology, College of Medicine and Hospital, National Taiwan University, Taipei, Taiwan
Graduate Institute of Medical Genomics and Proteomics, College of Medicine, National Taiwan University, Taipei, Taiwan

**Feng-Po Tsai**
Poyuan Women Clinic, Changhua, Taiwan

**Chi Chiu**
Department of Medical Genetics, National Taiwan University Hospital, Taipei, Taiwan

**Susana Isabel Ferreira, Luís Miguel Pires, José Ferrão, Ana Jardim, Alexandra Mascarenhas, Marta Pinto, Nuno Lavoura, Cláudia Pais, Patrícia Paiva and Lúcia Simões**
Laboratório de Citogenética e Genómica - Faculdade de Medicina, Universidade de Coimbra, Pólo Ciências da Saúde, Sub-Unidade 1 - Piso 2, Azinhaga de Santa Comba, 3000-354 Coimbra, Portugal

**Isabel Marques Carreira and Joana Barbosa de Melo**
Laboratório de Citogenética e Genómica - Faculdade de Medicina, Universidade de Coimbra, Pólo Ciências da Saúde, Sub-Unidade 1 - Piso 2, Azinhaga de Santa Comba, 3000-354 Coimbra, Portugal
CIMAGO - Centro de Investigação em Meio Ambiente, Genética e Oncobiologia, Faculdade de Medicina, Universidade de Coimbra, Coimbra, Portugal
Faculdade de Medicina, Universidade de Coimbra, Coimbra, Portugal
CNC, IBILI - Faculdade de Medicina, Universidade de Coimbra, Coimbra, Portugal

**Eunice Matoso**
CIMAGO - Centro de Investigação em Meio Ambiente, Genética e Oncobiologia, Faculdade de Medicina, Universidade de Coimbra, Coimbra, Portugal
Laboratório de Citogenética, Hospital Pediátrico de Coimbra, Coimbra, Portugal

**Margarida Venâncio, Fabiana Ramos and Jorge Saraiva**
Faculdade de Medicina, Universidade de Coimbra, Coimbra, Portugal
Serviço de Genética Médica, Hospital Pediátrico-Centro Hospitalar e Universitário de Coimbra, Coimbra, Portugal

**Francisco Caramelo and Lina Ramos**
Laboratório de Bioestatística e Informática Médica, IBILI - Faculdade de Medicina, Universidade de Coimbra, Coimbra, Portugal

**Ana Beleza and Joaquim Sá**
Serviço de Genética Médica, Hospital Pediátrico-Centro Hospitalar e Universitário de Coimbra, Coimbra, Portugal

# Index